CLINICAL COMPANION TO

MEDICAL-SURGICAL NURSING

Assessment and Management of Clinical Problems

NINTH EDITION

Prepared by
Shannon Ruff Dirksen, RN, PhD, FAAN
Associate Professor
College of Nursing and Health Innovation
Arizona State University
Phoenix, Arizona

Sharon L. Lewis, RN, PhD, FAAN
Margaret McLean Heitkemper, RN, PhD, FAAN
Linda Bucher, RN, PhD, CEN, CNE

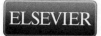

ELSEVIER
MOSBY

3251 Riverport Lane
St. Louis, Missouri 63043

CLINICAL COMPANION TO
MEDICAL-SURGICAL NURSING

ISBN: 978-0-323-09143-5

Notices

Knowledge and best practice in this field are constantly changing. As new research and experience broaden our understanding, changes in research methods, professional practices, or medical treatment may become necessary.

Practitioners and researchers must always rely on their own experience and knowledge in evaluating and using any information, methods, compounds, or experiments described herein. In using such information or methods they should be mindful of their own safety and the safety of others, including parties for whom they have a professional responsibility.

With respect to any drug or pharmaceutical products identified, readers are advised to check the most current information provided (i) on procedures featured or (ii) by the manufacturer of each product to be administered, to verify the recommended dose or formula, the method and duration of administration, and contraindications. It is the responsibility of practitioners, relying on their own experience and knowledge of their patients, to make diagnoses, to determine dosages and the best treatment for each individual patient, and to take all appropriate safety precautions.

To the fullest extent of the law, neither the Publisher nor the authors, contributors, or editors, assume any liability for any injury and/or damage to persons or property as a matter of products liability, negligence or otherwise, or from any use or operation of any methods, products, instructions, or ideas contained in the material herein.

Previous editions copyrighted 2011, 2007, 2004, 2000, 1996

Library of Congress Cataloging-in-Publication Data

Dirksen, Shannon Ruff, author.
Clinical companion to Medical-surgical nursing: assessment and management of clinical problems / prepared by Shannon Ruff Dirksen, Sharon L. Lewis, Margaret McLean Heitkemper, Linda Bucher. — Ninth edition.
    p. ; cm.
Complemented by: Medical-surgical nursing / Sharon L. Lewis, Shannon Ruff Dirksen, Margaret McLean Heitkemper, Linda Bucher. Ninth edition. [2014].
Preceded by: Clinical companion for Medical-surgical nursing / prepared by Shannon Ruff Dirksen . . . [et al.]. 8th ed. c2011.
Includes bibliographical references and index.
ISBN 978-0-323-09143-5 (pbk. : alk. paper)
I. Lewis, Sharon Mantik, author. II. Heitkemper, Margaret M. (Margaret McLean), author. III. Bucher, Linda, author. IV. Lewis, Sharon Mantik. Medical-surgical nursing. Complemented by (work): V. Title.
[DNLM: 1. Perioperative Nursing- -Handbooks. 2. Nursing Process- -Handbooks. WY 49]
RT41
610.73- -dc23

2013042735

Executive Content Strategist: Kristin Geen
Content Manager: Jamie Randall
Publishing Services Manager: Jeff Patterson
Senior Project Manager: Mary G. Stueck
Design Direction: Maggie Reid

Printed in the United States of America

Last digit is the print number: 9 8 7 6 5 4 3 2 1

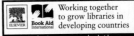

Working together
to grow libraries in
developing countries

www.elsevier.com • www.bookaid.org

The *Clinical Companion* to Lewis, Dirksen, Heitkemper, and Bucher's *Medical-Surgical Nursing: Assessment and Management of Clinical Problems,* ninth edition, has been revised and updated as a condensed reference of essential information on almost 200 medical-surgical patient problems and clinically related topics. The ninth edition of this pocket-sized book provides nurses and nursing students with quick access to current, concise, and important information when caring for patients.

The *Clinical Companion* can be used separately as a standalone reference or in conjunction with *Medical-Surgical Nursing: Assessment and Management of Clinical Problems,* ninth edition.

The book is divided into three sections. Part One contains commonly encountered medical-surgical patient problems that are arranged alphabetically and organized in an easy-to-use format. The disorders are extensively cross-referenced to *Medical-Surgical Nursing,* ninth edition, for the reader who desires additional information. Part Two contains brief explanations of common medical-surgical treatments and procedures (e.g., pacemakers, oxygen therapy) in which the role of the nurse is emphasized. Part Three contains reference material that is frequently used in clinical nursing practice (e.g., heart and breath sounds, medication administration, and blood and urine laboratory values). An extensive index is provided for easy location of information. Content updates may be found at http://evolve.elsevier.com/Lewis/medsurg.

We strongly believe the *Clinical Companion* is an invaluable source of information and will serve as an important resource in helping nurses meet the challenges and opportunities in caring for patients and their caregivers during states of altered health and well-being.

Shannon Ruff Dirksen
Sharon L. Lewis
Margaret McLean Heitkemper
Linda Bucher

"The little things are infinitely the most important."
-Sir Arthur Conan Doyle

CONTENTS

Contents

Part Two: Treatments and Procedures

Part Three: Reference Appendix

PART ONE

Disorders

ABDOMINAL PAIN, ACUTE

Description

Acute abdominal pain is pain of recent onset. It may signal a life-threatening problem and therefore requires immediate attention. Causes include damage to organs in the abdomen and pelvis, which leads to inflammation, infection, obstruction, bleeding, and perforation. The most common causes of acute abdominal pain are listed in Table 1.

Clinical Manifestations

Pain is the most common symptom of an acute abdominal problem. Patients may also complain of nausea, vomiting, diarrhea, constipation, flatulence, fatigue, fever, and bloating.

Diagnostic Studies

Diagnosis begins with a complete history and physical examination. Description of the pain (frequency, timing, duration, location), accompanying symptoms, and sequence of symptoms (e.g., pain before or after vomiting) provide vital clues about the problem. Physical examination should include both a rectal and pelvic examination in addition to an abdominal examination.

- Complete blood count (CBC), urinalysis, abdominal x-ray, and an electrocardiogram (ECG) are done initially, along with an ultrasound or computed tomography (CT) scan.
- A pregnancy test is performed in women of childbearing age to rule out ectopic pregnancy.

Collaborative Care

The goal of management is to identify and treat the cause and monitor and treat complications, especially shock. Table 43-10 in

Table 1	Causes of Acute Abdominal Pain
- Abdominal compartment syndrome	- Gastroenteritis
- Acute pancreatitis	- Pelvic inflammatory disease
- Appendicitis	- Perforated gastric or duodenal ulcer
- Bowel obstruction	- Peritonitis
- Cholecystitis	- Ruptured abdominal aneurysm
- Diverticulitis	- Ruptured ectopic pregnancy

Lewis et al., *Medical-Surgical Nursing,* ed 9, p. 971, outlines emergency management of the patient with acute abdominal pain.

- A minimally invasive diagnostic laparoscopy may be performed to inspect the surface of abdominal organs, obtain biopsy specimens, perform laparoscopic ultrasounds, and remove organs.
- A laparotomy is used when laparoscopic techniques are inadequate. If the cause of the acute abdomen can be surgically removed (e.g., inflamed appendix) or surgically repaired (e.g., ruptured abdominal aneurysm), surgery is considered definitive therapy.

Nursing Management

Goals

The patient will have resolution of inflammation, relief of abdominal pain, freedom from complications (especially hypovolemic shock), and normal nutritional status.

Nursing Interventions

General care involves management of fluid and electrolyte imbalances, pain, and anxiety. Assess the quality and intensity of pain at regular intervals, and provide medication and other comfort measures. Maintain a calm environment and provide information to help allay anxiety. Conduct ongoing assessments of vital signs, intake and output, and level of consciousness, which are key indicators of hypovolemic shock.

Preoperative care includes the emergency care of the patient and general care of the preoperative patient (Chapter 18 and Table 43-10 Lewis et al., *Medical-Surgical Nursing,* ed 9, p. 971).

Postoperative care depends on the type of surgical procedure performed. Laparoscopic procedures result in lower rates of postoperative complications (e.g., poor wound healing, paralytic ileus), earlier diet advancement, and shorter hospital stays compared with open surgical procedures. A general nursing care plan (eNCP 20-1) for the postoperative patient is presented on the website for Chapter 20.

A nasogastric (NG) tube with low suction may be used to empty the stomach and prevent gastric dilation. If the upper gastrointestinal (GI) tract has been entered, drainage from the NG tube may be dark brown to dark red for the first 12 hours. Later it should be light yellowish brown or greenish. If a dark red color continues or if bright red blood is observed, notify the surgeon because of the possibility of hemorrhage. "Coffee ground" granules in the drainage indicate blood that has been modified by acidic gastric secretions.

- Nausea and vomiting are common after a laparotomy and may be caused by the surgery, decreased peristalsis, or pain medication

Antiemetics such as prochlorperazine (Compazine), ondansetron (Zofran), or trimethobenzamide (Tigan) may be ordered (see Nausea and Vomiting, p. 432).

- Monitor fluid and electrolyte status along with blood pressure, heart rate, and respirations.
- Swallowed air and decreased peristalsis from decreased mobility, manipulation of abdominal organs during surgery, and anesthesia can lead to abdominal distention and gas pains. Early ambulation helps restore peristalsis and eliminate flatus and gas pain. Gradually, as intestinal activity increases, distention and gas pain disappear.

▼ **Patient and Caregiver Teaching**

Preparation for discharge begins soon after surgery. Teach the patient and caregiver about any modifications in activity, care of the incision, diet, and drug therapy.

- Clear liquids are given initially after surgery, and if tolerated, the patient progresses to a regular diet.
- Normal activities should be resumed gradually with planned rest periods.
- The patient and caregiver should be aware of possible complications after surgery and should be taught to notify the surgeon immediately if fever, pain, weight loss, incisional drainage, or changes in bowel function occur.

ACUTE CORONARY SYNDROME

Description

Acute coronary syndrome (ACS) develops when ischemia is prolonged and not immediately reversible. ACS encompasses the spectrum of unstable angina (UA), non–ST-segment-elevation myocardial infarction (NSTEMI), and ST-segment-elevation myocardial infarction (STEMI) (Fig. 1). Although each remains a distinct diagnosis, this nomenclature (ACS) reflects the relationships among the pathophysiology, presentation, diagnosis, prognosis, and interventions for these disorders.

Pathophysiology

ACS is associated with deterioration of a once-stable atherosclerotic plaque. The plaque then ruptures, exposing the intima to blood and stimulating platelet aggregation and vasoconstriction with thrombus formation. This unstable lesion may be partially occluded by a thrombus (manifesting as UA or NSTEMI) or totally occluded by a thrombus (manifesting as STEMI).

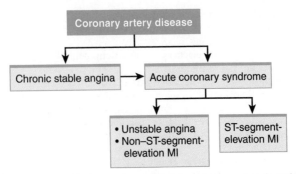

Fig. 1. Relationships among coronary artery disease, chronic stable angina, and acute coronary syndrome.

What causes a coronary plaque to suddenly become unstable is not well understood, but systemic inflammation is thought to play a role.

Unstable Angina

The patient with chronic stable angina may develop UA, or UA may be the first clinical manifestation of CAD. Unlike chronic stable angina, UA is unpredictable and represents an emergency.

- The patient with previously diagnosed chronic stable angina describes a significant change in the pattern of angina. It occurs with increasing frequency and is easily provoked by minimal or no exertion, during sleep, or even at rest.
- The patient without previously diagnosed angina describes anginal pain that has progressed rapidly in the past few hours, days, or weeks, often culminating in pain at rest.

Myocardial Infarction

A myocardial infarction (MI) occurs because of sustained ischemia, causing irreversible myocardial cell death (necrosis). Thrombus formation is responsible for 80% to 90% of all acute MIs. When a thrombus develops, perfusion to the myocardium distal to the occlusion is blocked, resulting in necrosis. Contractile function of the heart stops in the necrotic areas. The degree of altered function depends on the area of the heart involved and the size of the infarction. Most MIs involve some portion of the left ventricle.

Cardiac cells can withstand ischemic conditions for approximately 20 minutes before cellular death (necrosis) begins. If ischemia persists, it takes approximately 4 to 6 hours for the entire thickness of the heart muscle to become necrosed.

- MIs are usually described by the location of damage (e.g., anterior, inferior, lateral, or posterior wall infarction). The location correlates with the involved coronary circulation. For

A

example, inferior wall infarctions result from occlusions in the right coronary artery. Damage can occur in more than one location (e.g., anterolateral MI, anteroseptal MI).

- The degree of preestablished collateral circulation also influences the severity of the infarction. An individual with a long history of CAD develops collateral circulation to provide the area surrounding the infarction site with a blood supply.

The body's response to cell death is the inflammatory process. Within 24 hours, leukocytes infiltrate the area. Enzymes are released from the dead cardiac cells and are important diagnostic indicators of MI. Proteolytic enzymes from neutrophils and macrophages remove all necrotic tissue by the fourth day.

- The necrotic zone is identifiable by ECG changes (e.g., ST-segment elevation, pathologic Q wave) and by nuclear scanning after the onset of symptoms.

At 10 to 14 days after an MI, the new scar tissue is still weak. The myocardium is vulnerable to increased stress because of the unstable state of the healing heart wall. Changes in the infarcted muscle also alter the unaffected myocardium. In an attempt to compensate for the infarcted muscle, the normal myocardium hypertrophies and dilates. Remodeling of normal myocardium can lead to the development of late heart failure (HF).

Clinical Manifestations

Unstable Angina

The chest pain associated with UA is new in onset, occurs at rest, or has a worsening pattern. Women seek medical attention for symptoms of UA more often than men. Despite national efforts to increase awareness, women's symptoms (fatigue, shortness of breath, indigestion, anxiety) continue to go unrecognized as related to heart problems.

Myocardial Infarction

Severe, immobilizing, and persistent chest pain not relieved by rest or nitrate administration is the hallmark of an MI.

- Pain is usually described as a heaviness, pressure, burning, crushing, tightness, or constriction. The persistent pain is unlike any other pain.
- Common locations are epigastric, substernal, or retrosternal. The pain may radiate to the neck, jaw, and arms or to the back. It may occur while the patient is active or at rest, asleep or awake, and commonly occurs in the early morning hours.
- The pain usually lasts for 20 minutes or more and is more severe than usual anginal pain. When epigastric pain is present, the patient may take antacids without relief.

- Some patients may not have pain but may report having "discomfort," weakness, fatigue, or shortness of breath. Women may experience atypical discomfort, shortness of breath, or fatigue.
- An older patient may experience a change in mental status (e.g., confusion), shortness of breath, pulmonary edema, dizziness, or a dysrhythmia.

Additional manifestations may include nausea and vomiting, diaphoresis, and the patient's skin may be ashen, clammy, and cool (cold sweat). Fever occurs within the first 24 hours (up to 100.4° F [38° C]) and may continue for 1 week. BP and pulse rate are also elevated initially. The BP may then drop, with decreased urine output, lung crackles, hepatic engorgement, and peripheral edema. Jugular veins may be distended with obvious pulsations.

Complications

- *Dysrhythmias* are the most common complication after an MI and are the most common cause of death in patients in the pre-hospital period. Dysrhythmias are caused by any condition that affects the myocardial cell's sensitivity to nerve impulses, such as ischemia, electrolyte imbalances, and sympathetic nervous system stimulation. The intrinsic rhythm of the heart is disrupted, causing either a very fast heart rate (HR) (tachycardia), a very slow HR (bradycardia), or irregular HR. Life-threatening dysrhythmias occur most often with anterior wall infarction, heart failure, and shock. Complete heart block is seen in a massive infarction (see Dysrhythmias, p. 202).
- *Ventricular fibrillation,* a common cause of sudden death, is a lethal dysrhythmia that most often occurs within the first 4 hours after the onset of pain. Premature ventricular contractions may precede ventricular tachycardia and fibrillation. Life-threatening ventricular dysrhythmias must be treated immediately.
- *Heart failure* occurs when the heart's pumping action is reduced. Depending on the severity and extent of the injury, HF occurs initially with subtle signs such as slight dyspnea, restlessness, agitation, or slight tachycardia. Other signs include pulmonary congestion on chest x-ray, S_3 or S_4 heart sounds on auscultation, crackles on auscultation of breath sounds, and jugular venous distention.
- *Cardiogenic shock* occurs when inadequate oxygen and nutrients are supplied to the tissues because of severe left ventricular failure. Cardiogenic shock requires aggressive management, including control of dysrhythmias, intraaortic balloon pump therapy, and support of contractility with vasoactive drugs.

A

Diagnostic Studies

In addition to the patient's history of pain, risk factors, and health history, the primary diagnostic studies used to determine whether a person has UA or an MI include an ECG and serum cardiac markers. Other diagnostic measures can include coronary angiography, exercise stress testing, and echocardiogram.

ECG

- Changes in the QRS complex, ST segment, and T wave caused by ischemia and infarction can help differentiate among UA, STEMI, and NSTEMI.
- Patients with STEMI tend to have a more extensive MI that is associated with prolonged and complete coronary occlusion. A pathologic Q wave is seen on the ECG.
- Patients with UA or NSTEMI usually have transient thrombosis or incomplete coronary occlusion and usually do not develop pathologic Q waves.
- Because an MI evolves with time, the ECG often reveals the time sequence of ischemia, injury, infarction, and resolution of the infarction.
- When the ECG is normal or nondiagnostic at the time the patient presents with chest pain, within a few hours the ECG may change to reflect the infarction process.

Cardiac Markers

Certain proteins, called *serum cardiac markers,* are released into the blood from necrotic heart muscle after an MI.

- Cardiac-specific troponin has two subtypes: cardiac-specific troponin T (cTnT) and cardiac-specific troponin I (cTnI). These markers are highly specific indicators of MI and have greater sensitivity and specificity for myocardial injury than creatine kinase (CK) MB.
- Myoglobin is released into the circulation within 2 hours after an MI and peaks in 3 to 15 hours. Although it is one of the first serum cardiac markers to appear after an MI, it lacks cardiac specificity.

Collaborative Care

It is extremely important that a patient with ACS is rapidly diagnosed and treated to preserve cardiac muscle. Initial management of the patient with chest pain most often occurs in the emergency department (ED). Emergency care of the patient with chest pain is presented in Table 34-12, Lewis et al, *Medical-Surgical Nursing,* ed 9, p. 750.

- Establish an IV line and give sublingual nitroglycerin and chewable aspirin if not given before arrival at the ED. Morphine sulfate is given IV for pain unrelieved by nitroglycerin.

- Obtain a 12-lead ECG and start continuous ECG monitoring. Position patient in an upright position unless contraindicated, and initiate O_2 by nasal cannula to keep oxygen saturation above 93%.
- The patient usually receives ongoing care in a critical care or telemetry unit where continuous ECG monitoring is available and dysrhythmias can be treated.
- Monitor vital signs, including pulse oximetry, frequently during the first few hours after admission and closely thereafter. Maintain bed rest and limit activity for 12 to 24 hours with a gradual increase in activity unless contraindicated.
- For patients with UA or NSTEMI with negative cardiac markers and ongoing angina, a combination of aspirin, heparin, and a glycoprotein IIb/IIIa inhibitor (e.g., eptifibatide [Integrilin]) is recommended.

The goal in treatment of acute MI is to salvage as much myocardial muscle as possible.

- Coronary angiography with possible *percutaneous coronary intervention* (PCI) is considered once the patient is stabilized and angina is controlled, or if angina returns and increases in severity.
- *Reperfusion therapy* is indicated for patients with STEMI or NSTEMI with positive cardiac markers. Reperfusion therapy can include emergent PCI or fibrinolytic (thrombolytic) therapy. Emergent PCI is recommended as the first line of treatment for patients with confirmed MI. The patient undergoes cardiac catheterization to evaluate the blockage, and stents may be placed (see Angina, Chronic Stable, p. 46).

Thrombolytic therapy aims to stop the infarction process by dissolving the thrombus in the coronary artery and reperfusing the myocardium. Thrombolytic therapy (e.g., reteplase [Retavase]) is given as soon as possible, ideally within the first hour and preferably within the first 6 hours after the onset of symptoms. Mortality is reduced by 25% if reperfusion occurs within 6 hours. Contraindications and complications with thrombolytic therapy are described in Lewis et al, *Medical-Surgical Nursing*, ed 9, p. 751.

Coronary artery bypass graft (CABG) surgery consists of the placement of conduits to transport blood between the aorta, or other major arteries, and the myocardium distal to the obstructed coronary artery (or arteries). It requires a sternotomy (opening of the chest cavity) and the use of cardiopulmonary bypass (CPB). It is a palliative treatment for CAD and not a cure. Newer techniques include minimally invasive direct coronary artery bypass and transmyocardial laser revascularization. These surgical procedures and related nursing care are further discussed in Lewis et al, *Medical-Surgical Nursing*, ed 9, pp. 752 to 753.

Drug therapy includes IV nitroglycerin (Tridil), aspirin, β-adrenergic blockers, and systemic anticoagulation with either low-molecular-weight heparin given subcutaneously or IV unfractionated heparin as initial drug treatments of choice. Angiotensin-converting enzyme (ACE) inhibitors are added for select patients following MI, and calcium channel blockers may be used if the patient is already taking adequate doses of β-blockers or does not tolerate these blockers.

Nursing Management

Goals

The patient with an MI will experience relief of pain, preservation of myocardium, immediate and appropriate treatment, effective coping with illness-associated anxiety, participation in a rehabilitation plan, and reduction of risk factors.

See NCP 34-1 for the patient with acute coronary syndrome, Lewis et al, *Medical-Surgical Nursing*, ed 9, pp. 755 to 756.

Nursing Diagnoses

- Acute pain
- Decreased cardiac output
- Anxiety
- Activity intolerance
- Ineffective self-health management

Nursing Interventions

Priorities for nursing interventions in the initial phase include pain assessment and relief, physiologic monitoring, promotion of rest and comfort, alleviation of stress and anxiety, and understanding of the patient's emotional and behavioral reactions. Proper management of these priorities decreases the O_2 needs of a compromised myocardium. In addition, you should institute measures to avoid the hazards of immobility while encouraging rest.

- Provide nitroglycerin, morphine, and O_2 as needed to eliminate or reduce chest pain.
- Maintain continuous ECG monitoring while the patient is in the ED and intensive care unit and after transfer to a step-down or general unit. Dysrhythmias need to be identified quickly and treated.
- In addition to taking frequent vital signs, evaluate intake and output at least once per shift, and perform physical assessment to detect deviations from the patient's baseline parameters. Assess lung and heart sounds and inspect for evidence of early heart failure (e.g., dyspnea, tachycardia, pulmonary congestion, distended neck veins).

- Assess the patient's oxygenation status, especially if the patient is receiving O_2. In addition, check the nares for irritation or dryness (see Oxygen Therapy, p. 717).
- It is important to plan nursing and therapeutic actions to ensure adequate rest periods free from interruption.
- It is important to promote rest and comfort with any degree of myocardial injury. Bed rest may be ordered for the first few days after an MI involving a large portion of the ventricle.
- Anxiety is present in various degrees in all patients with ACS. Your role is to identify the source of anxiety and assist the patient in reducing it. If the patient is afraid of being alone, allow a caregiver to sit quietly by the bedside or to check in frequently with the patient. If a source of anxiety is fear of the unknown, you should explore these concerns with the patient.

▼ **Patient and Caregiver Teaching**

Patient teaching needs to occur at every stage of the patient's hospitalization and recovery (e.g., ED, telemetry unit, home care). The purpose of teaching is to give the patient and caregiver the tools they need to make informed health decisions (Table 2).

- Anticipatory guidance involves preparing the patient and caregiver for what to expect in the course of recovery and rehabilitation. By learning what to expect during treatment and recovery, the patient gains a sense of control over his or her life.
- Teach the patient the parameters within which to exercise and how to check pulse rate. Tell the patient the maximum HR that should be present at any point. If the HR exceeds this level or does not return to the rate of the resting pulse within a few minutes, instruct the patient to stop. Also instruct the patient to stop exercising if pain or shortness of breath occurs. Basic physical activity guidelines following ACS are presented in Table 34-20, Lewis et al, *Medical-Surgical Nursing*, ed 9, p. 761.
- Discuss participation in an outpatient cardiac rehabilitation program with all patients. These programs are beneficial, but not all patients choose or are able to participate in them (e.g., location). Home-based cardiac rehabilitation programs can be an alternative.
- It is important to include sexual counseling for cardiac patients and their partners. Tell the patient that resumption of sex depends on the patient and his or her partner's emotional readiness and on the physician's assessment of the extent of recovery. It is generally safe to resume sexual activity 7 to 10 days after an uncomplicated MI.

Table 2	Patient and Caregiver Teaching Guide *Acute Coronary Syndrome*	A

Include the following information in the teaching plan for the patient with acute coronary syndrome and the caregiver.

- Signs and symptoms of angina and MI and what to do should they occur (e.g., take nitroglycerin)*
- When and how to seek help (e.g., contact EMS)
- Anatomy and physiology of the heart and coronary arteries
- Cause and effect of CAD
- Definition of terms (e.g., CAD, angina, MI, sudden cardiac death, heart failure)
- Identification of and plan to decrease risk factors* (see Tables 34-2, 34-3, and 34-4, Lewis et al, *Medical-Surgical Nursing*, ed 9, pp. 736 and 737)
- Rationale for tests and treatments (e.g., ECG monitoring, blood tests, angiography), activity limitations and rest, diet, and medications*
- Appropriate expectations about recovery and rehabilitation (anticipatory guidance)
- Resumption of work, physical activity, sexual activity
- Measures to promote recovery and health
- Importance of the gradual, progressive resumption of activity*

*Identified by patients as most important to learn before discharge.

ACUTE RESPIRATORY DISTRESS SYNDROME

Description

Acute respiratory distress syndrome (ARDS) is a sudden and progressive form of acute respiratory failure in which the alveolar-capillary membrane becomes damaged and more permeable to intravascular fluid. The alveoli fill with fluid, resulting in severe dyspnea, hypoxemia refractory to supplemental oxygen (O_2), reduced lung compliance, and diffuse pulmonary infiltrates.

Incidence of ARDS in the United States is estimated at more than 150,000 cases annually. Despite supportive therapy, mortality from ARDS is approximately 50%. Patients who have both gram-negative septic shock and ARDS have a mortality rate of 70% to 90%.

- Table 3 lists conditions that predispose patients to the development of ARDS. The most common cause is sepsis. Patients with multiple risk factors are three or four times more likely to develop ARDS.

Table 3	Conditions Predisposing Patients to Acute Respiratory Distress Syndrome	
Direct Lung Injury	**Indirect Lung Injury**	

Direct Lung Injury	Indirect Lung Injury
Common Causes	
▪ Aspiration of gastric contents or other substances	▪ Sepsis (especially gram-negative infection)
▪ Viral or bacterial pneumonia	▪ Severe massive trauma
▪ Sepsis	
Less Common Causes	
▪ Chest trauma	▪ Acute pancreatitis
▪ Embolism: fat, air, amniotic fluid, thrombus	▪ Anaphylaxis
▪ Inhalation of toxic substances	▪ Cardiopulmonary bypass
▪ Near-drowning	▪ Disseminated intravascular coagulation
▪ O_2 toxicity	▪ Nonpulmonary systemic diseases
▪ Radiation pneumonitis	▪ Opioid drug overdose (e.g., heroin)
	▪ Severe head injury
	▪ Shock states
	▪ Transfusion-related acute lung injury (e.g., multiple blood transfusions)

▪ Direct lung injury may cause ARDS, or ARDS may develop as a consequence of the systemic inflammatory response syndrome (SIRS). ARDS may also develop as a result of multiple organ dysfunction syndrome (MODS) (see Systemic Inflammatory Response Syndrome and Multiple Organ Dysfunction Syndrome, p. 614).

Pathophysiology

An exact cause for damage to the alveolar-capillary membrane is not known. However, many changes are thought to be caused by stimulation of the inflammatory and immune systems, which causes an attraction of neutrophils to the pulmonary interstitium. The neutrophils cause a release of biochemical, humoral, and cellular mediators that produce changes in the lung, including increased pulmonary capillary membrane permeability, destruction of elastin and collagen, formation of pulmonary microemboli, and pulmonary artery vasoconstriction. Pathophysiologic changes in

ARDS are divided into three phases: injury or exudative, reparative or proliferative, and fibrotic.

The *injury* or *exudative phase* occurs approximately 1 to 7 days (usually 24 to 48 hours) after the initial direct lung injury or host insult. The primary changes of this phase are interstitial and alveolar edema (noncardiogenic pulmonary edema) and atelectasis.

- Initially, there is engorgement of the peribronchial and perivascular interstitial space, which produces interstitial edema. An intrapulmonary shunt develops because the alveoli fill with fluid, and blood passing through them cannot be oxygenated.
- Alveolar cells that produce surfactant are damaged by the changes caused by ARDS. This damage, in addition to further fluid and protein accumulation, results in surfactant dysfunction. Widespread atelectasis further decreases lung compliance, compromises gas exchange, and contributes to hypoxemia.
- Hyaline begins to line the alveolar membrane. Hyaline membranes contribute to fibrosis and atelectasis, leading to a decrease in gas exchange capability and lung compliance.
- Severe ventilation-perfusion (V/Q) mismatch and shunting of pulmonary capillary blood result in hypoxemia unresponsive to increasing concentrations of O_2 *(refractory hypoxemia)*.

The *reparative* or *proliferative phase* begins 1 to 2 weeks after the initial lung injury. During this phase there is an influx of granulocytes, monocytes, and lymphocytes and fibroblast proliferation.

- Increased pulmonary vascular resistance and pulmonary hypertension may occur in this stage because fibroblasts and inflammatory cells destroy the pulmonary vasculature.
- Lung compliance continues to decrease, and hypoxemia worsens because of the thickened alveolar membrane.
- If this phase persists, widespread fibrosis results. If this phase is stopped, the lesions resolve.

The *fibrotic phase* occurs approximately 2 to 3 weeks after the initial lung injury. This phase is also called the chronic or late phase of ARDS. By this time the lung is completely remodeled by collagenous and fibrous tissues. Diffuse scarring and fibrosis result in decreased lung compliance and decreased surface area for gas exchange. Pulmonary hypertension results from fibrosis.

Progression of ARDS varies among patients. Some patients survive the acute phase of lung injury, pulmonary edema resolves, and complete recovery occurs in a few days. Others go on to the fibrotic (late or chronic) phase requiring long-term mechanical ventilation, with a poor chance of survival.

Clinical Manifestations

At the time of initial injury and for several hours to 1 to 2 days afterward, the patient may not exhibit respiratory symptoms.

- The patient may exhibit tachypnea, dyspnea, cough, and restlessness. Chest auscultation may be normal or reveal fine, scattered crackles. Arterial blood gases (ABGs) usually indicate mild hypoxemia and respiratory alkalosis. Chest x-ray may be normal or exhibit evidence of minimal scattered interstitial infiltrates. Edema may not manifest until there is a 30% increase in lung fluid content.

As ARDS progresses, symptoms worsen because of increased fluid accumulation in the lungs and decreased lung compliance. Tachycardia, diaphoresis, changes in sensorium with decreased mentation, cyanosis, and pallor may be present. Chest auscultation usually reveals scattered to diffuse crackles and rhonchi.

- Hypoxemia, despite increased fraction of inspired oxygen concentration (FIO_2) by mask, cannula, or endotracheal tube, is a hallmark of ARDS. Hypercapnia signifies that respiratory muscle fatigue and hypoventilation are occurring, and the patient is no longer able to maintain the level of ventilation needed to provide optimum gas exchange.
- As ARDS progresses, profound respiratory distress occurs, requiring endotracheal intubation and positive pressure ventilation (PPV). The chest x-ray reveals *whiteout* or *white lung* because consolidation and coalescing infiltrates pervade the lungs, leaving few recognizable air spaces.
- Pleural effusions may be present. Severe hypoxemia, hypercapnia, and metabolic acidosis, with symptoms of target organ or tissue hypoxemia, may develop if therapy is not promptly started.

Complications may develop as a result of ARDS itself or its treatment. The major cause of death in ARDS is MODS, often accompanied by sepsis. The vital organs most commonly involved are the kidneys, liver, and heart. The organ systems most often involved are the central nervous system (CNS) and hematologic and gastrointestinal systems.

Diagnostic Studies

No precise criteria define ARDS. Findings that support a diagnosis of ARDS are the patient presents with refractory hypoxemia, a chest x-ray with new bilateral interstitial or alveolar infiltrates, and a pulmonary artery wedge pressure of 18 mm Hg or less with no evidence of heart failure.

Nursing and Collaborative Management

Goals

With appropriate therapy, the overall goals for the patient with ARDS include a partial pressure of oxygen in arterial blood (PaO_2) of at least 60 mm Hg and adequate lung volume to maintain normal pH. A patient recovering from ARDS will experience a PaO_2 within limits of normal for age or baseline values on room air, oxygen saturation in arterial blood (SaO_2) greater than 90%, a patent airway, and clear lungs on auscultation.

Nursing Diagnoses

Nursing diagnoses for the patient with ARDS may include, but are not limited to, those described under Respiratory Failure, Acute (p. 534).

Collaborative Care

The collaborative care for acute respiratory failure is applicable to ARDS (see Respiratory Failure, Acute, pp. 538 to 541). Patients with ARDS are commonly cared for in critical care units.

O_2 *Administration.* The goal of O_2 therapy is to correct hypoxemia (see Oxygen Therapy, p. 717). Initially use masks with high-flow systems that deliver higher O_2 concentrations to maximize O_2 delivery. The general standard for O_2 administration is to give the lowest concentration that results in a PaO_2 of 60 mm Hg or greater. When FIO_2 exceeds 60% for more than 48 hours, the risk for O_2 toxicity increases. Patients with ARDS need intubation with mechanical ventilation (see Artificial Airways: Endotracheal Tubes, p. 679) because the PaO_2 cannot otherwise be maintained at acceptable levels.

Mechanical Ventilation. Endotracheal intubation and positive pressure ventilation provide additional respiratory support. In patients with ARDS, positive expiratory-end pressure (PEEP) is often used. When PEEP is applied, the lung is kept partially expanded, which prevents the alveoli from totally collapsing. If hypoxemic failure persists in spite of high levels of PEEP, alternative modes and therapies may be used. These include airway pressure release ventilation, pressure-control inverse ratio ventilation, high-frequency ventilation, and permissive hypercapnia (low tidal volumes that allow $PaCO_2$ to increase slowly).

Extracorporeal membrane oxygenation (ECMO) and extracorporeal carbon dioxide (CO_2) removal pass blood across a gas-exchanging membrane outside the body and then return oxygenated blood back to the body.

Positioning. Some patients with ARDS have a marked improvement in PaO_2 when turned from the supine to the prone position (e.g., PaO_2 70 mm Hg supine, PaO_2 90 mm Hg prone) with no change in inspired O_2 concentration. The response may be sufficient to allow a reduction in inspired O_2 concentration or PEEP.

Another positioning strategy that you can consider for patients with ARDS is continuous lateral rotation therapy, which provides continuous, slow, side-to-side turning of the patient by rotating the actual bed frame. You should maintain the lateral movement of the bed for 18 of every 24 hours to stimulate postural drainage and help to mobilize pulmonary secretions. In addition, the bed may also contain a vibrator pack that can provide chest physiotherapy to assist with secretion mobilization and removal.

Medical Supportive Therapy

Patients on PPV and PEEP frequently experience decreased cardiac output. Hemodynamic monitoring is essential to see trends, detect changes, and adjust therapy as needed. An arterial catheter is inserted for continuous monitoring of blood pressure (BP) and sampling of blood for ABGs. Use of inotropic drugs, such as dobutamine (Dobutrex) or dopamine (Intropin), may also be necessary. Packed red blood cells are used to increase hemoglobin and thus the O_2-carrying capacity of the blood.

Maintenance of nutrition and fluid balance is challenging in the patient with ARDS. Parenteral or enteral feedings are started to meet the high energy requirements of these patients. Increasing pulmonary capillary permeability results in fluid in the lungs and causes pulmonary edema. At the same time, the patient may be volume depleted and therefore prone to hypotension and decreased cardiac output from mechanical ventilation and PEEP. Controversy exists as to the benefits of fluid replacement with crystalloids versus colloids. The patient is usually placed on fluid restriction, and diuretics are used as necessary.

▼ **Patient and Caregiver Teaching**

Fear of suffocation or death is not uncommon in patients with ARDS.

- Providing reassurance, spending time with the patient, and ensuring that help can be received immediately (e.g., call light is readily available) may help to decrease patient anxiety level. Anxiety also may be reduced through instruction and use of progressive relaxation, guided imagery, and music therapy.
- It is helpful to explain to the patient any possible sensations that may be encountered with each new experience (e.g., suctioning, drawing ABGs) so that coping strategies can be purposefully selected.

ADDISON'S DISEASE

Description

Addison's disease is a primary adrenocortical insufficiency in which all three classes of adrenal steroids (glucocorticoids, mineralocorticoids, and androgens) are reduced because of hypofunction of the adrenal cortex.

In secondary adrenocortical insufficiency, which is caused by a lack of pituitary adrenocorticotropic hormone (ACTH) secretion, corticosteroids and androgens are deficient but mineralocorticoids rarely are.

The most common cause of Addison's disease in the United States is an autoimmune response in which adrenal tissue is destroyed by antibodies against the patient's own adrenal cortex. Often other endocrine conditions are present and Addison's disease is considered a component of autoimmune polyglandular syndrome. Other causes include infarction, fungal infections (e.g., histoplasmosis), acquired immunodeficiency syndrome (AIDS), and metastatic cancer.

Addison's disease may be caused by adrenal hemorrhage (often related to anticoagulant therapy), antineoplastic chemotherapy, ketoconazole therapy for AIDS, or bilateral adrenalectomy.

Clinical Manifestations

Manifestations have a slow (insidious) onset and include progressive weakness, fatigue, weight loss, and anorexia. Skin hyperpigmentation, a striking feature due to increased ACTH, is seen primarily in sun-exposed areas of the body, at pressure points, over joints, and in creases, especially palmar creases.

- Other frequent manifestations are orthostatic hypotension, hyponatremia, hyperkalemia, nausea and vomiting, and diarrhea.

Patients with adrenocortical insufficiency are at risk for acute adrenal insufficiency *(addisonian crisis),* which is a life-threatening emergency caused by insufficient adrenocortical hormones or a sudden, sharp decrease in these hormones.

- The most dangerous feature is hypotension, which may cause shock, especially during stress. Circulatory collapse is often unresponsive to the usual treatment (vasopressors and fluid replacement).
- Addisonian crisis may be triggered by stress (e.g., from infection, surgery, trauma, or psychologic distress), sudden withdrawal of corticosteroid hormone therapy (often done by a patient who lacks knowledge regarding replacement therapy), adrenal surgery, or sudden pituitary gland destruction.

Diagnostic Studies

- Plasma cortisol levels are subnormal or fail to rise over basal levels with an ACTH stimulation test. A positive response to ACTH stimulation indicates a functioning adrenal gland and points to pituitary disease rather than adrenal disease.
- Urine levels of free cortisol and aldosterone are low.
- Serum electrolytes show hyperkalemia, hypochloremia, and hyponatremia.
- CT and MRI are used to localize causes other than autoimmune, including tumors, fungal infections, or tuberculosis.

Collaborative Care

Treatment is focused on management of the underlying cause when possible. The mainstay of treatment is hormone therapy with corticosteroids (e.g., hydrocortisone) with glucocorticoid and mineralocorticoid activity. Mineralocorticoid replacement with fludrocortisone acetate (Florinef) is administered daily with increased salt in the diet.

- During stressful situations, the glucocorticoid dosage is increased to prevent addisonian crisis. The patient usually is instructed to take 2 to 3 times the usual dose.

The patient in addisonian crisis requires immediate aggressive management. Treatment must be directed toward shock management and high-dose hydrocortisone replacement. Large volumes of 0.9% saline solution and 5% dextrose are administered to reverse hypotension and electrolyte imbalances until BP returns to normal.

Nursing Management

When the patient with Addison's disease is hospitalized, nursing management focuses on monitoring the patient while correcting fluid and electrolyte balance.

- Assess vital signs and signs of fluid volume deficit and electrolyte imbalance. Monitor trends in serum glucose, sodium, and potassium.
- Nursing interventions include daily weights, protection against exposure to infection (reverse isolation), and assistance with daily hygiene.
- Protect the patient from noise, light, and environmental temperature extremes. The patient cannot cope with these stresses because corticosteroids cannot be produced.
- If hospitalization was due to an adrenal crisis, patients usually respond by the second day and can start oral corticosteroid replacement.

- Because discharge frequently occurs before the usual maintenance dose of corticosteroids is reached, the patient should be instructed on the importance of keeping scheduled follow-up appointments.

▼ **Patient and Caregiver Teaching**

The serious nature of the disease and the need for lifelong hormone therapy necessitate a comprehensive teaching plan (Table 4).

- Patients must be taught the signs and symptoms of corticosteroid deficiency and excess and to report these to their health care provider so that the dosage can be adjusted.
- It is critical that the patient wear an identification bracelet (Medic Alert) and carry a wallet card stating the patient has Addison's disease so that appropriate therapy can be initiated in case of an emergency.
- Patients should carry an emergency kit with 100 mg of intramuscular (IM) methylprednisolone (Solu-Medrol), syringes, and instructions for use. Instruct the patient and significant others to give an IM injection if hormone therapy cannot be taken orally. Have the patient verbalize instructions, practice IM injections with saline, and have written instructions on when the dosage should be changed.

Table 4	Patient and Caregiver Teaching Guide *Addison's Disease*

Include the following information in the teaching plan for Addison's disease.
- Names, dosages, and actions of drugs
- Symptoms of overdosage and underdosage
- Conditions requiring increased medication (e.g., trauma, infection, surgery, emotional crisis)
- Course of action to take relative to changes in medication
  - Increase in dose of corticosteroid
  - Administration of large dose of corticosteroid intramuscularly, including demonstration and return demonstration
  - Consultation with health care provider
  - Prevention of infection and need for prompt and vigorous treatment of existing infections
- Need for lifelong replacement therapy
- Need for lifelong medical supervision
- Need for medical identification device
- Prevention of falls
- Adverse effects of corticosteroid therapy and prevention techniques
- Special instruction for patients who are diabetics and management of blood glucose when taking corticosteroids

ALZHEIMER'S DISEASE

Description

Alzheimer's disease (AD) is a chronic, progressive, degenerative disease of the brain. It is the most common form of dementia, accounting for about 60% to 80% of all cases of dementia (see Dementia, p. 171). Approximately 5.2 million people in the United States have AD. Ultimately the disease is fatal, with death typically occurring 4 to 8 years after diagnosis, although some patients live for 20 years. AD is the sixth leading cause of death in the United States.

Pathophysiology

The exact etiology of AD is unknown. AD is not a normal part of aging. When AD develops in someone younger than 60 years, it is referred to as *early-onset AD*. AD that becomes evident in individuals after the age of 60 years is called *late-onset AD*.

Characteristic findings in AD relate to changes in the brain's structure and function, including amyloid plaques, neurofibrillary tangles, loss of connections between neurons, and neuron death.

- *Amyloid plaques* consist of insoluble deposits of a protein called β-amyloid, other proteins, remnants of neurons, non-nerve cells such as microglia, and other cells. In AD the plaques develop first in brain areas used for memory and cognitive function. Eventually the cerebral cortex, especially the areas responsible for language and reasoning, is affected.
- *Neurofibrillary tangles* are abnormal collections of twisted protein threads inside nerve cells. The main component of these structures is a protein called *tau*. Normally tau proteins maintain cellular structure by holding intracellular microtubules together. In AD the tau protein is altered, and as a result, the microtubules twist together in a helical fashion, ultimately forming neurofibrillary tangles.

Plaques and neurofibrillary tangles are not unique to patients with AD or dementia. They are also found in the brains of individuals without evidence of cognitive impairment. However, they are more abundant in the brains of individuals with AD.

The other features of AD are the loss of connections between neurons and neuron death. These processes result in structural damage. Affected parts of the brain begin to shrink in a process called *brain atrophy*. By the final stage of AD, brain tissue has shrunk significantly.

Genetic factors may play a critical role in the way that the brain processes the β-amyloid protein. Overproduction of β-amyloid appears to be an important risk factor for AD. Abnormally high levels of β-amyloid cause cell damage either directly or through eliciting an inflammatory response and ultimately neuron death.

Diabetes mellitus, hypertension, current smoking, hypercholesterolemia, obesity, and trauma are associated with an increased risk of dementia including AD.

Clinical Manifestations

Pathologic changes often precede clinical manifestations of dementia by 5 to 20 years. (Early warning signs of AD are listed in Table 5.) The rate of progression from mild to severe is highly variable and ranges from 3 to 20 years.

Initial manifestations are usually related to changes in cognitive functioning. Patients may have complaints of memory loss, mild disorientation, and/or trouble with words and numbers. Often it is

Table 5	Patient and Caregiver Teaching Guide *Early Warning Signs of Alzheimer's Disease*

Include the following information in the teaching plan for the patient with Alzheimer's disease and the family caregiver.

Warning Sign	Description
1. Memory loss that affects job skills	▪ Frequent forgetfulness or unexplainable confusion at home or in the workplace may signal that something is wrong. ▪ This type of memory loss goes beyond forgetting an assignment, colleague's name, deadline, or phone number.
2. Difficulty performing familiar tasks	▪ It is normal for most people to become distracted and to forget something (e.g., leave something on the stove too long). ▪ People with AD may cook a meal but then forget not only to serve it but also that they made it.

Continued

Table 5	Patient and Caregiver Teaching Guide *Early Warning Signs of Alzheimer's Disease*—cont'd

Warning Sign	Description
3. Problems with language	▪ Most people have trouble finding the "right" word from time to time. ▪ People with AD may forget simple words or substitute inappropriate words, making their speech difficult to understand.
4. Disorientation to time and place	▪ Most individuals occasionally forget the day of the week or what they need from the store. ▪ People with AD can become lost on their own street, not knowing where they are, how they got there, or how to get back home.
5. Poor or decreased judgment	▪ Many individuals from time to time may choose not to dress appropriately for the weather (e.g., not bringing a coat or sweater on a cold evening). ▪ A person with AD may dress inappropriately in more noticeable ways, such as wearing a bathrobe to the store or a sweater on a hot day.
6. Problems with abstract thinking	▪ For the person with AD, this goes beyond challenges such as balancing a checkbook. ▪ A person with AD may have difficulty recognizing numbers or doing even basic calculations.
7. Misplacing things	▪ For many individuals, temporarily misplacing keys, purses, or wallets is a normal albeit frustrating event. ▪ A person with AD may put items in inappropriate places (e.g., eating utensils in clothing drawers) but have no memory of how they got there.
8. Changes in mood or behavior	▪ Most individuals experience mood changes. ▪ A person with AD tends to exhibit more rapid mood swings for no apparent reason.

Table 5	Patient and Caregiver Teaching Guide *Early Warning Signs of Alzheimer's Disease*—cont'd	A

Warning Sign	Description
9. Changes in personality	■ As most individuals age, they may demonstrate some change in personality (e.g., become less tolerant). ■ A person with AD can change dramatically, either suddenly or over time. For example, someone who is generally easygoing may become angry, suspicious, or fearful.
10. Loss of initiative	■ A person with AD may become and remain uninterested and uninvolved in many or all of his or her usual pursuits.

Adapted from Alzheimer's Association: *Early warning signs,* Chicago, The Association.

a family member, in particular the spouse, who reports the patient's declining memory to the health care provider.
■ Memory loss initially relates to recent events, with remote memories still intact. With time and progression of AD, memory loss includes both recent and remote memory and ultimately affects the ability to perform self-care.
■ Behavioral manifestations (e.g., agitation, aggression) result from changes that take place within the brain. The person's behaviors are neither intentional nor controllable by the individual with the disease. Some patients develop delusions and hallucinations.

As AD progresses, the individual may develop additional cognitive impairments such as *dysphasia* (difficulty comprehending language and oral communication), *apraxia* (inability to manipulate objects or perform purposeful acts), *visual agnosia* (inability to recognize objects by sight), and *dysgraphia* (difficulty communicating via writing).
■ Later in the disease, long-term memories cannot be recalled, patients lose the ability to recognize family members, and eventually the ability to communicate and perform activities of daily living (ADLs) is lost.
■ In the late or final stages, the patient is unresponsive and incontinent and requires total care.

Diagnostic Studies

The diagnosis of AD is primarily a diagnosis of exclusion. When all other possible conditions that can cause mental impairment have been ruled out and manifestations of dementia persist, the diagnosis of AD can be made.

- Comprehensive health history, physical examination, neurologic and mental status assessments, and laboratory tests are done.
- Brain imaging tests include CT or MRI scan, which may show brain atrophy in the later stages. However, this finding occurs in other diseases and in people without cognitive impairment.
- Positron emission tomography (PET) scanning can be used to differentiate AD from other forms of dementia.
- Definitive diagnosis of AD usually requires examination of brain tissue and the presence of neurofibrillary tangles and neuritic plaques at autopsy.

Collaborative Care

At this time there is no cure for AD. No treatment is available to stop the deterioration of brain cells in AD. Management of AD is aimed at controlling the undesirable behavioral manifestations that the patient may exhibit and providing support for the family caregiver. Table 60-10, Lewis et al, *Medical-Surgical Nursing*, ed 9, p. 1452, details drug therapy for AD. These drugs have no effect on overall disease progression.

- Cholinesterase inhibitors block cholinesterase, the enzyme responsible for the breakdown of acetylcholine in the synaptic cleft. Cholinesterase inhibitors include donepezil (Aricept), rivastigmine (Exelon), and galantamine (Razadyne). Rivastigmine is available as a patch.
- Memantine (Namenda) protects brain nerve cells by blocking the damaging effects of glutamate, which is released in large amounts by cells damaged by AD.
- Although antipsychotic drugs are approved for treating psychotic conditions (e.g., schizophrenia), they have been used for the management of behavioral problems (e.g., agitation, aggressive behavior) that occur in patients with AD. However, these drugs have been shown to increase the risk of death in older dementia patients.
- Treating the depression associated with AD may improve the patient's cognitive ability. These medications include selective serotonin reuptake inhibitors (SSRIs) such as fluoxetine (Prozac), sertraline (Zoloft), fluvoxamine (Luvox), and citalopram (Celexa).

Nursing Management

Goals

The patient with AD will maintain functional ability for as long as possible, be maintained in a safe environment with a minimum of injuries, have personal care needs met, and have dignity maintained.

Nursing Diagnoses

- Impaired memory
- Self-neglect
- Risk for injury
- Wandering

Nursing Interventions

You are in an important position to assess for depression. Antidepressant drugs and counseling may be indicated. Family caregivers may also be in denial and may not seek medical attention early in the disease. Along with patient assessment, assess family caregivers and their ability to accept and cope with the diagnosis.

Although there is no current treatment for reversing AD, there is a need for ongoing monitoring of both the patient and patient's caregiver. An important nursing responsibility is to work collaboratively with the patient's health care provider to manage symptoms effectively as they change over time. You are often responsible for teaching the caregiver to perform the many tasks that are required to manage the patient's care. You must consider both the patient with AD and the caregiver as patients with overlapping but unique problems.

Hospitalization of the patient with AD can be a traumatic event and can precipitate a worsening of the disease. Patients with AD hospitalized in the acute care setting will need to be observed more closely because of concerns for safety, frequently oriented to place and time, and given reassurance. Anxiety or disruptive behavior may be reduced through the use of consistent nursing staff.

- Adult day care is one of the options available to the person with AD. Common goals of all day-care programs are to provide respite for the family and a protective environment for the patient.
- As the disease progresses, the demands on the caregivers eventually exceed the resources. The person with AD may need to be placed in a long-term care facility, where special units to care for people with AD are becoming increasingly common.
- Support groups for caregivers and family members can provide an atmosphere of understanding and give current information about the disease itself and related topics such as safety, legal, ethical, and financial issues. The Alzheimer's Association has educational and support systems available to help family caregivers including the booklet *Caring for a Person with Alzheimer's Disease (www.nia.nih.gov/Alzheimers/Publications/CaringAD).*

A family and caregiver teaching guide based on the disease stages is provided in Table 6.

| Table 6 | **Family and Caregiver Teaching Guide** *Alzheimer's Disease* |

Include the following instructions when teaching families and care-givers the management of the patient with Alzheimer's disease.

Mild Stage

- Many treatable (and potentially reversible) conditions can mimic dementia (see Table 60-2, Lewis et al, *Medical-Surgical Nursing*, ed 9, p. 1444). Try to get a definitive diagnosis.
- Get the person to stop driving. Confusion and poor judgment can impair driving skills and potentially put others at risk.
- Encourage activities such as visiting with friends and family, listening to music, participating in hobbies, and exercising.
- Provide cues in the home, establish a routine, and determine a specific location where essential items (e.g., glasses) need to be kept.
- Do not correct misstatements or faulty memory.
- Register with MedicAlert + Alzheimer's Association Safe Return, a program established by the MedicAlert Foundation and the Alzheimer's Association to locate individuals who wander from their homes.
- Make plans for the future in terms of advance directives, care options, financial concerns, and personal preference for care.

Moderate Stage

- Install door locks for patient safety.
- Provide protective wear for urinary and fecal incontinence.
- Ensure that the home has good lighting, install handrails in stairways and bathroom, and remove area rugs.
- Label drawers and faucets (hot and cold) to ensure safety.
- Develop strategies such as distraction and diversion to cope with behavioral problems. Identify and reduce potential triggers (e.g., reduce stress, extremes in temperature) for disruptive behavior.
- Provide memory triggers, such as pictures of family and friends.

Severe Stage

- Provide a regular schedule for toileting to reduce incontinence.
- Provide care to meet needs, including oral care and skin care.
- Monitor diet and fluid intake to ensure their adequacy.
- Continue communication through talking and touching.
- Consider placement in a long-term care facility when providing total care becomes too difficult.

AMYOTROPHIC LATERAL SCLEROSIS

Amyotrophic lateral sclerosis (ALS) is a rare, progressive neurologic disease characterized by loss of motor neurons. This disease became known as Lou Gehrig's disease when the famous baseball player was stricken with it in the early 1940s. The onset is between the ages of 40 and 70 years, and twice as many men as women are affected. ALS usually leads to death within 2 to 6 years of diagnosis.

- For unknown reasons, motor neurons in the brainstem and spinal cord gradually degenerate in ALS. Consequently, chemical and electrical messages originating in the brain never reach the muscles to activate them.
- Typical symptoms are limb weakness, dysarthria, and dysphagia. Muscle wasting and fasciculations result from denervation of the muscles and lack of stimulation and use.
- Other symptoms include pain, sleep disorders, spasticity, drooling, emotional lability, depression, constipation, and esophageal reflux.
- Death usually results from respiratory infection secondary to compromised respiratory function.

There is no cure for ALS. This illness is devastating because the patient remains cognitively intact while wasting away.

- Riluzole (Rilutek) slows the progression of ALS. This drug works to decrease the amount of glutamate (an excitatory neurotransmitter) in the brain.

Nursing interventions include (1) facilitating communication, (2) reducing risk of aspiration, (3) facilitating early identification of respiratory insufficiency, (4) decreasing pain secondary to muscle weakness, (5) decreasing risk of injury related to falls, and (6) providing diversional activities such as reading and human companionship. Guide the patient in the use of moderate-intensity, endurance-type exercises for the trunk and limbs, as this may help to reduce ALS spasticity.

Support the patient's cognitive and emotional functions. Help the patient and family manage the disease process, including grieving related to the loss of motor function, and ultimately death. Discuss with the patient and caregiver issues such as artificial methods of ventilation and advance directives.

ANAL CANCER

Anal cancer is uncommon in the general population, but the incidence is increasing. Human papillomavirus (HPV) is associated with about 80% of the cases of anal cancer. The American Cancer Society estimates that about 6230 people are diagnosed with anal cancer each year in the United States, with more women diagnosed than men.

Risk factors include having many sexual partners, genital warts (which are caused by HPV), smoking, receptive anal sex, and HIV infection. The average age at diagnosis is 60. Anal cancer is more common in African Americans than in whites.

- Frequently the initial symptom is rectal bleeding. Other symptoms include rectal pain and sensation of a rectal mass. Some patients have no symptoms, which leads to delayed diagnosis and treatment.

It is especially important to screen high-risk individuals. A swab of the anal mucosa can be obtained during a digital rectal examination with identification of cell changes (e.g., dysplasia, neoplasia). High-resolution anoscopy allows for visualization of the mucosa and biopsy. An endo-anal (endorectal) ultrasound may also be done.

The use of condoms to reduce the transmission of HPV is recommended. The HPV vaccine Gardasil is used for the prevention of anal cancer and associated precancerous lesions caused by HPV types 6, 11, 16, and 18. Another HPV vaccine, Cervarix, may also be useful in the prevention of HPV-associated anal cancer. After vaccination with HPV vaccine, patients at risk need to continue the recommended screening program.

Treatment of anal cancer depends on the size and depth of the lesions. Topical therapy with bichloroacetic or trichloroacetic acid may be used to kill the HPV virus. Imiquimod (Aldara), an immunomodulator, is also used as a topical agent. Therapy also includes surgery, radiation, and chemotherapy. Chemotherapy may include mitomycin, cisplatin (Platinol), and 5 fluorouracil (5-FU).

ANEMIA

Description

Anemia is a deficiency in the number of red blood cells (RBCs) or erythrocytes, the quantity of hemoglobin (Hgb), and/or the volume of packed RBCs (hematocrit). It is a prevalent condition with many diverse causes such as blood loss, impaired production of erythrocytes, or increased destruction of erythrocytes.

- Because RBCs transport oxygen (O_2), erythrocyte disorders can lead to tissue hypoxia. This hypoxia accounts for many of the signs and symptoms of anemia.
- Anemia is not a specific disease; it is a manifestation of a pathologic process.

- Anemia can result from primary hematologic problems or can develop as a secondary consequence of defects in other body systems.

The various types of anemias can be classified according to morphology (cell characteristics) or etiology. Although the morphologic system is the most accurate means of classifying anemia, it is easier to discuss patient care by focusing on the etiology of the anemia.

- *Morphologic classification* is based on erythrocyte size and color (Table 7).
- *Etiologic classification* is related to clinical conditions causing the anemia (Table 8).

Diagnostic Studies

- Anemia is diagnosed using a complete blood count (CBC), reticulocyte count, and peripheral blood smear. Once anemia is identified, further investigation is done to determine its specific cause.
- Although the Hgb level is decreased in all types of anemias, other laboratory findings are characteristic of specific types of anemias (Table 9).

Clinical Manifestations

Manifestations of anemia are caused by the body's response to tissue hypoxia (Table 10). Specific manifestations vary depending on

| Table 7 | Morphology and Etiology of Anemia |

Morphology	Etiology
Normocytic, normochromic (normal size and color) MCV 80-100 fL, MCH 27-34 pg	Acute blood loss, hemolysis, chronic kidney disease, chronic disease, cancers, sideroblastic anemia, endocrine disorders, starvation, aplastic anemia, sickle cell anemia, pregnancy
Microcytic, hypochromic (small size, pale color) MCV <80 fL, MCH <27 pg	Iron-deficiency anemia, vitamin B_6 deficiency, copper deficiency, thalassemia, lead poisoning
Macrocytic (megaloblastic), normochromic (large size, normal color) MCV >100 fL, MCH >34 pg	Cobalamin (vitamin B_{12}) deficiency, folic acid deficiency, liver disease (including effects of alcohol abuse), postsplenectomy

MCH, Mean corpuscular hemoglobin; *MCV,* mean corpuscular volume.

Table 8	Classification of Anemia

Decreased RBC Production
Decreased Hemoglobin Synthesis
- Iron deficiency
- Thalassemias (decreased globin synthesis)
- Sideroblastic anemia (decreased porphyrin)

Defective DNA Synthesis
- Cobalamin (vitamin B_{12}) deficiency
- Folic acid deficiency

Decreased Number of RBC Precursors
- Aplastic anemia and inherited disorders (e.g., Fanconi syndrome)
- Anemia of myeloproliferative diseases (e.g., leukemia) and myelodysplasia
- Chronic diseases or disorders
- Medications and chemicals (e.g., chemotherapy, lead)
- Radiation

Blood Loss
Acute
- Trauma
- Blood vessel rupture
- Splenic sequestration crisis

Chronic
- Gastritis
- Menstrual flow
- Hemorrhoids

Increased RBC Destruction (Hemolytic Anemias)
Hereditary (Intrinsic)
- Abnormal hemoglobin (sickle cell disease)
- Enzyme deficiency (G6PD)
- Membrane abnormalities (paroxysmal nocturnal hemoglobinuria, hereditary spherocytosis)

Acquired (Extrinsic)
- Macroangiopathic: physical trauma (prosthetic heart valves, extracorporeal circulation)
- Microangiopathic: disseminated intravascular coagulopathy (DIC), thrombotic thrombocytopenic purpura (TTP)
- Antibodies (isoimmune and autoimmune)
- Infectious agents (e.g., malaria) and toxins

G6PD, Glucose-6-phosphate dehydrogenase.

Laboratory Study Findings in Anemias

Etiology of Anemia	Hgb/Hct	MCV	Reticulocytes	Serum Iron	TIBC	Transferrin	Ferritin	Bilirubin	Serum B$_{12}$	Folate
Iron deficiency	↓	↓	N or slight ↑	↓	↑	N or ↑	↓	N or ↓	N	N
Thalassemia major	↓	N or ↓	↑	↑	↓	↓	N or ↑	↑	N	↓
Cobalamin deficiency	↓	↑	N or ↓	N or ↑	N	Slight ↑	↑	N or slight ↑	↓	N
Folic acid deficiency	↓	↑	N or ↓	N or ↑	N	Slight ↑	↑	N or slight ↑	N	↓
Aplastic anemia	↓	N or slight ↑	↓	N or ↑	N or ↓	N or ↓	N	N	N	N
Chronic disease	↓	N or ↓	N or ↓	N or ↓	↓	N	N or ↑	N	N	N
Acute blood loss	↓	N or ↓	N or ↑	N	N or ↓	N	N	N	N	N
Chronic blood loss	↓	↓	N or ↓	↓	↑	N	N	N or ↓	N	N
Sickle cell anemia	↓	↑	↑	N or ↑	N or ↑	N	N	↑	N	↓
Hemolytic anemia	↓	N or ↑	↑	N or ↑	N or ↑	N	N or ↑	↑	N	N

MCV, Mean corpuscular volume; *N*, normal; *TIBC*, total iron-binding capacity.

Table 10   Manifestations of Anemia

Body System	Severity of Anemia		
	Mild (Hgb 10-12 g/dL [100-120 g/L])	Moderate (Hgb 6-10 g/dL [60-100 g/L])	Severe (Hgb <6 g/dL [<60 g/L])
Integument	None	None	Pallor, jaundice,* pruritus*
Eyes	None	None	Icteric conjunctiva and sclera,* retinal hemorrhage, blurred vision
Mouth	None	None	Glossitis, smooth tongue
Cardiovascular	Palpitations	Increased palpitations, "bounding pulse"	Tachycardia, increased pulse pressure, systolic murmurs, intermittent claudication, angina, heart failure, MI
Pulmonary	Exertional dyspnea	Dyspnea	Tachypnea, orthopnea, dyspnea at rest
Neurologic	None	"Roaring in the ears"	Headache, vertigo, irritability, depression, impaired thought processes
Gastrointestinal	None	None	Anorexia, hepatomegaly, splenomegaly, difficulty swallowing, sore mouth
Musculoskeletal	None	None	Bone pain
General	None or mild fatigue	Fatigue	Sensitivity to cold, weight loss, lethargy

*Caused by hemolysis.

the rate at which the anemia has evolved, its severity, and any co-existing disease. Hgb levels may determine the severity of anemia.

- *Mild anemia* (Hgb 10 to 14 g/dL [100 to 140 g/L]) may exist without causing symptoms. If symptoms develop, they are usually caused by an underlying disease or a compensatory response to heavy exercise. These symptoms include palpitations, dyspnea, and mild fatigue.
- In *moderate anemia* (Hgb 6 to 10 g/dL [60 to 100 g/L]), cardiopulmonary symptoms (e.g., increased heart rate) may be present with rest as well as activity.
- In *severe anemia* (Hgb <6 g/dL [60 g/L]) patients display many clinical manifestations involving multiple body systems.

Nursing Management
Goals
The patient with anemia will assume normal activities of daily living (ADLs), maintain adequate nutrition, and develop no complications related to anemia. See NCP 31-1 for the patient with anemia, Lewis et al, *Medical-Surgical Nursing,* ed 9, pp. 635 to 636.

Nursing Diagnoses
- Fatigue
- Imbalanced nutrition: less than body requirements
- Ineffective self-health management

Nursing Interventions
The numerous causes of anemia necessitate different nursing interventions specific to the type of anemia and the patient's needs. General components of care for all patients with anemia may include:

- Dietary and lifestyle changes that may reverse some causes of anemia.
- Acute interventions such as blood or blood product transfusions, drug therapy (e.g., erythropoietin, vitamin supplements), volume replacement, and O_2 therapy.
- Assessing the patient's knowledge regarding adequate nutritional intake and adherence to safety precautions to prevent falls and injury.
- Specific types of anemias are listed under separate headings.

ANEMIA, APLASTIC

Description
Aplastic anemia is a disease in which the patient has peripheral blood *pancytopenia* (decrease of all blood cell types—RBCs,

white blood cells [WBCs], and platelets) and hypocellular bone marrow. The spectrum of the anemia can range from a chronic condition managed with erythropoietin or blood transfusions to a critical condition with hemorrhage and sepsis.

Pathophysiology

Aplastic anemia has various etiologic classifications but is divided into two major groups: congenital or acquired.

- *Congenital (idiopathic)* aplastic anemia is caused by chromosomal alterations.
- *Acquired* aplastic anemia is a result of exposure to radiation, chemical agents and toxins (e.g., benzene, insecticides, arsenic, alcohol), viral and bacterial infections (e.g., hepatitis, parvovirus), and drugs (e.g., alkylating agents, antiseizure medications, antimetabolites, antimicrobials, gold). Approximately 75% of acquired aplastic anemias are idiopathic and thought to have an autoimmune basis.

Clinical Manifestations

Aplastic anemia can manifest abruptly over days or insidiously over weeks and months. It can vary from mild to severe. Clinically the patient may have symptoms caused by suppression of any or all bone marrow elements.

- General manifestations of anemia such as fatigue and dyspnea, as well as cardiovascular and cerebral signs, may be seen (see Table 10).
- The patient with neutropenia (low neutrophil count) is susceptible to infection and is at risk for septic shock and death. Even a low-grade temperature ($>100.4°$ F) should be considered a medical emergency.
- Thrombocytopenia may be manifested by a predisposition to bleeding (e.g., petechiae, ecchymoses, epistaxis).

Diagnostic Studies

Diagnosis is confirmed by laboratory studies.

- All marrow elements are affected (RBC, WBC, and platelet) with values often decreased (see Table 9).
- Reticulocyte count is low and bleeding time is prolonged.
- Serum iron and total iron-binding capacity (TIBC) may be elevated as initial signs of erythroid suppression.
- Bone marrow examination may be done for any anemic state, but it is especially important in aplastic anemia. Findings indicate a hypocellular marrow with increased yellow marrow (fat content).

Nursing and Collaborative Management

Management of aplastic anemia is based on identifying and removing the causative agent (when possible) and providing supportive care until pancytopenia reverses.

Nursing interventions appropriate for the patient with pancytopenia from aplastic anemia are presented in the nursing care plans for patients with anemia (see NCP 31-1, pp. 635 to 636), thrombocytopenia (eNCP 31-1 on the website), and neutropenia (eNCP 31-2 on the website). Nursing actions are directed at preventing complications from infection and hemorrhage.

- Prognosis of severe untreated aplastic anemia is poor. However, advances in medical management, including hematopoietic stem cell transplant (HSCT) and immunosuppressive therapy with antithymocyte globulin (ATG) and cyclosporine or high-dose cyclophosphamide (Cytoxan) have significantly improved outcomes.
- Treatment of choice for adults younger than 55 years old who do not respond to immunosuppressive therapy and who have a human leukocyte antigen (HLA)–matched donor is HSCT. Best results occur in younger patients who have not had previous blood transfusions. Prior transfusions increase the risk of graft rejection.

For the older adults without an HLA-matched donor, the treatment of choice is immunosuppression with ATG or cyclosporine or high-dose cyclophosphamide. This therapy may be only partially beneficial.

ANEMIA, COBALAMIN (VITAMIN B$_{12}$) DEFICIENCY

Description

Anemia resulting from a cobalamin (vitamin B$_{12}$) deficiency is a type of megaloblastic anemia caused by impaired DNA synthesis. When DNA synthesis is impaired, defective red blood cell (RBC) maturation results in large, abnormal RBCs. Normally a protein known as intrinsic factor (IF) is secreted by parietal cells of the gastric mucosa. IF is required for cobalamin (extrinsic factor) absorption in the distal ileum. Therefore if IF is not secreted, cobalamin will not be absorbed.

- In *pernicious anemia,* the most common cause of cobalamin deficiency, the gastric mucosa does not secrete IF.

Pathophysiology

Cobalamin deficiency can occur in patients who have had GI surgery, such as gastrectomy; patients who have had a small bowel resection involving the ileum; and patients with Crohn's disease, ileitis, diverticuli of the small intestine, and/or chronic atrophic gastritis. In these cases, cobalamin deficiency results from the loss of IF-secreting gastric mucosal surface or impaired absorption of cobalamin in the distal ileum. Cobalamin deficiency is also found in long-term users of histamine (H_2)-receptor blockers and proton pump inhibitors and those who are strict vegetarians.

Pernicious anemia is caused by an absence of IF, either from gastric mucosal atrophy or autoimmune destruction of parietal cells. This results in a decrease of HCl acid secretion by the stomach.

Clinical Manifestations

Manifestations of anemia related to cobalamin deficiency develop because of tissue hypoxia (see Table 10).

- GI manifestations include a sore tongue, anorexia, nausea, vomiting, and abdominal pain.
- Neuromuscular manifestations include weakness, paresthesias of feet and hands, reduced vibratory and position senses, ataxia, muscle weakness, and impaired thought processes ranging from confusion to dementia.

Diagnostic Studies

Laboratory data reflective of cobalamin deficiency anemia are presented in Table 9.

- Erythrocytes appear large (macrocytic) and have abnormal shapes. This structure contributes to erythrocyte destruction because the cell membrane is fragile.
- Serum cobalamin levels are reduced.
- If serum folate levels are normal and cobalamin levels are low, it suggests that megaloblastic anemia is due to a cobalamin deficiency.
- A serum test for anti-IF antibodies may be done that is specific for pernicious anemia.
- An upper GI endoscopy and biopsy of the gastric mucosa may also be done.

Collaborative Care

Regardless of how much cobalamin is ingested, the patient is not able to absorb it if IF is lacking or if absorption in the ileum is impaired, so dietary management is not used for cobalamin replacement.

- Lifelong administration of cobalamin is needed. It can be given parenterally (cyanocobalamin or hydroxocobalamin) or intranasally (Nascobal, CaloMist). A typical treatment schedule consists of 1000 mg cobalamin intramuscularly (IM) daily for 2 weeks, then weekly until hematocrit is normal, and then monthly for life. Regular supplemental cobalamin can reverse the anemia, but long-standing neuromuscular complications may not be reversible.

- High-dose oral cobalamin and sublingual cobalamin are also available for those in whom GI absorption is intact.

Nursing Management

- Nursing interventions for the patient with anemia are appropriate for the patient with cobalamin deficiency (see Anemia, p. 35). In addition to these measures, ensure that the patient is protected from burns and trauma because of a diminished sensation to heat and pain as a result of neurologic impairment.
- Ongoing care is primarily related to ensuring good patient compliance with treatment. There must be careful follow-up evaluation to assess for neurologic difficulties that were not fully corrected by cobalamin replacement therapy. Because the potential for gastric cancer is increased in patients with atrophic gastritis-related pernicious anemia, the patient should have frequent and appropriate screening for gastric cancer.

ANEMIA, FOLIC ACID DEFICIENCY

Folic acid (folate) deficiency can cause megaloblastic anemia. Folic acid is required for deoxyribonucleic acid (DNA) synthesis leading to the formation and maturation of red blood cells (RBCs). Common causes of folic acid deficiency are (1) dietary deficiency, especially a lack of leafy green vegetables and citrus fruits; (2) malabsorption syndromes; (3) drugs that interfere with absorption/or use of folic acid (e.g., methotrexate); antiseizure medications (e.g., phenobarbital, phenytoin [Dilantin]); (4) alcohol abuse and anorexia; and (5) hemodialysis treatments, because folic acid is lost during dialysis.

Clinical Manifestations

Clinical manifestations of folic acid deficiency are similar to those of cobalamin deficiency. The disease develops insidiously, and the patient's symptoms may be attributed to other coexisting problems, such as cirrhosis or esophageal varices.

- GI disturbances include dyspepsia and a smooth, beefy red tongue.
- Absence of neurologic problems is an important diagnostic finding and differentiates folic acid deficiency from cobalamin deficiency.

- Diagnostic findings for folic acid deficiency are presented in Table 9. The serum folate level is low (normal is 3 to 25 mg/mL [7 to 57 mol/L]), and the serum cobalamin is normal.

Nursing and Collaborative Management

Folic acid deficiency is treated by replacement therapy with the usual dosage of 1 mg/day by mouth. In malabsorption states, up to 5 mg/day may be required. The duration of treatment depends on the reason for the deficiency. Encourage the patient to eat foods containing large amounts of folic acid (e.g., breakfast cereals, breads, pasta).

Nursing interventions for the patient with anemia are appropriate for the patient with folic acid deficiency (see Anemia, p. 40).

ANEMIA, IRON-DEFICIENCY

Description

Iron-deficiency anemia, one of the most common chronic hematologic disorders, is found in 2% to 5% of adult men and postmenopausal women in developed countries. Those most susceptible to iron-deficiency anemia are the very young, those on poor diets, and women in their reproductive years.

Pathophysiology

Iron deficiency may develop from inadequate dietary intake, malabsorption, blood loss, or hemolysis. Dietary iron is adequate to meet the needs of men and older women, but it may be inadequate for those individuals who have higher iron needs (e.g., menstruating or pregnant women).

Iron absorption occurs in the duodenum, and absorption can be altered after surgical procedures that involve removal of or bypass of the duodenum. Malabsorption syndromes may also involve disease of the duodenum, affecting iron absorption.

Blood loss is a major cause of iron deficiency in adults. Major sources of chronic blood loss are from the GI and genitourinary (GU) systems.

- GI bleeding is often not apparent and therefore may exist for a considerable time before the problem is identified. Loss of 50 to 75 mL of blood from the upper GI tract is required to cause stools to appear black (melena). This color results from iron in the red blood cells (RBCs).
- Common causes of GI blood loss are peptic ulcer, esophagitis, diverticula, hemorrhoids, and neoplasia. GU blood loss occurs primarily from menstrual bleeding. The average monthly menstrual

blood loss is about 45 mL, which causes a loss of about 22 mg of iron.

- In addition to anemia of chronic kidney disease, dialysis treatment may induce iron-deficiency anemia because of the blood lost in the dialysis equipment and frequent blood sampling.

Clinical Manifestations

In the early course of iron-deficiency anemia, the patient may be free of symptoms. As the disease becomes chronic, general manifestations of anemia may develop (see Table 10). In addition, specific clinical symptoms related to iron-deficiency anemia may occur.

- Pallor is the most common finding, and glossitis (inflammation of the tongue) is the second most common; another finding is cheilitis (inflammation of the lips).
- In addition, the patient may report headache, paresthesias, and a burning sensation of the tongue, all of which are caused by lack of iron in the tissues.

Diagnostic Studies

Laboratory abnormalities characteristic of iron-deficiency anemia are presented in Table 9. Other diagnostic studies are done to determine the cause of iron deficiency. Endoscopy and colonoscopy may be used to detect GI bleeding.

Collaborative Care

The main goal is to treat the underlying cause of reduced intake (e.g., malnutrition, alcoholism) or absorption of iron. Efforts are directed toward replacing iron.

- Teach the patient which foods are good sources of iron. If nutrition is adequate, increasing iron intake by dietary means may not be practical. Consequently, oral or occasionally parenteral iron supplements are used.
- Drug therapy with iron supplements requires special considerations related to administration and side effects (see Drug Therapy, Iron Deficiency Anemia, Lewis et al, *Medical-Surgical Nursing,* ed 9, p. 638).
- If iron deficiency is from acute blood loss, transfusion of packed RBCs may be required.

Nursing Management

Consider groups of individuals who are at increased risk for development of iron-deficiency anemia, including premenopausal and pregnant women, people from low socioeconomic backgrounds, older adults, and individuals experiencing blood loss. Diet teaching, with an emphasis on foods high in iron and ways to maximize absorption, is important for these groups.

Appropriate nursing measures are presented in NCP 31-1, Lewis et al, *Medical-Surgical Nursing,* ed 9, pp. 635 to 636.

▼ **Patient and Caregiver Teaching**

- Discuss with the patient the need for diagnostic studies to identify the cause of anemia. Reassess the hemoglobin level (Hgb) and RBC counts to evaluate response to therapy.
- Emphasize adherence with dietary and drug therapy. To replenish the body's iron stores, the patient needs to take iron therapy for 2 to 3 months after the Hgb level returns to normal.
- Monitor patients who require lifelong iron supplementation for potential liver problems related to the iron storage.

ANEURYSM, AORTIC

Description

An *aneurysm* is a localized outpouching or dilation of the blood vessel wall. It is one of the most common problems affecting the aorta. About 1.1 million adults between 55 and 84 years of age have an *abdominal aortic aneurysm* (AAA).

Aneurysms occur in men more often than in women, and the incidence increases with age. Aneurysms may occur in more than one location. Peripheral artery aneurysms can also develop but are not common.

Aortic aneurysms may involve the aortic arch, thoracic aorta, and/or abdominal aorta. Most aneurysms are found in the abdominal aorta below the level of the renal arteries. Over time, the dilated aortic wall becomes lined with thrombi that can embolize, leading to acute ischemia in distal arteries.

Pathophysiology

A variety of disorders are associated with aortic aneurysms. The primary causes are classified as degenerative, congenital, mechanical (e.g., penetrating or blunt trauma), inflammatory (e.g., aortitis [Takayasu's arteritis]), or infectious (e.g., aortitis [*Chlamydia pneumoniae,* human immunodeficiency virus]). Growth rates are unpredictable, but the larger the aneurysm, the greater the risk of rupture.

- Male gender, older age, and tobacco use are the major risk factors. Other risk factors include coronary or peripheral artery disease, high BP, previous stroke, being overweight, and high cholesterol.
- The development of aortic aneurysm and dissection has a strong genetic component. The familial tendency is related to congenital

anomalies such as bicuspid aortic valve, coarctation of the aorta, Turner syndrome, and autosomal dominant polycystic kidney disease.

Aneurysms are classified as true and false aneurysms.

- A *true aneurysm* is one in which the wall of the artery forms the aneurysm, with at least one vessel layer still intact. True aneurysms are further subdivided into fusiform and saccular dilations. A fusiform aneurysm is circumferential and relatively uniform in shape. A saccular aneurysm is pouchlike, with a narrow neck connecting the bulge to one side of the arterial wall.
- A *false aneurysm,* or *pseudoaneurysm,* is not an aneurysm but a disruption of all layers of all wall layers with bleeding that is contained by surrounding anatomic structures. False aneurysms may result from trauma, infection, after peripheral artery bypass graft surgery at the site of the graft-to-artery anastomosis, or arterial leakage after removal of cannulae (e.g., upper or lower extremity arterial catheters, intraaortic balloon pump devices).

Clinical Manifestations

Thoracic aorta aneurysms are usually asymptomatic. When present, the most common symptom is deep, diffuse chest pain that may extend to the interscapular area.

Aneurysms in the ascending aorta and aortic arch can produce angina from decreased blood flow to the coronary arteries and hoarseness from pressure on the recurrent laryngeal nerve. Pressure on the esophagus can cause dysphagia. If the aneurysm presses on the superior vena cava, it can cause distended neck veins and face and arm edema.

AAAs also are often asymptomatic and frequently found during routine physical examinations or evaluations for an unrelated problem (e.g., abdominal x-ray). A pulsatile mass in the periumbilical area slightly to the left of midline may be present. Bruits may be auscultated over the aneurysm. Physical findings may be more difficult to detect in obese individuals.

- AAA symptoms may mimic pain associated with any abdominal or back disorders. Compression of nearby anatomic structures may cause symptoms such as back pain from lumbar nerve compression or epigastric discomfort and/or altered bowel elimination from bowel compression.
- Occasionally aneurysms spontaneously embolize plaque causing "blue toe syndrome," in which patchy mottling of the feet and toes occurs in the presence of peripheral pulses.

Complications

The most serious complication of an aortic aneurysm is rupture.

- If rupture occurs into the retroperitoneal space, bleeding may be controlled by surrounding structures, preventing exsanguination and death. In this case the patient has severe back pain and may have back and/or flank ecchymosis *(Grey Turner's sign)*.
- If rupture occurs into the thoracic or abdominal cavity, most patients die from massive hemorrhage. The patient who reaches the hospital will be in hypovolemic shock with tachycardia; hypotension; pale, clammy skin; decreased urine output; altered sensorium; and abdominal tenderness. In this situation, simultaneous resuscitation and immediate surgical repair are necessary.

Diagnostic Studies

- Chest x-rays reveal abnormal widening of the thoracic aorta. Abdominal x-rays may show calcification within the aortic wall.
- Echocardiography assesses the function of the aortic valve.
- Ultrasound is useful for aneurysm screening and to monitor aneurysm size.
- CT is the most accurate test to determine the length and cross-sectional diameter and the presence of thrombus in the aneurysm.
- MRI may be useful to diagnose and assess the location and severity of aneurysms.

Collaborative Care

The goal of management is to prevent aneurysm rupture. Early detection and prompt treatment are essential.

Conservative therapy of small, asymptomatic AAAs (4.0 to 5.5 cm) is the best practice. This consists of risk factor modification (ceasing tobacco use, decreasing BP, optimizing lipid profile) and annual monitoring of aneurysm size using ultrasound, CT, or MRI. Growth rates may be lowered with β-adrenergic blocking agents (e.g., propranolol [Inderal]), statins (e.g., simvastatin), and antibiotics (e.g., doxycycline).

Surgical repair is done for aneurysms 5.5 cm in diameter or larger. Surgical intervention may occur sooner if the patient has a genetic disorder (e.g., Marfan's), the aneurysm expands rapidly, it becomes symptomatic, or the risk of rupture is high.

- The open aneurysm repair (OAR) involves a large abdominal incision through which the surgeon (1) cuts into the diseased aortic segment, (2) removes any thrombus or plaque, (3) sutures a synthetic graft to the aorta proximal and distal to the aneurysm, and (4) sutures the native aortic wall around the graft to act as a protective cover.

Surgical repair of an AAA is presented in Fig. 38-6 in Lewis et al, *Medical-Surgical Nursing,* ed 9, pp. 842 to 843.

- An alternative to OAR is the minimally invasive endovascular grafting technique. This technique involves placement of a sutureless aortic graft into the abdominal aorta inside the aneurysm via a femoral artery cutdown.
- Endovascular aneurysm repair (EVAR) is less invasive than OAR. However, over time both techniques have similar rates of morbidity and mortality.

The most common complication is *endoleak,* the seepage of blood back into the old aneurysm. This may be due to an inadequate seal at either graft end, a tear through the graft fabric, or leakage between overlapping graft segments. Repair may require coil embolization (insertion of beads) for hemostasis.

Nursing Management

Goals

The patient undergoing aortic surgery will have normal tissue perfusion, intact motor and sensory function, and no complications related to surgical repair, such as infection, rupture, or thrombosis.

Nursing Diagnoses

- Ineffective peripheral tissue perfusion
- Risk for infection

Nursing Interventions

Encourage the patient to reduce cardiovascular risk factors, including controlling BP, smoking cessation, increasing physical activity, and maintaining normal body weight and serum lipid levels.

- During the preoperative period, provide emotional support and teaching to the patient and caregiver. Preoperative teaching includes a brief explanation of the disease process, the planned surgical procedure(s), preoperative routines, what to expect immediately after surgery (e.g., recovery room, tubes/drains), and usual postoperative timelines.
- In the postoperative period, in addition to the usual goals of care for a postoperative patient (e.g., maintaining adequate respiratory function, fluid and electrolyte balance, pain control), check for graft patency and renal perfusion. Also watch for and intervene to limit or treat dysrhythmias, ischemia, venous thromboembolism, infections, and neurologic complications.

▼ Patient and Caregiver Teaching

Instruct the patient and caregiver to gradually increase activities once home. Fatigue, poor appetite, and irregular bowel habits are common.

- Teach the patient to avoid heavy lifting for 6 weeks after surgery. Any redness, swelling, increased pain, drainage from incisions, or fever greater than 100° F (37.8° C) should be reported to a health care provider.
- Teach the patient and caregiver to observe for changes in color or warmth of the extremities. Patients and caregivers can learn to palpate peripheral pulses to assess changes in their quality.
- Sexual dysfunction in male patients is common after aortic surgery. Preoperatively, document baseline sexual function and recommend counseling as appropriate. A referral to a urologist may be useful if erectile dysfunction occurs.

ANGINA, CHRONIC STABLE

Description
Chronic stable angina refers to chest pain that occurs intermittently over a long period with the same pattern of onset, duration, and intensity of symptoms. Chronic stable angina is a clinical manifestation of coronary artery disease (CAD).

Angina, or chest pain, is a result of reversible myocardial ischemia that occurs when the demand for myocardial oxygen exceeds the ability of the coronary arteries to supply the heart muscle with oxygen. The primary cause of myocardial ischemia is insufficient blood flow to the myocardium through coronary arteries narrowed by atherosclerosis (see Coronary Artery Disease, p. 160).

Variants of chronic stable angina include:
- *Silent ischemia,* in which ischemia occurs in the absence of any subjective symptoms
- *Nocturnal ischemia and angina decubitus* occur only at night but not necessarily when the person is lying down or sleeping.
- *Prinzmetal's angina* (variant angina) often occurs at rest, usually in response to spasm of a major coronary artery. It is a rare form of angina and frequently seen in patients with a history of migraine headaches and Raynaud's phenomenon. Calcium channel blockers and/or nitrates are used to control the angina.
- *Microvascular angina* occurs in the absence of significant coronary atherosclerosis or coronary spasm, especially in women. In these patients chest pain is related to myocardial ischemia associated with abnormalities of the coronary microcirculation. This is known as coronary microvascular disease (MVD). Prevention and treatment of MVD follow the same recommendations as for CAD.

Pathophysiology

On the cellular level the myocardium becomes hypoxic within the first 10 seconds of coronary occlusion. Myocardial cells are deprived of oxygen and glucose needed for aerobic metabolism and contractility. Anaerobic metabolism begins, and lactic acid accumulates. Lactic acid irritates myocardial nerve fibers and transmits a pain message to the cardiac nerves and upper thoracic posterior nerve roots. This accounts for referred cardiac pain to the shoulders, neck, lower jaw, and arms.

- In ischemic conditions, cardiac cells are viable for about 20 minutes. With restoration of blood flow, aerobic metabolism resumes, and cellular repair begins.

Clinical Manifestations

When questioned, some patients may deny feeling pain but describe a pressure or ache in the chest. It is an unpleasant feeling, often described as a constrictive, squeezing, heavy, choking, or suffocating sensation (Table 11). Many people complain of severe indigestion or burning. Although most angina pain appears substernally, the sensation may occur in the neck or radiate to various locations, including the jaw, shoulders, and down the arms.

- Often people will complain of pain between the shoulder blades and dismiss it as not being related to the heart.

Table 11	PQRST Assessment of Angina

Use the following memory aid to obtain information from the patient who has chest pain.

	Factor	Questions to Ask Patient
P	Precipitating events	What events or activities precipitated the pain (e.g., argument, exercise, resting)?
Q	Quality of pain	What does the pain feel like (e.g., pressure, dull, aching, tight, squeezing, heaviness)?
R	Radiation of pain	Where is the pain located? Does the pain radiate to other areas (e.g., back, neck, arms, jaw, shoulder, elbow)?
S	Severity of pain	On a scale of 0 to 10, with 0 indicating no pain and 10 being the most severe pain you could imagine, what number would you give the pain?
T	Timing	When did the pain begin? Has the pain changed since this time? Have you had pain like this before?

- Relief of chronic stable angina pectoris is usually obtained with rest or relief of the precipitating factor.

The pain usually lasts for only a few minutes (5 to 15 minutes) and commonly subsides when the precipitating factor is relieved. Pain at rest is unusual.

- An ECG usually reveals ST-segment depression and/or T wave inversion, indicating ischemia.

Diagnostic Studies

Diagnostic studies used to evaluate angina are the same as those used to diagnose CAD (see Coronary Artery Disease, pp. 162 to 163). For patients with known CAD and chronic stable angina, common diagnostic studies include 12-lead ECG, echocardiogram, exercise stress testing, and pharmacologic nuclear imaging.

Collaborative Care

The treatment of chronic stable angina is aimed at decreasing oxygen demand and/or increasing oxygen supply. The reduction of CAD risk factors is a priority. In addition to antiplatelet and cholesterol-lowering drug therapy, the most common interventions for chronic stable angina are nitrates, angiotensin-converting enzyme (ACE) inhibitors, β-adrenergic blockers, and calcium channel blockers.

Emergency care of the patient with chest pain is presented in Table 34-12, Lewis et al, *Medical-Surgical Nursing*, ed 9, p. 750.

Drug Therapy

- Aspirin is given in the absence of contraindications.
- Short-acting nitrates are first-line therapy for the treatment of angina. Nitrates produce their principal effects by dilating peripheral blood vessels, coronary arteries, and collateral vessels. Sublingual nitroglycerin will usually relieve pain in approximately 3 minutes and has a duration of approximately 30 to 60 minutes. If symptoms are unchanged or worse after 5 minutes, the patient should activate the emergency medical services system. Nitroglycerin sublingually can be used prophylactically before undertaking an activity that the patient knows may precipitate an anginal attack.
- Long-acting nitrates such as isosorbide dinitrate (Isordil) and isosorbide mononitrate (Imdur) can be used to reduce the incidence of anginal attacks. Longer-acting nitrates are available in oral preparations, ointments, and transdermal controlled-release patches.
- Angiotensin-converting enzyme (ACE) inhibitors (e.g., captopril [Capoten]) are given for patients with chronic stable angina who are considered high risk for a cardiac event (e.g., ejection

fraction [EF] 40% or less, history of diabetes). These drugs result in vasodilation and reduced blood volume. Most important, they can prevent or reverse ventricular remodeling

- Patients with left ventricular dysfunction, elevated BP, or those who have had a myocardial infarction (MI) should start and continue taking β-adrenergic blockers. These medications decrease myocardial contractility, heart rate, systemic vascular resistance (SVR), and BP, all of which reduce myocardial oxygen demand.

- Calcium channel blockers, such as nifedipine (Procardia), verapamil (Calan), diltiazem (Cardizem), and nicardipine (Cardene), are used if β-adrenergic blocking agents are contraindicated, are poorly tolerated, or do not control symptoms. Calcium channel blockers cause smooth muscle relaxation and relative vasodilation of coronary and systemic arteries, thus increasing blood flow.

Cardiac Catheterization

For patients with increasing symptoms or with a significant amount of myocardium that is ischemic under stress, a cardiac catheterization is ordered. Cardiac catheterization and coronary angiography provide images of the coronary circulation and identify the location and severity of any blockage. If a coronary blockage is amenable to an intervention, coronary revascularization with an elective percutaneous coronary intervention (PCI) is done.

- During this procedure, which is called *balloon angioplasty,* a catheter equipped with a balloon tip is inserted into the appropriate coronary artery. When the blockage is located, the catheter is passed through, the balloon is inflated, and the atherosclerotic plaque is compressed, resulting in vessel dilation.

Intracoronary stents are often inserted in conjunction with balloon angioplasty. Stents are used to treat abrupt or threatened abrupt closure and restenosis after balloon angioplasty. A stent is an expandable, meshlike structure designed to keep the vessel open by compressing the arterial walls. Because stents are thrombogenic, unfractionated heparin (UH) or low-molecular-weight heparin (LMWH) is started to maintain the open vessel. After PCI, the patient is treated with dual antiplatelet agents (e.g., ticagrelor [Brilinta] and aspirin) until the intimal lining can grow over the stent and provide a smooth vascular surface.

- Many stents are coated with a drug (e.g., paclitaxel, sirolimus) that prevents the overgrowth of new intima, which is the primary cause of stent restenosis.

- The most serious complications from stent placement are abrupt closure and vascular injury. Other less common complications include acute MI, stent embolization, coronary spasm, and emergent coronary artery bypass graft (CABG) surgery. The possibility of dysrhythmias during and after the procedure is always present.

Nursing Management

Goals and Nursing Diagnoses

Goals and nursing diagnoses for the patient with chronic stable angina are the same as those used for ACS (see Acute Coronary Syndrome, pp. 11 to 12).

Nursing Interventions

If your patient experiences angina, institute the following measures: (1) position patient upright unless contraindicated and administer supplemental oxygen, (2) assess vital signs, (3) obtain a 12-lead ECG, (4) provide prompt pain relief first with a nitrate followed by an opioid analgesic if needed, and (5) auscultate heart and breath sounds.

- The patient is often distressed and may have pale, cool, clammy skin. BP and HR may be elevated. Auscultation of the heart may reveal an atrial (S_4) or a ventricular (S_3) gallop.
- Ask the patient to describe the pain and to rate it on a scale of 0 to 10 before and after treatment to evaluate the effectiveness of the interventions (see Table 11).
- Some patients may not report pain. Assess for other manifestations of pain, such as restlessness; ECG changes; elevated HR, respiratory rate, or BP; clutching of the bed linens; or other nonverbal cues.
- Supportive and realistic assurance and a calm approach help reduce the patient's anxiety during an anginal attack.

▼ Patient and Caregiver Teaching

Reassure the patient with a history of chronic stable angina that a long, productive life is possible.

- Teaching tools such as DVDs or CDs, heart models, and written information are important components of patient and caregiver teaching.
- Assist the patient to identify factors that precipitate angina and how to avoid or control these factors.
- Assist the patient to identify personal risk factors in CAD. Then discuss the various methods of decreasing any modifiable risk factors.
- Teach the patient and caregiver about diets that are low in sodium and have reduced saturated fats. Maintaining ideal body weight is important in controlling angina, because excess weight increases myocardial workload.
- Adhering to a regular, individualized exercise program that conditions the myocardium rather than overstressing it is important.

For example, advise patients to walk briskly on a flat surface at least 30 minutes a day, most days of the week, if not contraindicated.

- It is important to teach the patient and caregiver the proper use of nitroglycerin.
- If needed, arrange for counseling to assess psychologic adjustment of the patient and caregiver to the diagnosis of CAD and resulting angina. Many patients feel a threat to their identity and self-esteem.

ANKYLOSING SPONDYLITIS

Description

Ankylosing spondylitis (AS) is a chronic inflammatory disease that primarily affects the axial skeleton, including the sacroiliac joints, intervertebral disk spaces, and costovertebral articulations. HLA-B27 antigen is found in approximately 90% of people with AS. The usual age of onset of AS is before 40 years old. Men are three to five times more likely to develop AS than women. The disease may go undetected in women because of a milder course.

Pathophysiology

The cause of AS is unknown. Genetic predisposition appears to play an important role in disease pathogenesis, but the precise mechanisms are unknown. Aseptic synovial inflammation in joints and adjacent tissue causes the formation of granulation tissue (pannus) and the development of dense fibrous scars that lead to fusion of articular tissues. Extraarticular inflammation can affect the eyes, lungs, heart, kidneys, and peripheral nervous system.

Clinical Manifestations

Symptoms of inflammatory spine pain are the first clues to a diagnosis of AS. The patient typically complains of lower back pain, stiffness, and limitation of motion that is worse during the night and in the morning but improves with mild activity. General symptoms such as fever, fatigue, anorexia, and weight loss are rarely present.

Uveitis (intraocular inflammation) is the most common nonskeletal symptom. It can appear as an initial presentation of the disease years before arthritic symptoms develop. Patients may also experience chest pain and sternal/costal cartilage tenderness.

Severe postural abnormalities and deformity can lead to significant disability. Aortic insufficiency and pulmonary fibrosis are frequent complications. Cauda equina syndrome can also result, contributing to lower extremity weakness and bladder dysfunction. The patient is also at risk for spinal fracture because of associated osteoporosis.

Diagnostic Studies

- X-rays are used to diagnose AS.
- MRI can be useful in assessing early cartilage abnormalities.
- However, radiographs are limited in detecting early sacroiliitis or subtle changes in posterior vertebrae.
- Laboratory testing is not specific, but an elevated erythrocyte sedimentation rate (ESR) and mild anemia may be seen.
- When the suspicion of AS is high, the presence of the HLA-B27 antigen improves the likelihood of this diagnosis.

Collaborative Care

Prevention of AS is not possible. However, families with other diagnosed HLA-B27–positive rheumatic diseases (e.g., acute anterior uveitis, juvenile spondyloarthritis) should be alert to signs of lower back pain and arthritis symptoms for early identification and treatment of AS.

Care of the patient is aimed at maintaining maximal skeletal mobility while decreasing pain and inflammation. Heat applications, nonsteroidal antiinflammatory drugs (NSAIDs) and salicylates, and disease-modifying antirheumatic drugs (DMARDs), such as sulfasalazine (Azulfidine) or methotrexate, can help in relieving symptoms. Etanercept (Enbrel), a biologic therapy, inhibits the action of tumor necrosis factor (TNF) and has been shown to reduce active inflammation and improve spinal mobility. Additional anti-TNF inhibitors (infliximab [Remicade], adalimumab [Humira], or golimumab [Simponi]) may also be effective.

Postural control with stretching exercises of the back, neck, and chest is important to minimize spinal deformity. Hydrotherapy has also been shown to decrease pain and facilitate spinal extension. Surgery may be indicated for severe deformity and mobility impairment. Spinal osteotomy and total joint replacement are the most commonly performed procedures.

Nursing Management

A key responsibility is to teach the patient about the nature of the disease and principles of therapy. The home management program consists of local moist heat, regular exercise, and knowledgeable use of drugs.

- Discourage excessive physical exertion during periods of active inflammation.

- Encourage smoking cessation to decrease the risk for lung complications in those with reduced chest expansion.
- Ongoing physical therapy should include gentle, graded stretching and strengthening exercises to preserve range of motion (ROM) and improve thoracolumbar flexion and extension.
- Proper positioning at rest is essential. The mattress should be firm, and the patient should sleep on the back with a flat pillow, avoiding positions that encourage flexion deformity.
- Postural training emphasizes avoiding spinal flexion (e.g., leaning over a desk), heavy lifting, and prolonged walking, standing, or sitting. Encourage sports that facilitate natural stretching, such as swimming and racquet games.
- Family counseling and vocational rehabilitation are important.

AORTIC DISSECTION

Description

Aortic dissection, often misnamed "dissecting aneurysm," is not a type of aneurysm. Rather, dissection results from the creation of a false lumen between the intima (inner layer) and media (middle layer) of the arterial wall. Classification is based on anatomic location (ascending versus descending aorta) and duration of onset (acute versus chronic).

- Approximately two thirds of dissections involve the ascending aorta and are acute in onset. Chronic dissections almost always involve the descending aorta.
- Aortic dissection affects men two to five times more often than women and occurs most frequently in the sixth and seventh decades of life. Predisposing factors include age, aortitis (e.g., syphilis), blunt trauma, congenital heart disease (e.g., bicuspid aortic valve, coarctation of the aorta), connective tissue disorders (e.g., Marfan's), prior aortic surgery, or recent trauma.

Pathophysiology

Most nontraumatic aortic dissections are attributed to the degeneration of the elastic fibers in the medial layer. Chronic hypertension accelerates the degradation process. In aortic dissection a tear develops in the inner wall of the aorta. Blood surges through this tear, causing the inner and middle layers to separate (dissect). If the blood-filled channel ruptures through the outside aortic wall, aortic dissection is often fatal.

As the heart contracts, each pulsation increases the pressure on the damaged area, which further increases dissection. Extension of the dissection may cut off blood supply to critical areas such as the brain, kidneys, spinal cord, and extremities. The false lumen may remain patent, become thrombosed (clotted), rejoin the true lumen by way of a distal tear, or rupture.

Clinical Manifestations and Complications

The majority of patients with an acute ascending aortic dissection reports sudden, severe onset of excruciating chest and/or back pain radiating to the neck or shoulders. Patients with acute descending aortic dissection are more likely to report pain in their back, abdomen, or legs. The pain is frequently described as "sharp" and "worst ever" followed less frequently by "tearing" or "ripping." Dissection pain can be differentiated from myocardial infarction (MI) pain, which is more gradual in onset and has increasing intensity.

- Older patients are less likely to have an abrupt onset of chest or back pain and more likely to have hypotension and vague symptoms. Some patients have a painless aortic dissection, emphasizing the importance of the physical examination.
- If the aortic arch is involved, the patient may exhibit neurologic deficits, including altered level of consciousness, dizziness, and weakened or absent carotid and temporal pulses.
- An ascending aortic dissection usually produces some disruption of coronary blood flow and aortic valvular insufficiency.
- When either subclavian artery is involved, pulse quality and blood pressure (BP) readings may differ between the left and right arms.
- As dissection progresses down the aorta, the abdominal organs and lower extremities demonstrate evidence of altered tissue perfusion.

A life-threatening complication of an acute ascending aortic dissection is cardiac tamponade, which occurs when blood from the dissection leaks into the pericardial sac. Clinical manifestations include hypotension, narrowed pulse pressure, distended neck veins, muffled heart sounds, and pulsus paradoxus.

- Because the aorta is weakened by dissection, it may rupture. Hemorrhage may occur into the mediastinal, pleural, or abdominal cavities.
- Dissection can lead to occlusion of the blood supply to vital organs, including the spinal cord, kidneys, and abdominal structures. Spinal cord ischemia leads to weakness and decreased sensation to complete lower extremity paralysis. Renal ischemia can lead to renal failure. Signs of abdominal ischemia include abdominal pain, decreased bowel sounds, and altered bowel elimination.

Diagnostic Studies

Studies to detect aortic dissection are similar to those performed for suspected aneurysms.

- Chest x-ray indicates widening of the mediastinum and pleural effusion.
- 3-D CT scanning and transesophageal echocardiography (TEE) have become the standard tests for a diagnosis of acute aortic dissection.
- CT scan can provide information on the presence and severity of the dissection.
- Although MRI has the highest accuracy for detecting aortic dissection, this modality is contraindicated in some patients (e.g., those with metal implants or who are hemodynamically unstable).

Collaborative Care

The patient with an acute or chronic descending aortic dissection without complications can be treated conservatively. Conservative treatment includes pain relief, heart rate (HR) and BP control, and cardiovascular disease risk factor modification. HR and BP control reduces aortic wall stress by decreasing systolic BP and myocardial contractility.

- An IV β-adrenergic blocker (e.g., esmolol) is often used to control the HR.
- Other antihypertensive agents, such as calcium channel blockers and angiotensin-converting enzyme (ACE) inhibitors, may also be used.
- Morphine is the preferred analgesic because it decreases sympathetic nervous system stimulation and relieves pain.
- Supportive treatment for an acute aortic dissection serves as a bridge to surgery.

Endovascular repair of acute descending aortic dissections with complications (e.g., hemodynamic instability) and chronic descending aortic dissection with complications (e.g., peripheral ischemia) is a treatment option.

An acute ascending aortic dissection is considered a surgical emergency. Otherwise, surgery is indicated when conservative therapy is ineffective or when complications (e.g., heart failure) occur. Because the aorta is fragile following dissection, surgical intervention is delayed for as long as possible to allow time for edema to decrease and to permit clotting of the blood in the false lumen.

- Surgery involves resection of the aortic segment containing the intimal tear and replacement with a synthetic graft.

Even with prompt surgical intervention, the in-hospital mortality rate of acute aortic dissection is high. Causes of death include aortic rupture, mesenteric ischemia, MI, sepsis, and multiorgan failure.

Nursing Management

Preoperatively, nursing management includes keeping the patient in bed in a semi-Fowler's position and maintaining a quiet environment. These measures help to keep the HR and systolic BP at the lowest possible level that maintains vital organ perfusion (typically HR <60 beats/minute; systolic BP <120 mm Hg). Administer opioids and sedatives as ordered. Manage pain and anxiety for patient comfort and because they can cause elevations in the systolic BP.

- IV administration of antihypertensive agents requires close supervision. This requires continuous ECG and intraarterial BP monitoring. Monitor vital signs frequently, sometimes as often as every 2 to 3 minutes until target HR and BP are reached. Observe for changes in peripheral pulses and signs of increasing pain, restlessness, and anxiety.

Postoperative care is similar to that after open aneurysm repair (see Aneurysm, Aortic, p. 45 in this book, and Nursing Management of Aortic Aneurysms in Lewis et al, *Medical-Surgical Nursing,* ed 9, pp. 844 to 845).

▼ **Patient and Caregiver Teaching**

- Instruct patients that they need to take antihypertensive drugs daily for the rest of their lives to control HR and BP.
- It is important for patients to understand the drug regimen and potential side effects (e.g., dizziness, depression, fatigue, erectile dysfunction). Tell the patient to discuss any side effects with the health care provider before discontinuing the drugs.
- Follow-up with regularly scheduled MRIs or CTs is essential.
- You must instruct patients that if the pain or other symptoms return, they should activate EMS for immediate care.

APPENDICITIS

Description

Appendicitis is an inflammation of the appendix, a narrow blind tube that extends from the inferior part of the cecum. It is most common in individuals 10 to 30 years of age. It is the most common cause of acute abdominal pain.

Pathophysiology

A common cause of appendicitis is obstruction of the lumen by a fecalith (accumulated feces). Obstruction results in distention; venous engorgement; and the accumulation of mucus and bacteria, which can lead to gangrene, perforation, and peritonitis.

Clinical Manifestations and Complications

Appendicitis typically begins with periumbilical pain, followed by anorexia, nausea, and vomiting. The pain is persistent and continuous, eventually shifting to the right lower quadrant and localizing at McBurney's point (halfway between the umbilicus and right iliac crest).

- Further assessment reveals localized and rebound tenderness with muscle guarding. Coughing, sneezing, and deep inhalation magnify the pain.
- The patient usually prefers to lie still, often with the right leg flexed. Low-grade fever may be present.

If diagnosis and treatment are delayed, the appendix can rupture, and the resulting peritonitis can be fatal.

Diagnostic Studies

- Differential white blood cell (WBC) count is usually elevated.
- Urinalysis is done to rule out genitourinary conditions that mimic manifestations of appendicitis.
- CT scan and ultrasound may be used.

Collaborative Care

Treatment is immediate surgical removal (appendectomy) if the inflammation is localized. If the appendix has ruptured and there is evidence of peritonitis or an abscess, antibiotic therapy and parenteral fluids are given for 6 to 8 hours before the appendectomy to prevent sepsis and dehydration.

Nursing Management

Encourage the patient with abdominal pain to see a health care provider and to avoid self-treatment, particularly the use of laxatives and enemas. Increased peristalsis from these procedures may cause perforation.

- Nothing should be taken by mouth (NPO) to ensure the stomach will be empty if surgery is needed.

Postoperative nursing management is similar to postoperative care of a patient after laparotomy (see Abdominal Pain, Acute, pp. 4 to 5). Ambulation begins the day of surgery or the first postoperative day. Diet is advanced as tolerated.

- The patient is usually discharged on the first or second postoperative day and resumes normal activities 2 to 3 weeks after surgery.

ASTHMA

Description

Asthma is a chronic inflammatory disease of the airways. The chronic inflammation leads to recurrent episodes of wheezing, breathlessness, chest tightness, and cough, especially at night and in the early morning. These episodes are associated with widespread but variable airflow obstruction that is usually reversible, either spontaneously or with treatment. The clinical course of asthma is unpredictable, ranging from periods of adequate control, to exacerbations with poor control of symptoms.

- Asthma affects an estimated 17.5 million adult Americans. Among adults, women are 76% more likely to have asthma than men. Despite a decline in the number of deaths from asthma over the past 8 years, more than 3400 people still die from asthma yearly.
- Risk factors for asthma and triggers of asthma attacks are in Table 12.

Pathophysiology

The primary pathophysiologic process in asthma is persistent but variable airway inflammation. The airflow is limited because the inflammation results in bronchoconstriction, airway hyperresponsiveness (hyperactivity), and airway edema. Exposure to allergens or irritants initiates the inflammatory cascade.

- As the inflammatory process begins, mast cells in the bronchial wall degranulate and release multiple inflammatory mediators including leukotrienes, histamine, cytokines, prostaglandins, and nitric oxide.
- The resulting inflammatory process causes vascular congestion; edema; production of thick, tenacious mucus; bronchial muscle spasm; thickening of airway walls; and increased bronchial hyperresponsiveness.
- This process can occur within 30 to 60 minutes after exposure to a trigger or irritant and is sometimes referred to as the *early-phase response* in asthma.

Symptoms can recur 4 to 6 hours after the early response because of the influx of many inflammatory cells and the further release of more inflammatory mediators.

- At this later time the patient may again develop symptoms or worsening of symptoms. This is called the *late-phase response,* which occurs in about 50% of individuals with asthma.

Table 12 Triggers of Asthma Attacks

Allergen Inhalation
- Animal dander (e.g., cats, mice, guinea pigs)
- House dust mites
- Cockroaches
- Pollens
- Molds

Air Pollutants
- Exhaust fumes
- Perfumes
- Oxidants
- Sulfur dioxides
- Cigarette smoke
- Aerosol sprays

Inflammation and Infection
- Viral upper respiratory tract infection
- Sinusitis, allergic rhinitis

Drugs
- Aspirin
- Nonsteroidal antiinflammatory drugs
- β-Adrenergic blockers

Occupational Exposure
- Agriculture, farming
- Paints, solvents
- Laundry detergents
- Metal salts
- Wood and vegetable dusts
- Industrial chemicals and plastics
- Pharmaceutical agents

Food Additives
- Sulfites (bisulfites and metabisulfites)
- Beer, wine, dried fruit, shrimp, processed potatoes
- Monosodium glutamate
- Tartrazine

Other Factors
- Exercise and cold, dry air
- Stress
- Hormones, menses
- Gastroesophageal reflux disease (GERD)

- Bronchoconstriction with symptoms persists for 24 hours or longer. Corticosteroids are effective in treating this inflammation.

Chronic inflammation may result in structural changes in the bronchial wall known as *remodeling*. A progressive loss of lung function occurs that is not prevented or fully reversed by therapy.

During an asthma attack, decreased perfusion and ventilation of the alveoli and increased alveolar gas pressure lead to ventilation-perfusion abnormalities in the lungs.

- The patient is hypoxemic early on with decreased $PaCO_2$ and increased pH (respiratory alkalosis) as a result of hyperventilation.
- As the airflow limitation worsens with air trapping, the $PaCO_2$ normalizes, and then it increases to produce respiratory acidosis, which is an ominous sign of respiratory failure.

Clinical Manifestations

Depending on an individual's response, asthma can rapidly progress from normal breathing to acute severe asthma. Recurrent episodes of wheezing, breathlessness, chest tightness, and cough, particularly at night and in the early morning, are typical in asthma. An attack of asthma may have an abrupt onset, but usually symptoms occur more gradually. Attacks may last for a few minutes to several hours.

- Characteristic manifestations are wheezing, cough, dyspnea, and chest tightness. Expiration may be prolonged with an inspiratory/expiratory (I/E) ratio of 1:3 or 1:4.
- Wheezing is an unreliable sign to gauge the severity of an attack because many patients with minor attacks wheeze loudly, whereas others with severe attacks do not wheeze.
- In some patients with asthma, cough is the only symptom. The cough may be nonproductive because secretions may be so thick, tenacious, and gelatinous that their removal is difficult.
- During an acute attack, the patient usually sits upright or slightly bent forward using accessory muscles of respiration. The more difficult the breathing becomes, the more anxious the patient feels.
- Signs of hypoxemia include restlessness, increased anxiety, inappropriate behavior, and increased pulse and BP.
- Percussion reveals hyperresonance of the lungs. Auscultation indicates inspiratory or expiratory wheezing.
- Diminished breath sounds may indicate a significant decrease in air movement. Severely diminished breath sounds or a "silent chest" is an ominous sign, indicating severe obstruction and impending respiratory failure.

Classification of Asthma

Asthma can be classified as intermittent, mild persistent, moderate persistent, or severe persistent (Table 13). The classification system is used to determine the treatment. Patients may move to different asthma classifications over the course of their disease.

Complications

Severe asthma exacerbations occur when the patient is dyspneic at rest and the patient talks in words, not sentences, because of the difficulty breathing. They are usually sitting forward to maximize the diaphragmatic movement with prominent wheezing and a respiratory rate >30 breaths/minute and pulse >120 beats/minute.

- Accessory muscles in the neck are straining to lift the chest wall and the patient is often agitated. The peak flow (PEFR [peak expiratory flow rate]) is 40% of the personal best or <150 mL.
- Neck vein distention may result. These patients usually are seen in emergency departments (EDs) or hospitalized.

A few patients perceive asthma symptoms poorly and may have a significant decrease in lung function without any change in symptoms. Patients with life-threatening asthma are typically too dyspneic to speak and will perspire profusely. The breath sounds may be difficult to hear, and no wheezing is apparent because the airflow is exceptionally limited.

- If the patient has been wheezing and then there is an absence of a wheeze (i.e., silent chest) and the patient is obviously struggling, this is a life-threatening situation that may require mechanical ventilation.

Diagnostic Studies

Underdiagnosis of asthma is common. In general, the health care provider should consider the diagnosis of asthma if various indicators (i.e., clinical manifestations, health history, peak flow variability or spirometry) are positive.

- Detailed history helps to identify asthma triggers.
- Pulmonary function tests determine the reversibility of bronchoconstriction and thus establish the diagnosis of asthma.
- Sputum specimen can be used to rule out bacterial infection.
- Serum IgE levels and eosinophil count, when elevated, are highly suggestive of allergic tendency.
- Chest x-ray during an attack shows hyperinflation.
- Pulmonary function tests (PFTs), oximetry, and arterial blood gases (ABGs) provide information about the severity of the attack and response to treatment.
- Allergy skin testing can be used to determine sensitivity to specific allergens.

Table 13 Classification of Asthma Severity

Components of Severity		Asthma Severity			
		Intermittent	Persistent		
			Mild	Moderate	Severe
Impairment					
Symptoms		≤2 days/wk	>2 days/wk, not daily	Daily	Continuous
Nighttime awakenings		≤2/mo	3-4/mo	>1/wk, not nightly	Often, 7/wk
SABA use for symptoms		≤2 days/wk	>2 days/wk, not daily	Daily	Several times per day
Interference with normal activity		None	Minor limitation	Some limitation	Extremely limited
Lung function*		Normal FEV$_1$ between exacerbations FEV$_1$ >80% FEV$_1$/FVC normal	FEV$_1$ >80% predicted FEV$_1$/FVC normal	FEV$_1$ 60%-80% predicted FEV$_1$/FVC reduced by 5%	FEV$_1$ >60% predicted FEV$_1$/FVC reduced by 5%
Risk					
Exacerbations requiring oral corticosteroids		0-1/yr	>2/yr even in the absence of impairment ‹————————————————›		
			Consider severity and interval since last exacerbation ‹—————————————————›		
			Frequency and severity may fluctuate over time ‹———————————————————————›		
			Relative annual risk of exacerbation may be related to FEV$_1$ ‹———————————›		

Recommended Step for Initiating Treatment	Step 1	Step 2	Step 3[†]	Step 4 or 5[†]
	Reevaluate asthma control in 2-6 wk and adjust therapy accordingly			

Guidelines for Using Table

- Patients should be assigned to the most severe step in which any feature occurs. Clinical features for individual patients may overlap across steps. Determine level of severity by assessment of both impairment and risk. Assess impairment by patient's recall of previous 2-4 wk and spirometry results.
- An individual's classification should change over time as treatment is initiated. After treatment, the focus switches to level of control, not the classification of severity.
- Patients at any level of severity of chronic asthma can have mild, moderate, or severe exacerbations of asthma. Some patients with intermittent asthma experience severe and life-threatening exacerbations separated by long periods of normal lung function and no symptoms.

Source: Adapted from National Asthma Education and Prevention Program, National Heart, Lung, and Blood Institute: *Expert Panel Report 3: guidelines for the diagnosis and management of asthma*, NIH pub no 08-4051, Bethesda, Md, 2007, National Institutes of Health. Retrieved from *www.nhlbi.nih.gov/guidelines*.

*Percent predicted values for FEV_1, or ratio of FEV_1/FVC. Normal FEV_1/FVC: 8-19 yr, 85%; 20-39 yr, 80%; 40-59 yr, 75%; 60-80 yr, 70%.

[†]Consider short-term corticosteroid therapy.

FEV_1, Forced expiratory volume in 1 sec; *FVC*, forced vital capacity; *SABA*, short-acting β_2-adrenergic agonist.

Collaborative Care

The goal of asthma treatment is to achieve and maintain control of the disease. Guidelines for the diagnosis and management of asthma are presented in Table 13 on pp. 62 to 63 and in Table 29-5 and Fig. 29-4, Lewis et al, *Medical-Surgical Nursing,* ed 9, pp. 567 and 568. The current guidelines focus on (1) assessing the severity of the disease at diagnosis and initial treatment and then (2) monitoring periodically to control the disease.

At initial diagnosis a patient may have severe asthma and require asthma medication. After treatment the patient is assessed for level of control (i.e., well controlled, not well controlled, or very poorly controlled). The health care provider steps down the medication as the patient achieves control of the symptoms or steps it up as the symptoms worsen.

- Achieving rapid control of the symptoms is the goal in order to return the patient to daily functioning at the best possible level. The level of control is determined by the patient's current peak flow or forced expiratory volume in 1 second (FEV_1) and any exacerbations or adverse treatment effects.

Intermittent and Persistent Asthma. The classification of severity of asthma at the initial diagnosis helps determine which types of medications are best suited to control the asthma symptoms (see Table 13).

- Patients in all classifications of asthma require a *short-term* (rescue or reliever) medication. The most effective ones are short-acting β_2-adrenergic agonists (SABAs) (e.g., albuterol). Patients with persistent asthma must also be on a long-term or controller medication.
- For *long-term* control of moderate to severe persistent asthma, long-acting β_2-adrenergic agonists (LABAs), including salmeterol (Serevent) and formoterol (Foradil), are added to a daily dose of inhaled corticosteroids (ICS) (e.g., fluticasone [Flovent]). ICS are the most effective class of drugs to treat the inflammation.

Acute Asthma Exacerbations. Asthma exacerbations may be mild to life threatening. With mild exacerbations, patients have difficulty breathing only with activity and may feel they "can't get enough air." Peak flow is >70% of their personal best, and symptoms often are relieved at home promptly with a SABA such as albuterol delivered via a nebulizer or metered dose inhaler (MDI) with a spacer.

- With a moderate exacerbation, dyspnea interferes with usual activities and peak flow is 40% to 60% of personal best. In this situation, the patient usually comes to the ED or a health care provider's office to get help. Relief is provided with the SABA delivered as in the mild exacerbation, and oral corticosteroids are needed. Symptoms may persist for several days even after corticosteroids are started. Oxygen can be used with both mild and moderate exacerbations.

Severe and Life-Threatening Asthma Exacerbations. Management of the patient with severe and life-threatening asthma focuses on correcting hypoxemia and improving ventilation. The goal is to keep the O_2 saturation $\geq 90\%$. Continuous monitoring of the patient is critical.

- Many therapeutic measures are the same as those for acute asthma. Repetitive or continuous SABA administration is provided in the ED. Initially three treatments of SABA (spaced 20 to 30 minutes apart) are given. Then more SABA is given depending on the patient's airflow, improvement, and side effects from the SABA.
- In life-threatening asthma, IV corticosteroids are administered and are usually tapered rapidly. IV corticosteroids (methylprednisolone) are administered every 4 to 6 hours. Adjunctive medications such as IV magnesium sulfate may be administered in certain patients with very low FEV_1 or peak flow (<40% of predicted or personal best at presentation) or those who fail to respond to initial treatment.
- Supplemental O_2 is given by mask or nasal prongs to achieve a PaO_2 of at least 60 mm Hg or an O_2 saturation >90%. An arterial catheter may be inserted to facilitate frequent ABG monitoring.

Occasionally asthma exacerbations are life threatening and respiratory arrest is pending or actually occurring. The patient requires intubation and mechanical ventilation if there is no response to treatment. The patient is provided with 100% oxygen, hourly or continuously nebulized SABA, IV corticosteroids, and possible other adjunctive therapies as noted above.

Drug Therapy

A stepwise approach to drug therapy is based initially on asthma severity and then on level of control. Persistent asthma requires daily long-term therapy in addition to appropriate medications to manage acute symptoms. Medications are divided into two general classifications:

- *Quick-relief or rescue medications* to treat symptoms and exacerbations, such as SABAs
- *Long-term control medications* to achieve and maintain control of persistent asthma such as ICS. Some of the controllers are used in combination to gain better asthma control (e.g., fluticasone/

salmeterol [Advair]) (see Table 29-7, Lewis et al, *Medical-Surgical Nursing,* ed 9, pp. 570 to 571).

Patient teaching about medications should include the name, purpose, dosage, method of administration, and schedule, taking into consideration activities of daily living (ADLs) (e.g., bathing) that require energy expenditure and thus oxygen.

- Information should also include side effects, appropriate action if side effects occur, how to properly use and clean devices, and consequences for breathing if not taking medications as prescribed.

Nursing Management

Goals

The patient with asthma will maintain greater than 80% of personal best PEFR or FEV_1 and will have minimal symptoms during the day and night, few or no adverse effects of therapy, acceptable activity levels (including exercise and other physical activity), no recurrent exacerbations of asthma, and adequate knowledge to participate in and carry out management.

See NCP 29-1 for the patient with asthma, Lewis et al, *Medical-Surgical Nursing,* ed 9, p. 576.

Nursing Diagnoses

- Ineffective airway clearance
- Anxiety
- Deficient knowledge

Nursing Interventions

A goal in asthma care is to maximize the patient's ability to safely manage acute asthma exacerbations via an asthma action plan developed in conjunction with the health care provider (see Table 29-12, Lewis et al, *Medical-Surgical Nursing,* ed 9, p. 578.

- The patient can take two to four puffs of a SABA every 20 minutes three times as a rescue plan. Depending on the response with alleviation of symptoms or improved peak flow, continued SABA use and/or oral corticosteroids may be a part of the home management plan at this point. If symptoms persist or if the patient's peak flow is <50% of the personal best, the health care provider or emergency medical services need to be immediately contacted.
- When the patient is in the health care facility with an acute exacerbation, it is important to monitor the patient's respiratory and cardiovascular systems. This includes auscultating lung sounds; taking the heart and respiratory rates and BP; and monitoring ABGs, pulse oximetry, and peak flow.

- An important nursing goal during an acute attack is to decrease the patient's sense of panic. A calm, quiet, reassuring attitude may help the patient relax. Position the patient comfortably (usually sitting) to maximize chest expansion. Stay with the patient and be available to provide additional comfort.
- In a firm, calm voice coach the patient to use pursed-lip breathing, which keeps the airways open by maintaining positive pressure, and abdominal breathing, which slows the respiratory rate and encourages deeper breaths.

▼ **Patient and Caregiver Teaching**
- Teach the patient to avoid known personal triggers for asthma (e.g., cigarette smoke, pet dander) and irritants (e.g., cold air, aspirin, foods, cats). If cold air cannot be avoided, dressing properly with a scarf or mask helps reduce the risk of an asthma attack. Aspirin and nonsteroidal antiinflammatory drugs (NSAIDs) should be avoided if they are known to precipitate an attack. Many over-the-counter (OTC) drugs contain aspirin, and the patient should be instructed to read labels carefully.
- Nonselective β-blockers (e.g., propranolol [Inderal]) are contraindicated because they inhibit bronchodilation.
- Prompt diagnosis and treatment of upper respiratory tract infections and sinusitis may prevent an exacerbation of asthma.
- If exercise is planned or if the patient has asthma only with exercise, the health care provider can suggest a medication regimen for pretreatment or long-term control of symptoms to prevent bronchospasm.

It is important to involve the patient's caregiver or family. These people should know where the patient's inhalers, oral medications, and emergency phone numbers are located. Instruct them on how to decrease the patient's anxiety if an asthma attack occurs. When the patient is stabilized or controlled, the caregiver can gently remind the patient about doing daily PEFR by asking questions such as, "What zone are you in? How's your peak flow today?"

A patient and caregiver teaching guide for the patient with asthma and the caregiver is presented in Table 14.

| Table 14 | Patient and Caregiver Teaching Guide |
| | *Asthma* |

Include the following information in the teaching plan for the patient with asthma and the caregiver.

Goal

To assist patient in improving quality of life through education, increased understanding, and promotion of lifestyle practices that support successful living with asthma

Teaching Topic	Resources
What Is Asthma? ▪ Basic anatomy and physiology of lung ▪ Pathophysiology of asthma ▪ Relationship of pathophysiology to signs and symptoms ▪ Measurement and correlation of pulmonary function tests and peak expiratory flow rate	*What Is Asthma?* (National Heart, Lung, and Blood Institute) Retrieved from *www.nhlbi.nih.gov/health/dci/Diseases/Asthma/Asthma_WhatIs.html.* *What Is Asthma?* (Global Initiative for Asthma). Retrieved from *www.ginasthma.org/q-a-general-information-about-asthma.html.* *Asthma: Overview* (National Jewish Health). Retrieved from *www.njhealth.org/healthinfo/conditions/asthma/index.aspx.*
What Is Good Asthma Control? ▪ Resource for patient on personal ideas of good control	*Asthma Control Test.* Retrieved from *www.qualitymetric.com/demos/TP_Launch.aspx?SID=52461.*
Hindrances to Asthma Treatment and Control ▪ Intermittent nature of symptoms ▪ Role of denial ▪ Poor perception of asthma severity by patient	Discussion with patient and caregiver about possible hindrances.

| Table 14 | Patient and Caregiver Teaching Guide *Asthma*—cont'd | A |

Environmental and Trigger Control

- Identifications of possible triggers and possible preventive measures
- Avoidance of allergens and other triggers
- Need to maintain good hydration

Environmental Management (National Jewish Health). Retrieved from *www. nationaljewish.org/ healthinfo/conditions/ asthma/lifestyle-management/environmental.*

Pollen Count Report (sign up for daily notification about a particular area) (American Academy of Asthma Allergy and Immunology). Retrieved from *www.aaaai. org/nab.*

Trigger diary kept by patient.

Medications

Types (include mechanism of action)

- β_2-Agonists
- Corticosteroids
- Methylxanthines
- Anti-IgE
- Leukotriene modifiers
- Combination drugs

Establishing medication schedule

Use of preventive and maintenance agents (e.g., antiinflammatory agents)

Asthma: Treatment (National Jewish Health). Available at *www.nationaljewish.org/ healthinfo/conditions/ asthma/treatment.*

Asthma Action Plan (see Table 29-12, Lewis et al, *Medical-Surgical Nursing,* ed 9, p. 578).

Write out medication list and schedule.

Continued

Table 14	Patient and Caregiver Teaching Guide *Asthma*—cont'd

Correct use of inhalers, spacer, and nebulizer	Demonstration–return demonstration with placebo devices (see Figs. 29-5 to 29-7 and Tables 29-8 to 29-10, Lewis et al, *Medical-Surgical Nursing,* ed 9, pp. 571 to 574). *Inhaled Medication Instructional Videos: Asthma and General Lung Disease* (National Jewish Health). Retrieved from *www. nationaljewish.org/ healthinfo/medications/ lung-diseases/devices/ instructional-videos.* Patient instructions for inhaled devices in English and Spanish (American College of Chest Physicians). Retrieved from *www. chestnet.org/accp/patient-guides/patient-instructions-inhaled-devices-english-and-spanish.*
Breathing Techniques Pursed-lip breathing	See Table 29-13, Lewis et al, *Medical-Surgical Nursing,* ed 9, p. 579.
Correct use of peak flow meter	See Table 29-14, Lewis et al, *Medical-Surgical Nursing,* ed 9, p. 579. *Measuring Your Peak Flow Rate (text and video)* (American Lung Association). Retrieved from *www.lung. org/lung-disease/asthma/ living-with-asthma/take-control-of-your-asthma/ measuring-your-peak-flow-rate.html.*

Table 14	Patient and Caregiver Teaching Guide *Asthma*—cont'd

Asthma Action Plan

- Peak flow zones
- Individualize plan
- Early recognition of infection
- Building a partnership with your health care provider
- Questions patients may have about asthma, but patient cannot reach the provider

See Table 29-12, Lewis et al, *Medical-Surgical Nursing*, ed 9, p. 578.

Patient completes asthma action plan and discusses it with health care provider.

Asthma Clinical Research Centers (American Lung Association). Retrieved from *www.lung.org/finding-cures/our-research/acrc*.

My Asthma Wallet Card (National Heart, Lung, and Blood Institute). Retrieved from *www.nhlbi.nih.gov/health/public/lung/asthma/asthma_walletcard.htm*.

Asthma Profiler (online decision support tool to assist patients in understanding treatment options and side effects; includes personalized questions to ask the provider and research reports) (American Lung Association). Retrieved from *www.lung.org/lung-disease/asthma/living-with-asthma/making-treatment-decisions*.

Lung Line (ask a specialized nurse questions about early detection, care, and prevention of respiratory diseases) (National Jewish Health). Telephone: 800-222-LUNG or *www.njhealth.org/about/contact/lung-line.aspx*.

BELL'S PALSY

Description

Bell's palsy (peripheral facial paralysis, acute benign cranial poly-neuritis) is a disorder characterized by inflammation of the facial nerve (CN VII) on one side of the face in the absence of any other disease, such as a stroke. Despite its good prognosis, Bell's palsy leaves more than 8000 people a year in the United States with permanent, potentially disfiguring facial weakness.

- Bell's palsy is considered benign, with full recovery in 3 to 6 months, especially if treatment is begun immediately.

Pathophysiology

Although the exact etiology is not known, it is believed that a viral infection such as viral meningitis or activation of herpes simplex virus 1 (HSV1), may trigger Bell's palsy. The viral infection causes inflammation, edema, ischemia, and eventual demyelination of the nerve, creating pain and alterations in motor and sensory function.

Clinical Manifestations

The onset of Bell's palsy is often accompanied by an outbreak of herpes vesicles in or around the ear. Patients may complain of pain around and behind the ear. Additional manifestations may include fever, tinnitus, and hearing deficit.

Paralysis of the motor branches of the facial nerve typically re-sults in a flaccidity of the affected side of the face, with drooping of the mouth accompanied by drooling. Inability to close the eyelid, with an upward movement of the eyeball when closure is attempted, is also evident.

- A widened palpebral fissure (opening between the eyelids); flat-tening of the nasolabial fold; unilateral loss of taste; and inabil-ity to smile, frown, or whistle are also common.
- Decreased muscle movement may alter chewing ability, and some patients may experience a loss of tearing or excessive tearing.

Complications can include psychologic withdrawal because of changes in appearance, malnutrition and dehydration, mucous membrane trauma, corneal abrasions, and facial spasms and con-tractures.

Diagnosis of Bell's palsy is one of exclusion. Diagnosis and prognosis are indicated by observation of the typical pattern of onset and the testing of percutaneous nerve excitability by electro-myogram (EMG).

Collaborative Care

Methods of treatment include moist heat, gentle massage, and electrical stimulation of the nerve. Stimulation may maintain muscle tone and prevent atrophy. Care is primarily focused on relief of symptoms, protection of the eye on the affected side, and prevention of complications.

- Corticosteroids (prednisone) are started immediately, with best results obtained if corticosteroids are initiated before paralysis is complete. When the patient improves to the point that corticosteroids are no longer necessary, they should be tapered off over 2 weeks.
- Because HSV is implicated in many cases of Bell's palsy, treatment with acyclovir (Zovirax) alone or in conjunction with prednisone may be used. Valacyclovir (Valtrex) and famciclovir (Famvir) have also been used.

Nursing Management

Mild analgesics can relieve pain. Hot wet packs can reduce discomfort of herpetic lesions, aid circulation, and relieve pain. Tell the patient to protect the face from cold and drafts because trigeminal hyperesthesia (extreme sensitivity to pain or touch) may occur.

- Maintenance of good nutrition is important. Teach the patient to chew on the unaffected side of the mouth to avoid trapping food and to improve taste. Thorough oral hygiene must be carried out after each meal to prevent development of parotitis, caries, and periodontal disease from accumulated residual food.
- Dark glasses may be worn for protective and cosmetic reasons. Artificial tears (methylcellulose) should be instilled frequently during the day to prevent corneal drying. Ointment and an impermeable eye shield can be used at night to retain moisture. In some patients taping the lids closed at night may be necessary to provide protection.
- A facial sling may be helpful to support affected muscles, improve lip alignment, and facilitate eating. Vigorous massage can break down tissues, but gentle upward massage has psychologic benefits. When function begins to return, active facial exercises are performed several times per day.

The change in physical appearance as a result of Bell's palsy can be devastating. Reassure the patient that a stroke did not occur and that chances for a full recovery are good. It is important to share with the patient that most patients recover within about 6 weeks of the onset of symptoms.

BENIGN PAROXYSMAL POSITIONAL VERTIGO

Benign paroxysmal positional vertigo (BPPV) is a condition where free-floating debris in the semicircular canal causes vertigo with specific head movements, such as getting out of bed, rolling over in bed, and sitting up from lying down. BPPV causes about 50% of cases of vertigo. The debris ("ear rocks") is composed of small crystals of calcium carbonate that may occur in the inner ear due to head trauma, infection, or the aging process. In many cases a cause cannot be found.

Symptoms are intermittent and include dizziness, vertigo, lightheadedness, loss of balance, and nausea. There is no hearing loss. The symptoms of BPPV may be confused with those of Ménière's disease. Diagnosis is based on auditory and vestibular testing results.

Although BPPV is a bothersome problem, it is rarely serious unless a person falls. Repositioning maneuvers and procedures may help in providing symptom relief for many patients. (See Lewis et al, *Medical-Surgical Nursing,* ed. 9, p. 406, for a description of these procedures.)

BENIGN PROSTATIC HYPERPLASIA

Description
Benign prostatic hyperplasia (BPH) is a benign enlargement of the prostate gland.
- BPH is the most common urologic problem in male adults, occurring in about 50% of all men in their lifetime. Of these men, almost half will have bothersome lower urinary tract symptoms.
- It is not clear if having BPH leads to an increased risk of developing prostate cancer.

Pathophysiology
Although the cause is not completely understood, it is thought that BPH results from endocrine changes associated with aging.
- Possible causes include (1) the excessive accumulation of dihydroxytestosterone (the principal intraprostatic androgen), which can lead to an overgrowth of prostate tissue, or (2) a decrease in testosterone, which occurs with aging, resulting in a greater proportion of estrogen. This imbalance may lead to prostatic cell growth.
- The enlargement of the gland gradually compresses the urethra, eventually leading to partial or complete obstruction. The location

of the enlargement rather than the size of the prostate is most significant in the development of obstructive symptoms.

- Risk factors for BPH include aging, obesity (in particular increased waist circumference), lack of physical activity, alcohol consumption, erectile dysfunction, smoking, and diabetes. A family history of BPH in first-degree relatives may also be a risk factor.

Clinical Manifestations

Early symptoms are often minimal because the bladder can compensate for a small amount of resistance to urine flow. Symptoms gradually worsen as the degree of urethral obstruction increases. Symptoms can be divided into two groups: obstructive and irritative.

- *Obstructive symptoms* of BPH due to urinary retention include a decrease in the caliber and force of the urinary stream, difficulty in initiating voiding, intermittency (stopping and starting stream several times while voiding), and dribbling at the end of urination.
- *Irritative symptoms*, including urinary frequency, urgency, dysuria, bladder pain, nocturia, and incontinence, are associated with inflammation and infection.

Complications

- Acute urinary retention is manifested as a sudden and painful inability to urinate. Treatment involves the insertion of a catheter to drain the bladder. Surgery may also be indicated.
- Urinary tract infections can result from incomplete bladder emptying, which provides a favorable environment for bacterial growth.
- Calculi may develop in the bladder because of alkalinization of the residual urine.
- Hydronephrosis and pyelonephritis caused by back pressure of urine in an obstructed system may lead to renal failure.

Diagnostic Studies

- Physical examination, including a digital rectal examination (DRE) to determine prostate size, symmetry, and consistency
- Urinalysis with culture to determine the presence of infection
- Postvoid residual urine volume to assess the degree of urine flow obstruction
- Prostate-specific antigen (PSA) blood test to rule out prostate cancer
- Uroflowmetry flow studies and transrectal ultrasound scan of prostate
- Cystoscopy to visualize the urethra and bladder

Collaborative Care

The goals of collaborative care are to restore bladder drainage, relieve the patient's symptoms, and prevent or treat the complications of BPH. Treatment is generally based on the degree to which the symptoms bother the patient or the presence of complications rather than the size of the prostate. Alternatives to surgical intervention for some patients include drug therapy and minimally invasive procedures.

Conservative treatment that may be recommended for some patients with BPH is referred to as active surveillance or "watchful waiting." When there are no symptoms or only mild ones, a wait-and-see approach is taken.

- Dietary changes (decreasing intake of caffeine and artificial sweeteners, limiting spicy or acidic foods), avoiding medications such as decongestants and anticholinergics, and restricting evening fluid intake may result in improvement of symptoms.
- A timed voiding schedule may reduce or eliminate symptoms, thus negating the need for further intervention.

If the patient begins to have signs or symptoms that indicate an increase in obstruction, further treatment is indicated.

Drug Therapy

Drugs are often used to treat BPH with variable results.

- 5α-Reductase inhibitors reduce the size of the prostate gland. Finasteride (Proscar) blocks the enzyme needed to convert testosterone to dihydroxytestosterone, the principal intraprostatic androgen. This results in a regression of hyperplastic tissue. Dutasteride (Avodart) has the same effect as finasteride and may also be used.
  - Patients who have an increased PSA level while taking these medications should be referred to their health care provider. The need for regular prostate cancer screening should also be discussed with the provider.
- α-Adrenergic receptor blockers cause smooth muscle relaxation in prostate tissue, which ultimately facilitates urinary flow through the urethra. α-Adrenergic receptor blockers, such as silodosin (Rapaflo), terazosin (Hytrin), and tamsulosin (Flomax), are currently being used.
- The combination of a 5α-reductase inhibitor (dutasteride) and an α-adrenergic receptor blocker (tamsulosin) in a single oral medication (Jalyn) is now available.
- Erectogenic drugs such as tadalafil (Cialis) have been used in men who have symptoms of BPH alone or in combination with erectile dysfunction (ED). The drug has shown to be effective in reducing symptoms for both of these conditions.

- Herbal preparations such as saxifrage, beta-sitosterol, *Pygeum africanum,* and Cernilton have shown some success in reducing symptoms of BPH. Emphasize to the patient that he should tell his health care provider about all herbal supplements that he uses.

Minimally Invasive Therapy

Minimally invasive therapies generally do not require hospitalization or catheterization and have few adverse events. Many minimally invasive therapies have shown outcomes comparable to invasive techniques. Advantages and disadvantages of the various minimally invasive and invasive treatment options are compared in Table 55-3, Lewis et al, *Medical-Surgical Nursing,* ed. 9, p. 1311.

Transurethral microwave thermotherapy (TUMT) is an outpatient procedure that involves the delivery of microwaves directly to the prostate through a transurethral probe. The temperature of the prostate tissue is raised to about 113° F (45° C), causing necrosis and thus relieving the obstruction.

Transurethral needle ablation (TUNA) is another outpatient procedure that increases the temperature of prostate tissue, thus causing localized necrosis. TUNA differs from TUMT in that only prostate tissue in direct contact with the needle is affected, allowing greater precision in removal of the target tissue.

There are a variety of laser procedures using different sources, wavelengths, and delivery systems. Retreatment rates are comparable to those of a transurethral resection of the prostate (TURP). The laser beam is delivered transurethrally through a fiber instrument and is used for cutting, coagulation, and vaporization of prostatic tissue. Examples of this technique include visual laser ablation, contact lasers, photovaporization, and interstitial laser coagulation.

Invasive (Surgical) Therapy

Invasive therapy is indicated when there is a decrease in urine flow sufficient to cause discomfort, persistent residual urine, acute urinary retention because of obstruction with no reversible precipitating cause, or hydronephrosis.

Transurethral resection of the prostate (TURP) is a surgical procedure involving removal of prostate tissue using a resectoscope inserted through the urethra. TURP has long been considered the "gold standard" surgical treatment for obstructing BPH. Although this procedure is still commonly performed, there has recently been a decrease in the number of TURP procedures because of the development of less invasive technologies.

- After the procedure, a large three-way indwelling catheter with a 30-mL balloon containing sterile water is usually inserted into the bladder to provide hemostasis and facilitate urinary drainage. The bladder is irrigated, either continuously

or intermittently, for at least 24 hours to prevent obstruction from mucous threads and blood clots.
- The outcome for 80% to 90% of patients is excellent, with marked improvements in symptoms and urinary flow rates. Postoperative complications include bleeding, clot retention, and dilutional hyponatremia associated with irrigation.

Transurethral incision of the prostate (TUIP) is performed with the patient under local anesthesia and is indicated for men with moderate to severe symptoms and small prostates who are poor surgical candidates. TUIP has outcomes similar to those of TURP in relieving symptoms.

Nursing Management
Because you will be most directly involved with the care of patients having prostatic surgery, the focus of nursing management is on preoperative and postoperative care.

Goals
Overall preoperative goals for the patient having prostatic surgery are to have restoration of urinary drainage, treatment of any urinary tract infection, and understanding of the upcoming surgery. Overall postoperative goals are that the patient will have no complications, restoration of urinary control, complete bladder emptying, and satisfying sexual expression.

Nursing Diagnoses
Preoperative
- Acute pain
- Risk for infection

Postoperative
- Acute pain
- Impaired urinary elimination
- Deficient knowledge

Nursing Interventions
The cause of BPH is largely attributed to the aging process. The focus of health promotion is on early detection and treatment. When symptoms of prostatic hyperplasia become evident, further diagnostic screening may be necessary.
- Some men find that ingestion of alcohol and caffeine tends to increase prostatic symptoms because of the diuretic effect that increases bladder distention.
- Advise patients with obstructive symptoms to urinate every 2 to 3 hours or when they first feel the urge to minimize urinary stasis and acute urinary retention.

Preoperative Care. Urinary drainage must be restored before surgery; a urethral catheter such as a coudé (curved-tip) catheter may be needed.

- Any infection of the urinary tract must be treated before surgery. Restoring drainage and encouraging a high fluid intake (2 to 3 L/day) are helpful.
- Patients are often concerned about the impact of impending surgery on sexual function. Provide an opportunity for the patient and his partner to express their concerns.

Postoperative Care. The plan of care should be adjusted to the type of surgery, reasons for surgery, and patient response to surgery.

- Postoperatively, bladder irrigation is typically done to remove clotted blood from the bladder and ensure drainage of urine. The bladder is irrigated either manually on an intermittent basis or more commonly as continuous bladder irrigation (CBI) with sterile normal saline solution or another prescribed solution. Monitor the inflow and outflow of the irrigant. The infusion of the continuous bladder irrigation fluid should be at a rate to keep the urine drainage light pink without clots.
- The catheter should be connected to a closed drainage system and not disconnected unless it is being removed, changed, or irrigated. On a daily basis, cleanse the secretions that accumulate around the meatus with soap and water.
- Blood clots are expected for the first 24 to 36 hours. However, large amounts of bright red blood in the urine can indicate hemorrhage.
- Painful bladder spasms occur as a result of irritation of the bladder mucosa from insertion of a resectoscope, presence of a catheter, or clots leading to obstruction of the catheter. Instruct the patient not to urinate around the catheter because this increases the likelihood of spasm. If bladder spasms develop, check the catheter for clots. If present, remove the clots by irrigation so urine can flow freely. Belladonna and opium suppositories, along with relaxation techniques, are used to relieve pain and decrease spasm.
- Sphincter tone may be poor immediately after catheter removal, resulting in urinary incontinence or dribbling. Sphincter tone can be strengthened by having the patient practice Kegel exercises (pelvic floor muscle technique). Continence can improve for up to 12 months.
- Observe the patient for signs of postoperative infection. If an external wound is present, the area should be observed for redness, heat, swelling, and purulent drainage. Rectal procedures, such as rectal temperatures and enemas (except insertion of well-lubricated belladonna and opium suppositories), should be avoided.
- Dietary intervention and stool softeners are important to prevent straining while having bowel movements. A diet high in fiber facilitates the passage of stool.

- Activities that increase abdominal pressure, such as sitting or walking for prolonged periods and straining to have a bowel movement (Valsalva maneuver), should be avoided.

▼ **Patient and Caregiver Teaching**

Discharge planning and home care issues are important aspects of care after prostate surgery.

- Instructions include (1) caring for an indwelling catheter, if one is in place; (2) managing urinary incontinence; (3) maintaining oral fluids between 2 and 3 L/day; (4) observing for signs and symptoms of urinary tract and wound infection; (5) preventing constipation; (6) avoiding heavy lifting (more than 10 lb [more than 4.5 kg]); and (7) refraining from driving or sexual intercourse as directed by the physician.
- Many men experience retrograde ejaculation because of trauma to the internal sphincter. Semen is discharged into the bladder at orgasm and may produce cloudy urine when the patient urinates after orgasm. Discuss these changes with the patient and his partner and allow them to ask questions and express their concerns.
- Sexual counseling and treatment options may be necessary if erectile dysfunction becomes a chronic or permanent problem.
- The bladder may take up to 2 months to return to its normal capacity. The patient should be instructed to drink at least 2 to 3 L of fluid per day and to urinate every 2 to 3 hours to flush the urinary tract. Teach the patient to avoid or limit the amounts of bladder irritants such as caffeine products, citrus juices, and alcohol.
- Advise the patient to have yearly digital rectal examinations (DREs) if he has had any procedure other than complete removal of the prostate. Hyperplasia or cancer can occur in the remaining prostatic tissue.

BLADDER CANCER

Description

The most frequent malignant tumor of the urinary tract is transitional cell carcinoma of the bladder, which accounts for nearly 1 in every 20 cancers diagnosed in the United States. Cancer of the bladder is most common between the ages of 60 and 70 years and is at least three times as common in men as in women.

Risk factors for bladder cancer include cigarette smoking, exposure to dyes used in the rubber and cable industries, and chronic abuse of phenacetin-containing analgesics. Individuals with chronic, recurrent renal calculi and chronic lower urinary tract infections have an increased risk of squamous cell bladder cancer. Women treated with radiation for cervical cancer, patients who received cyclophosphamide, and patients who take the diabetes drug pioglitazone (Actos) also have an increased risk for bladder cancer.

Clinical Manifestations

Microscopic or gross, painless hematuria (chronic or intermittent) is the most common clinical finding. Dysuria, frequency, and urgency may also occur because of bladder irritability.

Diagnostic Studies

- When cancer is suspected, obtain urine specimens to identify neoplastic or atypical cells.
- Ultrasound, CT, or MRI may be used to detect bladder cancer.
- Cystoscopy and biopsy are used to confirm a diagnosis of bladder cancer.

Pathologic grading systems are used to classify the malignant potential of tumor cells, indicating a scale ranging from well differentiated to undifferentiated (anaplastic).

Nursing and Collaborative Management

The majority of bladder cancers are diagnosed at an early stage when the cancer is treatable. Low-stage, low-grade, superficial bladder cancers are most common and most responsive to treatment. Periodic surveillance is important as 30% of patients have tumor recurrence within 5 years and nearly 95% have recurrence by 15 years.

Surgical therapies include a variety of procedures.

- *Transurethral resection of the bladder tumor* (TURBT) is used for superficial lesions of the bladder's inner lining. This procedure is also used to control bleeding in patients who are poor operative risks or who have advanced tumors.
- *A partial or radical cystectomy with urinary diversion* is the treatment of choice when the tumor is invasive or involves the trigone (area where ureters insert into the bladder) and the patient is free from metastases beyond the pelvic area.
- *A partial cystectomy* includes resection of that portion of the bladder wall containing the tumor, along with a margin of normal tissue.
- *A radical cystectomy* involves removal of the bladder, prostate, and seminal vesicles in men and the bladder, uterus, cervix, urethra, and ovaries in women.

Postoperative management for any of these surgical procedures includes instructions to drink large amounts of fluid each day for the first week after the procedure, avoid alcoholic beverages, use opioid analgesics and stool softeners if necessary, and take sitz baths to promote muscle relaxation and reduce urinary retention. Administer opioid analgesics for a brief period after the procedure, along with stool softeners.

Radiation therapy is used with cystectomy or as the primary therapy when the cancer is inoperable or when the patient refuses surgery. Chemotherapy drugs used in treating invasive cancer include cisplatin (Platinol), vinblastine (Velban), doxorubicin (Adriamycin), and methotrexate.

Chemotherapy with local instillation of chemotherapeutic or immune-stimulating agents can be delivered into the bladder through a urethral catheter, usually at weekly intervals for 6 to 12 weeks. Intravesical agents are instilled directly into the patient's bladder and retained for about 2 hours. The position of the patient may be changed every 15 minutes for maximum contact in all areas of the bladder.

- Bacille Calmette-Guérin (BCG), a weakened strain of *Mycobacterium bovis,* is the treatment of choice for carcinoma in situ. When BCG fails, α-interferon, thiotepa (Thioplex), and valrubicin (Valstar) may be used.
- After intravesical therapy most patients have irritative voiding symptoms and hemorrhagic cystitis. Encourage patients to increase daily fluid intake and to quit smoking. Assess the patient for a secondary urinary tract infection (UTI) and stress the need for routine urologic follow-up care. The patient may have fears or concerns about sexual activity or bladder function that will need to be addressed.

BONE TUMORS

Description
Primary bone tumors, both benign and malignant, are relatively rare in adults. They account for only about 3% of all tumors. Metastatic bone cancer in which the cancer has spread from another site is a more common problem.

- Benign bone tumors are more common than primary malignant tumors. These types of tumors, which include osteochondroma, osteoclastoma, and endochroma, are often removed by surgery.
- Primary malignant bone cancer is called *sarcoma*. The more common types of primary bone cancer are osteosarcoma, chondrosarcoma, Ewing's sarcoma, and chordoma. Primary malignant tumors occur most often during childhood and young

adulthood. They are characterized by their rapid metastasis and bone destruction.

Osteochondroma

Osteochondroma is the most common primary benign bone tumor. It is characterized by an overgrowth of cartilage and bone near the end of the bone at the growth plate. It is more commonly found in the long bones of the leg, pelvis, or scapula.

- Clinical manifestations of osteochondroma include a painless, hard, and immobile mass; lower-than-normal-height for age; soreness of muscles in close proximity to the tumor; one leg or arm longer than the other; and pressure or irritation with exercise. Patients may also be asymptomatic.
- Diagnosis is confirmed using x-ray, CT scan, and MRI.
- No treatment is necessary for asymptomatic osteochondroma. If the tumor is causing pain or neurologic symptoms due to compression, surgical resection is usually done. Patients should have regular screening examinations for early detection of malignant transformation.

Osteosarcoma

Osteosarcoma is a primary malignant bone tumor that is extremely aggressive and rapidly metastasizes to distant sites. It usually occurs in the metaphyseal region of long bones of the extremities, particularly in regions of the distal femur, proximal tibia, and proximal humerus, as well as the pelvis. It is the most common malignant bone tumor affecting children and young adults and is most often associated with Paget's disease and prior radiation.

- Clinical manifestations of osteosarcoma are usually associated with a gradual onset of pain and swelling, especially around the knee. A minor injury does not cause the tumor but rather serves to bring the preexisting condition to medical attention.
- Diagnosis is confirmed from tissue biopsy, elevation of serum alkaline phosphatase and calcium levels, x-ray, CT or positron emission tomography (PET) scans, and MRI.
- Metastasis is present in 10% to 20% of individuals when they are diagnosed with osteosarcoma.

Preoperative chemotherapy may be used to decrease tumor size before surgery. Limb-salvage surgical procedures are usually considered when there is a clear (no cancer present) 6- to 7-cm margin surrounding the lesion. Adjunct chemotherapy after surgery has increased the 5-year survival rate to 70% in patients without metastasis.

Metastatic Bone Cancer

Metastatic bone cancer is the most common type of malignant bone tumor. It occurs as a result of metastasis from a primary tumor. Common sites for the primary tumor include the breast, prostate, lungs, kidney, and thyroid. Metastatic bone lesions are commonly found in the vertebrae, pelvis, femur, humerus, or ribs.

- Pathologic fractures at the site of metastasis are common because of a weakening of the involved bone. High serum calcium levels result as calcium is released from damaged bones.
- Once a primary lesion has been identified, radionuclide bone scans are often done to detect metastatic lesions before they are visible on x-ray. Metastatic bone lesions may occur at any time (even years later) following diagnosis and treatment of the primary tumor.
- Metastasis to the bone should be suspected in any patient who has local bone pain and a history of cancer.
- Treatment may be palliative and consists of radiation and pain management. Surgical stabilization of the fracture may be indicated if there is a fracture or pending fracture. Prognosis depends on the primary type of cancer and if other sites of metastasis are present.

Nursing Management: Bone Cancer

Nursing care of the patient with a malignant bone tumor does not differ significantly from care provided to the patient with a malignant disease of any other body system. However, special attention is required to reduce complications associated with prolonged bed rest and to prevent pathologic fractures. It is important to prevent fractures by careful handling and support of the affected extremity and logrolling for those on bed rest.

- Weakness caused by anemia and decreased mobility may also be noted. Monitor the site of the tumor for swelling, changes in circulation, and decreased movement, sensation, or joint function.
- The pain associated with bone cancer can be very severe. The pain is often caused by the tumor pressing against nerves and other organs near the bone. You need to carefully monitor the patient's pain and ensure that they have adequate pain medication. Sometimes radiation therapy is used as a palliative therapy to shrink the tumor and decrease the pain.
- The patient is often reluctant to participate in therapeutic activities because of weakness and fear of pain. Provide regular rest periods between activities.
- Assist the patient and family in accepting substitute "accepting" with "adjusting to" the guarded prognosis associated with bone cancer. Inability to accomplish age-specific developmental

tasks can increase the frustrations with this condition. Special attention is necessary for problems of pain and dysfunction, chemotherapy, and specific surgery, such as spinal cord decompression or amputation.

B

BRAIN TUMORS

Description

Brain tumors may be primary, arising from tissues within the brain, or secondary, resulting from a metastasis from a malignant neoplasm elsewhere in the body. Secondary brain tumors are the most common type.

Brain tumors are generally classified according to the tissue from which they arise. *Meningiomas* comprise 34% of all primary brain tumors, making them the most common primary brain tumor. *Gliomas* (e.g., astrocytoma, glioblastoma multiforme) account for 30% of all brain tumors and 80% of all malignant tumors. *Glioblastoma multiforme* is the most common form of glioma.

- More than half of brain tumors are malignant. They infiltrate the brain tissue and are not amenable to complete surgical removal. Other tumors may be histologically benign but are located such that complete removal is not possible.
- Brain tumors rarely metastasize outside the central nervous system (CNS) because they are contained by structural (meninges) and physiologic (blood-brain) barriers. (For a comparison of the most common brain tumors, see Table 57-12, Lewis et al, *Medical-Surgical Nursing,* ed. 9, p. 1375.)
- Unless treated, all brain tumors eventually cause death from increasing tumor volume leading to increased intracranial pressure (ICP).

Clinical Manifestations

Manifestations depend on the location and size of the tumor. A wide range of clinical manifestations are associated with brain tumors.

- Headache is a common problem. Tumor-related headaches tend to be worse at night and may awaken the patient. The headaches are usually dull and constant but occasionally throbbing.
- Seizures are common in patients with gliomas and brain metastases. Brain tumors can cause nausea and vomiting from increased ICP.
- Cognitive dysfunction, including memory problems and mood or personality changes, is common in patients with brain metastases. As the tumor expands, it may produce signs of increased ICP, cerebral edema, or obstruction of the cerebrospinal fluid (CSF) pathways.

Diagnostic Studies

- Extensive history and a comprehensive neurologic examination are essential in the diagnostic workup.
- MRI and positron emission tomography (PET) scans allow for detection of very small tumors.
- CT and brain scanning assist in tumor location.
- Other tests include angiography, magnetic resonance spectroscopy, functional MRI, PET scans, and single-photon emission computed tomography (SPECT).

Correct diagnosis of a brain tumor is made by obtaining tissue for histologic study. In most patients, tissue is obtained at time of surgery.

Collaborative Care

Treatment goals are aimed at identifying the tumor type and location, removing or decreasing tumor mass, and preventing or managing increased ICP.

Surgical removal is the preferred treatment for brain tumors (see section on cranial surgery in Chapter 57, Lewis et al, *Medical-Surgical Nursing*, ed. 9, pp. 1375 to 1379). Surgical outcome depends on the type, size, and location of the tumor. Meningiomas and oligodendrogliomas can usually be completely removed, whereas more invasive gliomas and medulloblastomas can be only partially removed. Even if complete surgical removal of the tumor is not possible, surgery can reduce tumor mass, which decreases ICP and provides relief of symptoms with an extension of survival time.

Radiation therapy is used as a follow-up measure after surgery. Radiation seeds can also be implanted into the brain. Cerebral edema and rapidly increasing ICP may be complications of radiation therapy, but they can be managed with high doses of corticosteroids (dexamethasone [Decadron], prednisone).

- Stereotactic radiosurgery delivers a highly concentrated dose of radiation precisely directed at a location within the brain. It may be used when conventional surgery has failed or is not an option because of the tumor location.

Normally the blood-brain barrier prohibits the entry of most drugs into brain tissue. The most malignant brain tumors cause a breakdown of the blood-brain barrier in the tumor area, thus allowing chemotherapy drugs to be used. Chemotherapy-laden biodegradable wafers implanted during surgery can deliver chemotherapy directly to the tumor site. Intrathecal administration also allows direct delivery of chemotherapeutic drugs to the central nervous system.

Bevacizumab (Avastin) is used to treat patients with glioblastoma multiforme when this type of brain cancer continues to progress following standard therapy. Bevacizumab is a targeted therapy that inhibits the action of vascular endothelial growth factor that helps form new blood vessels.

- Although progress in treatment has increased the length and quality of survival of patients with gliomas, outcomes remain poor. The 5-year survival rate for these brain tumors is approximately 36%.

Nursing Management

Goals

The patient with a brain tumor will maintain normal ICP, maximize neurologic functioning, achieve control of pain and discomfort, and be aware of the long-term implications with respect to prognosis and cognitive and physical functioning.

Nursing Diagnoses/Collaborative Problems

- Risk for ineffective cerebral tissue perfusion
- Acute pain (headache)
- Self-care deficits
- Anxiety
- Potential complication: seizures
- Potential complication: increased ICP

Nursing Interventions

Behavioral changes associated with a frontal lobe lesion, such as loss of emotional control, confusion, memory loss, and depression, are often not perceived by the patient but can be very disturbing and frightening to the family. Assist the caregiver and family in understanding what is happening.

- The confused patient with behavioral instability can be a challenge. Close supervision of activity, use of side rails, padding of rails, and a calm, reassuring approach are all essential care techniques.
- Minimize environmental stimuli, create a routine, and use reality orientation for the confused patient.
- Seizures often occur with brain tumors, and seizure precautions should be instituted for the protection of the patient (see Seizure Disorders, p. 556).
- Motor and sensory dysfunctions are problems that interfere with the activities of daily living. Alterations in mobility must be managed, and encourage the patient to provide as much self-care as physically possible. Self-image often depends on the patient's ability to participate in care within the limitations of the physical deficits.
- Motor (expressive) or sensory (receptive) dysphasia may occur. Disturbances in communication can be frustrating for the patient and may interfere with your ability to meet patient

needs. Make attempts to establish a communication system that can be used by both the patient and staff.

- Nutritional intake may be decreased because of the patient's inability to eat, loss of appetite, or loss of desire to eat. Assessing the nutritional status of the patient and ensuring adequate nutritional intake are important aspects of care. The patient may need encouragement to eat or, in some cases, may need enteral or parenteral nutrition (see Enteral Nutrition, p. 709, and Parenteral Nutrition, p. 728).

Social workers and home health nurses may be needed to assist the caregiver with discharge planning and to help the family adjust to role changes and psychosocial and socioeconomic factors. Issues related to palliative and end-of-life care need to be discussed with both the patient and family.

BREAST CANCER

Description

Breast cancer is the most common malignancy in women in the United States except for skin cancer and is second only to lung cancer as the leading cause of death from cancer in women. In the United States over 230,480 new cases of invasive breast cancer and over 57,650 cases of in situ breast cancer are diagnosed annually. About 2100 new cases of breast cancer are diagnosed in men annually.

Patients diagnosed with localized breast cancer with no axillary node involvement have a 5-year survival rate of 98%. Conversely, only 23% of patients diagnosed with advanced-stage breast cancer with metastases to distant sites will survive 5 years or more.

Pathophysiology

Although the etiology is not completely understood, a number of factors are related to breast cancer. Risk factors appear to be cumulative and interactive (Table 15). A breast cancer risk assessment tool for health care providers is available through the National Cancer Institute *(www.cancer.gov/bcrisk tool)*.

- The use of combined hormone therapy (estrogen plus progesterone) increases the risk of breast cancer and also the risk of having a larger, more advanced breast cancer at diagnosis. The use of estrogen therapy alone for longer than 10 years (for women with a prior hysterectomy) increases a woman's long-term risk for breast cancer.
- About 5% to 10% of all breast cancers are hereditary and are associated with mutations in two genes: *BRCA1* and *BRCA2*.

| Table 15 | Risk Factors for Breast Cancer |

Risk Factor	Comments
Female	Women account for 99% of breast cancer cases.
Age ≥50 yr	Majority of breast cancers are found in postmenopausal women. After age 60, increase in incidence.
Hormone use	Use of estrogen and/or progesterone as hormone therapy, especially in postmenopausal women.
Family history	Breast cancer in a first-degree relative, particularly when premenopausal or bilateral, increases risk.
Genetic factors	Gene mutations *(BRCA1* or *BRCA2)* play a role in 5%-10% of breast cancer cases.
Personal history of breast cancer, colon cancer, endometrial cancer, ovarian cancer	Personal history significantly increases risk of breast cancer, risk of cancer in other breast, and recurrence.
Early menarche (before age 12), late menopause (after age 55)	A long menstrual history increases the risk of breast cancer.
First full-term pregnancy after age 30, nulliparity	Prolonged exposure to unopposed estrogen increases risk for breast cancer.
Benign breast disease with atypical epithelial hyperplasia, lobular carcinoma in situ	Atypical changes in breast biopsy increase the risk of breast cancer.
Dense breast tissue	Mammograms harder to read and interpret. Dense tissue may be associated with more aggressive tumors.
Weight gain and obesity after menopause	Fat cells store estrogen, which increases the likelihood of developing breast cancer.

B

Continued

Table 15	Risk Factors for Breast Cancer—cont'd

Risk Factor	Comments
Exposure to ionizing radiation	Radiation damages DNA (e.g., prior treatment for Hodgkin's lymphoma).
Alcohol consumption	Women who drink ≥1 alcoholic beverage per day have an increased risk of breast cancer.
Physical inactivity	Breast cancer risk is decreased in physically active women.

In general, breast cancer arises from the epithelial lining of the ducts *(ductal carcinoma)* or from the epithelium of the lobules *(lobular carcinoma)*. Breast cancers may be *in situ* (within the duct) or invasive (arising from the duct and invading through the wall of the duct).

Breast cancer can be classified as noninvasive or invasive, and ductal or lobular (Table 16).

- Factors that affect cancer prognosis are tumor size, axillary node involvement (the more nodes involved, the worse the prognosis), tumor differentiation (morphology of malignant cells), estrogen and progesterone receptor status, and human epidermal growth factor receptor 2 (HER-2) status, which is a genetic marker.

Table 16	Types of Breast Cancer

Type	Frequency of Occurrence
Noninvasive	20%
▪ Ductal carcinoma in situ	
Invasive/infiltrating ductal carcinoma	70%-75%
▪ Medullary	
▪ Tubular	
▪ Colloid (mucinous)	
▪ Inflammatory	
▪ Paget's disease	
Invasive/infiltrating lobular carcinoma	5%-10%

Clinical Manifestations

Breast cancer is usually detected as a lump in the breast or mammographic abnormality. It occurs most often in the upper outer quadrant of the breast because that is the location of most of the glandular tissue.

- If palpable, breast cancer is characteristically hard, and may be irregularly shaped, poorly delineated, nonmobile, and nontender.
- A small percentage of breast cancers cause nipple discharge. The discharge is usually unilateral and may be clear or bloody. Nipple retraction may occur.
- Plugging of the dermal lymphatics can cause skin thickening and exaggeration of the usual skin markings, giving skin the appearance of an orange peel (peau d'orange).
- In large cancers, infiltration, induration, and dimpling (pulling in) of the overlying skin may occur.

Recurrence may be local or regional (skin or soft tissue near mastectomy site, axillary lymph nodes) or distant (most commonly bone, lung, brain, and liver).

Diagnostic Studies

Screening

- Physical examination of breast and lymphatics
- Mammography and ultrasound
- Breast MRI
- Biopsy including fine-needle aspiration and stereotactic core biopsy

Post-Diagnosis

- *Axillary node dissection* is often performed. An examination of the nodes is often performed to determine if cancer has spread to the axilla on the side of the breast cancer. The more nodes involved, the greater the risk of recurrence.
- *Lymphatic mapping and sentinel lymph node dissection* (SLND) helps the surgeon identify the lymph node(s) that drain from the tumor site (sentinel node). Assessment of this node can be used to determine the extent of tumor spread to axillary lymph nodes.
- Tumor size is a prognostic variable: the larger the tumor, the poorer the prognosis. In general, poorly differentiated tumors appear morphologically disorganized and are more aggressive.
- Estrogen and progesterone receptor status helps to determine treatment decisions and prognosis. Receptor-positive tumors commonly (1) show histologic evidence of being well differentiated, (2) have a lower chance for recurrence, and (3) are

frequently responsive to hormonal therapy. Receptor-negative tumors (1) are often poorly differentiated histologically, (2) frequently recur, and (3) are usually unresponsive to hormonal therapy.

- DNA content (ploidy status) correlates with tumor aggressiveness. Diploid tumors have been shown to have a significantly lower risk of recurrence than aneuploid tumors.
- Overexpression of the HER-2 receptor has been associated with a greater risk for recurrence and a poorer prognosis in patients with breast cancer. About 25% of metastatic breast cancers produce excessive HER-2.
- Genomic assays (MammaPrint and Oncotype DX) are used to analyze the activity of a group of genes.

A patient whose breast cancer tests negative for all three receptors (estrogen, progesterone, and HER-2) has *triple-negative breast cancer*. The incidence of triple-negative breast cancer is higher in Hispanics, African Americans, women who are younger, and women with a *BRCA1* mutation. These patients tend to have a more aggressive tumor with a poorer prognosis.

Collaborative Care

Prognostic factors are considered in treatment decisions, and tumor size (T), nodal involvement (N), and presence of metastasis (M) are used to stage breast cancer with the TNM system (see TNM Classification System, p. 777).

Surgical Therapy

The most common surgical options for resectable breast cancer are (1) breast-conserving surgery (lumpectomy) and (2) modified radical mastectomy. Most women diagnosed with early-stage breast cancer (tumors smaller than 4 to 5 cm) are candidates for either treatment choice.

Breast-conserving surgery (lumpectomy) usually involves removal of the entire tumor along with a margin of normal tissue. An axillary lymph node dissection (ALND) is usually done along with a lumpectomy. Following surgery, radiation therapy is delivered to the entire breast, ending with a boost to the tumor bed. If evidence exists that the risk for recurrence is high, chemotherapy may be administered before radiation therapy.

- A typical ALND generally involves the removal of 12 to 20 nodes. Recently, sentinel lymph node dissection (SLND) has become the standard of care with ALND reserved for patients when clinically indicated (evidence of disease in the axilla).
- One of the main advantages of breast-conserving surgery and radiation is that it preserves the breast, including the nipple.

The goal of combined surgery and radiation is to maximize the benefits of both cancer treatment and cosmetic outcome while minimizing risks.

Modified radical mastectomy includes removal of the breast and axillary lymph nodes but preserves the pectoralis major muscle. This surgery would be selected over breast-conserving therapy if the tumor were too large to excise with good margins and attain a reasonable cosmetic result. Some patients may select this procedure over lumpectomy when presented with the choice of either procedure. See Table 52-7, Lewis et al, *Medical-Surgical Nursing,* ed. 9, p. 1248, for treatment options, side effects, complications, and patient issues related to surgical procedures for breast cancer.

Radiation Therapy

Radiation therapy may be used for breast cancer as treatment to (1) prevent local breast recurrences after breast-conserving surgery, (2) prevent local and nodal recurrences following mastectomy, or (3) palliate pain caused by local, regional, and distant recurrence.

- The MammoSite system is a minimally invasive method of delivering internal radiation therapy. The technique uses a balloon catheter to insert radioactive seeds into the breast after the tumor is removed.

Chemotherapy

Cytotoxic drugs are used to destroy cancer cells. Many breast cancers are responsive to chemotherapy. In some patients, chemotherapy is given preoperatively. The use of a combination of drugs is most often superior to the use of a single drug. The incidence and severity of the side effects that accompany chemotherapy are influenced by the specific drug combinations, drug schedule, and dose of the drugs (see Chemotherapy, p. 694).

Hormonal Therapy

Estrogen can promote growth of breast cancer cells if cells are estrogen-receptor positive. Hormonal therapy can block the source of estrogen, thus promoting tumor regression. It may be used as an adjuvant to primary treatment or in patients with recurrent or metastatic cancer.

Hormone receptor assays can identify women who are likely to respond to hormone therapy. Hormonal therapy can block estrogen receptors or suppress estrogen synthesis through inhibiting aromatase, an enzyme needed for estrogen synthesis (Table 17).

- Antiestrogens include tamoxifen (Nolvadex), toremifene (Fareston), and fulvestrant (Faslodex).
- Aromatase inhibitor drugs include anastrozole (Arimidex), letrozole (Femara), and exemestane (Aromasin) and are used in the treatment of breast cancer in postmenopausal women.

Table 17	Drug Therapy *Breast Cancer*	

Drug Class	Mechanism of Action	Indications
Hormone Therapy		
Estrogen Receptor Blockers		
tamoxifen (Nolvadex)	Blocks estrogen receptors (ERs)	ER-positive breast cancer in premenopausal and postmenopausal women Used as a preventive measure in high-risk premenopausal and postmenopausal women
toremifene (Fareston)	Blocks ERs	ER-positive breast cancer in postmenopausal women only
fulvestrant (Faslodex)	Blocks ERs	ER-positive breast cancer in postmenopausal women only
Aromatase Inhibitors		
anastrozole (Arimidex) letrozole (Femara) exemestane (Aromasin)	Prevents production of estrogen by inhibiting aromatase	ER-positive breast cancer in postmenopausal women only
Estrogen Receptor Modulator		
raloxifene (Evista)	In breast, blocks the effect of estrogen In bone, promotes effect of estrogen and prevents bone loss	Postmenopausal women

EGFR, Epidermal growth factor receptor; *HER-2,* human epidermal growth factor receptor 2.

Table 17	Drug Therapy *Breast Cancer*—cont'd	
Drug Class	**Mechanism of Action**	**Indications**
Biologic and Targeted Therapy		
trastuzumab (Herceptin) pertuzumab (Perjeta)	Blocks HER-2 receptor	HER-positive breast cancer in postmenopausal women only
lapatinib (Tykerb)	Inhibits HER-2 tyrosine kinase and EGFR tyrosine kinase	HER-positive breast cancer in postmenopausal women only

B

Aromatase inhibitors do not block the production of estrogen by the ovaries. Thus they are of little benefit and may be harmful in premenopausal women.

Biologic and Targeted Therapy

Trastuzumab (Herceptin) is a monoclonal antibody to HER-2. After the antibody attaches to the antigen, it is taken into the cells and eventually kills them. It can be used alone or in combination with other chemotherapy to treat patients with breast cancer whose tumors overexpress the HER-2 gene.

Lapatinib (Tykerb) may be used in combination with capecitabine (Xeloda) for patients with advanced, metastatic disease who are HER-2 positive. Pertuzumab (Perjeta) is a new anti–HER-2 therapy that is used for patients who have not received prior treatment for metastatic breast cancer with an anti–HER-2 therapy or chemotherapy. Pertuzumab is combined with trastuzumab and docetaxel.

Follow-Up and Survivorship Care

After treatment for breast cancer, the patient will have ongoing survivorship care.

- Recommended follow-up examinations generally occur every 3 to 6 months for the first 5 years, and then annually thereafter.
- Advise women to perform monthly self-examinations of the breast and chest wall and report any changes to their health care provider. The most common site of local recurrence of breast cancer is at the surgical site.
- The woman should have appropriate breast imaging done at regular intervals (usually 6 months to 1 year) as determined by her risk of recurrence and breast cancer history.

Nursing Management

Goals

The patient with breast cancer will actively participate in the decision-making process related to treatment, adhere to the therapeutic plan, communicate about and manage the side effects of adjuvant therapy, and access and benefit from the support provided by significant others and health care providers.

Nursing Diagnoses

After a diagnosis of breast cancer and before a treatment plan has been selected, the following diagnoses apply:

- Decisional conflict
- Fear and/or anxiety
- Disturbed body image

If the patient undergoes a lumpectomy or modified radical mastectomy, nursing diagnoses may include:

- Acute pain
- Disturbed body image
- Impaired physical mobility

Nursing Interventions

The time between the diagnosis of breast cancer and the selection of a treatment plan is a difficult period for the woman and her family. Although the health care provider discusses treatment options, the woman often relies on you to clarify and expand on these options.

- Appropriate nursing interventions are to explore the woman's usual decision-making processes, help her to evaluate the advantages and disadvantages of the options, provide information relevant to the decision(s), and support the patient and family once the decision is made.
- Regardless of the surgery planned, provide the patient with sufficient information to ensure informed consent. Teaching in the preoperative phase includes turning and deep breathing, a review of postoperative exercises, and an explanation of the recovery period from the time of surgery until the first postoperative visit.

The woman who has breast-conserving surgery usually has an uncomplicated postoperative course with variable pain intensity. If an axillary lymph node dissection (ALND) has been done or if a woman has had a mastectomy, drains are generally left in place and patients are discharged home with them. Teach the patient and family (including a return demonstration) how to manage the drains at home.

- Restoring arm function on the affected side after mastectomy and axillary lymph node dissection is a key nursing goal.
- Place the woman in a semi-Fowler's position with the arm on the affected side elevated on a pillow. Flexing and extending the

fingers should begin in the recovery room, with progressive increases in activity.

- Postoperative arm and shoulder exercises are instituted gradually.
- Postoperative discomfort can be minimized by administering analgesics about 30 minutes before initiating exercises. When able to shower, the warm water on the affected shoulder often has a muscle-relaxing effect and reduces joint stiffness.

Lymphedema (accumulation of lymph in soft tissue) can occur as a result of excision or radiation of the lymph nodes. The patient may experience heaviness, pain, impaired motor function in the arm, and numbness and paresthesia of the fingers. Help the patient to understand that she is at risk of developing lymphedema for the rest of her life. Teach measures to prevent or reduce lymphedema including:

- No blood pressure readings, venipunctures, or injections on the affected arm.
- The affected arm should not be dependent for long periods of time and caution should be used to prevent infection, burns, or compromised circulation on the affected side.
- If trauma to the arm occurs, the area should be washed thoroughly with soap and water and observed. A topical antibiotic ointment and a bandage or other sterile dressing may be applied.

Frequent and sustained elevation of the arm, regular use of a custom-fitted pressure sleeve, and treatment with an inflatable sleeve (pneumomassage) may also be helpful.

It is important to remain sensitive to the complex psychologic impact that a diagnosis of cancer and subsequent breast surgery can have on a woman and her family. Help to meet the woman's psychologic needs by the following:

- Help her identify sources of support and strength to her, such as her partner, family, and spiritual practices.
- Provide a safe environment for the expression of the full range of feelings.
- Encourage her to identify and learn individual coping strengths.
- Promote communication between the patient and her family and/or friends.
- Provide accurate and complete answers to questions about the disease, treatment options, and reproductive or lactation issues (if appropriate).
- Make resources available for mental health counseling.
- Offer information about community resources, such as Reach to Recovery or local breast cancer organizations.
- Breast reconstruction is discussed in Chapter 52, Lewis et al, *Medical-Surgical Nursing,* ed. 9.

▼ **Patient and Caregiver Teaching**

- Explain the specific follow-up plan to the patient and emphasize the importance of ongoing monitoring and self-care.
- Immediately after surgery, advise the patient of symptoms to report to the health care provider including fever, inflammation at the surgical site, erythema, postoperative constipation, and unusual swelling.
- For women who have had a mastectomy without breast reconstruction, a variety of garment choice products are available, including camisoles with soft breast prosthetic inserts as well as a fitted prosthesis with bra.
- A preoperative sexual assessment provides baseline data that can be used to plan postoperative interventions. Often the husband, sexual partner, or family members may need assistance in dealing with their emotional reactions to the diagnosis and surgery so that they can act as effective means of support for the patient.
- Depression and anxiety may occur with the continued stress and uncertainty of a cancer diagnosis. The support of family and friends and participation in a cancer support group are important aspects of care that are often helpful in improving quality of life and have a significant impact on survival.

BRONCHIECTASIS

Description

Bronchiectasis is characterized by permanent, abnormal dilation of medium-sized bronchi as a result of inflammatory changes that destroy elastic and muscular structures supporting the bronchial wall. Infection is the primary reason for the continuing cycle of inflammation, airway damage, and remodeling.

Stasis of thickened mucus occurs along with impaired clearance by the cilia resulting in a reduced ability to clear mucus from the lungs.

Cystic fibrosis is the main cause of bronchiectasis in children. In adults the main cause is bacterial infections of the lungs that are either not treated or receive delayed treatment. Other causes include obstruction of an airway with mucus plugs or generalized impairment of pulmonary defenses, inflammatory bowel disease, rheumatoid arthritis, or immune disorders (e.g., acquired immunodeficiency syndrome [AIDS]).

Clinical Manifestations

The hallmark of bronchiectasis is persistent cough with consistent production of purulent, thick sputum. However, some patients with severe disease and upper lobe involvement may have no sputum production and little cough. Recurrent infections injure blood vessels, and hemoptysis occurs.

- Other manifestations are pleuritic chest pain, dyspnea, wheezing, clubbing of digits, weight loss, and anemia.
- Lung auscultation reveals a variety of adventitious sounds (e.g., crackles, wheezes, rhonchi).

Diagnostic Studies

An individual with a chronic productive cough with copious purulent sputum (which may be blood streaked) should be suspected of having bronchiectasis.

- Chest x-ray shows some nonspecific abnormalities.
- High-resolution CT (HRCT) scan of the chest is the preferred method for diagnosing bronchiectasis.
- Bronchoscopy may be used with localized bronchiectasis to diagnose obstruction.
- Sputum may provide additional information regarding severity of impairment and presence of active infection. Patients are frequently found to have *H. influenzae* or *P. aeruginosa.*
- Pulmonary function studies usually show an obstructive pattern including a decrease in forced expiratory volume in 1 second (FEV_1) and the ratio of FEV_1 to forced vital capacity (FVC).

Collaborative Care

Bronchiectasis is difficult to treat. Therapy is aimed at treating acute flare-ups and preventing a decline in lung function. Antibiotics are the mainstay of treatment. Concurrent bronchodilator therapy or anticholinergics are given to prevent bronchospasm and stimulate mucociliary clearance.

- Maintaining good hydration is important to liquefy secretions. Chest physiotherapy and other airway clearance techniques facilitate expectoration of sputum. Teach the patient to reduce exposure to excessive air pollutants and irritants, avoid cigarette smoking, and obtain pneumococcal and influenza vaccinations.
- For selected patients who are disabled in spite of maximal therapy, lung transplantation is an option.

Nursing Management

Early detection and treatment of lower respiratory tract infections helps prevent complications such as bronchiectasis. Any obstructing lesion or foreign body should be removed promptly.

An important nursing goal is to promote drainage and removal of bronchial mucus. Various airway clearance techniques can be effectively used to facilitate secretion removal.

- The patient needs to understand the importance of taking the prescribed regimen of drugs to obtain maximum effectiveness.
- If hemoptysis occurs in the acute care setting, contact the health care provider immediately,
- Elevate the head of the bed and place the patient in a side-lying position with the suspected bleeding side down.
- Good nutrition is important and may be difficult to maintain because the patient is often anorexic. Oral hygiene to cleanse the mouth and remove dried sputum crusts may improve the patient's appetite.
- Unless there are contraindications, instruct the patient to drink at least 3 L of fluid daily.
- Direct hydration of the respiratory system may be beneficial in expectorating secretions. Often nebulized hypertonic saline may be ordered for a more aggressive effect. At home, a steamy shower can prove effective.
- Teach the patient and caregiver to recognize significant clinical manifestations to report to the health care provider. These manifestations include increased sputum production, bloody sputum, increasing dyspnea, fever, chills, and chest pain.

BURNS

Description

Burns are tissue injuries caused by heat, chemicals, electric current, or radiation. An estimated 450,000 Americans seek medical care each year for burns. The highest fatality rates occur in children ages 4 years and younger and adults over age 65.

Pathophysiology

Immediately after the burn injury occurs, there is increased blood flow to the area surrounding the wound. This is followed by the release of various vasoactive substances from burned tissue, which results in increased capillary permeability. Fluid then shifts from the intravascular compartment to the interstitial space, producing edema, hypovolemia, and (potentially) shock. After several days, diuresis from fluid mobilization occurs and healing begins.

Types of Burn Injury

Various types of burns may be seen alone or in combination with other burns.

- *Thermal burns* are caused by flame, flash, scald, or contact with hot objects. Severity depends on the temperature of the burning agent and the duration of contact.
- *Chemical burns* are the result of tissue injury and destruction from acids, alkalis (e.g., fertilizer, oven cleaners), and organic compounds such as petroleum products.
- *Smoke and inhalation injury* results from inhalation of hot air or noxious chemicals that can cause damage to the respiratory tract. These injuries include metabolic asphyxiation, upper airway injury, and lower airway injury.
- *Electrical burns* result from the intense heat of an electric current.

Classification of Burn Injury

The treatment of burns is related to the severity of injury. A variety of methods exist for determining burn severity.

1. *Depth of burn* is described according to the depth of skin destruction (epidermis, dermis, or subcutaneous tissue). Table 18 compares the various burn classifications according to the depth of injury.
2. Extent of the burn wound is calculated as the percent of total body surface area (TBSA) affected. Two common methods for determining the extent of a burn include:
- *Lund-Browder chart,* which is considered the most accurate because it takes into account patient age in proportion to relative body area size.
- *Rule of Nines chart,* which is often used for initial assessment because it is easy to remember (Fig. 2).
3. Severity of the burn injury is also determined by the location of the burn wound. For example, face and neck burns may inhibit respiratory function. Hands, feet, joint, and eye burns may limit self-care and functioning.
4. Preexisting disorders such as cardiovascular, pulmonary, or renal disease reduce the patient's ability to recover from the tremendous demands of burn injury. The patient with diabetes mellitus or peripheral vascular disease is at high risk for poor healing, especially with foot and leg burns.

The American Burn Association (ABA) has established referral criteria to determine which burn injuries should be treated in burn centers with specialized facilities (Table 19 on p. 104).

Table 18 Classification of Burn Injury Depth

Classification	Appearance	Possible Cause	Structures Involved
Partial-Thickness Skin Destruction			
Superficial (first-degree) burn	Erythema, blanching on pressure, pain and mild swelling, no vesicles or blisters (although after 24 hr skin may blister and peel).	Superficial sunburn Quick heat flash	Superficial epidermal damage with hyperemia. Tactile and pain sensation intact.
Deep (second-degree) burn	Fluid-filled vesicles that are red, shiny, wet (if vesicles have ruptured). Severe pain caused by nerve injury. Mild to moderate edema.	Flame Flash Scald Contact burns Chemical Tar Electric current	Epidermis and dermis involved to varying depths. Skin elements, from which epithelial regeneration occurs, remain viable.
Full-Thickness Skin Destruction			
Third- and fourth-degree burns	Dry, waxy white, leathery, or hard skin; visible thrombosed vessels. Insensitivity to pain because of nerve destruction. Possible involvement of muscles, tendons, and bones.	Flame Scald Chemical Tar Electric current	All skin elements and local nerve endings destroyed. Coagulation necrosis present. Surgical intervention required for healing.

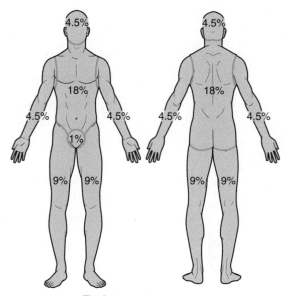

Fig. 2. Rule of Nines chart.

Clinical Manifestations

Burns can be organized chronologically into three phases: emergent (resuscitative), acute (wound healing), and rehabilitative (restorative).

Emergent Phase

Patient is likely to be in shock from hypovolemia. Shivering (a result of heat loss or anxiety) and a paralytic ileus (if the burn area is large) may also be present. Frequently full-thickness and deep partial-thickness burns are initially anesthetic because nerve endings have been destroyed. Superficial to moderate partial-thickness burns are very painful. Blisters are common in partial-thickness burns. Unconsciousness or altered mental status is the result of smoke inhalation or head trauma. Complications may include dysrhythmias, venous thromboembolism, respiratory distress, and acute tubular necrosis.

Acute Phase

Partial-thickness wounds form eschar. When eschar is removed, reepithelialization begins at wound margins and appears as red or pink scar tissue. Wound closure and healing usually occur within 10 to 21 days. Separation of eschar from full-thickness wounds

| Table 19 | Burn Center Referral Criteria |

Burn injuries that should be referred to a burn center include the following:

1. Partial-thickness burns >10% of total body surface area (TBSA).
2. Burns that involve the face, hands, feet, genitalia, perineum, or major joints.
3. Third-degree burns in any age-group.
4. Electrical burns, including lightning injury.
5. Chemical burns.
6. Inhalation injury.
7. Burn injury in patients with preexisting medical disorders that could complicate management, prolong recovery, or affect mortality risk (e.g., heart or kidney disease).
8. Any patients with burns and concomitant trauma (e.g., fractures) in which the burn injury poses the greatest risk of morbidity or mortality. In such cases, if the trauma poses the greater immediate risk, the patient may be initially stabilized in a trauma center before being transferred to a burn center. The health care provider will need to use his or her judgment, in consultation with the regional medical control plan and triage protocols.
9. Burn injury in children in hospitals without qualified personnel or equipment needed to care for them.
10. Burn injury in patients who will require special social, emotional, or long-term rehabilitative intervention.

Source: Guidelines for the operation of burn centers. In American College of Surgeons, Committee on Trauma: *Resources for optimal care of the injured patient*, 2006. Retrieved from *www.ameriburn.org/Chapter14.pdf*.

takes longer, and these wounds require surgical debridement and skin grafting for healing. Wound infection is a serious complication. Other complications include acute transient neurologic reactions (including extreme disorientation and delirium), contractures, Curling's ulcer, and stress diabetes.

Rehabilitative Phase

Mature healing occurs in about 12 months. New scar tissue will shorten, causing a contracture if adequate range of motion (ROM) is not performed. The healing site, which is extremely sensitive to trauma, may itch. Complications are skin and joint contractures and hypertrophic scarring.

Diagnostic Studies
- Serum electrolytes, especially sodium (Na^+) and potassium (K^+), to monitor fluid and electrolyte shifts
- Chest x-ray, arterial blood gases (ABGs), and sputum for inhalation injury
- Urine output and specific gravity to evaluate fluid replacement and detect acute tubular necrosis and/or renal ischemia
- Complete blood count (CBC) to detect anemia and immunologic response to injury
- White blood cell (WBC) count and wound cultures if infection is suspected

Nursing and Collaborative Management
Burn management can be classified into three phases: emergent, acute, and rehabilitative (Table 20).

Emergent Phase

Patient survival depends on rapid and thorough assessment and intervention.
- Assess adequacy of airway management and fluid therapy, provide pain medication and wound care, and offer support to patient and family. Begin feeding patient by most appropriate route as soon as possible.

Acute Phase

Predominant interventions are wound care, excision and grafting, pain management, physical and occupational therapy, nutritional therapy, and psychosocial care.
- Wound care consists of ongoing observation, assessment, cleansing, debridement, and dressing reapplication.
- A critical function is pain assessment and management.

Rehabilitative Phase

Encourage the patient and caregiver to actively participate in care.
- Water-based creams that penetrate the dermis (e.g., Vaseline Intensive Rescue) should be used routinely on healed areas to keep skin supple and moisturized. Occasionally low-dose antihistamines may be used at bedtime if itching persists.
- Continue to encourage patient to perform physical and occupational therapy routines.
- Assist patients in adapting to a realistic, yet positive appraisal of their particular situation, emphasizing what they *can* do instead of what they *cannot* do.

▼ **Patient and Caregiver Teaching**
- Describe to the patient and caregiver the burn injury process and the expected signs and symptoms related to phases of burn management.

Table 20 Collaborative Care
Burn Injury

Emergent Phase	Acute Phase	Rehabilitation Phase
Fluid Therapy	**Fluid Therapy**	■ Continue to counsel and teach patient and caregiver.
■ Assess fluid needs.	■ Continue to replace fluids, depending on patient's clinical response.	■ Continue to encourage and assist patient in resuming self-care.
■ Begin IV fluid replacement (see Table 25-11, Lewis et al, *Medical-Surgical Nursing*, ed 9, p. 460).	**Wound Care**	■ Continue to prevent or minimize contractures and assess likelihood for scarring (surgery, physical and occupational therapy, splinting, pressure garments).
■ Insert urinary catheter.	■ Continue daily shower and wound care.	
■ Monitor urine output.	■ Continue debridement (if necessary).	■ Discuss possible reconstructive surgery.
Wound Care	■ Assess wound daily and adjust dressing protocols as necessary.	■ Prepare for discharge home or transfer to rehabilitation hospital.
■ Start daily shower and wound care.	■ Observe for complications (e.g., infection).	
■ Debride as necessary.	**Early Excision and Grafting**	
■ Assess extent and depth of burns.	■ Provide temporary allografts.	
■ Administer tetanus toxoid or tetanus antitoxin.	■ Provide permanent autografts.	
Pain and Anxiety	■ Care for donor sites.	
■ Assess and manage pain and anxiety.	**Pain and Anxiety**	
Physical and Occupational Therapy	■ Continue to assess for and treat pain and anxiety.	
■ Place patient in position that prevents contracture formation and reduces edema.		
■ Assess need for splints.		

Nutritional Therapy
- Assess nutritional needs and begin feeding patient by most appropriate route as soon as possible.

Respiratory Therapy
- Assess oxygenation needs.
- Provide supplemental O_2 as needed.
- Intubate if necessary.
- Monitor respiratory status.

Psychosocial Care
- Provide support to patient and caregiver during initial crisis phase.

Physical and Occupational Therapy
- Begin daily therapy program for maintenance of range of motion.
- Assess need for splints and anticontracture positioning.
- Encourage and assist patient with self-care as possible.

Nutritional Therapy
- Continue to assess diet to support wound healing.

Respiratory Therapy
- Continue to assess oxygenation needs.
- Continue to monitor respiratory status.
- Monitor for signs of complications (e.g., pneumonia).

Psychosocial Care
- Provide ongoing support, counseling, and teaching to patient and caregiver about physical and emotional aspects of care and recovery.
- Begin to anticipate discharge needs.

Drug Therapy (see Table 25-13, Lewis et al, *Medical-Surgical Nursing*, ed 9, p. 463)
- Assess need for medications (e.g., antibiotics).
- Continue to monitor effectiveness and adjust dosage as needed.

- Explain therapeutic interventions, precautionary measures, gowning and hand washing, and institution visiting policy to elicit cooperation and decrease anxiety.
- Teach the patient to watch for injuries to new skin.
- Instruct the patient and caregiver about the signs and symptoms of infection so early treatment can be initiated.
- Teach caregivers how to perform dressing changes to ensure proper technique and increase their sense of control.
- Emphasize the importance of exercise and appropriate physical therapy to the patient and caregiver. Plan a daily program with the patient, and offer appropriate resources to provide a continuing activity program as needed.
- Help the patient and caregiver in setting realistic future expectations because anticipatory guidance decreases anxiety and inaccurate perceptions. In addition, they will need anticipatory guidance to know what to expect physiologically as well as psychologically during recovery.
- Assist the patient and caregivers to establish contact with family and patient support groups, such as the Phoenix Society *(www.phoenix-society.org)*.

CARDIOMYOPATHY

Description

Cardiomyopathy (CMP) is a group of diseases that directly affect myocardial structure or function. CMP can be classified as primary or secondary:
- *Primary CMP* refers to those conditions in which the etiology of the heart disease is unknown. The heart muscle in this case is the only portion of the heart involved, and other cardiac structures are unaffected.
- In *secondary CMP* the cause of the myocardial disease is known and is secondary to another disease process. Common causes of secondary CMP are coronary artery disease (CAD), myocarditis, hypertension, cardiotoxic agents (alcohol, cocaine), valve disease, and metabolic and autoimmune disorders.

Three major types of CMP are *dilated, hypertrophic,* and *restrictive.* Each type has its own pathogenesis, clinical presentation, and treatment protocols (Table 21). CMP can lead to cardiomegaly and heart failure (HF). CMP is the primary reason why heart transplants are performed.

Table 21	Comparison of Types of Cardiomyopathy		
Dilated	**Hypertrophic**	**Restrictive**

	Dilated	Hypertrophic	Restrictive
Major Manifestations			
	Fatigue, weakness, palpitations, dyspnea	Exertional dyspnea, fatigue, angina, syncope, palpitations	Dyspnea, fatigue
Cardiomegaly			
	Moderate to severe	Mild to moderate	Mild
Contractility			
	Decreased	Increased or decreased	Normal or decreased
Valvular Incompetence			
	Atrioventricular (AV) valves, especially mitral	Mitral valve	AV valves
Dysrhythmias			
	Sinus tachycardia, atrial and ventricular dysrhythmias	Atrial and ventricular dysrhythmias	Atrial and ventricular dysrhythmias
Cardiac Output			
	Decreased	Normal or decreased	Normal or decreased
Outflow Tract Obstruction			
	None	Increased	None

C

Dilated Cardiomyopathy

Pathophysiology

Dilated cardiomyopathy is the most common type of CMP. It is characterized by diffuse inflammation and rapid degeneration of myocardial fibers that results in ventricular dilation, impairment of systolic function, atrial enlargement, and stasis of blood in the left ventricle. The ventricular walls do not hypertrophy.

- Dilated CMP often follows an infectious myocarditis. Other common causes include alcohol and cocaine, hypertension, and CAD.

Clinical Manifestations

Signs and symptoms of dilated CMP may develop acutely after a systemic infection or slowly over time. Most people eventually develop HF. Symptoms can include fatigue, dyspnea at rest, paroxysmal nocturnal dyspnea, and orthopnea. Dry cough, abdominal bloating, and anorexia may occur as the disease progresses. Signs can include an irregular heart rate with an abnormal S_3 and/or S_4, pulmonary crackles, edema, pallor, hepatomegaly, heart murmurs, dysrhythmias, and jugular venous distention.

Diagnostic Studies

A diagnosis is made on the basis of patient history and exclusion of other causes of HF.

- Doppler echocardiography is the basis for the diagnosis of dilated CMP.
- Chest x-ray may show cardiomegaly with pulmonary venous hypertension and pleural effusion.
- ECG may reveal tachycardia, bradycardia, and dysrhythmias with conduction disturbances.
- Serum levels of b-type natriuretic peptide (BNP) are elevated in the presence of HF.
- Cardiac catheterization confirms or excludes CAD, and multiple gated acquisition (MUGA) nuclear scan determines ejection fraction (EF).

Nursing and Collaborative Management

Interventions focus on controlling HF by enhancing myocardial contractility and decreasing preload and afterload.

- Nitrates and loop diuretics decrease preload, and angiotensin-converting enzyme (ACE) inhibitors reduce afterload.
- β-Adrenergic blockers (e.g., metoprolol [Lopressor]) and aldosterone antagonists (e.g., spironolactone [Aldactone]) control the neurohormonal stimulation that occurs in HF.
- Antidysrhythmics (e.g., amiodarone) and anticoagulants are used as indicated.
- Drug and nutritional therapy and cardiac rehabilitation may help alleviate symptoms of HF and improve cardiac output (CO) and quality of life.
- A patient with secondary dilated CMP must be treated for the underlying disease process. For example, the patient with alcohol-induced dilated CMP must abstain from all alcohol.
- The use of statins (e.g., atorvastatin [Lipitor]) in ischemic and idiopathic dilated CMP improves survival and cardiac function while reducing inflammatory markers.
- Patients may also benefit from nondrug therapies. A ventricular assist device (VAD) allows the heart to rest and recover from acute HF. It may also serve as a bridge to heart transplantation.

In addition, cardiac resynchronization therapy and an implantable cardioverter-defibrillator are used in appropriate patients.

- The patient with terminal or end-stage CMP may consider heart transplantation. Currently, approximately 50% of heart transplantations are performed for treatment of CMP. Cardiac transplant recipients have a good prognosis.

- Observe for signs and symptoms of worsening HF, dysrhythmias, embolic formation, and drug responsiveness. The goals of therapy are to keep the patient at an optimal level of functioning and out of the hospital.

- Encourage caregivers to learn cardiopulmonary resuscitation (CPR). Instruct them on when and how to access emergency care.

Hypertrophic Cardiomyopathy
Pathophysiology
Hypertrophic cardiomyopathy (HCM) is asymmetric left ventricular hypertrophy without ventricular dilation. HCM occurs less commonly than dilated CMP and is more common in men than in women. It is usually diagnosed in young adulthood and is often seen in active, athletic individuals. Hypertrophic CMP is the most common cause of sudden cardiac death (SCD) in otherwise healthy young people.

- The main characteristics of HCM are massive ventricular hypertrophy; rapid, forceful contraction of the left ventricle; impaired relaxation (diastole); and obstruction to aortic outflow (not present in all patients). The primary defect is diastolic dysfunction from left ventricular stiffness. Decreased ventricular filling and obstruction to outflow result in decreased CO, especially during exertion.

Clinical Manifestations
Patients may be asymptomatic. The most common symptom is dyspnea, which is caused by an elevated left ventricular diastolic pressure. Other manifestations include fatigue, angina, syncope (especially during exertion), and dysrhythmias.

- Common dysrhythmias include atrial fibrillation, ventricular tachycardia, and ventricular fibrillation. Any of these dysrhythmias may lead to syncope or SCD.

Diagnostic Studies
Clinical findings on examination may be unremarkable. The following diagnostic studies may be used:

- Echocardiogram is the primary diagnostic tool to confirm HCM, which is hypertrophy of the left ventricle (LV).

- Auscultation may reveal an S_4 and a systolic murmur between the apex and the sternal border at the fourth intercostal space.

- Cardiac catheterization and nuclear stress testing may be helpful in diagnosing and guiding treatment.

Nursing and Collaborative Management

Goals of care are to improve ventricular filling by reducing ventricular contractility and relieving LV outflow obstruction. This can be done with the use of β-adrenergic blockers (e.g., metoprolol) or calcium channel blockers (e.g., verapamil [Calan]).

- Amiodarone or sotalol (Betapace) are effective antidysrhythmia medications. However, their use does not prevent SCD. For patients at risk for SCD, a cardioverter-defibrillator is needed.
- Atrioventricular pacing can reduce the degree of outflow obstruction by causing the septum to move away from the left ventricular wall.
- Patients with severe symptoms unresponsive to therapy with marked obstruction to aortic outflow may be candidates for surgical treatment (ventriculomyotomy and myectomy) of their hypertrophied septum. Most patients have an improvement in symptoms and exercise tolerance after surgery.
- An alternative nonsurgical procedure to reduce symptoms is alcohol-induced, percutaneous transluminal septal myocardial ablation (PTSMA), in which alcohol is used to cause ischemia and septal wall infarction. Ablation of the septal wall decreases the obstruction to flow, and the patient's symptoms decrease.

Nursing interventions focus on relieving symptoms, observing for and preventing complications, and providing emotional support.

- Teaching should focus on helping the patients to adjust their lifestyle to avoid strenuous activity and dehydration. Any activity that causes an increase in systemic vascular resistance (thus increasing obstruction to forward blood flow) is dangerous and should be avoided.
- Rest and elevation of the feet to improve venous return to the heart can manage chest pain in these patients. Vasodilators such as nitroglycerin may worsen the chest pain by decreasing venous return and further increasing obstruction of blood flow from the heart.

Restrictive Cardiomyopathy

Pathophysiology

Restrictive cardiomyopathy is the least common type of cardiomyopathic condition. It is a disease of the heart muscle that impairs diastolic filling and stretch.

- A number of pathologic processes may be involved, including myocardial fibrosis, hypertrophy, and infiltration, which produce stiffness of the ventricular wall.

- The ventricles are resistant to filling and therefore demand high diastolic filling pressures to maintain CO.

Clinical Manifestations

Classic symptoms of restrictive CMP are fatigue, exercise intolerance, and dyspnea. Other manifestations may include angina, orthopnea, syncope, palpations, and signs of HF.

Diagnostic Studies

Chest x-ray may be normal or show cardiomegaly with pleural effusions and pulmonary congestion.

- ECG may reveal mild tachycardia at rest. The most common dysrhythmias are atrial fibrillation or atrioventricular block.
- Echocardiography may reveal a left ventricle that is normal size with a thickened wall, a slightly dilated right ventricle, and dilated atria.
- Endomyocardial biopsy, CT scan, and nuclear imaging may help to determine a diagnosis.

Nursing and Collaborative Management

Currently, no specific treatment for restrictive CMP exists. Interventions are aimed at improving diastolic filling and the underlying disease process. Treatment includes conventional therapy for HF and dysrhythmias. Heart transplant may also be a consideration.

Nursing care is similar to the care of a patient with HF. As in the treatment of patients with HCM, teach patients to avoid situations such as strenuous activity and dehydration that impair ventricular filling and increase systemic vascular resistance.

CARPAL TUNNEL SYNDROME

Description

Carpal tunnel syndrome (CTS) is a condition caused by compression of the median nerve, which enters the hand through the narrow confines of the carpal tunnel. The carpal tunnel is formed by ligaments and bones. This condition is often caused by pressure from trauma or edema caused by inflammation of a tendon (tenosynovitis), neoplasm, rheumatoid arthritis, or soft tissue masses such as ganglia. CTS is the most common compression neuropathy in the upper extremities.

- This syndrome is associated with hobbies or occupations that require continuous wrist movement (e.g., musicians, carpenters, computer users).
- Women are affected more than men, possibly because of a smaller carpal tunnel.

Clinical Manifestations

Manifestations are weakness (especially of the thumb), pain and numbness, impaired sensation in the distribution of the median nerve, and clumsiness in performing fine hand movements. Numbness and tingling may awaken the patient at night. Shaking the hands will often relieve these symptoms. Physical signs of CTS include Tinel's sign and Phalen's sign.

- *Tinel's sign* can be elicited by tapping over the median nerve as it passes through the carpal tunnel in the wrist. A positive response is a sensation of tingling in the distribution of the median nerve over the hand.
- *Phalen's sign* can be elicited by allowing the wrists to fall freely into maximum flexion and maintain the position for more than 60 seconds. A positive response is a sensation of tingling in the distribution of the median nerve over the hand.

In late stages, there is atrophy of the thenar muscles around the base of the thumb, resulting in recurrent pain and eventual dysfunction of the hand.

Nursing and Collaborative Management

Teach employees and employers about risk factors for CTS to prevent its occurrence. Adaptive devices such as wrist splints may be worn to relieve pressure on the median nerve. Special keyboard pads and mice are available for computer users. Other ergonomic changes include workstation modifications, change in body positions, and frequent breaks from work-related activities.

Early symptoms of CTS can usually be relieved by stopping the aggravating movement and by resting the hand and wrist by immobilizing them in a hand splint. Splints worn at night help keep the wrist in a neutral position and may reduce night pain and numbness. Injection of a corticosteroid drug directly into the carpal tunnel may provide short-term relief.

If symptoms persist for more than 6 months, surgery is generally recommended, which involves severing the band of tissue around the wrist to reduce pressure on the median nerve. Surgery is done in the outpatient setting under local anesthesia. Endoscopic carpal tunnel release is performed through a small puncture incision(s) in the wrist and palm.

- After surgery, assess the neurovascular status of the hand regularly.
- Instruct the patient about wound care and the appropriate assessments to perform at home.

Although symptoms may be relieved immediately after surgery, full recovery may take months.

CATARACT

Description

A *cataract* is an opacity within the lens of one or both eyes, causing a gradual decline in vision. Almost 22 million Americans ages 40 years and older have cataracts, and by age 80 more than 50% have cataracts. Cataract removal is the most common surgical procedure in the United States.

Pathophysiology

Although most cataracts are age related (senile cataracts), they can be associated with other factors including trauma, congenital factors such as maternal rubella, radiation or ultraviolet (UV) light exposure, certain drugs such as systemic corticosteroids or long-term topical corticosteroids, and ocular inflammation. The patient with diabetes mellitus tends to develop cataracts at a younger age.

- In senile cataract formation, altered metabolic processes within the lens cause water accumulation and alterations in the lens fiber structure. These changes affect lens transparency, causing vision changes.

Clinical Manifestations

- Patient may complain of decreased vision, abnormal color perception, and glare.
- Visual decline is gradual, with the rate of cataract development varying from patient to patient.

Diagnostic Studies

- Opacity directly observable by ophthalmoscopic or slit lamp microscopic examination
- Visual acuity measurement
- Glare testing
- Keratometry and A-scan ultrasound if surgery is planned

Collaborative Care

The presence of a cataract does not necessarily indicate a need for surgery. For many patients the diagnosis is made long before they actually decide to have surgery. Currently no treatment is available to "cure" cataracts other than surgical removal.

- Helpful palliative measures include a change in eyeglass prescription, strong reading glasses or magnifiers, an increased amount of light for reading, and avoidance of nighttime driving if glare is worse at night.

- When palliative measures no longer provide an acceptable level of visual function, the patient is a candidate for surgery. Removal of the lens may also be medically necessary in patients with increased intraocular pressure and diabetic retinopathy. In these cases the cataract may be removed to allow visualization of the retina and adequate management of the problem.

Almost all patients have an intraocular lens (IOL) implanted at the time of cataract extraction surgery. Depending on the type of anesthesia, the patient's eye may be covered with a patch or protective shield, which is usually worn overnight and removed during the first postoperative visit. Most patients experience little visual impairment after surgery. IOL implants provide immediate visual rehabilitation, and many patients achieve a usable level of visual acuity within a few days after surgery.

Nursing Management

Goals
- Preoperatively, the patient will make an informed decision and experience minimal anxiety.
- Postoperatively, the patient will understand and comply with therapy, maintain an acceptable level of physical and emotional comfort, and remain free of infection and other complications.

Nursing Diagnoses
- Self-care deficits
- Anxiety

Nursing Interventions
For the patient who chooses not to have surgery, suggest vision enhancement techniques and a modification of activities and lifestyle to accommodate the visual deficit.

For the patient who elects surgery, provide information, support, and reassurance about the surgical and postoperative experience to reduce or alleviate patient anxiety. Postoperatively, offer mild analgesics for slight scratchiness or mild eye pain. The physician needs to be notified if severe pain, increased or purulent drainage, increased redness, or decreased visual acuity is present.

▼ Patient and Caregiver Teaching
- Written and verbal discharge teaching should include postoperative eye care, activity restrictions, medications, follow-up visit schedule, and signs of possible complications (Table 22).
- Include the patient's caregiver in the teaching because some patients may have difficulty with self-care activities, especially if vision in the unoperated eye is poor. Provide an opportunity for the patient and caregiver to do return demonstrations of any self-care activities.

Table 22	Patient and Caregiver Teaching Guide *After Eye Surgery*

Include the following information in the teaching plan for the patient and the caregiver after eye surgery.

- Proper hygiene and eye care techniques to ensure that medications, dressings, and/or surgical wound is not contaminated during eye care
- Signs and symptoms of infection and when and how to report these to allow for early recognition and treatment of possible infection
- Importance of complying with postoperative restrictions on head positioning, bending, coughing, and Valsalva maneuver to optimize visual outcomes and prevent increased intraocular pressure
- How to instill eye medications using aseptic techniques and adherence with prescribed eye medication routine to prevent infection
- How to monitor pain, take pain medication, and report pain not relieved by medication
- Importance of continued follow-up as recommended to maximize potential visual outcomes

Source: Lamb P, Simms-Eaton S: *Core curriculum for ophthalmic nursing,* ed. 3, Dubuque, Iowa, 2008, Kendall-Hunt.

- Suggest ways the patient and caregiver can modify activities and environment to maintain an adequate level of safe functioning. Suggestions may include getting assistance with steps, removing area rugs and other potential obstacles, preparing meals for freezing before surgery, and obtaining audio books for diversion until visual acuity improves.

CELIAC DISEASE

Description

Celiac disease is an autoimmune disease characterized by damage to the small intestinal mucosa from the ingestion of wheat, barley, and rye in genetically susceptible individuals. It is a relatively common disease that occurs at all ages and has a wide variety of symptoms.

Celiac disease is not the same as the disease *tropical sprue,* a chronic disorder acquired in tropical areas that is characterized by progressive disruption of jejunal and ileal tissue resulting in nutritional difficulties. Tropical sprue is treated with folic acid and tetracycline.

The incidence of celiac disease is thought to be about 1% of the U.S. population. High-risk groups include first- or second-degree relatives of someone with celiac disease and people with disorders associated with the disease such as migraine and myocarditis. It is slightly more common in women, and symptoms often begin in childhood. Many people seek treatment for nonspecific complaints for years before celiac disease is diagnosed.

Pathophysiology

Three factors necessary for the development of celiac disease are a genetic predisposition, gluten ingestion, and an immune-mediated response.

- About 90% to 95% of patients with celiac disease have human leukocyte antigen (HLA) allele HLA-DQ2, and the other 5% to 10% have HLA-DQ8. However, not everyone with these genetic markers develops the disease.
- Tissue destruction that occurs with celiac disease is the result of chronic inflammation activated by the ingestion of gluten found in wheat, rye, and barley.
- Damage is most severe in the duodenum, probably because it is the site of the highest concentration of gluten. The inflammation lasts as long as gluten ingestion continues.

Clinical Manifestations

Classic manifestations of celiac disease include foul-smelling diarrhea, steatorrhea, flatulence, abdominal distention, and symptoms of malnutrition. Some people may instead have atypical symptoms such as decreased bone density and osteoporosis, dental enamel hypoplasia, iron and folate deficiencies, peripheral neuropathy, and reproductive problems.

- A pruritic, vesicular skin lesion, called dermatitis herpetiformis, is sometimes present and occurs as a rash on the buttocks, scalp, face, elbows, and knees.
- Weight loss, muscle wasting, and other signs of malnutrition may be present. Patients may exhibit lactose intolerance.
- Iron-deficiency anemia is common.
- Celiac disease is also associated with other autoimmune diseases, particularly rheumatoid arthritis, type 1 diabetes mellitus, and thyroid disease.

Diagnostic Studies

Celiac disease is confirmed by (1) histologic evidence when a biopsy is taken from the small intestine and (2) the symptoms and histologic evidence disappearing when the person eats a gluten-free diet.

Nursing and Collaborative Management

Treatment with a gluten-free diet halts the process. Most patients recover completely within 3 to 6 months of treatment, but they need to maintain a gluten-free diet for life. If the disease is untreated, chronic inflammation and hyperplasia continue. Individuals with celiac disease have an increased risk of non-Hodgkin's lymphoma and gastrointestinal cancers.

- Dietary gluten comes from wheat, barley, rye, and oats (oats do not contain gluten but can become contaminated with gluten during milling). Gluten is also found in some medications, food additives, preservatives, and stabilizers.
- In patients with refractory celiac disease who do not respond to the gluten-free diet alone, corticosteroids may be used.

▼ **Patient and Caregiver Teaching**
- Maintenance of a gluten-free diet is difficult. Dietary consultation is imperative. The patient needs to know where to purchase gluten-free products and may need financial assistance because gluten-free products are more expensive than regular foods.
- The Celiac Sprue Association website *(www.csaceliacs.info)* and the Celiac Disease Foundation *(www.celiac.org)* provide suggestions for maintaining a gluten-free diet and living with celiac disease.
- Continually encourage and motivate patients to continue the gluten-free diet. Reinforce that nonadherence to the diet will result in chronic inflammation, which can lead to complications such as anemia and osteoporosis.

CERVICAL CANCER

Description

Approximately 12,000 women in the United States are diagnosed annually with cervical cancer. Noninvasive cervical cancer (in situ) is about four times more common than invasive cervical cancer.

- The number of deaths from cervical cancer has fallen steadily over the past 50 years. This is because of earlier and better diagnosis with widespread use of the Papanicolaou (Pap) test. In addition to cancer, the Pap test detects precancerous changes. By treating precancerous lesions, progression to cervical cancer can be prevented.
- An increased risk of cervical cancer is associated with low socioeconomic status, early sexual activity (before 17 years old), multiple sexual partners, infection with human papillomavirus (HPV), immunosuppression, and smoking.

Pathophysiology

The progression from normal cervical cells to dysplasia and on to cervical cancer appears to be related to repeated injuries to the cervix. The progression occurs slowly over years rather than months. There is a strong relationship between dysplasia and HPV infections. HPV types 16 and 18 together cause about 70% of cervical cancers. Cancer rates are expected to decline further with vaccines (e.g., Gardasil, Cervarix) now being used for the prevention of HPV.

Clinical Manifestations

Early cervical cancer is generally asymptomatic, but leukorrhea and intermenstrual bleeding eventually occur.

- A vaginal discharge that is usually thin and watery becomes dark and foul smelling as the disease advances.
- Vaginal bleeding is initially only spotting, but as the tumor enlarges, it becomes heavier and more frequent.
- Pain is a late symptom and is followed by weight loss, anemia, and cachexia.

Diagnostic Studies

- Pap test, colposcopy, and biopsy

Collaborative Care

Vaccines against HPV reduce the incidence of both cervical-related neoplasia and cervical cancer due to infection from HPV types 16 and 18. Vaccination against HPV is recommended for females and males at ages 11 or 12 years.

The treatment of cervical cancer is guided by the patient's age, general health, and stage of the tumor (see Table 54-11, Lewis et al, *Medical-Surgical Nursing,* ed. 9, p. 1293).

Four procedures can preserve fertility. Conization may be the only therapy needed for noninvasive cervical cancer if analysis of removed tissue indicates that a wide area of normal tissue surrounds the excised tissue. Laser treatments can be used to destroy abnormal tissue. Cautery and cryosurgery may also be used.

Invasive cancer of the cervix is treated with surgery, chemotherapy, and/or radiation.

- Surgical procedures include hysterectomy, radical hysterectomy, and, rarely, pelvic exenteration (Table 23).
- Radiation may be external (e.g., cobalt) or internal (e.g., cesium or radium). Standard radiation treatment is 4 to 6 weeks of external radiation followed by one or two treatments with internal implants (brachytherapy).
- Cisplatin-based chemotherapy regimens benefit patients with cancer spread beyond the cervix.

Table 23	Surgical Procedures Involving the Female Reproductive System

Type of Surgery	Description
Abdominal Hysterectomy	
Total hysterectomy	Uterus and cervix removed using large abdominal incision (bikini cut).
Total abdominal hysterectomy and bilateral salpingo-oophorectomy (TAH-BSO)	Uterus, cervix, fallopian tubes, and ovaries removed using large abdominal incision.
Radical hysterectomy	Panhysterectomy, partial vaginectomy, and dissection of lymph nodes in pelvis.
Vaginal Hysterectomy	Uterus and cervix removed through a cut in the top of vagina.
Laparoscopic Hysterectomy	Uses laparoscope (video camera and small surgical instruments).
Laparoscopic-assisted vaginal hysterectomy (LAVH)	Incision made at top of vagina. Uterus and cervix removed through the vagina. Laparoscope inserted into abdomen to assist in the procedure.
Laparoscopic supracervical hysterectomy	Uterus removed using only laparoscopic instruments. Cervix is left intact.
Robotic-Assisted Surgery	Robot (special machine) used to do surgery through small abdominal incisions. Most often used when a patient has cancer or is very overweight and vaginal surgery is not safe.
Vulvectomy	Surgical procedure to remove part or all of the vulva.
Skinning vulvectomy	Removal of top layer of vulvar skin where the cancer is found. Skin grafts from other parts of the body may be needed to cover the area.
Simple vulvectomy	Entire vulva is removed.

Continued

C

Table 23	Surgical Procedures Involving the Female Reproductive System—cont'd
Type of Surgery	**Description**
Radical vulvectomy	Entire vulva, including clitoris, labia majora and minora, and nearby tissue, is removed. Nearby lymph nodes may also be removed.
Vaginectomy	Removal of vagina.
Pelvic Exenteration	Radical hysterectomy, total vaginectomy, removal of bladder with diversion of urinary system, and resection of colon and rectum with colostomy.

Nursing Management: Cervical Cancer and Other Cancers of the Female Reproductive System

In addition to cervical cancer, malignant tumors of the female reproductive system can be found in the endometrium, ovaries, vagina, and vulva. Management of the patient with any cancer of the female reproductive system includes many similar interventions.

Goals

The patient with a malignant tumor of the female reproductive system will actively participate in treatment decisions, achieve satisfactory pain and symptom management, recognize and report problems promptly, maintain preferred lifestyle as long as possible, and continue to practice cancer detection strategies.

Nursing Diagnoses

- Anxiety
- Acute pain
- Disturbed body image
- Ineffective sexuality patterns
- Grieving

Nursing Interventions

Through your contact with women in a variety of settings, teach women the importance of routine screening for cancers of the reproductive system. Cancer can be prevented when screening reveals precancerous conditions of the vulva, cervix, endometrium, and rarely the ovaries. Assist women to view routine cancer screening as an important self-care activity and recommend vaccination against cervical cancer.

- Teaching women about risk factors for cancers of the reproductive system is important. Limiting sexual activity during adolescence, using condoms, having fewer sexual partners, and not smoking reduce the risk of cervical cancer.

Hysterectomy. Preoperatively, the patient is prepared for surgery with the standard perineal or abdominal preparation. A vaginal douche and enema may be given according to surgeon preference. The bladder should be emptied before the patient is sent to the operating room. An indwelling catheter is often inserted.

Postoperatively, the patient who has had a hysterectomy will have an abdominal dressing (abdominal hysterectomy) or a sterile perineal pad (vaginal hysterectomy).

- The dressing should be observed frequently for any sign of bleeding during the first 8 hours after surgery. A moderate amount of serosanguineous drainage on the perineal pad is expected after a vaginal hysterectomy.
- Urinary retention may occur postoperatively because of temporary bladder atony resulting from edema or nerve trauma. An indwelling catheter may be used for 1 or 2 days to maintain bladder drainage and prevent strain on the suture line.
- Food and fluids may be restricted if the patient is nauseated. Ambulation is encouraged to relieve abdominal flatus.
- Special care must be taken to prevent the development of deep vein thrombosis (DVT). Frequent position changes and avoidance of high Fowler's position minimize blood flow stasis and pooling. Encourage leg exercises to promote circulation.

The loss of the uterus may bring about grief responses similar to any great personal loss. The ability to bear children may be essential to a woman's image of being a female. Elicit the woman's feelings and concerns about her surgery.

Teach the patient what to expect after surgery (e.g., she will not menstruate). Instructions should include specific activity restrictions. Intercourse should be avoided until the wound is healed (about 4 to 6 weeks). If a vaginal hysterectomy is performed, inform the patient that there may be a temporary loss of vaginal sensation.

- Physical restrictions are limited for a short time. Heavy lifting should be avoided for 2 months. Activities that may increase pelvic congestion, such as dancing and brisk walking, should be avoided for several months, whereas activities such as swimming may be both physically and mentally helpful.

Salpingectomy and Oophorectomy. Postoperative care of the woman who has undergone removal of a fallopian tube (salpingectomy) or an ovary (oophorectomy) is similar to that for any patient having abdominal surgery. When both ovaries are removed (bilateral oophorectomy), surgical menopause results. Symptoms are similar to those of regular menopause but may be more severe because of the sudden withdrawal of hormones.

Pelvic Exenteration. When other forms of therapy are ineffective in controlling cancer spread and no metastases have been found outside the pelvis, pelvic exenteration may be performed. This radical surgery usually involves removal of the uterus, ovaries, fallopian tubes, vagina, bladder, urethra, and pelvic lymph nodes. In some situations the descending colon, rectum, and anal canal may also be removed. Postoperative care involves that of a patient who has had a radical hysterectomy, an abdominal perineal resection, and an ileostomy or colostomy. Physical, emotional, and social adjustments to life on the part of the woman and her family are great. There are urinary or fecal diversions in the abdominal wall, a reconstructed vagina, and the onset of menopausal symptoms.

- Much understanding and support are needed from the nursing staff during a long recovery period. Gently encourage the patient to regain her independence.

CHLAMYDIAL INFECTIONS

Description

Chlamydia trachomatis is a gram-negative bacterium recognized as a genital pathogen responsible for a variety of illnesses. In the United States and Canada, chlamydial infections are the most commonly reported sexually transmitted infection (STI). Infection rates have increased over the past 20 years, with more than 1.3 million cases reported in 2010. This increase may be due in part to better and more intensive screening for the infection. Underreporting is significant because many people are asymptomatic and do not seek testing.

Pathophysiology

Chlamydia can be transmitted during vaginal, anal, or oral sex. Numerous different strains of *C. trachomatis* cause urogenital infections (e.g., nongonococcal urethritis [NGU] in men and cervicitis in women), ocular trachoma, and lymphogranuloma venereum. As with gonorrhea, chlamydial infections result in a superficial mucosal infection that can become more invasive.

Risk factors include women and adolescents, new or multiple sex partners, sexual partners who have had multiple partners, history of STIs and cervical ectopy, coexisting STIs, and inconsistent or incorrect use of a condom.

Clinical Manifestations

Symptoms may be absent or minor in most infected women and many men.

Men

Signs and symptoms in men include urethritis (dysuria, urethral discharge), epididymitis (unilateral scrotal pain, swelling, tenderness, fever), and proctitis (rectal discharge and pain during defecation).

Women

Signs and symptoms in women include cervicitis (mucopurulent discharge and hypertrophic ectopy [area that is edematous and bleeds easily]), urethritis (dysuria, pyuria, and frequent urination), dyspareunia (painful intercourse), bartholinitis (purulent exudate), and menstrual abnormalities.

- Chlamydial infections are closely associated with gonococcal infections, making clinical differentiation difficult. Therefore both infections are usually treated concurrently even without diagnostic evidence.

Complications

Complications often develop from poorly managed, inaccurately diagnosed, or undiagnosed chlamydial infections.

- In men, rare complications may result in epididymitis with possible infertility and reactive arthritis.
- In women, chlamydial infections may result in pelvic inflammatory disease, which can lead to chronic pelvic pain.

Diagnostic Studies

Chlamydial infections in men and women can be diagnosed by urine or collecting swab specimens from the endocervix or vagina (women) and urethra (men). Rectal swab specimens are tested in people engaging in anal sex. Cell culture can be used to detect *Chlamydia* organisms.

The most common diagnostic tests include the nucleic acid amplification test (NAAT), direct fluorescent antibody (DFA) test, and enzyme immunoassay (EIA). These tests can be used with urine samples rather than urethral and cervical swabs.

Collaborative Care

The Centers for Disease Control and Prevention (CDC) recommends that all sexually active females 25 years of age or younger

C

be routinely screened for *Chlamydia*. Annual screening of all women older than 25 years of age with one or more risk factors for the infection is also advised.

Doxycycline (Vibramycin) or azithromycin (Zithromax) are used to treat patients and their partners. Treatment of pregnant women usually prevents transmission to the fetus.

- Patients treated for chlamydial infections should abstain from sexual intercourse for 7 days after treatment and until all sexual partners have completed a full course of treatment.
- Follow-up care includes advising the patient to return if symptoms persist or recur, treating sexual partners, and encouraging condom use during all sexual contacts.

The high incidence of recurrence may be due to failure to treat the sexual partners of infected people. Because of the high prevalence of asymptomatic infections, screening of high-risk populations is needed to identify those who are infected.

Nursing Management

See Nursing Management: Sexually Transmitted Infections, p. 564.

CHOLELITHIASIS/CHOLECYSTITIS

Description

The most common disorder of the biliary system is *cholelithiasis* (stones in the gallbladder). The stones may be lodged in the neck of the gallbladder or in the cystic duct. *Cholecystitis* (inflammation of the gallbladder) may be acute or chronic, and it is usually associated with cholelithiasis.

Gallbladder disease is a common health problem in the United States. Approximately 8% to 10% of American adults have cholelithiasis.

- The incidence of cholelithiasis is higher in women, especially multiparous women, and people over 40 years old. Other factors that seem to increase the incidence of gallbladder disease are sedentary lifestyle, familial tendency, and obesity.
- The incidence of gallbladder disease is especially high in the Native American population, especially in the Navajo and Pima tribes.

Pathophysiology

The cause of gallstones is unknown. Cholelithiasis develops when the balance that keeps cholesterol, bile salts, and calcium in solution is altered so that these substances precipitate. Conditions that upset this balance include infection and disturbances in the metabolism of cholesterol. Mixed cholesterol stones, which are predominantly cholesterol, are the most common gallstones.

The stones may remain in the gallbladder or migrate to the cystic duct or common bile duct. They cause pain as they pass through the ducts and may lodge in the ducts and cause obstruction. Stasis of bile in the gallbladder can lead to cholecystitis.

Cholecystitis is most commonly associated with obstruction resulting from gallstones or biliary sludge. Cholecystitis in the absence of obstruction occurs most frequently in older adults and in patients who are critically ill. Bacteria reaching the gallbladder by the vascular or lymphatic route or chemical irritants in the bile can also produce cholecystitis. *Escherichia coli,* streptococci, and salmonellae are common causative bacteria. Other etiologic factors include adhesions, neoplasms, anesthesia, and opioids.

- During an acute attack of cholecystitis, the gallbladder is edematous and hyperemic and it may be distended with bile or pus. The cystic duct is also involved and may become occluded.
- The wall of the gallbladder becomes scarred after an acute attack. Decreased functioning occurs if large amounts of tissue are fibrosed.

Clinical Manifestations

Cholelithiasis may produce severe symptoms or none at all. Many patients have "silent cholelithiasis." Severity of symptoms depends on whether the stones are stationary or mobile and whether obstruction is present.

- When a stone is lodged in the ducts or when stones are moving through the ducts, spasms may result. This sometimes produces severe pain, which is termed *biliary colic*. The pain can be accompanied by tachycardia, diaphoresis, and prostration. The severe pain may last up to 1 hour, and when it subsides there is residual tenderness in the right upper quadrant.
- The attacks of pain frequently occur 3 to 6 hours after a high-fat meal or when the patient lies down.
- When total obstruction occurs, symptoms related to bile blockage are manifested. These include steatorrhea, pruritus, dark amber urine, bleeding tendencies, and jaundice.

Manifestations of cholecystitis vary from indigestion to moderate to severe pain, fever, and jaundice. Initial symptoms include indigestion and pain and tenderness in the right upper quadrant, which may be referred to the right shoulder and scapula. Pain may be acute and is accompanied by restlessness, diaphoresis, and nausea and vomiting.

- Symptoms of chronic cholecystitis include a history of fat intolerance, dyspepsia, heartburn, and flatulence.

Complications

Complications of cholecystitis include gangrenous cholecystitis, subphrenic abscess, pancreatitis, *cholangitis* (inflammation of biliary ducts), biliary cirrhosis, fistulas, and rupture of the gallbladder, which can produce bile peritonitis.

Diagnostic Studies

- Ultrasonography is used to diagnose gallstones.
- Endoscopic retrograde cholangiopancreatography (ERCP) allows for visualization of the gallbladder, cystic duct, common hepatic duct, and common bile duct. Bile taken during ERCP is sent for culture to identify any possible infecting organism.
- Percutaneous transhepatic cholangiography may be used to locate stones within the bile ducts.
- Laboratory tests reveal elevated serum enzymes and pancreatic enzymes, increased white blood cell (WBC) count, elevated direct and indirect bilirubin levels, and urinary bilirubin.

Collaborative Care

The treatment of gallstones in cholelithiasis depends on the stage of disease. Bile acids (cholesterol solvents) such as ursodeoxycholic (ursodiol) and chenodeoxycholic (chenodiol) are used to dissolve stones. ERCP with sphincterotomy (papillotomy) may be used for stone removal. ERCP allows for visualization of the biliary system and placement of stents and sphincterotomy (if warranted).

Extracorporeal shock-wave lithotripsy (ESWL) may be used to treat cholelithiasis. In this procedure a lithotriptor uses high-energy shock waves to disintegrate gallstones.

Drug therapy for gallbladder disease includes analgesics, anticholinergics (antispasmodics), fat-soluble vitamins, and bile salts. Morphine may be used initially for pain management. Cholestyramine, which may be used to provide relief from pruritus, is a resin that binds bile salts in the intestine, increasing their excretion in the feces.

During an acute episode of cholecystitis, treatment focuses on pain control, control of possible infection with antibiotics, and maintenance of fluid and electrolyte balance. Treatment is mainly supportive and symptomatic. A cholecystostomy may be used to drain purulent material from the obstructed gallbladder.

- If nausea and vomiting are severe, nasogastric (NG) tube insertion and gastric decompression may be used to prevent further gallbladder stimulation.
- Anticholinergics may be administered to decrease secretions and counteract smooth muscle spasms. Nonsteroidal antiinflammatory drugs (NSAIDs) (e.g., ketorolac [Toradol]) are given to decrease pain.

Laparoscopic cholecystectomy is the preferred surgical procedure for symptomatic cholelithiasis. In this procedure, the gallbladder is removed through one of four small punctures in the abdomen. Most patients experience minimal postoperative pain and are discharged the day of surgery or the day after. In most cases they are able to resume normal activities and return to work within 1 week.

After surgery people have fewer problems if they eat smaller, more frequent meals with some fat at each meal to promote gallbladder emptying. If obesity is a problem, a reduced-calorie diet is indicated. The diet should be low in saturated fats and high in fiber and calcium.

Nursing Management

Goals

The patient with gallbladder disease will have relief of pain and discomfort, no postoperative complications, and no recurrent attacks of cholecystitis or cholelithiasis.

Nursing Diagnoses
- Acute pain
- Ineffective self-health management

Nursing Interventions

Nursing goals for the patient undergoing conservative therapy include relieving pain, relieving nausea and vomiting, providing comfort and emotional support, maintaining fluid and electrolyte balance and nutrition, making accurate assessments to ensure effective treatment, and observing for complications.

The patient with acute cholecystitis or cholelithiasis is frequently experiencing severe pain. Medications ordered to relieve pain should be given as required before it becomes more severe.

Assess what drugs relieve the pain and how much medication is required. Observe for signs of obstruction of the ducts by stones, including jaundice; clay-colored stools; dark, foamy urine; steatorrhea; fever; and increased white blood cell (WBC) count.

Postoperative nursing care after a laparoscopic cholecystectomy includes monitoring for complications such as bleeding, making the patient comfortable, and preparing the patient for discharge.

- A common postoperative problem is referred pain to the shoulder because of the CO_2 that was not released or absorbed by the body. CO_2 can irritate the phrenic nerve and the diaphragm, causing some difficulty breathing. Placing the patient in Sims' position (left side with right knee flexed) helps move the gas pocket away from the diaphragm. Deep breathing should be encouraged, along with movement and ambulation. The pain can usually be relieved by NSAIDs or codeine.

Table 24	Patient and Caregiver Teaching Guide *Postoperative Laparoscopic Cholecystectomy*

Include the following instructions in the patient's postoperative teaching plan.
- Remove the bandages on the puncture site the day after surgery and you can shower.
- Notify your surgeon if any of the following signs and symptoms occurs:
  - Redness, swelling, bile-colored drainage or pus from any incision
  - Severe abdominal pain, nausea, vomiting, fever, chills
- You can gradually resume normal activities.
- Return to work within 1 wk of surgery.
- You can resume your usual diet, but a low-fat diet is usually better tolerated for several weeks after surgery.

- If the patient has a T tube, you need to maintain bile drainage and observe for T tube functioning and drainage.

▼ **Patient and Caregiver Teaching**
- When the patient has conservative therapy, dietary teaching is usually necessary. The diet is often low in fat, and sometimes a weight-reduction diet is also recommended. The patient may need to take fat-soluble vitamin supplements.
- Instruct the patient on manifestations that may indicate obstruction (stool and urine changes, jaundice, and pruritus).
- The patient who undergoes a laparoscopic cholecystectomy is discharged soon after the surgery, so home care and teaching are important (Table 24).

CHRONIC FATIGUE SYNDROME

Description
Chronic fatigue syndrome (CFS) is a disorder characterized by debilitating fatigue and a variety of associated complaints. An estimated 1 million people in the United States have CFS, but fewer than 20% of them have been diagnosed. CFS affects women more often than men and occurs in all ethnic and socioeconomic groups.

Pathophysiology
Despite numerous attempts to determine the etiology and pathology of CFS, the precise mechanisms remain unknown. There are many theories about the etiology of CFS.

- Neuroendocrine abnormalities have been implicated involving a hypofunction of the hypothalamic-pituitary-adrenal (HPA) axis and hypothalamic-pituitary-gonadal axis, which together regulate the stress response and reproductive hormone levels.
- Several microorganisms have been investigated as etiologic agents, including herpes viruses (e.g., Epstein-Barr virus [EBV], cytomegalovirus [CMV]), retroviruses, enteroviruses, *Candida albicans,* and mycoplasma).
- Because cognitive deficits such as decreased memory, attention, and concentration occur in many of the patients, it has been proposed that CFS is caused by changes in the central nervous system.

Clinical Manifestations

It is often difficult to distinguish between CFS and fibromyalgia because many clinical features are similar (Table 25).

In about half of cases, CFS develops insidiously, or the patient may have intermittent episodes that gradually become chronic.

Table 25	Commonalities Between Fibromyalgia and Chronic Fatigue Syndrome

Commonality	Description
Occurrence	Previously healthy, young, and middle-aged women.
Etiology (theories)	Infectious trigger, dysfunction in HPA axis, alteration in CNS.
Clinical manifestations	Generalized musculoskeletal pain, malaise and fatigue, cognitive dysfunction, headaches, sleep disturbances, depression, anxiety, fever.
Course of disease	Variable intensity of symptoms, fluctuates over time.
Diagnosis	No definitive laboratory tests or joint and muscle examinations; mainly a diagnosis of exclusion.
Collaborative therapy	Treatment is symptomatic and may include antidepressant drugs such as amitriptyline (Elavil) and fluoxetine (Prozac). Other measures are heat, massage, regular stretching, biofeedback, stress management, and relaxation training. Patient and caregiver teaching is essential.

HPA, Hypothalamic-pituitary-adrenal.

- Incapacitating fatigue is the most common symptom that causes the patient to seek health care. Associated symptoms (Table 26) may fluctuate in intensity over time.
- The patient may become angry and frustrated with the inability of health care providers to diagnose a problem. The disorder may have a major impact on work and family responsibilities.

Diagnostic Studies

Physical examination and diagnostic studies can rule out other possible causes of the patient's symptoms. No laboratory test can diagnose CFS or measure its severity. The Centers for Disease Control and Prevention (CDC) has helped develop diagnostic criteria based on the patient's symptoms (see Table 26). In general, CFS remains a diagnosis of exclusion.

Nursing and Collaborative Management

Because no definitive treatment exists for CFS, supportive management is essential. Tell the patient what is known about the disease. All complaints should be taken seriously.

- Nonsteroidal antiinflammatory drugs (NSAIDs) can be used to treat headaches, muscle and joint aches, and fever. Antihistamines

Table 26	Diagnostic Criteria for Chronic Fatigue Syndrome*

Major Criterion
- Unexplained, persistent, or relapsing chronic fatigue of new and definite onset (not lifelong). Not due to ongoing exertion. Not substantially alleviated by rest. Results in substantial reduction in occupational, educational, social, or personal activities.

Minor Criteria
- Impaired memory or concentration
- Frequent or recurring sore throat
- Tender cervical or axillary lymph nodes
- Muscle pain
- Multijoint pain without joint swelling or redness
- Headaches of a new type, pattern, or severity
- Unrefreshing sleep
- Postexertional malaise

Adapted from Centers for Disease Control and Prevention: Chronic fatigue syndrome: revised case definition. Retrieved from *www.cdc.gov/cfs/cfsdefinitionHCP.htm.*

*For a diagnosis to be made, the patient must demonstrate the major criterion, plus four or more of the minor criteria for ≥6 mo. These criteria were prepared by the Centers for Disease Control and Prevention, National Institutes of Health, and International Chronic Fatigue Syndrome Study Group.

and decongestants can be used to treat allergic symptoms. Tricyclic antidepressants (e.g., doxepin [Sinequan], amitriptyline [Elavil]) and selective serotonin reuptake inhibitors (e.g., fluoxetine [Prozac], paroxetine [Paxil]) can improve mood and sleep disorders. Clonazepam (Klonopin) can also be used to treat sleep disturbances and panic disorders.

- Total rest is not advised, because it can potentiate the self-image of being an invalid, whereas strenuous exertion can exacerbate the exhaustion. Therefore it is important to plan a carefully graduated exercise program.
- Behavioral therapy may be used to promote a positive outlook, as well as improve overall disability, fatigue, and other symptoms.
- One of the major problems facing many CFS patients is financial instability. When the illness strikes, they cannot work or must decrease the amount of time working.

CFS does not appear to progress. Although most patients recover or at least gradually improve over time, some do not show substantial improvement. Recovery is more common in individuals with a sudden onset of CFS.

CHRONIC OBSTRUCTIVE PULMONARY DISEASE

Description

Chronic obstructive pulmonary disease (COPD) is a disease state characterized by persistent airflow limitation that is slowly progressive. COPD is associated with an enhanced inflammatory response of the airways and lungs to noxious particles or gases, primarily caused by cigarette smoking. Previous definitions of COPD encompassed two types of obstructive airway disease, emphysema and chronic bronchitis.

- *Emphysema* is an abnormal permanent enlargement of the air spaces distal to the terminal bronchioles, accompanied by destruction of their walls and without obvious fibrosis.
- *Chronic bronchitis* is the presence of chronic productive cough for 3 months in each of 2 consecutive years in a patient in whom other causes of chronic cough have been excluded.
- Patients with COPD may have a predominance of one of these conditions, but the conditions usually coexist, and COPD is considered one disease state in terms of pathophysiology and management.
- It is sometimes difficult to distinguish COPD from asthma, especially if the individual has a history of cigarette smoking.

More than 12.7 million people in the United States have COPD, and it is the third leading cause of death in the United States.

Etiology

Cigarette smoking is the major risk factor for developing COPD. It affects about 15% of smokers.

- The irritating effect of cigarette smoke causes hyperplasia of cells, which subsequently results in increased mucus production. Hyperplasia reduces airway diameter and increases the difficulty in clearing secretions. Smoking reduces ciliary activity and produces abnormal dilation of the distal air space with destruction of alveolar walls.
- If a person has intense or prolonged exposure to various dusts, vapors, irritants, or fumes in the workplace, symptoms of lung impairment consistent with COPD can develop. If a person has occupational exposure and smokes, the risk of COPD increases.
- High levels of urban air pollution are harmful to people with existing lung disease; however, the effect of outdoor air pollution as a risk factor for the development of COPD is unclear.
- Severe recurring respiratory tract infections in childhood have been associated with reduced lung function and increased respiratory symptoms in adulthood. It is unclear whether the development of COPD can be related to recurrent infections in adults.
- Although the evidence is not conclusive, asthma may be a risk factor for COPD development.
- The fact that a relatively small percentage of smokers get COPD strongly suggests that genetic factors influence which smokers get the disease.

α_1-Antitrypsin (AAT) deficiency is a genetic risk factor for COPD. AAT is a serum protein produced by the liver and normally found in the lungs. The main function of AAT, an α_1-protease inhibitor, is to protect normal lung tissue from attack by proteases during inflammation related to cigarette smoking and infections.

Pathophysiology

COPD is characterized by chronic inflammation of the airways, lung parenchyma (respiratory bronchioles and alveoli), and pulmonary blood vessels. The pathogenesis of COPD is complex and involves many mechanisms. The defining features of COPD are irreversible airflow limitation during forced exhalation caused by loss of elastic recoil and airflow obstruction caused by mucus hypersecretion, mucosal edema, and bronchospasm.

The inflammatory process starts with inhalation of noxious particles (e.g., cigarette smoke) that causes the release of inflammatory mediators that damage lung tissue. This process causes tissue destruction and disrupts the normal defense mechanisms and repair process of the lung.

- The predominant inflammatory cells are neutrophils, macrophages, and lymphocytes. These cells attract other inflammatory mediators (e.g., leukotrienes) and proinflammatory cytokines (e.g., tumor necrosis factor). The end result of the inflammatory process is structural changes in the lungs.

- After the inhalation of oxidants in tobacco or air pollution, protease activity (which breaks down the connective tissue of the lungs) increases and antiproteases (which protect against the breakdown) are inhibited.

- Inability to expire air is the main characteristic of COPD. As the peripheral airways become obstructed, air is progressively trapped during expiration. The chest hyperexpands and becomes barrel shaped since the respiratory muscles are not able to function effectively.

- Gas exchange abnormalities result in hypoxemia and hypercapnia (increased CO_2). As air trapping increases and alveoli are destroyed, bullae (large air spaces in the parenchyma) and blebs (air spaces adjacent to pleurae) can form. There is a significant ventilation/perfusion (V/Q) mismatch, and hypoxemia results.

- Excess mucus production, resulting in a chronic productive cough, is due to an increased number of mucus-secreting goblet cells and enlarged submucosal glands.

- Pulmonary vascular changes resulting in mild to moderate pulmonary hypertension may occur late in the course of COPD.

In addition to lung disease, COPD is a systemic disease. Chronic inflammation is an underlying etiology for these systemic effects. Cardiovascular diseases commonly occur in COPD (smoking is a primary risk factor for both of them.) Other common systemic diseases include cachexia (skeletal muscle wasting), osteoporosis, diabetes, and metabolic syndrome, which cannot be readily related to smoking.

Clinical Manifestations

Manifestations of COPD typically develop slowly, but COPD should be considered in all patients over age 40 with 10 or more pack-years of cigarette smoking.

- A diagnosis of COPD should be considered in any patient who has symptoms of cough, sputum production, or dyspnea, and/or a history of exposure to risk factors for the disease.

- A chronic intermittent cough, which is often the first symptom to develop, may later be present every day as the disease progresses.

- Dyspnea is often progressive and usually occurs with exertion. In the late stages of COPD, dyspnea may be present at rest. Wheezing and chest tightness may be present, but may vary by time of the day or from day to day, especially in patients with more severe disease.
- Even when the patient with advanced COPD has adequate caloric intake, weight loss is still experienced. Fatigue is a prevalent symptom that affects the patient's activities of daily living.
- During physical examination a prolonged expiratory phase of respiration, wheezes, or decreased breath sounds are noted in all lung fields. The anterior-posterior diameter of the chest is increased *(barrel chest)* from chronic air trapping. The patient may assume a tripod position and use pursed-lip breathing.
- Over time, hypoxemia may develop with hypercapnia. The bluish-red color of the skin results from polycythemia and cyanosis. Polycythemia develops as a result of increased production of red blood cells as the body attempts to compensate for chronic hypoxemia.

Complications

Cor pulmonale results from pulmonary hypertension. In COPD, pulmonary hypertension is caused primarily by constriction of pulmonary vessels in response to alveolar hypoxia, with acidosis further potentiating vasoconstriction. Chronic hypoxia also stimulates erythropoiesis, which causes polycythemia. This results in increased viscosity of the blood. When pulmonary hypertension develops, the pressures on the right side of the heart must increase to push blood into the lungs. Eventually right-sided heart failure develops (see Cor Pulmonale, p. 159).

A *COPD exacerbation* is an acute event in the natural course of the disease characterized by an acute change in the patient's baseline dyspnea, cough, and/or sputum. The primary causes of exacerbations are bacterial or viral infection. Exacerbations are typical and increase in frequency (average one or two a year) as the disease progresses.

- Other complaints include malaise, insomnia, increased wheezing, fatigue, depression, confusion, or decreased exercise tolerance. Exacerbations are managed with short-acting bronchodilators, oral systemic corticosteroids, and antibiotics.
- Teach the patient and caregiver early recognition of the three cardinal symptoms of exacerbations (increase in dyspnea, sputum volume, or sputum purulence) to promote early treatment and thus prevent hospitalization and possible respiratory failure.

Acute respiratory failure may occur in patients with severe COPD who have exacerbations (see Acute Respiratory Distress Syndrome, p. 13). Frequently COPD patients wait too long to contact their health care provider when they first develop symptoms suggestive of an exacerbation. Discontinuing bronchodilator or corticosteroid medication may also precipitate respiratory failure. Indiscriminate use of sedatives, benzodiazepines, and opioids, especially in the preoperative or postoperative patient who retains CO_2, may suppress the ventilatory drive and lead to respiratory failure.

Depression and anxiety are other complications of COPD. A consult to a mental health specialist may be needed for proper screening and diagnosis of depression or other mental health problems. Cognitive and behavioral therapy along with COPD teaching can improve quality of life. Medications may be used to treat both depression and anxiety.

Diagnostic Studies

- A forced expiratory volume/forced vital capacity (FEV_1/FVC) <70% along with the appropriate symptoms can help to diagnose COPD. The value of FEV_1 provides a guideline for the degree of severity of COPD. The lower the FEV_1, the sicker the patient.
- A history and physical examination are extremely important in a diagnostic workup.
- Chest x-rays are not diagnostic but may show a flat diaphragm due to hyperinflated lungs.
- ECG can be used to determine right- and left-sided ventricular failure.
- Sputum culture and sensitivity are done if an acute exacerbation is present.
- Arterial blood gases (ABGs) in later stages usually indicate low PaO_2, elevated $PaCO_2$, decreased or low normal pH, and increased bicarbonate (HCO_3^-) levels.

Collaborative Care

Most patients with COPD are treated as outpatients. They are hospitalized for exacerbations and potential complications when respiratory failure, pneumonia, and cor pulmonale occur.

Evaluate the patient's exposure to environmental or occupational irritants, and determine ways to control or avoid them. The patient with COPD and anyone who smokes should receive an influenza virus vaccine yearly. The pneumococcal vaccine (Pneumovax) is recommended for all smokers ages 19 or older and all patients with COPD.

- Exacerbations of COPD should be treated as soon as possible, especially if the patient is in the severe stages. Some patients are given a prescription for antibiotics and are instructed to begin taking them when the first symptoms or signs of an exacerbation occur.
- Cessation of cigarette smoking in any stage of COPD is the intervention that can have the biggest impact on reducing the risk of developing COPD and decreasing progression of the disease. Smoking cessation techniques are discussed in Lewis et al, *Medical-Surgical Nursing,* ed. 9, pp. 156 to 159, and in Tables 11-4 to 11-6, pp. 156 to 158.

Medications for COPD can reduce symptoms, increase exercise capacity, improve overall health, and reduce the number and severity of exacerbations.

- Bronchodilator medications commonly used are β_2-adrenergic agonists, anticholinergic agents, and methylxanthines (see Table 29-7, Lewis et al, *Medical-Surgical Nursing,* ed. 9, pp. 570 to 571). When the patient has mild COPD or intermittent symptoms, a short-acting bronchodilator is used as needed. In the moderate stage of COPD, a long-acting bronchodilator is used in addition to a short-acting bronchodilator. Inhaled corticosteroids are beneficial for patients with severe or very severe COPD because they reduce the frequency of COPD exacerbations.

Long-term continuous (more than 15 hr/day) O_2 therapy (LTOT) increases survival and improves exercise capacity and mental status in hypoxemic patients with COPD (see Oxygen Therapy, p. 717).

The main types of breathing exercises commonly taught are pursed-lip breathing and diaphragmatic breathing. However, patients with moderate to severe COPD with marked hyperinflation may be poor candidates for diaphragmatic breathing.

Airway clearance techniques loosen mucus and secretions so they can be cleared by coughing. A variety of treatments can be used to achieve airway clearance. Respiratory therapy, physical therapy, and nurses are involved in performing these techniques. See Lewis et al, *Medical-Surgical Nursing,* ed. 9, pp. 594 to 595, for further information on respiratory care.

- Weight loss and muscle wasting are common in the patient with severe COPD. To decrease dyspnea and conserve energy, the patient should rest at least 30 minutes before eating and use a bronchodilator before meals. Fluid intake should be at least 3 L/day unless contraindicated by other medical conditions. A diet high in calories and protein, moderate in carbohydrates, and moderate to high in fat is recommended and can be divided into five or six small meals a day.

Surgical Therapy

Three different surgical procedures have been used in severe COPD. One type of surgery is lung volume reduction surgery, which is done to reduce the size of the lungs by removing the most diseased lung tissue so the remaining healthy lung tissue can perform better. Another surgical procedure is a bullectomy, which is used for patients with emphysematous COPD who have large bullae (>1 cm). The bullae are usually resected via thoracoscope. A third surgical procedure is lung transplantation, which benefits carefully selected patients with advanced COPD.

Nursing Management

Goals

The overall goals are that the patient with COPD will have prevention of disease progression, ability to perform activities of daily living (ADLs) and improved exercise tolerance, relief from symptoms, no complications related to COPD, knowledge and ability to implement a long-term treatment regimen, and overall improved quality of life.

See NCP 29-2 for specific goals related to the nursing diagnoses for the patient with COPD (Lewis et al, *Medical-Surgical Nursing,* ed. 9, p. 598).

Nursing Diagnoses
- Ineffective airway clearance
- Ineffective breathing pattern
- Impaired gas exchange

Nursing Interventions

Counseling the patient in smoking cessation is vital, because it is the only way to slow the progression of COPD. Avoiding or controlling exposure to occupational and environmental pollutants and irritants is another preventive measure to maintain healthy lungs. Early diagnosis and treatment of respiratory tract infections and exacerbations of COPD help prevent progression of the disease.

- People with COPD should avoid people who are sick, practice good hand-washing techniques, take medications as prescribed, exercise regularly, and maintain a healthy weight. Influenza and pneumococcal pneumonia vaccines are recommended for patients with COPD.
- The patient with COPD requires acute intervention for complications such as exacerbations of COPD, pneumonia, cor pulmonale, and acute respiratory failure. Once the crisis in these situations has been resolved, assess the degree and severity of the underlying respiratory problem. The information obtained will help in planning nursing care.

▼ **Patient and Caregiver Teaching**
The most important aspect in long-term care of the patient with COPD is teaching (Table 27).

Pulmonary rehabilitation (PR) is an evidence-based intervention that includes many disciplines working together to individualize treatment of the patient with COPD.

Table 27	Patient and Caregiver Teaching Guide *Chronic Obstructive Pulmonary Disease*

Include the following information in the teaching plan.

Goal
To assist the patient and caregiver in improving quality of life through education and promotion of lifestyle practices that support successful living with chronic obstructive pulmonary disease (COPD)

Teaching Topic	Resources
Overall Guide	*Patient Guide: What You Can Do About a Lung Disease Called COPD* (Global Initiative for Lung Disease). Retrieved from *www.goldcopd.org/ uploads/users/files/GOLD_ Patient_RevJan10.pdf.* (Also available in other languages.)
What Is COPD? ■ Basic anatomy and physiology of lung ■ Basic pathophysiology of COPD ■ Signs and symptoms of COPD, exacerbation, cold, flu, pneumonia ■ Tests to assess breathing	*COPD Statement: Patient Education Section* (American Thoracic Society [ATS]). Retrieved from *www. thoracic.org.* (Also available in Spanish.) *How Lungs Work* (American Lung Association [ALA]). Available under "Your Lungs" at *www.lung.org/your-lungs.*
Breathing and Airway Clearance Exercises ■ Pursed-lip breathing	See Table 29-13, Lewis et al, *Medical-Surgical Nursing*, ed. 9, p. 579.
■ Airway clearance technique—huff cough	See Table 29-23, Lewis et al, *Medical-Surgical Nursing*, ed. 9, p. 594.

Table 27	Patient and Caregiver Teaching Guide *Chronic Obstructive Pulmonary Disease*—cont'd

Teaching Topic	Resources
Energy Conservation Techniques	
▪ Daily activities (e.g., waking up, bathing, grooming, shopping, traveling)	Consult with physical therapist and occupational therapist. *09143-5_Chronic Obstructive Pulmonary Disease_formatted. doc* *COPD: Lifestyle Management* (National Jewish Health). Retrieved from *www. nationaljewish.org/healthinfo/ conditions/copd-chronic-obstructive-pulmonary-disease/lifestyle-management*.
Medications	
Types (include mechanism of action and types of devices) ▪ Methylxanthines ▪ β_2-Adrenergic agonists ▪ Corticosteroids ▪ Anticholinergics ▪ Antibiotics ▪ Other medications Establishing medication schedule	*COPD Statement: Patient Education Section: Medications and Other Treatments* OR *Patient Information Series: Medicines to Treat COPD* (ATS). Retrieved from *www.thoracic.org.* OR *COPD Medicines* (ALA). Retrieved from *www.lungusa.org.* OR *COPD Medications* (National Jewish Health). Search "COPD medications." Also has link to medication chart to take to provider. Retrieved from *www.nationaljewish. org/healthinfo.*
Correct use of inhalers, spacer, and nebulizer	See Figs. 29-5 to 29-7, Lewis et al, *Medical-Surgical Nursing*, ed. 9, pp. 571, 573, and 574. See Tables 29-8 to 29-10, Lewis et al, *Medical-Surgical Nursing*, ed. 9, p. 574. See Table 29-15, Lewis et al, *Medical-Surgical Nursing*, ed. 9, p. 581 for links to videos on medication devices.

C

Continued

Table 27   Patient and Caregiver Teaching Guide
Chronic Obstructive Pulmonary Disease—cont'd

Teaching Topic	Resources
Home Oxygen	
Explanation of rationale for use	*Oxygen Therapy* (National Jewish Health). Retrieved from *www.nationaljewish. org/healthinfo/medications/ lung-diseases/treatments/ oxygen-therapy.*
Guide for home O_2 use and equipment	*Traveling With Oxygen* (American College of Chest Physicians). Retrieved from *www.chestnet. org/accp/patient-guides/ traveling-oxygen.*
Psychosocial/Emotional Issues	
Concerns about interpersonal relationships	Open discussion (sharing with patient, significant other, and family). *Living With COPD: Get Social Support* (ALA help line, Better Breathers Club, and printed materials). Retrieved from *www.lung. org/lung-disease/copd/ living-with-copd/get-social-support.html.*
▪ Dependency	
▪ Intimacy	
Problems with emotions	
▪ Depression, anxiety, panic	
Treatment decisions	
▪ Support and rehabilitation groups	*Questions About Pulmonary Rehabilitation* (ATS). Retrieved from *patients. thoracic.org/materials/ index.php.* (Available in English and Spanish.)
End-of-life issues	
COPD Management Plan	
▪ Focus on self-management	Nurse and patient develop and write up COPD management plan that meets individual needs.
▪ Need to report changes	
▪ Cause of flare-ups or exacerbation	
▪ Recognition of signs and symptoms of respiratory infection, heart failure	*COPD Management Tools* (ALA). Retrieved from *www.lung. org/lung-disease/copd/ living-with-copd/copd-management-tools.html.*
▪ Reduce risk factors, especially smoking cessation	
▪ Exercise program of walking and arm strengthening	
▪ Yearly follow-up	

Table 27	Patient and Caregiver Teaching Guide *Chronic Obstructive Pulmonary Disease*—cont'd

Teaching Topic	Resources
Healthy Nutrition	
▪ Strategies to lose weight (if overweight) ▪ Strategies to gain weight (if underweight)	Consultation with dietitian. See Table 29-24, Lewis et al, *Medical-Surgical Nursing*, ed. 9, p. 596. *Nutrition* (ALA). Retrieved from *www.lung.org/lung-disease/copd/living-with-copd/nutrition.html*.

C

- Components of PR vary, but usually include exercise training, smoking cessation, nutrition counseling, and education. A mandatory component is exercise that focuses on the muscles used in ambulation.
- Other important topics include health promotion, psychologic counseling, and vocational rehabilitation. Smoking cessation is critical.

Energy conservation is an important component in COPD rehabilitation. Exercise training of the upper extremities may improve muscle function and reduce dyspnea. Alternative energy-saving practices for ADLs and scheduled rest periods should be planned.

- Walking or other endurance exercises (e.g., cycling) combined with strength training are likely the best interventions to strengthen muscles and improve the patient's endurance. Teach the patient coordinated walking with slow, pursed-lip breathing. Encourage the patient to walk 15 to 20 minutes per day at least three times a week with gradual increases.
- Modifying but not abstaining from sexual activity can also contribute to a healthy psychologic well-being. Using an inhaled bronchodilator before sexual activity can help ventilation.
- Adequate sleep is extremely important. The patient who is a restless sleeper, snores, stops breathing while asleep, and has a tendency to fall asleep during the day may need to be tested for sleep apnea.
- Healthy coping is a challenge for the COPD patient and family. People with COPD frequently have to deal with many lifestyle changes that may involve decreased ability to care for themselves, decreased energy for social activities, and loss of a job. Support groups at local chapters of the American Lung Association, hospitals, and clinics may be helpful.

CIRRHOSIS

Description

Cirrhosis is a chronic progressive disease of the liver characterized by extensive degeneration and destruction of liver cells. It is the eighth leading cause of death in the United States and is twice as common in men as women. The most common causes of cirrhosis are chronic hepatitis C infection and alcohol-induced liver disease. Environmental factors and genetic predisposition may also lead to the development of cirrhosis, regardless of dietary or alcohol intake.

Pathophysiology

Damaged liver cells with chronic disease attempt to regenerate, but the regenerative process is disorganized, resulting in abnormal blood vessel and bile duct architecture. The overgrowth of new and fibrous connective tissue distorts the liver's normal lobular structure, resulting in lobules of irregular size and shape with impeded blood flow.

Eventually, irregular and disorganized liver regeneration, poor cellular nutrition, and hypoxia (from inadequate blood flow and scar tissue) result in decreased functioning of the liver. The development of cirrhosis is an insidious, prolonged course, usually after decades of chronic liver disease.

Biliary causes of cirrhosis include primary biliary cirrhosis and primary sclerosing cholangitis. *Primary sclerosing cholangitis* is a chronic inflammatory condition affecting the liver and bile ducts. The etiology of primary sclerosing cholangitis is unknown. However, it is strongly associated with ulcerative colitis. The chronic inflammation can ultimately progress to cirrhosis and end-stage liver disease.

Clinical Manifestations

The onset of cirrhosis is usually insidious. Early symptoms can include anorexia, dyspepsia, flatulence, nausea and vomiting, and change in bowel habits (diarrhea or constipation). In addition, fever and abdominal pain may occur.

Later manifestations may be severe and result from liver failure and portal hypertension. Jaundice, peripheral edema, and ascites develop gradually. Other late symptoms include skin lesions, hematologic disorders, endocrine disturbances, and peripheral neuropathies. In advanced stages, the liver becomes small and nodular (see Fig. 44-6, Lewis et al, *Medical-Surgical Nursing,* ed. 9, p. 1019, for systemic clinical manifestations of cirrhosis).

- *Jaundice* occurs as a result of the decreased ability of the liver to conjugate and excrete bilirubin.
- *Skin lesions* such as *spider angiomas* that occur on the nose, cheeks, upper trunk, and neck and a redness of the palms of the hands, known as *palmar erythema,* result from an increase in circulating estrogen because the liver cannot metabolize steroid hormones.
- *Hematologic disorders* such as anemia, leukopenia, and thrombocytopenia are probably caused by splenomegaly that results from backup of blood from the portal vein into the spleen (portal hypertension). Coagulation problems result from the liver's inability to produce prothrombin and other factors essential for clotting.
- *Endocrine problems* result because adrenocortical hormones, estrogen, and testosterone cannot be metabolized and inactivated by a damaged liver. Men lose masculine sex characteristics as a result of increased estrogen levels, and amenorrhea may occur in younger women. Sodium and water retention and potassium loss occur as a result of hyperaldosteronism.
- *Peripheral neuropathy* is probably caused by a dietary deficiency of thiamine, folic acid, and cobalamin.

Complications

Major complications of cirrhosis are portal hypertension with resultant esophageal and/or gastric varices, peripheral edema and ascites, hepatic encephalopathy (coma), and hepatorenal syndrome.

Portal hypertension and *esophageal* and *gastric varices* result because of structural liver changes from cirrhosis. There is compression and destruction of the portal and hepatic veins and sinusoids. Portal hypertension is characterized by increased venous pressure in the portal circulation, splenomegaly, large collateral veins, ascites, and gastric and esophageal varices. Collateral circulation develops in an attempt to reduce high portal pressure and the increased plasma volume and lymphatic flow.

- Collateral channels commonly form in the lower esophagus, anterior abdominal wall, parietal peritoneum, and rectum.
- Varicosities may develop in areas where collateral and systemic circulations communicate, resulting in esophageal and gastric varices, *caput medusae* (ring of varices around the umbilicus), and hemorrhoids.

Esophageal varices are a complex of tortuous veins at the end of the esophagus, which are enlarged and swollen as a result of portal hypertension. *Gastric varices* are located in the upper portion (cardia, fundus) of the stomach. These collateral vessels contain little elastic tissue and are fragile. They tolerate high pressure poorly, and as a result bleed easily.

- Bleeding esophageal varices are the most life-threatening complication of cirrhosis. Patients may have melena or hematemesis. There may be slow oozing or massive bleeding, which is a medical emergency.

Peripheral edema results from decreased colloidal osmotic pressure from impaired liver synthesis of albumin and increased portacaval pressure from portal hypertension. Peripheral edema occurs as ankle and presacral edema.

Ascites is the accumulation of serous fluid in the peritoneal or abdominal cavity. With portal hypertension, proteins move from the blood vessels by way of larger pores of the sinusoids (capillaries) into the lymph space. When the lymphatic system is unable to carry off excess proteins and water, proteins leak into the peritoneal cavity. A second mechanism is hypoalbuminemia and decreased colloidal oncotic pressure resulting from the liver's inability to synthesize albumin. A third mechanism is hyperaldosteronism, which results when aldosterone is not metabolized by damaged hepatocytes, causing increased renal reabsorption of sodium and water.

- Ascites is manifested by abdominal distention with weight gain. If ascites is severe, the umbilicus may be everted. Abdominal striae with distended abdominal wall veins may be present.
- The patient has signs of dehydration (e.g., dry tongue and skin, sunken eyeballs, muscle weakness) and decreased urinary output.
- Hypokalemia is common and is caused by an excessive loss of potassium from hyperaldosteronism and the use of diuretic therapy to treat ascites.

Hepatic encephalopathy is a neuropsychiatric manifestation of liver disease. When blood is shunted past the liver by way of collateral vessels or the liver is unable to convert ammonia to urea, the levels of ammonia in the systemic circulation rise. Ammonia crosses the blood-brain barrier and produces neurologic toxic manifestations.

- Factors that increase ammonia in the circulation include GI hemorrhage, constipation, infection, hypokalemia, hypovolemia, dehydration, and metabolic alkalosis.
- Hepatic encephalopathy is manifested by changes in neurologic and mental responsiveness, ranging from sleep disturbance to lethargy to deep coma. A characteristic symptom is *asterixis* (flapping tremors), a rapid flexion and extension movement of the hands when the arms and hands are held stretched out.

Hepatorenal syndrome is a type of renal failure with advancing azotemia, oliguria, and intractable ascites.

- There is no structural abnormality of the kidneys. The etiology is complex, but the final common pathway is usually portal hypertension along with liver decompensation that results in splanchnic and systemic vasodilation and decreased arterial blood volume. As a result, renal vasoconstriction occurs and renal failure follows.
- In the patient with cirrhosis, this syndrome frequently follows diuretic therapy, GI hemorrhage, or paracentesis.

Diagnostic Studies

- Liver function studies demonstrate an elevation in alkaline phosphatase, aspartate aminotransferase (AST), alanine aminotransferase (ALT), and γ-glutamyl transferase (GGT).
- Prothrombin time is prolonged.
- Serum albumin and protein levels are decreased, and bilirubin and globulin levels are increased.
- Liver ultrasound and biopsy (percutaneous needle) are done to determine severity of cirrhosis.
- Differential analysis of ascitic fluid may help to confirm the cause.

Collaborative Care

The goal of treatment is to slow the progress of cirrhosis and prevent and treat any complications. Management of ascites focuses on sodium restriction (250 to 500 mg/day for severe ascites), diuretic therapy (e.g., a potassium-sparing diuretic combined with a loop diuretic), and fluid removal (paracentesis) for those patients with impaired respiration or abdominal pain. Transjugular intrahepatic portosystemic shunt (TIPS) is also used to alleviate ascites.

The main therapeutic goal related to esophageal varices is to prevent bleeding and hemorrhage. The patient who has esophageal varices should avoid ingesting alcohol, aspirin, and nonsteroidal antiinflammatory drugs (NSAIDs). Patients with varices at risk of bleeding are started on a nonselective β-blocker (nadolol [Corgard] or propranolol [Inderal]) to reduce the incidence of hemorrhage. β-Blockers decrease high portal pressure.

- When variceal bleeding occurs, the first step is to stabilize the patient and manage the airway. IV therapy is initiated and may include administration of blood products. Management that involves a combination of drug therapy and endoscopic therapy is more successful than either approach alone. Drug therapy may include somatostatin analog octreotide (Sandostatin) or vasopressin (VP).

- Balloon tamponade may be used in patients with acute variceal hemorrhage that cannot be controlled on initial endoscopy. Balloon tamponade controls the hemorrhage by mechanical compression of the varices.
- Supportive measures during an acute variceal bleed include administration of fresh frozen plasma and packed red blood cells (RBCs), vitamin K (AquaMEPHYTON), and proton pump inhibitors (e.g., pantoprazole [Protonix]). Lactulose (Cephulac) and rifaximin (Xifaxan) may be administered to prevent hepatic encephalopathy from breakdown of blood and the release of ammonia in the intestine. Antibiotics are given to prevent bacterial infection.
- Nonsurgical (e.g., TIPS) and surgical methods of shunting blood away from the varices are available. Shunting procedures tend to be used more after a second major bleeding episode than during an initial bleeding episode.

The goal of management in hepatic encephalopathy is the reduction of ammonia formation. Lactulose discourages bacterial growth, traps ammonia in the gut, and expels ammonia from the colon. Antibiotics such as rifaximin may also be given, particularly in patients who do not respond to lactulose. Constipation should be prevented. Control of hepatic encephalopathy also involves treating GI bleeding and removing blood from the GI tract to decrease protein in the intestine.

A number of medications may be used to treat symptoms and complications of advanced liver disease (see Table 44-13, Lewis et al, *Medical-Surgical Nursing,* ed. 9, p. 1024). Specific nutritional therapy varies with the degree of liver damage and the danger of encephalopathy; generally, the diet is high in calories (3000 cal/day) and carbohydrates with sodium restricted. Protein restriction is rarely justified in patients with persistent hepatic encephalopathy. Malnutrition is a more serious clinical problem than hepatic encephalopathy for many of these patients.

Nursing Management
Goals
The patient with cirrhosis will have relief of discomfort, have minimal to no complications (ascites, esophageal varices, hepatic encephalopathy), and return to as normal a lifestyle as possible.
Nursing Diagnoses
- Imbalanced nutrition: less than body requirement
- Excess fluid volume
- Impaired skin integrity

Nursing Interventions

Prevention and early treatment of cirrhosis focus on reducing or eliminating risk factors.

- Alcoholism must be treated. Adequate nutrition, especially for the alcoholic and other individuals at risk for cirrhosis, is essential to promote liver regeneration.
- Identify and treat acute hepatitis early so that it does not progress to chronic hepatitis and cirrhosis.

Nursing care for the patient with cirrhosis focuses on conserving the patient's strength while maintaining muscle strength and tone. Modify the activity and rest schedule according to signs of clinical improvement (e.g., decreasing jaundice, improvement in liver function studies).

- Anorexia, nausea and vomiting, pressure from ascites, and poor eating habits all interfere with adequate intake of nutrients. Make between-meal snacks available so the patient can eat them at times when he or she can best tolerate them. Provide food preferences whenever possible.
- The patient's physiologic response to cirrhosis should be assessed, including the presence and progression of jaundice, any pruritus, and urine and stool color.
- Accurate recordings of intake and output, daily weights, and measurements of extremities and abdominal girth help in the ongoing assessment of edema.
- A semi-Fowler's or Fowler's position allows for maximal respiratory efficiency when dyspnea is a problem. Use pillows to support arms and chest to increase patient comfort and ability to breathe.
- When the patient is taking diuretics, monitor the serum levels of sodium, potassium, chloride, and bicarbonate.
- Meticulous skin care is essential because edematous tissues are subject to breakdown. Use an alternating air pressure mattress or other special mattress. A turning schedule (minimum of every 2 hours) must be adhered to rigidly. Support the abdomen with pillows.
- When a paracentesis is done, have the patient void immediately before the procedure to prevent puncture of the bladder. After the procedure, monitor for hypovolemia and electrolyte imbalances, and check the dressing for bleeding and leakage.
- If the patient has esophageal or gastric varices, observe for any signs of bleeding from varices, such as hematemesis and melena. If hematemesis occurs, assess the patient for hemorrhage, call the physician, and be ready to assist with treatments to control bleeding.

Nursing care of the patient with hepatic encephalopathy focuses on maintaining a safe environment, sustaining life, and assisting with measures to reduce the formation of ammonia.

▼ **Patient and Caregiver Teaching**

The patient and caregiver need to understand the importance of continuous health care and medical supervision. Teach the patient and caregiver about symptoms of complications and when to seek medical attention.

- Abstinence from alcohol is important and results in improvement in most patients. Provide information regarding community support programs such as Alcoholics Anonymous for help with alcohol abuse.
- Explain both verbally and in writing information about fluid or possible dietary changes.
- Instruct on the importance of adequate rest periods, skin care, drug therapy precautions, observation for bleeding, and protection from infection.
- Referral to a community or home health nurse may be helpful to ensure adequate adherence to prescribed therapy.

COLORECTAL CANCER

Description

Colorectal cancer is the third most common form of cancer and is responsible for 9% of cancer deaths. Colorectal cancer is more common in men than in women. Mortality rates are highest among African American men and women. The risk of colorectal cancer increases with age, with about 90% of new cases detected in people older than 50.

Pathophysiology

Risk factors include a diet high in red or processed meat, obesity, physical inactivity, alcohol, long-term smoking, and low intake of fruits and vegetables. Genetic conditions such as familial adenomatous polyposis (FAP) and a personal history of irritable bowel syndrome place an individual at risk for colorectal cancer. About one third of cases of colorectal cancer occur in patients with a family history of colorectal cancer.

- Physical exercise and a diet with large amounts of fruits, vegetables, and grains may decrease the risk. Long-term use of nonsteroidal antiinflammatory drugs (NSAIDs) (e.g., aspirin) is also associated with reduced risk.

Adenocarcinoma is the most common type of colorectal cancer. Typically it begins as adenomatous polyps. As the tumor grows, the cancer invades and penetrates the muscularis mucosae. Eventually tumor cells gain access to the regional lymph nodes and vascular system and spread to distant sites. Because venous blood leaving the colon and the rectum flows through the portal vein and the inferior rectal vein, the liver is a common site of metastasis. The cancer spreads from the liver to other sites, including the lungs, bones, and brain.

Clinical Manifestations and Complications

Manifestations are usually nonspecific or do not appear until the disease is advanced (Fig. 3). Symptoms may include iron-deficiency anemia, rectal bleeding, abdominal pain, change in bowel habits, and intestinal obstruction or perforation.

- Additional findings for early disease may include fatigue and weight loss. In advanced disease, an abdominal mass, hepatomegaly, and ascites may be present.
- Right-sided lesions are more likely to bleed and cause diarrhea, whereas left-sided tumors are usually detected later and could present with bowel obstruction.
- Complications include obstruction, bleeding, perforation, peritonitis, and fistula formation.

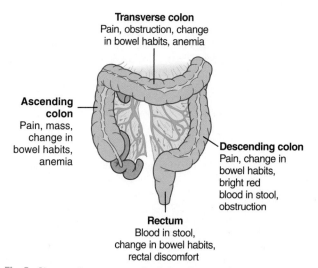

Transverse colon
Pain, obstruction, change
in bowel habits, anemia

Ascending colon
Pain, mass,
change in
bowel habits,
anemia

Descending colon
Pain, change in
bowel habits,
bright red
blood in stool,
obstruction

Rectum
Blood in stool,
change in bowel habits,
rectal discomfort

Fig. 3. Signs and symptoms of colorectal cancer by location of primary cancer.

Diagnostic Studies

Because cancer symptoms do not become evident until the disease is advanced, regular screening is advocated to detect and remove polyps before they become cancerous. Beginning at age 50, both men and women at average risk for developing colorectal cancer should have screening tests to detect both polyps and cancer.

- Colonoscopy is the screening procedure of choice to examine the entire colon, obtain biopsy specimens, and remove polyps.
- Fecal occult blood tests are done to detect blood.
- Complete blood count (CBC), coagulation studies, and liver function tests are done when the diagnosis is confirmed by colonoscopy and biopsy.
- CT scan or MRI of abdomen and pelvis is used to detect liver metastases.
- Carcinoembryonic antigen (CEA) serum test is used as a baseline to follow the progress of the patient after surgery or chemotherapy.

Collaborative Care

Prognosis and treatment correlate with the pathologic staging of the disease. The TNM staging system is the most commonly used method to stage the tumor (see p. 777). As with other cancers, prognosis worsens with greater size and depth of tumor, lymph node involvement, and metastasis.

Surgical Therapy

Surgical goals include complete resection of the tumor with adequate margins of healthy tissue, a thorough exploration of the abdomen to detect spread, removal of all lymph nodes that drain the cancer area, restoration of bowel continuity so that normal bowel function will return, and prevention of surgical complications.

- Polypectomy during colonoscopy can be used to resect colorectal cancer in situ.
- The site of the tumor determines the site of the resection (e.g., right hemicolectomy, left hemicolectomy).
- Surgery for stage I cancer includes removal of the tumor and at least 5 cm of intestine on either side of the tumor, plus removal of nearby lymph nodes. The remaining cancer-free ends are sewn back together. Laparoscopic surgery is sometimes used for stage I tumors, especially those in the left colon.
- Low-risk stage II tumors are treated with wide resection and reanastomosis, but chemotherapy is used in addition to surgery for high-risk stage II tumors.
- Stage III tumors are treated with surgery and chemotherapy.

In rectal cancer the surgeon has three major options: (1) local excision, (2) abdominal-perineal resection (APR) with a permanent colostomy, and (3) low anterior resection (LAR) to preserve sphincter function. The surgical decision is based on the location and staging of the cancer and ability to restore normal bowel function and continence. Most patients with rectal cancer require an APR or LAR.

Chemotherapy and Targeted Therapy

Chemotherapy can be used to shrink the tumor before surgery, as adjuvant therapy after colon resection, and as palliative treatment for nonresectable disease (see Chemotherapy, p. 694). Current chemotherapy protocols include 5-fluorouracil (5-FU) and folinic acid (leucovorin) alone or in combination with oxaliplatin (Eloxatin). The preferred protocol includes oxaliplatin, but it may be omitted for patients who have too many side effects. Oral fluoropyrimidines (e.g., capecitabine [Xeloda]) have been found as effective as 5-FU/folinic acid monotherapy and can also be given in combination with oxaliplatin.

A variety of targeted therapies are used to treat metastatic disease. Angiogenesis inhibitors, which inhibit the blood supply to tumors, include bevacizumab (Avastin) and ziv-aflibercept (Zaltrap). Regorafenib (Stivarga) is a multikinase inhibitor that blocks several enzymes that promote cancer growth. Cetuximab (Erbitux) and panitumumab (Vectibix) block the epidermal growth factor receptor.

Radiation Therapy

Radiation may be used postoperatively as an adjuvant to surgery and chemotherapy or as a palliative measure for patients with metastatic cancer. As a palliative measure, its primary objective is to reduce tumor size and provide symptomatic relief (see Radiation Therapy, p. 730).

Nursing Management

Goals

The patient with colorectal cancer will have normal bowel elimination patterns, quality of life appropriate to disease progression, relief of pain, and feelings of comfort and well-being.

Nursing Diagnoses

- Diarrhea or constipation
- Fear and anxiety
- Ineffective coping

Nursing Interventions

Encourage all patients over 50 to have regular colorectal cancer screening. Help identify those at high risk who need screening at an earlier age.

Preoperative Care. Nursing care for patients with a colon resection is similar to the care of the patient having a laparotomy (see Abdominal Pain, Acute, pp. 4 to 5). Patients who have an APR will have a permanent ostomy and need emotional support to cope with their prognosis and the radical change in body appearance and function.

Postoperative Care. Many patients have immediate reanastomosis of bowel and require general postoperative care. Patients with more extensive surgery (e.g., APR) may have an open wound and drains (e.g., Jackson-Pratt, Hemovac) and a permanent stoma.

Postoperative care includes sterile dressing changes, care of drains, and patient and caregiver teaching about the stoma. Consult with a wound, ostomy, and continence care nurse before surgery to select the ostomy site on the abdomen, and then provide follow-up care and teaching.

- A patient who has open and packed wounds requires meticulous postoperative care. Reinforce dressings and change them frequently during the first several hours postoperatively. Carefully assess all drainage for amount, color, and consistency. Examine the wound regularly and record bleeding, excessive drainage, and unusual odor.
- The patient may experience phantom rectal sensation because the sympathetic nerves responsible for rectal control are not severed during the surgery. Be astute in distinguishing phantom sensations from perineal abscess pain.
- Sexual dysfunction is a possible complication of an APR. Although the likelihood of sexual dysfunction depends on the surgical technique used, the surgeon should discuss the possibility with the patient.

▼ **Patient and Caregiver Teaching**
- The patient and caregiver should be aware of community resources and services available for assistance.
- Patients with colostomies need to know how to care for them.
- Patients and caregivers need to know about diet, incontinence products, and strategies for managing bloating, diarrhea, and bowel evacuation.
- Patients with sphincter-sparing surgery may need antidiarrheal drugs or bulking agents to control diarrhea. A dietitian should help the patient choose foods that are less likely to cause diarrhea.

CONJUNCTIVITIS

Description
Conjunctivitis is an inflammation or infection of the conjunctiva. Conjunctivitis may be caused by bacteria or viruses, and inflammation can result from exposure to allergens or chemical irritants. The tarsal conjunctiva (lining of the lid's interior surface) may become inflamed as a result of a long-term foreign body in the eye, such as a contact lens. See Table 28 for a comparison of clinical manifestations and management of the different types of conjunctivitis.

C

Table 28 Types of Conjunctivitis

Description	Clinical Manifestations	Management
Bacterial		
■ Acute bacterial conjunctivitis (pinkeye) ■ More common in children ■ *Staphylococcus aureus* is most common cause	Discomfort, pruritis, redness, mucopurulent drainage. Generally spreads to unaffected eye	Usually self-limiting, but antibiotic drops will shorten course
Viral		
■ Caused by many different viruses ■ Adenovirus conjunctivitis contracted by direct contact with infected person and in contaminated swimming pools	Tearing, foreign body sensation, redness, mild photophobia. Usually mild and self-limiting but can be severe with increased discomfort and subconjunctival hemorrhaging	■ Treatment usually palliative ■ Topical corticosteroids provide temporary relief if patient is severely symptomatic, but have no benefit in outcome ■ Antiviral drops ineffective

Continued

Table 28 Types of Conjunctivitis—cont'd

Description	Clinical Manifestations	Management
Chlamydial	Mucopurulent ocular discharge, irritation, redness, lid swelling. AIC does not lead to blindness as does trachoma	▪ Antibiotic therapy usually effective for both trachoma and AIC
▪ *Chlamydia trachomatis* (serotypes A-C) causes trachoma, a chronic conjunctivitis that is a major cause of blindness worldwide		▪ Patients with AIC have a high risk of concurrent chlamydial genital infection and other sexually transmitted infections
▪ Adult inclusion conjunctivitis (AIC) caused by *Chlamydia trachomatis* (serotypes D-K) is increasing with rise in chlamydial infections		▪ Teaching about ocular condition and sexual implications of condition necessary
Allergic	Itching (defining symptom), burning, redness, and tearing	▪ Artificial tears to dilute allergen and wash from eye
▪ Conjunctivitis may develop in response to exposure to pollens, animal dander, ocular solutions, contact lenses, or other allergens		▪ Effective topical medications include antihistamines and corticosteroids
		▪ Teach to avoid allergen if known

CONSTIPATION

Description

Constipation is characterized by absent or infrequent stools and hard, dry stools that are difficult to defecate. Normal bowel movements are formed and easy to pass. Frequency varies from three bowel movements daily to one bowel movement every 3 days. Because individuals vary, it is important to compare the current symptoms with the patient's normal pattern of elimination.

Common causes of constipation include taking in insufficient dietary fiber or fluids, decreasing physical activity, and ignoring the defecation urge. Many drugs, especially opioids, cause constipation. Constipation occurs with diseases that slow GI transit and hamper neurologic function, such as diabetes mellitus, Parkinson's disease, and multiple sclerosis. Emotions, including anxiety, depression, and stress, affect the GI tract and can contribute to constipation.

Clinical Manifestations

Constipation may vary from a chronic discomfort to an acute event mimicking an acute abdomen. Stools are absent or hard, dry, and difficult to pass. Abdominal distention, bloating, increased flatulence, and increased rectal pressure may also be present.

- Hemorrhoids are the most common complication of chronic constipation. They result from venous engorgement resulting from repeated Valsalva maneuvers (straining) and venous compression from hard impacted stool (see Hemorrhoids, p. 295).
- In the presence of obstipation (fecal impaction secondary to constipation), colonic perforation may occur. Perforation, which is life threatening, causes abdominal pain, nausea, vomiting, fever, and an elevated white blood cell (WBC) count.

Diagnostic Studies

Perform a thorough history and physical examination so that the underlying cause can be identified.

- Abdominal x-rays, barium enema, colonoscopy, sigmoidoscopy, and anorectal manometry may be performed.

Collaborative Care

Most cases of constipation can be prevented by increasing dietary fiber, fluid intake, and exercise. Laxatives and enemas may be used to treat acute constipation but are used cautiously because overuse leads to chronic constipation.

- Methylnaltrexone (Relistor) is a peripheral μ-opiate receptor that reduces constipation caused by opioid use. It is administered subcutaneously.
- Enemas are fast acting and beneficial for immediate treatment of constipation, but must be used cautiously. Soap suds enemas produce inflammation of colon mucosa, tap water enemas can lead to water intoxication, and sodium phosphate (e.g., Fleet) enemas may cause electrolyte imbalances in some patients.
- Biofeedback therapy may benefit patients who are constipated as a result of anismus (uncoordinated contraction of the anal sphincter during straining).

A patient with severe constipation related to a motility or mechanical disorder may require more intensive treatment. In a patient with unrelenting constipation, a subtotal colectomy with ileorectal anastomosis may be performed.

Many patients experience improved symptoms when they increase their intake of dietary fiber and fluids. The diet should include fluid intake of at least 2 L/day unless contraindicated by cardiac or renal disease.

Nursing Management

Goals

The patient with constipation will increase dietary intake of fiber and fluids; increase physical activity; pass soft, formed stools; and not have any complications, such as bleeding hemorrhoids.

Nursing Diagnosis

- Constipation

Nursing Interventions

Interventions should be based on the patient's symptoms and assessment. Defecation is easiest when the person is sitting on a commode with the knees higher than the hips. The sitting position allows gravity to aid defecation, and flexing the hips straightens the angle between the anal canal and the rectum so that stool flows out more easily.

Place a footstool in front of the toilet to promote flexion of the thighs. It is challenging to defecate while sitting on a bedpan. For a patient in bed, elevate the head of the bed as high as the patient can tolerate.

Encourage patients to exercise the abdominal muscles and contract the abdominal muscles several times each day. Sit-ups and straight-leg raises can also improve abdominal muscle tone.

▼ **Patient and Caregiver Teaching**

- Teach the patient the importance of diet in the prevention of constipation. Emphasize the maintenance of a high-fiber diet, increased fluid intake, and a regular exercise program.

- Teach the patient to establish a regular time to defecate and not suppress the urge to defecate.
- Discourage the patient from using laxatives and enemas to achieve fecal elimination.
- Teach patients taking bulking products to follow product recommendations in terms of fluid intake.

COR PULMONALE

C

Description

Cor pulmonale is enlargement of the right ventricle (RV) caused by a primary disorder of the respiratory system. Pulmonary hypertension is usually a preexisting condition in cor pulmonale. Cor pulmonale may be present with or without overt cardiac failure.

- The most common cause of cor pulmonale is chronic obstructive pulmonary disease (COPD) (see p. 133). Almost any disorder that affects the respiratory system can cause cor pulmonale.

Clinical Manifestations

- Manifestations are subtle and often masked by the symptoms of the pulmonary condition. Common symptoms include exertional dyspnea, tachypnea, cough, and fatigue.
- Physical signs include evidence of right ventricular hypertrophy on ECG and an increase in intensity of the second heart sound. Chronic hypoxemia leads to polycythemia and increased total blood volume and viscosity of the blood.
- If heart failure accompanies cor pulmonale, additional manifestations include peripheral edema; weight gain; distended neck veins; full, bounding pulse; and enlarged liver.

Diagnostic tests may include arterial blood gases (ABGs), SpO_2, b-type natriuretic peptide (BNP) level, ECG, chest x-ray, CT scan, MRI, and cardiac catheterization.

Collaborative Care

Management is directed at treating the underlying pulmonary problem. Long-term, low-flow oxygen (O_2) therapy to correct the hypoxemia reduces vasoconstriction and pulmonary hypertension.

- If fluid, electrolyte, and acid-base imbalances are present, they must be corrected. Diuretics and a low-sodium diet will help to decrease the plasma volume and reduce the workload on the heart.
- Bronchodilator therapy is indicated if the underlying respiratory problem is due to an obstructive disorder.

- Theophylline may help because of its weak inotropic effect on the heart.
- Other treatments include those for pulmonary hypertension such as vasodilator therapy, calcium channel blockers, and anticoagulants.
- With end-stage lung disease, lung transplantation may be an option.

Nursing management of chronic cor pulmonale resulting from COPD is similar to that described for COPD (see p. 139).

CORONARY ARTERY DISEASE

Description

Coronary artery disease (CAD) is a type of blood vessel disorder that is included in the general category of atherosclerosis. *Atherosclerosis* is derived from two Greek words: *athero,* meaning "fatty mush," and *skleros,* meaning "hard." Atherosclerosis is often referred to as "hardening of the arteries." Although this condition can occur in any artery in the body, the atheromas (fatty deposits) prefer the coronary arteries.

- Arteriosclerotic heart disease, cardiovascular heart disease, ischemic heart disease, coronary heart disease, and CAD all describe this disease process.
- Cardiovascular disease is the major cause of death in the United States. CAD is the most common type of cardiovascular disease and accounts for the majority of these deaths.
- Patients with CAD may be asymptomatic or develop *chronic stable angina (chest pain).*
- Unstable angina (UA) and myocardial infarction (MI) are more serious manifestations of CAD and are termed *acute coronary syndrome* (ACS).

Figure 1 on p. 6 illustrates the relationship among the clinical manifestations of CAD.

Risk factors for CAD can be categorized as nonmodifiable and modifiable (Table 29).

Pathophysiology

Atherosclerosis is characterized by a deposit of lipids within the intima of the artery. Inflammation and endothelial injury play a central role in the development of atherosclerosis.

- The endothelial lining can be injured as a result of tobacco use, hyperlipidemia, hypertension, diabetes, hyperhomocystinemia, and infection causing a local inflammatory response.

| Table 29 | Risk Factors for Coronary Artery Disease |

Nonmodifiable Risk Factors	Modifiable Risk Factors
Increasing age	**Major**
Gender (more common in men than in women until 65 yr of age)	Serum lipids:
	Total cholesterol >200 mg/dL
	Triglycerides ≥150 mg/dL*
Ethnicity (more common in whites than in African Americans)	LDL cholesterol >160 mg/dL
	HDL cholesterol <40 mg/dL in men or <50 mg/dL in women*
Genetic predisposition and family history of heart disease	BP: ≥140/90 mm Hg*
	Diabetes mellitus
	Tobacco use
	Physical inactivity
	Obesity: Waist circumference ≥102 cm (≥40 inches) in men and ≥88 cm (≥35 inches) in women*
	Contributing
	Fasting blood glucose ≥100 mg/dL*
	Psychosocial risk factors (e.g., depression, hostility, anger, stress)
	Elevated homocysteine levels

*Three or more of these risk factors meet the criteria for metabolic syndrome (as defined by the National Cholesterol Education Program Adult Treatment Panel III). Metabolic syndrome is discussed in Chapter 41 of Lewis et al, *Medical-Surgical Nursing,* ed. 9, p. 921.
HDL, High-density lipoprotein; *LDL,* low-density lipoprotein.

- C-reactive protein (CRP), a protein produced by the liver, is a nonspecific marker of inflammation. It is increased in many patients with CAD, with the level rising when there is systemic inflammation.
- CAD takes many years to develop. When it becomes symptomatic, the disease process is usually well advanced. Stages of development in atherosclerosis are (1) fatty streak, (2) fibrous plaque resulting from smooth muscle cell proliferation, and (3) complicated lesion.

Figure 34-1, Lewis et al., *Medical-Surgical Nursing,* ed. 9, p. 731 illustrates the progression of atherosclerosis.

Normally some arterial anastomoses or connections, termed *collateral circulation,* exist within the coronary circulation.

- When occlusion of the coronary arteries occurs slowly over a long period, there is a greater chance of adequate collateral circulation developing, and the myocardium may still receive an adequate amount of blood and oxygen. However, with rapid-onset CAD (e.g., familial hypercholesterolemia) or coronary spasm, time is inadequate for collateral development, and a diminished arterial flow results in a more severe ischemia or infarction.

Clinical Manifestations

CAD is a progressive disease, and patients may be asymptomatic for many years or may develop chronic stable angina. When the demand for myocardial oxygen exceeds the ability of the coronary arteries to supply the heart with oxygen, myocardial ischemia occurs.

- *Angina,* or chest pain, is the clinical manifestation of reversible myocardial ischemia. The primary reason for insufficient blood flow is narrowing of coronary arteries by atherosclerosis.
- Chronic stable angina refers to chest pain that occurs intermittently over a long period with the same pattern of onset, duration, and intensity of symptoms (see Angina, Chronic Stable, p. 46).

When ischemia is prolonged and not immediately reversible, ACS develops and encompasses the spectrum of UA, non–ST-segment-elevation myocardial infarction (NSTEMI), and ST-segment-elevation myocardial infarction (STEMI) (see Fig. 1 on p. 6).

Diagnostic Studies

- Chest x-ray is used to detect cardiac enlargement, cardiac calcifications, and pulmonary congestion.
- 12-lead ECG detects heart rhythm, pacemaker activity, conduction abnormalities, position of heart, size of atria and ventricles, and presence of ischemia/injury/infarction.
- Serum lipid levels are used to screen for risk factors.
- Exercise or stress testing is used to detect ST-segment and T-wave changes that indicate ischemia with exercise.
- Ambulatory 24- to 48-hour ECG monitoring can help to identify silent ischemia.
- Nuclear imaging studies are used to determine myocardial perfusion, contractility, and ejection fraction.
- Positron emission tomography (PET) is used to identify and quantify ischemia and infarction.

- Angiography studies are used to visualize coronary arteries and help to determine treatment and prognosis.
- Echocardiography with exercise is used to diagnose coronary artery stenosis.

See Chapter 32 and Table 32-6 for a discussion of these studies, including nursing considerations, in Lewis et al, *Medical-Surgical Nursing,* ed. 9, pp. 699 to 703.

Nursing and Collaborative Management

Management of CAD involves modification of risk factors to prevent, modify, or slow disease progression. People who have modifiable risk factors should be encouraged to make lifestyle changes to reduce their risk of CAD. You can play a major role in teaching health-promoting behaviors. For highly motivated people, knowing how to reduce this risk may be the information they need to get started.

Lifestyle changes, including a low-saturated-fat, high-fiber diet; avoidance of tobacco; and increase in physical activity, can promote regression in the course of coronary atherosclerosis and a reduction in coronary events.

- A physical activity program should be designed to improve physical fitness by following the FITT formula: Frequency (how often), Intensity (how hard), Type (isotonic), and Time (how long). Everyone should aim for at least 30 minutes of moderate physical activity on most days of the week.
- Specific diet recommendations and plans are presented in Tables 34-3 and 34-4 in Lewis et al, *Medical-Surgical Nursing,* ed. 9, p. 737.

Drug Therapy

People with serum cholesterol levels higher than 200 mg/dL are at risk for CAD and should be treated. Treatment usually begins with dietary caloric restriction (if overweight), decreased dietary fat and cholesterol intake, and increased physical activity. Guidelines for the treatment of high cholesterol focus on low-density lipoprotein (LDL) levels. Serum lipid levels are reassessed after 6 weeks of diet therapy. If they remain elevated, additional dietary options and drug therapy may be considered.

The statin drugs are the most widely used lipid-lowering drugs. These drugs inhibit the synthesis of cholesterol in the liver by blocking hydroxy-methyl-glutaryl coenzyme A (HMG-CoA) reductase. Examples include lovastatin (Mevacor), pravastatin (Pravachol), simvastatin (Zocor), fluvastatin (Lescol), atorvastatin (Lipitor), and rosuvastatin (Crestor). These drugs primarily lower LDL cholesterol and also cause an increase in high-density lipoprotein (HDL). Niacin (Nicobid), a water-soluble

B vitamin, also interferes with the synthesis of LDL and triglyceride levels.

Fibric acid derivatives such as gemfibrozil (Lopid) are effective in lowering very-low-density lipoprotein (VLDL) levels and triglycerides, while increasing HDL levels. Drugs that increase lipoprotein removal by increasing conversion of cholesterol to bile acids include cholestyramine (Questran), colestipol (Colestid), and colesevelam (Welchol) and are commonly used. Ezetimibe (Zetia) inhibits the absorption of dietary and biliary cholesterol across the intestinal wall and may be combined with a statin to promote greater reductions in LDL.

- Drug therapy for hyperlipidemia often continues for a lifetime. It is essential that diet modification be used to minimize the need for drug therapy. The patient must fully understand the rationale and goals of treatment as well as drug safety and side effects.

Antiplatelet therapy with low-dose aspirin (e.g., 81 mg) is recommended for most people at risk for CAD unless contraindicated (e.g., history of GI bleeding). For high-risk women who are aspirin intolerant, clopidogrel (Plavix) can be considered.

Nursing Management

Regardless of the health care setting, it is extremely important to identify the person at risk for CAD. Risk screening involves obtaining a thorough health history. Question the patient about a family history of heart disease in parents and siblings. Note the presence of any cardiovascular symptoms.

Assess environmental factors, such as eating habits, type of diet, and level of exercise to elicit lifestyle patterns. Include a psychosocial history to determine tobacco use, alcohol ingestion, recent life-stressing events (e.g., loss of a spouse), and the presence of any negative psychologic states (e.g., anxiety, depression, anger). The place and type of employment provide important information on the kind of activity performed, exposure to pollutants or noxious chemicals, and the degree of stress associated with work.

- Identify patient attitudes and beliefs about health and illness. This information can give some indication of how disease and lifestyle changes may affect the patient and can reveal possible misconceptions about heart disease.
- Knowledge of the patient's educational background is helpful in deciding the level to begin teaching.
- If the patient is taking medications, it is important to know the names and dosage, and whether the patient is compliant with the drug regimen.

CROHN'S DISEASE

Description

Crohn's disease is an autoimmune disorder that, along with ulcerative colitis, is referred to as *inflammatory bowel disease* (IBD). See Inflammatory Bowel Disease, p. 352, for a discussion of the disorder.

C

CUSHING SYNDROME

Description

Cushing syndrome is a clinical condition that results from chronic exposure to excess corticosteroids, particularly glucocorticoids. Several conditions can cause Cushing syndrome, with the most common being iatrogenic administration of exogenous corticosteroids (e.g., prednisone). Approximately 85% of the cases of endogenous Cushing syndrome result from an adrenocorticotropic hormone (ACTH)–secreting pituitary tumor *(Cushing disease)*. Other causes of Cushing syndrome include adrenal tumors and ectopic ACTH production by tumors outside the hypothalamic-pituitary-adrenal axis.

Clinical Manifestations

Manifestations can be seen in most body systems and are related to excess levels of corticosteroids (see Table 50-13, Lewis et al, *Medical-Surgical Nursing,* ed. 9, p. 1208). Although signs of glucocorticoid excess usually predominate, symptoms of mineralocorticoid and androgen excess may also be seen.

- Corticosteroid excess causes pronounced changes in physical appearance. Weight gain, the most common feature, results from an accumulation of adipose tissue in the trunk, face, and cervical neck area. Hyperglycemia occurs because of glucose intolerance (associated with cortisol-induced insulin resistance) and increased gluconeogenesis by the liver.
- Muscle wasting leads to muscle weakness, especially in the extremities. Loss of bone protein matrix leads to osteoporosis with pathologic fractures (e.g., vertebral compression fractures) and bone and back pain. Loss of collagen makes the skin weaker, thinner, and easier to bruise.
- Mineralocorticoid excess may cause hypertension, whereas adrenal androgen excess may cause pronounced acne, virilization in women, and feminization in men.

The first indication of Cushing syndrome may be the clinical presentation, including (1) centripetal (truncal) obesity or generalized obesity; (2) *"moon face"* (fullness of the face) with facial plethora; (3) purplish red striae (usually depressed below the skin surface) on the abdomen, breast, or buttocks); (4) hirsutism in women; (5) menstrual disorders in women; (6) hypertension; and (7) unexplained hypokalemia.

Diagnostic Studies

- Plasma cortisol levels may be elevated with loss of diurnal variation.
- A 24-hour urine collection for free cortisol is done. Urine cortisol levels beyond the normal range of 80 to 120 mcg/24 hr in adults indicate Cushing syndrome. If these results are borderline, a low-dose dexamethasone suppression test is done.
- Plasma ACTH levels may be low, normal, or elevated depending on the underlying cause of Cushing syndrome.
- Other findings on diagnostic tests associated with, but not diagnostic of, Cushing syndrome include hyperglycemia, hypokalemia, glycosuria, hypercalciuria, and osteoporosis.
- CT scan and MRI of the pituitary and adrenal glands may be done.

Collaborative Care

The primary goal is to normalize hormone secretion. The standard treatment for a pituitary adenoma is surgical removal of the pituitary tumor using the transsphenoidal approach. Radiation therapy may be used for patients who are not good surgical candidates. Adrenalectomy is indicated for adrenal tumors or hyperplasia. Patients with ectopic ACTH-secreting tumors are best managed by removing the tumor (usually lung or pancreas).

- Drug therapy may be attempted when the patient is a poor surgical candidate or prior surgery has failed. The goal of drug therapy is inhibition of adrenal function *(medical adrenalectomy)*. Drugs that inhibit corticosteroid synthesis include ketoconazole (Nizoral), and aminoglutethimide (Cytadren).

If Cushing syndrome has developed during the course of prolonged administration of corticosteroids (e.g., prednisone), the following alternatives may be tried: (1) gradual discontinuance of corticosteroid therapy, (2) reduction of corticosteroid dose, and (3) conversion to an alternate-day regimen.

Nursing Management

Goals

The patient with Cushing syndrome will experience relief of symptoms with no serious complications, maintain a positive self-image, and actively participate in the therapeutic plan.

Nursing Diagnoses
- Risk for infection
- Imbalanced nutrition: more than body requirements
- Disturbed body image
- Impaired skin integrity

Nursing Interventions

Because the therapy for Cushing syndrome has many side effects, assessment focuses on signs and symptoms of hormone and drug toxicity and complicating conditions (e.g., cardiovascular disease, diabetes mellitus, infection).

- Assess and monitor vital signs, glucose, and daily weights.
- Signs and symptoms of inflammation (e.g., fever, redness) may be minimal or absent, so assess for pain, loss of function, and purulent drainage.
- Monitor for signs of abnormal thromboembolic phenomena, such as sudden chest pain, dyspnea, and tachypnea.

Another important focus of nursing care is the provision of emotional support. Changes in appearance, such as centripetal obesity, multiple bruises, hirsutism in females, and gynecomastia in males, can be distressing. You can help by remaining sensitive to the patient's feelings and offering respect and unconditional acceptance. Reassure the patient that the physical changes and much of the emotional lability will resolve when hormone levels return to normal.

If treatment involves surgical removal of a pituitary adenoma, an adrenal tumor, or one or both adrenal glands, nursing care will have an additional focus on preoperative and postoperative care.

Preoperative Care. Before surgery, hypertension and hyperglycemia need to be controlled, with hypokalemia corrected by diet and potassium supplements. A high-protein meal plan helps correct protein depletion. Preoperative teaching depends on the type of surgical approach (hypophysectomy or adrenalectomy), but should include information regarding the anticipated postoperative care.

Postoperative Care. Because of hormone fluctuations, the patient's BP, fluid balance, and electrolyte levels tend to be unstable after surgery. High doses of corticosteroids (hydrocortisone) are administered IV during surgery and for several days afterward to ensure adequate responses to the stress of the procedure.

- Report any rapid or significant changes in BP, respirations, or HR.
- Carefully monitor fluid intake and output and assess for potential imbalance.

- If corticosteroid dosage is tapered too rapidly after surgery, acute adrenal insufficiency may develop. Vomiting, increased weakness, dehydration, and hypotension may indicate hypocortisolism. In addition, the patient may complain of painful joints, pruritus, or peeling skin and may experience severe emotional disturbances.
- Patients may have a nasogastric (NG) tube, urinary catheter, IV therapy, central venous pressure monitoring, and leg sequential compression devices to prevent emboli.

After surgery the patient is usually maintained on bed rest until the BP stabilizes. Be alert for subtle signs of postoperative infections. Provide meticulous care when changing the dressing and during any other procedures that involve access to body cavities, circulation, or areas under skin.

▼ **Patient and Caregiver Teaching**

Discharge instructions are based on the patient's lack of endogenous cortisol and resulting inability to react to stressors physiologically.

- Instruct patients to wear a Medic Alert bracelet at all times and carry medical identification and instructions in a wallet or purse. Teach the patient to avoid exposure to extreme temperatures, infections, and emotional disturbances.
- Stress may produce or precipitate acute adrenal insufficiency because the remaining adrenal tissue cannot meet an increased hormonal demand. Teach patients to adjust their corticosteroid replacement therapy in accordance with stress levels.
- If the patient cannot adjust his or her own medication or if weakness, fainting, fever, or nausea and vomiting occur, the patient should contact the health care provider for a possible adjustment in corticosteroid dosage.

Lifetime replacement therapy is required by many patients, but it may take several months to satisfactorily adjust the hormone dose.

CYSTIC FIBROSIS

Description

Cystic fibrosis (CF) is an autosomal recessive, multisystem disease characterized by altered function of the exocrine glands involving primarily the lungs, pancreas, biliary tract, and reproductive tract.

Severity and progression of the disease vary. With early diagnosis and improvements in therapy, the prognosis has been significantly improved. The median predicted survival in 1970 was 16 years, but has currently increased to more than 38 years.

Pathophysiology

CF results from mutations in a gene located on chromosome 7 that produces a protein called CF transmembrane regulator (CFTR). CFTR regulates sodium and chloride channels in the epithelial surface of the airways, pancreatic ducts, and sweat gland ducts. Mutations in the CFTR gene alter this protein in such a way that the channel is blocked.

- Cells that line the passageways of the lungs, pancreas, and other organs produce abnormally thick, sticky mucus. This mucus plugs up the glands in these organs and causes the glands to atrophy, ultimately resulting in organ failure.
- The hallmark of respiratory involvement is its effect on the airways. The disease progresses from being a disease of the small airways *(chronic bronchiolitis)* to involvement of the larger airways, and finally causes destruction of lung tissue. CF is also characterized by chronic airway infection that cannot be eradicated. Lung disorders include chronic bronchiolitis and bronchitis that eventually lead to bronchiectasis, blebs, large cysts, and hemoptysis from erosion of pulmonary arteries.
- Individuals with CF secrete normal volumes of sweat, but are unable to absorb sodium chloride from sweat as it moves through the sweat duct. Therefore they excrete four times the normal amount of sodium and chloride in sweat. This abnormality rarely affects the person's general health, but it is the main diagnostic test for CF.
- Pancreatic insufficiency is caused primarily by mucus plugging the pancreatic duct, which results in atrophy of the gland and progressive fibrotic cyst formation. Because the pancreatic digestive enzymes cannot reach the intestine, malabsorption of fat, protein, and fat-soluble vitamins occurs.
- Fat malabsorption results in steatorrhea, and protein malabsorption results in failure to grow and gain weight.
- CF-related diabetes mellitus results from fibrotic scarring of the pancreas.

Clinical Manifestations

Manifestations vary depending on the disease severity. Carriers are not affected by the gene mutation. Median age of diagnosis of CF is 5 months of age. An initial finding of meconium ileus in the newborn infant may prompt a diagnosis of CF. Other signs may include acute or persistent respiratory symptoms (wheezing, coughing, frequent pneumonia), failure to thrive or malnutrition, steatorrhea, and family history.

- In the adult, a common symptom is frequent cough that becomes persistent and produces viscous, purulent sputum.

- Over time exacerbations (increased cough and sputum, weight loss) become frequent, bronchiectasis worsens, and the recovery of lost lung function is less complete, which may ultimately lead to respiratory failure.
- Affected males and females both have delayed puberty, and some affected women are infertile.

Pneumothorax is an uncommon but serious complication caused by the formation of bullae and blebs. CF-related diabetes, bone disease, and liver disease are additional complications.

Diagnostic Studies

- Sweat chloride test (pilocarpine iontophoresis method) is the gold standard for a diagnosis of CF.
- A genetic test is often used if the results from a sweat test are unclear.

Collaborative Care

An interdisciplinary team should be involved in the care of a patient with CF, including a nurse, physician, respiratory and physical therapists, dietitian, and social worker.

- Management of pulmonary problems is focused on relieving airway obstruction and controlling infection. Drainage of thick bronchial mucus is assisted by aerosol and nebulization treatments that dilate the airways, liquefy mucus, and facilitate clearance.
- Airway clearance techniques include chest physiotherapy (CPT), positive expiratory pressure (PEP) devices, and breathing exercises.
- More than 95% of CF patients die of complications resulting from lung infection. Standard treatment includes antibiotics for exacerbations and chronic suppressive therapy. The use of antibiotics should be carefully guided by sputum culture results.

Management of pancreatic insufficiency includes pancreatic enzyme replacement (e.g., Pancreaze, Zenpep, Creon) administered before each meal and snack. Fat-soluble vitamins need to be supplemented. Added dietary salt is indicated whenever sweating is excessive, such as during hot weather, in the presence of fever, or from intense physical activity. Hyperglycemia may require treatment with insulin.

- Aerobic exercise also seems to be effective in clearing airways.
- More than 20% of adults with CF have depression because CF imposes a significant burden on the individual and family. Issues such as fertility, decreased life expectancy, costs of health care, and career choices may lead to depression.

Nursing Management

Goals

The patient with CF will have adequate airway clearance, reduced risk factors associated with respiratory infections, adequate nutritional support to maintain appropriate body mass index (BMI), ability to perform activities of daily living (ADLs), recognition and treatment of complications related to CF, and active participation in planning and implementing a therapeutic regimen.

Nursing Diagnoses

- Ineffective airway clearance
- Ineffective breathing pattern
- Impaired gas exchange
- Imbalanced nutrition: less than body requirements
- Ineffective coping

Nursing Interventions

You and other health care professionals can assist young adults to gain independence by helping them assume responsibility for their care and vocational or school goals. For a couple considering children, genetic counseling may be suggested.

Acute intervention for the patient with CF includes relief of bronchoconstriction, airway obstruction, and airflow limitation. Interventions include aggressive CPT, antibiotics, and O_2 therapy in severe disease.

▼ Patient and Caregiver Teaching

- Sexuality is an important issue that should be discussed with the young adult. Delayed or irregular menstruation is not uncommon. There may also be delayed development of secondary sex characteristics, such as breasts in girls.
- Because most CF patients now live to childbearing age, family planning and genetic counseling are important.
- The burden of living with a chronic disease at a young age can be emotionally overwhelming. Community resources are often available to help the family. In addition, the Cystic Fibrosis Foundation can be of assistance.

DEMENTIA

Description

Dementia is a syndrome characterized by dysfunction or loss of memory, orientation, attention, language, judgment, and reasoning. Personality changes and behavioral problems such as agitation, delusions, and hallucinations may occur. Ultimately these problems result in alterations in the individual's ability to work, fulfill social and family responsibilities, and perform activities of daily living.

- Fifteen percent of older Americans have dementia. In the United States, about half of all patients in long-term care facilities have Alzheimer's disease (AD) or a related dementia.
- About 60% to 80% of patients with dementia have a diagnosis of AD.

Pathophysiology

The two most common causes of dementia are neurodegenerative conditions (e.g., AD) and vascular disorders. Dementia is sometimes caused by treatable conditions that initially may be reversible, such as vitamin B_1 and B_{12} deficiencies, thyroid disorders, subarachnoid hemorrhage, prescribed drugs (e.g., anticholinergics, hypnotics, cocaine), alcoholism, and head injury. However, with prolonged exposure or disease, irreversible changes may occur.

Vascular dementia is loss of cognitive function resulting from ischemic or hemorrhagic brain lesions caused by cardiovascular disease. Vascular dementia may be caused by a single stroke (infarct) or by multiple strokes.

- The greatest risk factor for dementia is aging, although it is not a normal part of aging. Family history is also an important risk factor, as those with a first-degree relative with dementia are more likely to develop the disease. Other risk factors include diabetes mellitus, obesity, smoking, cardiac dysrhythmias (e.g., atrial fibrillation), hypertension, hypercholesterolemia, and coronary artery disease.

Clinical Manifestations

- Dementia associated with neurologic degeneration is often gradual and progressive over time. Causes of vascular dementia often result in more abrupt symptoms or symptoms that progress in a more stepwise pattern.
- An acute (days to weeks) or subacute (weeks to months) pattern of change may be indicative of an infectious or metabolic cause, including encephalitis, meningitis, hypothyroidism, or drug-related dementia.
- Depression is often mistaken for dementia in older adults, and, conversely, dementia for depression. Manifestations of depression (especially in the older adult) include sadness, difficulty thinking and concentrating, fatigue, apathy, feelings of despair, and inactivity.

Other clinical manifestations of dementia are discussed with Alzheimer's disease (p. 23).

Diagnostic Studies

- Comprehensive medical, neurologic, and psychologic histories are important in determining the presence and cause of dementia.
- Physical examination is performed to rule out other medical conditions.
- Dementia is often diagnosed when two or more brain functions are significantly impaired (e.g., memory loss, impaired language skills).

Diagnosis of dementia related to vascular causes is based on the presence of cognitive loss, the presence of vascular brain lesions demonstrated by neuroimaging techniques (CT or MRI), and the exclusion of other causes of dementia (e.g., AD).

Nursing and Collaborative Management

Management of dementia is similar to management of the patient with AD (see Alzheimer's Disease, p. 27). One form of dementia, vascular dementia, can often be prevented. Preventive measures include treatment of risk factors such as hypertension, diabetes, smoking, hypercholesterolemia, and cardiac dysrhythmias. Drugs that are used for patients with AD are also useful in patients with vascular dementia.

DIABETES INSIPIDUS

Description

Diabetes insipidus (DI) is caused by a deficiency of production or secretion of antidiuretic hormone (ADH) or a decreased renal response to ADH. The decrease in ADH results in fluid and electrolyte imbalances caused by increased urine output and increased plasma osmolality. Depending on the cause, DI may be transient or a lifelong condition.

There are several types of DI. *Central DI* (also known as *neurogenic DI*) results from an interference with ADH synthesis, transport, or release. Causes include brain tumor or surgery, central nervous infections, and head injury. It is the most common form of DI.

Nephrogenic DI occurs when there is adequate ADH, but there is a decreased response to ADH in the kidney. Causes include drug therapy (especially lithium), renal damage, and hereditary renal disease.

Psychogenic DI, a less common condition, is associated with excessive water intake. This can be caused by a structural lesion in the thirst center or a psychologic disorder.

Clinical Manifestations

The primary characteristic of DI is excretion of large quantities of urine (2 to 20 L/day) with a very low specific gravity (<1.005) and urine osmolality (<100 mOsm/kg). Serum osmolality is elevated as a result of hypernatremia, which is caused by pure water loss in the kidney.

- Most patients compensate for fluid loss by drinking great amounts of water (polydipsia) so that serum osmolality is normal or only moderately elevated. The patient may be fatigued from nocturia and may experience generalized weakness.
- Central DI is usually acute and accompanied by excessive fluid loss. Central DI that results from head trauma is usually self-limiting and improves with treatment of the underlying problem. DI following cranial surgery is more likely to be permanent.
- Although the clinical manifestations of nephrogenic DI are similar, the onset and amount of fluid losses are less dramatic than with central DI.
- If oral fluid intake cannot keep up with urinary losses, severe dehydration results. This is manifested by poor tissue turgor, hypotension, tachycardia, and hypovolemic shock.
- The patient may also show central nervous system (CNS) manifestations ranging from irritability and mental dullness to coma, which are related to rising serum osmolality and hypernatremia.

Diagnostic Studies

- Water deprivation test differentiates central DI from nephrogenic DI. Patients with central DI exhibit a dramatic increase in urine osmolality with this test, from 100 to 600 mOsm/kg, and a significant decrease in urine volume. The patient with nephrogenic DI will not be able to increase urine osmolality to >300 mOsm/kg.
- Measuring ADH levels after an analog of ADH (e.g., desmopressin) is given also differentiates central DI from nephrogenic DI. If the cause is central DI, the kidneys will respond to the hormone by concentrating urine. If the kidneys do not respond in this way, then the cause is nephrogenic.

Nursing and Collaborative Management

Management of the patient with DI includes early detection, maintenance of adequate hydration, and patient teaching for long-term management. A therapeutic goal is the maintenance of fluid and electrolyte balance.

For central DI, fluid and hormone therapy is necessary. Fluids are replaced orally or IV, depending on the patient's condition and ability to drink copious amounts of fluids. If IV glucose solutions are used, monitor serum glucose levels because hyperglycemia and glucosuria can lead to osmotic diuresis, which increases the fluid volume deficit.

- Monitor BP, heart rate, and urine output and specific gravity hourly in the patient who is acutely ill.
- Monitor level of consciousness and assess for signs of acute dehydration by assessing alertness, mucous membranes, tachycardia, and skin turgor.
- Maintain an accurate record of intake and output and daily weights to determine fluid volume status.
- DDAVP, an analog of ADH, is the hormone replacement of choice for central DI. Other ADH replacement drugs include aqueous vasopressin (Pitressin) or lysine vasopressin (Diapid). Assess response to DDAVP (e.g., weight gain, headache, depression, restlessness, hyponatremia).

Treatment for nephrogenic DI revolves around dietary measures (low-sodium diet) and thiazide diuretics. Limiting sodium intake to no more than 3 g/day often helps decrease urine output. When a low-sodium diet and thiazide drugs are not effective, indomethacin (Indocin) may be prescribed. Indomethacin, a nonsteroidal antiinflammatory drug (NSAID), helps increase renal responsiveness to ADH.

DIABETES MELLITUS

Description

Diabetes mellitus (DM) is a chronic multisystem disease related to abnormal insulin production, impaired insulin utilization, or both. Currently in the United States an estimated 25.8 million people, or 8.3% of the population, have diabetes mellitus. Approximately 7 million people with diabetes mellitus have not been diagnosed and are unaware that they have the disease.

- Diabetes is the leading cause of adult blindness, end-stage kidney disease, and nontraumatic lower limb amputations. It is also a major contributing factor to heart disease and stroke.
- The two most common types of diabetes are classified as type 1 or type 2 diabetes mellitus (Table 30).

Type 1 Diabetes Mellitus

Type 1 diabetes, formerly known as "juvenile onset" or "insulin-dependent" diabetes, accounts for approximately 5% of all people with diabetes. This type generally affects people younger than 40 years of age, and 40% develop it before 20 years of age.

Table 30 Comparison of Type 1 and Type 2 Diabetes Mellitus

Factor	Type 1 Diabetes Mellitus	Type 2 Diabetes Mellitus
Age at onset	More common in young people but can occur at any age.	Usually age 35 yr or older but can occur at any age. Incidence is increasing in children.
Type of onset	Signs and symptoms abrupt, but disease process may be present for several years.	Insidious, may go undiagnosed for years.
Prevalence	Accounts for 5%-10% of all types of diabetes.	Accounts for 90%-95% of all types of diabetes.
Environmental factors	Virus, toxins.	Obesity, lack of exercise.
Primary defect	Absent or minimal insulin production.	Insulin resistance, decreased insulin production over time, and alterations in production of adipokines.
Islet cell antibodies	Often present at onset.	Absent.
Endogenous insulin	Absent.	Initially increased in response to insulin resistance. Secretion diminishes over time.
Nutritional status	Thin, normal, or obese.	Frequently overweight or obese. May be normal.
Symptoms	Polydipsia, polyuria, polyphagia, fatigue, weight loss.	Frequently none, fatigue, recurrent infections. May also experience polyuria, polydipsia, and polyphagia.
Ketosis	Prone at onset or during insulin deficiency.	Resistant except during infection or stress.
Nutritional therapy	Essential.	Essential.
Insulin	Required for all.	Required for some. Disease is progressive and insulin treatment may need to be added to treatment regimen.
Vascular and neurologic complications	Frequent.	Frequent.

Pathophysiology. Type 1 diabetes is an immune-mediated disease caused by autoimmune destruction of the pancreatic β cells, the site of insulin production. This eventually results in a total absence of insulin production. Autoantibodies to the islet cells cause a reduction of 80% to 90% of normal function before hyperglycemia and other manifestations occur.

- A genetic predisposition and exposure to a virus are factors that may contribute to the pathogenesis of immune-related type 1 diabetes.

In type 1 diabetes the islet cell autoantibodies responsible for β cell destruction are present for months to years before the onset of symptoms. Manifestations develop when the person's pancreas can no longer produce sufficient amounts of glucose to maintain normal glucose. Once this occurs, the onset of symptoms is usually rapid.

- The patient usually has a history of recent and sudden weight loss and the classic symptoms of *polydipsia* (excessive thirst), *polyuria* (frequent urination), and *polyphagia* (excessive hunger).
- The individual with type 1 diabetes requires a supply of insulin from an outside source *(exogenous insulin)* to sustain life. Without insulin, the patient develops *diabetic ketoacidosis* (DKA), a life-threatening condition resulting in metabolic acidosis.

Type 2 Diabetes Mellitus

Type 2 diabetes mellitus was formerly known as "adult-onset diabetes (AODM)" or "non–insulin-dependent diabetes (NIDDM)." This type is the most prevalent type of diabetes, accounting for greater than 90% of patients with diabetes.

Pathophysiology. In type 2 diabetes, the pancreas usually continues to produce some endogenous (self-made) insulin. However, the insulin that is produced either is insufficient for the body's needs or is poorly used by the tissues. The presence of endogenous insulin is the major pathophysiologic distinction between type 1 and type 2 diabetes.

- Risk factors for developing type 2 diabetes include being overweight or obese, being older, and having a family history of type 2 diabetes. The incidence is increasing in children because of the increasing prevalence of obesity in these individuals.

Four major metabolic abnormalities play a role in the development of type 2 diabetes.

- The first factor is *insulin resistance,* which describes a condition in which body tissues do not respond to the action of insulin because insulin receptors are unresponsive, insufficient in number, or both. Entry of glucose into the cell is impeded, resulting in hyperglycemia.

- A second factor is a marked decrease in the ability of the pancreas to produce insulin as the β cells become fatigued from the compensatory overproduction of insulin or when β cell mass is lost.
- A third factor is inappropriate glucose production by the liver. Instead of properly regulating the release of glucose in response to blood levels, the liver does so in a haphazard way that does not correspond to the body's needs at the time.
- A fourth factor is alteration in the production of hormones and cytokines by adipose tissue (adipokines). Adipokines appear to play a role in glucose and fat metabolism and likely contribute to pathophysiology of type 2 diabetes.

Individuals with metabolic syndrome are at an increased risk for the development of type 2 diabetes (see Metabolic Syndrome, p. 415).

Disease onset in type 2 diabetes is usually gradual. The person may go for many years with undetected hyperglycemia that might produce few, if any, symptoms. Many people are diagnosed on routine laboratory testing or when they undergo treatment for other conditions and elevated glucose or glycosylated hemoglobin (A1C) levels are found.

Prediabetes

Individuals diagnosed with prediabetes are at increased risk for the development of type 2 diabetes. It is an intermediate stage between normal glucose homeostasis and diabetes where the blood glucose levels are elevated, but not high enough to meet the diagnostic criteria for diabetes. *Prediabetes* is defined as impaired glucose tolerance (IGT), impaired fasting glucose (IFG), or both.

- A diagnosis of IGT is made if the 2-hour oral glucose tolerance test (OGTT) values are 140 to 199 mg/dL (7.8 to 11.0 mmol/L). IFG is diagnosed when fasting blood glucose levels are 100 to 125 mg/dL (5.56 to 6.9 mmol/L).

People with prediabetes usually do not have symptoms. However, long-term damage to the body, especially the heart and blood vessels, may already be occurring. It is important for you to encourage patients to undergo screening and to provide teaching about managing risk factors for diabetes.

- Those with prediabetes should have their blood glucose and A1C tested regularly and monitor for symptoms of diabetes, such as polyuria, polyphagia, and polydipsia.
- Maintaining a healthy weight, exercising regularly, and eating a healthy diet have all been found to reduce the risk of developing overt diabetes in people with prediabetes.

Clinical Manifestations

Type 1 Diabetes

Because the onset of type 1 DM is rapid, the initial manifestations are usually acute. The osmotic effect of glucose produces polydipsia and polyuria. Polyphagia is a consequence of cellular malnourishment when insulin deficiency prevents use of glucose for energy. Weight loss, weakness, and fatigue may also occur.

Type 2 Diabetes

Manifestations of type 2 diabetes are often nonspecific, including fatigue, recurrent infections, prolonged wound healing, and visual changes. Polydipsia, polyuria, and polyphagia may also occur.

Acute Complications

Acute complications arise from events associated with hyperglycemia and hypoglycemia (also referred to as *insulin reaction*). It is important for the health care provider to distinguish between hyperglycemia and hypoglycemia because hypoglycemia worsens rapidly and constitutes a serious threat if action is not immediately taken. Table 31 compares hyperglycemia and hypoglycemia.

Table 31   Comparison of Hyperglycemia and Hypoglycemia

Hyperglycemia	Hypoglycemia
Manifestations*	
▪ Elevated blood glucose[†]	▪ Blood glucose <70 mg/dL (3.9 mmol/L)
▪ Increase in urination	
▪ Increase in appetite followed by lack of appetite	▪ Cold, clammy skin
	▪ Numbness of fingers, toes, mouth
	▪ Rapid heart rate
▪ Weakness, fatigue	▪ Emotional changes
▪ Blurred vision	▪ Headache
▪ Headache	▪ Nervousness, tremors
▪ Glycosuria	▪ Faintness, dizziness
▪ Nausea and vomiting	▪ Unsteady gait, slurred speech
▪ Abdominal cramps	▪ Hunger
▪ Progression to DKA or HHS	▪ Changes in vision
	▪ Seizures, coma

*There is usually a gradual onset of symptoms in hyperglycemia and a rapid onset in hypoglycemia.
[†]Specific clinical manifestations related to elevated levels of blood glucose vary according to the patient.
DKA, Diabetic ketoacidosis; *HHS,* hyperosmolar hyperglycemic syndrome.

Continued

| Table 31 | Comparison of Hyperglycemia and Hypoglycemia—cont'd |

Hyperglycemia	Hypoglycemia
Causes	
▪ Illness, infection ▪ Corticosteroids ▪ Too much food ▪ Too little or no diabetes medication ▪ Inactivity ▪ Emotional, physical stress ▪ Poor absorption of insulin	▪ Alcohol intake without food ▪ Too little food—delayed, omitted, inadequate intake ▪ Too much diabetic medication ▪ Too much exercise without adequate food intake ▪ Diabetes medication or food taken at wrong time ▪ Loss of weight without change in medication ▪ Use of β-adrenergic blockers interfering with recognition of symptoms
Treatment	
▪ Get medical care ▪ Continue diabetes medication as ordered ▪ Check blood glucose frequently and check urine for ketones; record results ▪ Drink fluids at least on an hourly basis ▪ Contact health care provider regarding ketonuria	▪ Immediately ingest 15 g of simple carbohydrates ▪ Wait 15 min. Then check blood glucose again. ▪ If blood glucose is < 70 mg/dL, repeat 15 g of carbohydrate ▪ Contact emergency medical service (EMS) if no relief obtained ▪ Discuss medication dosage with health care provider
Preventive Measures	
▪ Take prescribed dose of medication at proper time ▪ Accurately administer insulin, noninsulin injectables, OA ▪ Maintain diet ▪ Adhere to sick-day rules when ill ▪ Check blood for glucose as ordered ▪ Wear diabetic identification	▪ Take prescribed dose of medication at proper time ▪ Accurately administer insulin, noninsulin injectables, OA ▪ Ingest all recommended foods at proper time ▪ Provide adequate food intake needed for calories for exercise ▪ Be able to recognize and know symptoms and treat them immediately ▪ Carry simple carbohydrates ▪ Teach family and caregiver about symptoms and treatment ▪ Check blood glucose as ordered ▪ Wear Medic Alert (diabetic) identification

OA, Oral agent.

Diabetic Ketoacidosis

Diabetic ketoacidosis (DKA) is caused by a profound deficiency of insulin and is characterized by hyperglycemia, ketosis, acidosis, and dehydration. Precipitating factors include illness and infection, inadequate insulin dosage, undiagnosed type 1 diabetes, poor self-management, and neglect.

- DKA is most likely to occur in type 1 diabetes, but may be seen in type 2 in conditions of severe illness or stress when the pancreas cannot meet the extra demand for insulin. If left untreated, death is inevitable.
- Manifestations of DKA include dehydration signs (e.g., poor skin turgor, dry mucous membranes), tachycardia, orthostatic hypotension with a weak and rapid pulse, vomiting, Kussmaul respirations, and a sweet fruity odor of acetone on the breath.
- Laboratory findings include a blood glucose level greater than or equal to 250 mg/dL (13.9 mmol/L), arterial blood pH less than 7.30, serum bicarbonate level less than 16 mEq/L (16 mmol/L), and moderate to large amount of ketones in the urine or serum.

Hyperosmolar Hyperglycemic Syndrome

Hyperosmolar hyperglycemic syndrome (HHS) is a life-threatening syndrome that can occur in the patient with DM who is able to produce enough insulin to prevent DKA but not enough to prevent severe hyperglycemia, osmotic diuresis, and extracellular fluid depletion.

- The main difference between HHS and DKA is that the patient with HHS usually has enough circulating insulin so that ketoacidosis does not occur. Because HHS produces fewer symptoms in the earlier stages, blood glucose levels can climb quite high before the problem is recognized. The higher blood glucose levels increase serum osmolality and produce more severe neurologic manifestations, such as somnolence, coma, seizures, hemiparesis, and aphasia.
- HHS is less common than DKA. It often occurs in patients greater than 60 years of age with type 2 diabetes. Common causes of HHS are urinary tract infections, pneumonia, sepsis, any acute illness, and newly diagnosed type 2 diabetes.
- Laboratory values include a blood glucose level above 600 mg/dL (33.33 mmol/L) and a marked increase in serum osmolality. Ketone bodies are absent or minimal in both blood and urine.

Hypoglycemia

Hypoglycemia, or low blood glucose, occurs when there is too much insulin in proportion to available glucose in the blood. This causes the blood glucose level to drop below 70 mg/dL. Manifestations include shakiness, palpitations, nervousness, diaphoresis, anxiety, hunger, and pallor. Untreated hypoglycemia can progress to loss of consciousness, seizures, coma, and death.

Chronic Complications

Chronic complications are primarily those of end-organ disease from damage to the blood vessels from chronic hyperglycemia. *Angiopathy,* or blood vessel disease, is one of the leading causes of diabetes-related deaths. These chronic blood vessel problems are divided into two categories: macrovascular complications and microvascular complications.

Macrovascular Complications

These complications are diseases of the large and medium-sized blood vessels that occur with greater frequency and an earlier onset in people with diabetes. Risk factors associated with macrovascular complications, such as obesity, smoking, hypertension, high fat intake, and sedentary lifestyle, can be reduced. Insulin resistance appears to play a role in the development of cardiovascular disease and is implicated in the pathogenesis of essential hypertension and dyslipidemia.

Microvascular Complications

These complications result from thickening of the vessel membranes in the capillaries and arterioles in response to chronic hyperglycemia. Although microangiopathy can be found throughout the body, the areas most noticeably affected are the eyes (retinopathy), kidneys (nephropathy), and skin (dermopathy).

Diabetic retinopathy is estimated to be the most common cause of new cases of adult blindness.

- In *nonproliferative retinopathy,* the most common form, partial occlusion of the small blood vessels in the retina, causes microaneurysms to develop in the capillary walls. The walls of these microaneurysms are so weak that capillary fluid leaks out, causing retinal edema and eventually hard exudates or intraretinal hemorrhages. Vision may be affected if the macula is involved.
- *Proliferative retinopathy* is more severe and involves the retina and vitreous. When retinal capillaries become occluded, new, fragile blood vessels are formed. Eventually light does not reach the retina as vessels tear and bleed. A tear or retinal detachment may then occur. If the macula is involved, vision is lost. Treatment involves laser photocoagulation.

Diabetic nephropathy is a microvascular complication associated with damage to the small blood vessels that supply the glomeruli of the kidney. It is the leading cause of end-stage kidney disease in the United States. Tight blood glucose control is critical in the prevention and delay of diabetic nephropathy. Hypertension significantly accelerates the progression of nephropathy. Therefore aggressive BP management is indicated for all patients with diabetes.

- Patients with diabetes are screened for nephropathy annually with a random spot urine collection to assess for albuminuria and measure the albumin-to-creatinine ratio. Serum creatinine is also measured to provide an estimation of the glomerular filtration rate and thus the degree of kidney function.

Neuropathy

Neuropathy is nerve damage that occurs because of the metabolic alterations associated with diabetes. About 60% to 70% of patients with diabetes have some degree of neuropathy. More than 60% of nontraumatic amputations in the United States occur in people with diabetes. Screening for neuropathy should begin at the time of diagnosis in patients with type 2 diabetes and 5 years after diagnosis in patients with type 1 diabetes.

Two major categories of diabetic neuropathy are *sensory neuropathy,* which affects the peripheral nervous system and is the more common type of neuropathy, and *autonomic neuropathy,* which can affect nearly all body systems.

- The most common form of sensory neuropathy is distal symmetric neuropathy, which affects the hands or feet bilaterally. Characteristics include loss of sensation, abnormal sensations, pain, and paresthesias. The pain, which is often described as burning, cramping, crushing, or tearing, is usually worse at night. The paresthesias may be associated with tingling, burning, and itching sensations.
- Autonomic neuropathy can lead to hypoglycemic unawareness, bowel incontinence and diarrhea, and urinary retention. Delayed gastric emptying *(gastroparesis),* a complication of autonomic neuropathy, can produce nausea, vomiting, gastroesophageal reflux, and persistent feelings of fullness. Cardiovascular abnormalities, such as postural hypotension, painless myocardial infarction, and resting tachycardia, can occur.

Control of blood glucose is the only treatment for diabetic neuropathy. It is effective in many but not all cases. Drug therapy may be used to treat neuropathic symptoms, particularly pain.

Diagnostic Studies

The diagnosis of diabetes can be made through one of the following four methods. In the absence of unequivocal hyperglycemia, criteria 1 to 3 should be confirmed by repeat testing.

1. Glycosylated hemoglobin (A1C) of 6.5% or greater.
2. Fasting plasma glucose (FPG) level at or above 126 mg/dL (7.0 mmol/L). *Fasting* is defined as no caloric intake for at least 8 hours.
3. Two-hour plasma glucose level at or above 200 mg/dL (11.1 mmol/L) during an oral glucose tolerance test (OGTT), using a glucose load of 75 g.

4. In a patient with classic symptoms of hyperglycemia (poly-uria, polydipsia, unexplained weight loss) or hyperglyce-mic crisis, a random plasma glucose of at least 200 mg/dL (11.1 mmol/L).

Collaborative Care

The goals of diabetes management are to reduce symptoms, promote well-being, prevent acute complications of hyperglyce-mia, and prevent or delay the onset and progression of long-term complications. Nutritional therapy, drug therapy, exercise, and self-monitoring of blood glucose are the tools used in the man-agement of diabetes. The major types of glucose-lowering agents (GLAs) used in the treatment of diabetes are insulin and oral and noninsulin injectable agents. For the majority of people, drug therapy is necessary.

Drug Therapy: Insulin

Exogenous (injected) insulin is needed when a patient has inade-quate insulin to meet specific metabolic needs. People with type 1 diabetes require exogenous insulin to survive. People with type 2 diabetes, who are usually controlled with diet, exercise, and/or OAs, may require exogenous insulin during periods of severe stress, such as illness or surgery. When patients with type 2 diabe-tes cannot maintain satisfactory blood glucose levels, exogenous insulin is added to the management plan.

Human insulin is prepared using genetic engineering. The insulin is derived from common bacteria (e.g., *Escherichia coli*) or yeast cells using recombinant DNA technology. Insulins differ by their onset, peak action, and duration and are categorized as rapid-acting, short-acting, intermediate-acting, and long-acting insulin (Table 32).

Examples of insulin regimens ranging from one to four injec-tions per day are presented in Table 49-4 in Lewis et al, *Medical-Surgical Nursing,* ed. 9, p. 1159.

- The insulin regimen that most closely mimics endogenous insu-lin production is a basal-bolus regimen that uses rapid and short-acting (bolus) insulin before meals and long-acting (basal) background insulin once or twice per day.
- In addition to mealtime insulin, people with type 1 diabetes must also use a long- or intermediate-acting (background) insulin to control blood glucose levels between meals and overnight.
- Combination insulin therapy involves the mixing of short- or rapid-acting insulin with intermediate-acting insulin to provide both mealtime and basal coverage with one injection. Pre-mixed formulas are available for this regimen, but optimal blood glucose control is not as likely because there is less flex-ibility in dosing.

Table 32	Drug Therapy *Types of Insulin*	

Classification	Examples	Clarity of Solution
Rapid-acting insulin	lispro (Humalog) aspart (NovoLog) glulisine (Apidra)	Clear
Short-acting insulin	regular (Humulin R, Novolin R)	Clear
Intermediate-acting insulin	NPH (Humulin N, Novolin N)	Cloudy
Long-acting insulin	glargine (Lantus) detemir (Levemir)	Clear
Combination therapy (premixed)	NPH/regular 70/30* (Humulin 70/30, Novolin 70/30) NPH/regular 50/50* (Humulin 50/50) lispro protamine/lispro 75/25* (Humalog Mix 75/25) lispro protamine/lispro 50/50* (Humalog Mix 50/50) aspart protamine/aspart 70/30* (NovoLog Mix 70/30)	Cloudy

*These numbers refer to percentages of each type of insulin.

The steps in administering a subcutaneous insulin injection are outlined in Table 49-5 in Lewis et al, *Medical-Surgical Nursing*, ed. 9, p. 1161.

Continuous subcutaneous insulin infusion can be administered through an insulin pump, a small battery-operated device that resembles a standard paging device in size and appearance. Every 2 or 3 days the insertion site is changed. A major advantage of the pump is the potential for tight glucose control.

Nursing Care Related to Insulin Therapy. Nursing responsibilities for the patient receiving insulin include proper administration, assessment of patient's response to insulin therapy, and teaching the patient regarding administration of, adjustment to, and side effects of insulin.

- Assess the patient who is new to insulin and evaluate his or her ability to manage insulin therapy safely. This includes the ability to understand the interaction of insulin, diet, and activity and to recognize and treat appropriately the symptoms of hypoglycemia.

- The patient or caregiver also must be able to prepare and inject the insulin (see Table 49-5, Lewis et al, *Medical-Surgical Nursing,* ed. 9, p. 1161). If the patient or caregiver lacks this ability, additional resources will be needed.
- Follow-up assessment of the patient who has been using insulin therapy includes inspection of insulin sites for lipodystrophy (atrophy of subcutaneous tissue) and other reactions, a review of the insulin preparation and injection technique, a history pertaining to the occurrence of hypoglycemic episodes, and assessment of the patient's method for handling hypoglycemic episodes.
- A review of the patient's record of urine and blood glucose tests is also important in assessing overall glycemic control.

Drug Therapy: Oral and Noninsulin Injectable Agents

Oral agents (OAs) and noninsulin injectable agents work to improve the mechanisms by which the body produces and uses insulin and glucose. These drugs work on the three defects of type 2 diabetes: insulin resistance, decreased insulin production, and increased hepatic glucose production. These drugs may be used in combination with agents from other classes or with insulin to achieve blood glucose targets.

Many types of OAs and noninsulin injectable agents are used in the treatment of type 2 diabetes:

- *Biguanides* primarily reduce glucose production by the liver, but they also enhance insulin sensitivity and improve glucose transport into cells. The most widely used agent is metformin. Forms of metformin include Glucophage (immediate release), Glucophage XR (extended release), Fortamet (extended release), and Riomet (liquid form of metformin).
- *Sulfonylureas* increase insulin production by the pancreas and include glipizide (Glucotrol, Glucotrol XL), glyburide (Micronase, DiaBeta, Glynase), and glimepiride (Amaryl).
- *Meglitinides* also increase insulin production from the pancreas, but they are more rapidly absorbed and eliminated than the sulfonylureas, decreasing the potential for hypoglycemia. Meglitinides include repaglinide (Prandin) and nateglinide (Starlix).
- *α-Glucosidase inhibitors* slow down the absorption of carbohydrate in the small intestine. Acarbose (Precose) and miglitol (Glyset) are the drugs in this class.
- *Thiazolidinediones* improve insulin sensitivity, transport, and utilization at target tissues. These agents include pioglitazone (Actos) and rosiglitazone (Avandia).
- *Dipeptidyl peptidase-4 (DDP) inhibitors* slow the inactivation of incretin hormones. Incretin hormones are released by the

intestines throughout the day, but levels increase in response to a meal. This class of drugs includes sitagliptin (Januvia), linagliptin (Tradjenta), saxagliptin (Onglyza), and alogliptin (Nesina).

- The *amylin analog* class of drugs, synthetic analogs of human amylin (a hormone secreted by the β cells of the pancreas), works to control diabetes by slowing gastric emptying, reducing postprandial glucagon secretion, and increasing satiety. The drug in this class is pramlintide (Symlin), which must be administered subcutaneously and cannot be mixed in the same syringe as insulin.

- *Glucagon-like peptide (GLP-1) receptor agonists* simulate GLP-1 glucagon-like peptide-1 (one of the incretin hormones), which is found to be decreased in type 2 diabetes. These drugs increase insulin synthesis and release from the pancreas, inhibit glucagon secretion, decrease gastric emptying, and reduce food intake by increasing satiety. These drugs are administered subcutaneously and may be used as monotherapy or adjunct therapy for patients with type 2 diabetes who have not achieved optimal glucose control on OAs. Drugs in this class include exenatide (Byetta), exenatide extended-release (Bydureon), and liraglutide (Victoza).

- *Sodium-glucose co-transporter 2 (SGLT2) inhibitors* are a new class of drugs that work by blocking the reabsorption of glucose by the kidney, increasing glucose excretion, and lowering blood glucose levels in diabetics. The first drug in this class is canagliflozin (Invokana).

Nursing Care Related to Oral and Noninsulin Injectable Agents. Your responsibilities for the patient taking oral and noninsulin injectable agents are similar to those for the patient taking insulin. Proper administration, assessment of the patient's use of and response to these drugs, and teaching the patient and family are all essential nursing actions.

- Your assessment is valuable in determining the most appropriate drug for a patient. This includes assessing the patient's mental status, eating habits, home environment, attitude toward diabetes, and medication history.

- The patient needs to understand the importance of diet and activity plans.

Nutritional Therapy

Nutritional therapy is a cornerstone of diabetes care. Guidelines from the American Diabetes Association (ADA) indicate that within the context of an overall healthy eating plan, a person with DM can eat the same foods as a person who does not have diabetes. This means that the same principles of good nutrition that apply to the general population also apply to the person with diabetes. See Table 49-8, which describes nutritional therapy for patients with diabetes, Lewis et al, *Medical-Surgical Nursing,* ed. 9, p. 1166.

- *Type 1 Diabetes.* Meal planning should be based on the individual's usual food intake and balanced with insulin and exercise patterns. For patients using conventional, fixed insulin regimens, day-to-day consistency in timing and amount of food eaten is important. Patients using rapid-acting insulin can adjust the dose before the meal based on current blood glucose level and the carbohydrate content of the meal. Intensified insulin therapy, such as multiple daily injections or the use of an insulin pump, allows considerable flexibility in food selection and can be adjusted for deviations from usual eating and exercise habits.
- *Type 2 Diabetes.* Nutritional therapy in type 2 diabetes should emphasize achieving glucose, lipid, and BP goals. Modest weight loss has been associated with improved insulin resistance and glycemic control.

Most often, the dietitian initially teaches the principles of the nutritional therapy regimen. Whenever possible, you should be prepared to work with dietitians as part of an interdisciplinary diabetes care team. Some patients who have limited insurance coverage or live in remote areas do not have access to a dietitian. In these cases, you may need to assume responsibility for teaching basic dietary management to patients with diabetes.

Exercise

Regular, consistent exercise is an essential part of diabetes and prediabetes management. The ADA recommends that people with diabetes perform at least 150 min/wk (30 minutes, 5 days/wk) of a moderate-intensity aerobic physical activity. Encourage people with type 2 diabetes to perform resistance training three times a week in the absence of contraindications.

Exercise decreases insulin resistance and can have a direct effect on lowering blood glucose levels. It also contributes to weight loss, which further decreases insulin resistance, and in addition it may help reduce triglyceride and low-density lipoprotein (LDL) cholesterol levels, increase high-density lipoprotein (HDL), reduce BP, and improve circulation. Additional information is provided in the patient and caregiver teaching guide (see Table 49-10, Lewis et al, *Medical-Surgical Nursing,* ed. 9, p. 1168).

Monitoring Blood Glucose

Self-monitoring of blood glucose is a critical part of diabetes management. By providing a current blood glucose reading, self-monitoring enables the patient to make decisions regarding food intake, activity patterns, and medication dosages.

Because errors in monitoring technique can cause errors in management strategies, comprehensive patient teaching is essential. Initial instruction should be followed up with regular reassessment. Table 49-11 in Lewis et al, *Medical-Surgical Nursing,* ed. 9, p. 1169, presents instructions for teaching the patient to perform self-monitoring of blood glucose.

Management of Acute Complications

Diabetic Ketoacidosis

DKA may be managed on an outpatient basis if fluid and electrolyte imbalances are not severe and blood glucose levels can be safely monitored at home. Emergency management of the DKA is needed when fluid imbalance is potentially life threatening. The initial goal of therapy is to establish IV access and begin fluid and electrolyte replacement. The aim of fluid and electrolyte therapy is to replace extracellular and intracellular water and to correct deficits of sodium, chloride, bicarbonate, potassium, phosphate, magnesium, and nitrogen.

- IV insulin administration is directed toward correcting hyperglycemia and hyperketonemia. Insulin is immediately started by a continuous infusion.

Hyperosmolar Hyperglycemic Syndrome

HHS constitutes a medical emergency and has a high mortality rate. Therapy is similar to that for DKA except that HHS requires greater fluid replacement.

- Insulin is given immediately by IV infusion.
- Electrolytes are monitored and replaced as needed. Assess vital signs, intake and output, tissue turgor, laboratory values, and cardiac monitoring to monitor the efficacy of fluid and electrolyte replacement.

Hypoglycemia

At the first sign of hypoglycemia, check the blood glucose if possible. If it is below 70 mg/dL (3.9 mmol/L), immediately begin treatment for hypoglycemia. If the patient has manifestations of hypoglycemia and monitoring equipment is not available or the patient has a history of chronic poor glycemic control, hypoglycemia should be assumed and treatment initiated.

- Hypoglycemia is treated by ingesting 15 g of a simple (fast-acting) carbohydrate, such as 4 to 6 ounces of fruit juice or regular soft drink. Avoid overtreatment with large quantities of quick-acting carbohydrates, such as candy bars, so that a rapid fluctuation to hyperglycemia does not occur.
- Re-check the blood glucose 15 minutes later. If the value is still below 70 mg/dL, have the patient ingest 15 g more of carbohydrate and recheck the blood glucose in 15 minutes. Because of

the potential for rebound hypoglycemia after an acute episode, have the patient ingest a complex carbohydrate after recovery to prevent another hypoglycemic attack.

- If no significant improvement occurs after two or three doses of 15 g of simple carbohydrate, contact the health care provider.

Once acute hypoglycemia has been reversed, you should explore with the patient the reasons why the situation developed. This assessment may indicate a need for additional teaching of the patient and caregiver to avoid future episodes of hypoglycemia.

Nursing Management

Goals

The patient with diabetes will engage in self-care behaviors to actively manage his or her diabetes, experience few or no episodes of acute hyperglycemic or hypoglycemic emergencies, maintain blood glucose levels at normal or near-normal levels, prevent or minimize chronic complications of diabetes, and adjust lifestyle to accommodate the diabetes regimen with a minimum of stress.

Nursing Diagnoses

- Ineffective self-health management
- Risk for unstable blood glucose levels
- Risk for injury
- Risk for peripheral neurovascular dysfunction

Nursing Interventions

Your role in health promotion is to identify, monitor, and teach the patient at risk for diabetes.

Management of Acute Illness and Surgery. Emotional and physical stress can increase blood glucose levels and result in hyperglycemia. Acute illness, injury, and surgery are situations that may evoke a counterregulatory hormone response resulting in hyperglycemia. When patients with diabetes are ill, they should check blood glucose at least every 4 hours. An acutely ill patient with type 1 diabetes with a blood glucose level above 240 mg/dL (13.3 mmol/L) should test his or her urine for ketones every 3 to 4 hours.

- Patients should report to the health care provider when glucose levels are above 300 mg/dL for two tests in a row or urine ketone levels are moderate to large.
- If patients are able to eat normally, they should continue with the regular meal plan while increasing the intake of noncaloric fluids, such as broth, water, diet gelatin, and other decaffeinated beverages, and continue taking oral agents and insulin as prescribed.
- If illness causes the patient to eat less than normal, drug therapy should be continued as prescribed while supplementing food

intake with carbohydrate-containing fluids. The health care provider should be notified if the patient is unable to keep down fluid or food.

- Adjustments in the diabetes regimen during the intraoperative period can be planned to ensure glycemic control. The patient is given IV fluids and insulin (if needed) immediately before, during, and after surgery when there is no oral intake.
- When caring for an unconscious surgical patient receiving insulin, you must be alert for hypoglycemic signs, such as sweating, tachycardia, and tremors.

Ambulatory and Home Care. Successful management of diabetes requires ongoing interaction among the patient, family, and health care team. It is important that a certified diabetes educator be involved in the care of the patient and family.

A diagnosis of diabetes affects the patient in many profound ways. Patients with diabetes must continually face lifestyle choices that affect the food they eat, their activities, and demands on their time and energy. In addition, they face the challenge of preventing or dealing with the devastating complications of diabetes. Careful assessment of what it means to the patient to have diabetes should be the starting point of patient teaching.

The potential for infection requires diligent skin and dental hygiene practices. Routine care includes tooth brushing and flossing and regular bathing, with particular emphasis given to foot care. If cuts, scrapes, or burns occur, they should be treated promptly and monitored carefully. If the injury does not begin to heal within 24 hours or signs of infection develop, the health care provider should be notified immediately.

▼ **Patient and Caregiver Teaching**

The goals of diabetes self-management education are to match the level of self-management to the patient's individual ability so he or she can become the most active participant possible. Patients who actively manage their diabetes care have better outcomes than those who do not. Guidelines for patient and caregiver teaching for management of diabetes are in Table 33.

Assess the patient's knowledge base frequently so that gaps in knowledge or incorrect or inaccurate ideas can be quickly corrected.

- Instruct the patient to carry medical identification at all times indicating that he or she has diabetes. An identification card can supply valuable information, such as the name of the health care provider and the type and dose of insulin or other drug therapy.

Table 33

Patient and Caregiver Teaching Guide
Management of Diabetes Mellitus

Include the following instructions when teaching the patient and caregiver how to manage diabetes mellitus.

Component	What to Teach
Disease process	■ Include an introduction about the pancreas and the islets of Langerhans. ■ Describe how insulin is made and what affects its production. ■ Discuss the relationship of insulin and glucose. ■ Explain the difference between type 1 and type 2 diabetes.
Physical activity	■ Discuss the effect of regular exercise on the management of blood glucose, improvement of cardiovascular function, and general health.
Menu planning	■ Stress the importance of a well-balanced diet as part of a diabetes management plan. ■ Explain the impact of carbohydrates on the glycemic index and blood glucose levels.
Medication adherence	■ Ensure that the patient understands the proper use of prescribed medication (e.g., insulin [see Table 49-5, Lewis et al, *Medical-Surgical Nursing*, ed. 9, p. 1161], OAs, and noninsulin injectables). ■ Account for a patient's physical limitations or inabilities for self-medication. If necessary, involve the family or caregiver in proper use of medication. ■ Discuss all side effects and safety issues regarding medication.
Monitoring blood glucose	■ Teach correct blood glucose monitoring. ■ Include when blood glucose levels should be checked, how to record them, and how to adjust insulin levels if necessary.
Risk reduction	■ Ensure that the patient understands and appropriately responds to the signs and symptoms of hypoglycemia and hyperglycemia (see Table 49-16, Lewis et al, *Medical-Surgical Nursing*, ed. 9, p. 1175). ■ Stress the importance of proper foot care (see Table 49-21, Lewis et al, *Medical-Surgical Nursing*, ed. 9, p. 1184), regular eye examinations, and consistent glucose monitoring. ■ Inform the patient about the effect that stress can have on blood glucose.
Psychosocial	■ Advise the patient of resources that are available to facilitate the adjustment and answer questions about living with a chronic condition such as diabetes (see Resources at end of Chapter 49).

OAs, Oral agents.

DIARRHEA

Description

Diarrhea is the passage of at least three loose or liquid stools per day. It may be acute, or it may be considered chronic if it lasts longer than 4 weeks.

Pathophysiology

Viruses cause most cases of infectious diarrhea in the United States. Bacterial infections are also common. *Escherichia coli* O157:H7 is the most common cause of bloody diarrhea in the United States. It is transmitted by inadequately cooked beef or chicken contaminated with the bacteria or in fruits and vegetables exposed to contaminated manure. *Giardia lamblia* is the most common intestinal parasite that causes diarrhea in the United States.

Infectious organisms attack the intestines in different ways. Some organisms (e.g., *Rotavirus, Norovirus, G. lamblia*) alter secretion and/or absorption of the enterocytes of the small intestine without causing inflammation. Other organisms (e.g., *Clostridium difficile*) impair absorption by destroying cells and producing inflammation in the colon.

Patients receiving broad-spectrum antibiotics (e.g., clindamycin [Cleocin], cephalosporins, or fluoroquinolones) are susceptible to pathogenic strains of *C. difficile.* Probiotics, in particular *Saccharomyces boulardii* and *Lactobacillus,* may be helpful in preventing antibiotic-induced diarrhea in some patients.

Clinical Manifestations

Infections that attack the upper GI tract (e.g., *Norovirus* organisms, *G. lamblia*) usually produce large-volume, watery stools; cramping; and periumbilical pain. Patients have either a low-grade or no fever and often experience nausea and vomiting before the diarrhea begins.

Infections of the colon and distal small bowel (e.g., *Shigella* or *Salmonella* organisms or *C. difficile)* produce fever and frequent bloody diarrhea with a small volume. Leukocytes, blood, and mucus may be present in the stool.

Severe diarrhea produces life-threatening dehydration, electrolyte disturbances (e.g., hypokalemia), and acid-base imbalances (metabolic acidosis). *C. difficile* infection can progress to fulminant colitis and intestinal perforation.

D

Diagnostic Studies

Because most cases of diarrhea resolve quickly, stool cultures are indicated only for patients who are very ill, have a significant fever, or have had diarrhea longer than 3 to 5 days.

- Stools are examined for blood, mucus, white blood cells (WBCs), and parasites, and cultures are done to identify infectious organisms.
- *C. difficile* is detected by enzyme immunoassay (EIA).
- In a patient with chronic diarrhea, measurement of stool electrolytes, pH, and osmolality may help determine whether diarrhea is related to decreased fluid absorption or increased fluid secretion.
- Measurement of stool fat and undigested muscle fibers may indicate fat and protein malabsorption conditions, including pancreatic insufficiency.

Collaborative Care

Treatment depends on the cause. Foods and drugs that cause diarrhea should be avoided. Acute infectious diarrhea is usually self-limiting. The major concerns are preventing transmission, replacing fluid and electrolytes, and protecting the skin. Oral solutions containing glucose and electrolytes (e.g., Gatorade, Pedialyte) may be sufficient to replace losses from mild diarrhea. In severe diarrhea, parenteral administration of fluids, electrolytes, vitamins, and nutrition may be necessary.

Antidiarrheal agents may be given to coat and protect mucous membranes, absorb irritating substances, inhibit GI motility, decrease intestinal secretions, or decrease central nervous system (CNS) stimulation to the GI tract. Antidiarrheal agents are contraindicated in the treatment of infectious diarrhea because they potentially prolong exposure to the organism.

- Antidiarrheal agents are contraindicated in the treatment of some infectious diarrheas because they potentially prolong exposure to the infectious agent. They are used cautiously in inflammatory bowel disease because of the danger of *toxic megacolon* (colonic dilation greater than 5 cm).
- Regardless of the cause, antidiarrheal medications should be given only for a short period. Antibiotics are rarely used to treat infectious diarrhea.

C. difficile is a particularly hazardous health care–associated infection. Its spores can survive for up to 70 days on objects, including commodes, telephones, thermometers, bedside tables, and floors. *C. difficile* can be transmitted from patient to patient by health care workers who do not adhere to infection control precautions.

- The infection is usually treated by stopping antibiotics and starting the patient on metronidazole (Flagyl) or vancomycin (Vancocin).

Nursing Management: Acute Infectious Diarrhea

Goals

The patient with diarrhea will have no transmission of the micro-organism causing the infectious diarrhea, cessation of diarrhea and resumption of normal bowel patterns, normal fluid and electrolyte and acid-base balance, normal nutritional status, and no perianal skin breakdown.

Nursing Diagnoses

- Diarrhea
- Deficient fluid volume

Nursing Interventions

Consider all cases of acute diarrhea infectious until the cause is known.

- Strict infection control precautions are necessary to prevent the illness from spreading to others. Wash your hands before and after contact with each patient and when handling body fluids of any kind.
- Provide private rooms for patients with *C. difficile* and ensure that visitors and health care providers wear gloves and gowns.

▼ Patient and Caregiver Teaching

- Teach the patient and caregiver the principles of hygiene, infection control precautions, and potential dangers of an illness that is infectious to themselves and others.
- Discuss proper food handling, cooking, and storage of food.

DISSEMINATED INTRAVASCULAR COAGULATION

Description

Disseminated intravascular coagulation (DIC) is a serious bleeding and thrombotic disorder that results from abnormally initiated and accelerated clotting. Subsequent decreases in clotting factors and platelets may lead to uncontrollable hemorrhage. The term *DIC* can be misleading because it suggests that blood is clotting. However, this condition is characterized by the profuse bleeding that results from depletion of platelets and clotting factors. DIC is always caused by an underlying disease that must be treated for DIC to resolve.

Pathophysiology

DIC is an abnormal response of the normal clotting cascade stimulated by a disease process or disorder. The diseases and disorders known to predispose patients to acute DIC are major physiologic assaults and include shock, septicemia, abruptio placentae, malignancies, severe head injury, heatstroke, and pulmonary emboli.

- DIC can occur as an acute, catastrophic condition, or it may exist at a subacute or chronic level. Each condition may have one or multiple triggering mechanisms to start the clotting cascade.

Tissue factor is released at the site of tissue injury and by some malignancies, such as leukemia, and enhances normal coagulation mechanisms. Abundant intravascular thrombin, the most powerful coagulant, is produced. It catalyzes the conversion of fibrinogen to fibrin and enhances platelet aggregation. There is widespread fibrin and platelet deposition in capillaries and arterioles, resulting in thrombosis. Excessive clotting activates the fibrinolytic system, which in turn breaks down newly formed clots, creating fibrin-split (fibrin-degradation) products (FSPs), which inhibit normal blood clotting. Ultimately the blood loses its ability to form a stable clot at injury sites, which predisposes the patient to hemorrhage.

- Chronic and subacute DIC is most commonly seen in patients with long-standing illnesses such as malignant disorders or autoimmune diseases. Occasionally these patients have sub-clinical disease manifested only by laboratory abnormalities.

Clinical Manifestations

Bleeding in a person with no previous history or obvious cause should be questioned because it may be one of the first manifestations of acute DIC. Other nonspecific manifestations include weakness, malaise, and fever. There are both bleeding and thrombotic manifestations in DIC (Fig. 4).

- *Bleeding manifestations* include petechiae, oozing blood, tachypnea, hemoptysis, tachycardia, hypotension, bloody stools, hematuria, dizziness, headache, changes in mental status, and bone and joint pain.
- *Thrombotic manifestations* are a result of fibrin or platelet deposition in the microvasculature. Manifestations include ischemic tissue necrosis (e.g., gangrene), acute respiratory distress syndrome (ARDS), cardiovascular and ECG changes, kidney damage, and paralytic ileus.

Diagnostic Studies

Diagnostic findings include:

- Prolonged prothrombin time and partial thromboplastin time
- Prolonged activated partial thromboplastin time and thrombin time
- Reduced fibrinogen, antithrombin III (AT III), and platelets

D

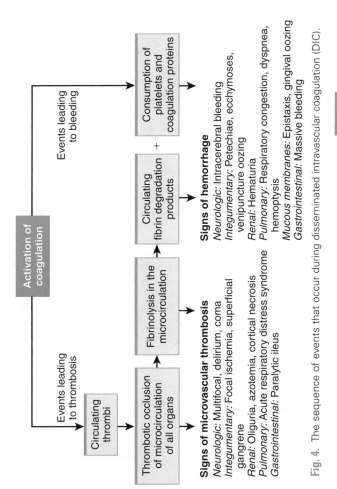

Fig. 4. The sequence of events that occur during disseminated intravascular coagulation (DIC).

Activation of coagulation

Events leading to thrombosis

Events leading to bleeding

Circulating thrombi

Thrombotic occlusion of microcirculation of all organs

Fibrinolysis in the microcirculation

Circulating fibrin degradation products

Consumption of platelets and coagulation proteins

Signs of microvascular thrombosis
Neurologic: Multifocal, delirium, coma
Integumentary: Focal ischemia, superficial gangrene
Renal: Oliguria, azotemia, cortical necrosis
Pulmonary: Acute respiratory distress syndrome
Gastrointestinal: Paralytic ileus

Signs of hemorrhage
Neurologic: Intracerebral bleeding
Integumentary: Petechiae, ecchymoses, venipuncture oozing
Renal: Hematuria
Pulmonary: Respiratory congestion, dyspnea, hemoptysis
Mucous membranes: Epistaxis, gingival oozing
Gastrointestinal: Massive bleeding

- Elevated FSPs and elevated D-dimers (cross-linked fibrin fragments)
- Reduced levels of factors V, VII, VIII, X, and XIII

Collaborative Care

It is important to diagnose DIC quickly, stabilize the patient if needed (e.g., oxygenation, volume replacement), treat the underlying causative disease or problem, and control the ongoing thrombosis and bleeding. Depending on its severity, a variety of different methods are used to manage DIC.

- If chronic DIC is diagnosed in a patient who is not bleeding, no therapy for DIC is necessary. Treatment of the underlying disease may be sufficient to reverse DIC (e.g., chemotherapy when DIC is caused by malignancy).
- When the patient with DIC is bleeding, therapy is directed toward providing support with necessary blood products while treating the primary disorder. Blood product support is usually reserved for a patient with life-threatening hemorrhage. Therapy stabilizes a patient, prevents exsanguination or massive thrombosis, and permits institution of definitive therapy to treat the underlying cause. Platelets are given to correct thrombocytopenia, cryoprecipitate replaces factor VIII and fibrinogen, and fresh frozen plasma (FFP) replaces all clotting factors except platelets and provides a source of antithrombin.
- A patient with manifestations of thrombosis is often treated by anticoagulation with heparin or low-molecular-weight heparin. Heparin is used in the treatment of DIC only when the benefit (reduce clotting) outweighs the risk of bleeding. Antithrombin III (AT III, ATnativ) may be useful in fulminant DIC, although it increases the risk of bleeding.
- Chronic DIC does not respond to oral anticoagulants, but it can be controlled with long-term use of heparin.

Nursing Management

Nursing Diagnoses

- Ineffective peripheral tissue perfusion
- Acute pain
- Decreased cardiac output
- Anxiety

Nursing Interventions

Be alert to the possible development of DIC. Remember that because DIC is secondary to an underlying disease, the causative problem needs to be managed while providing supportive care for the manifestations of DIC.

- Early detection of bleeding, both occult and overt, must be a primary goal. Assess for signs of external bleeding (e.g., petechiae, oozing at IV or injection sites) and internal bleeding (e.g., changes in mental status, increasing abdominal girth, pain) and any indications that microthrombi may be causing clinically significant organ damage (e.g., decreased renal output).

- Minimize tissue damage and protect the patient from additional foci of bleeding.
- An additional nursing responsibility is to administer blood products and medications correctly.

DIVERTICULOSIS/DIVERTICULITIS

Description

Diverticula are saccular dilations or outpouchings of the mucosa that develop in the colon. In *diverticulosis,* multiple noninflamed diverticula are present. *Diverticulitis* is inflammation of the diverticula, resulting in perforation into the peritoneum. Clinically, diverticular disease covers a spectrum from asymptomatic, uncomplicated diverticulosis to diverticulitis with complications such as perforation, abscess, fistula, and bleeding.

- Diverticula are common, especially in older adults, but most people never develop diverticulitis.
- The disease is more prevalent in Western, industrialized populations that consume diets low in fiber and high in refined carbohydrates. Diverticula are uncommon in vegetarians.

Pathophysiology

Diverticula may occur anywhere in the gastrointestinal (GI) tract but are most commonly found in the left (descending, sigmoid) colon. The etiology of diverticulosis of the sigmoid colon is thought to be associated with high luminal pressures from a deficiency in dietary fiber intake.

Inadequate dietary fiber slows transit time, and more water is absorbed from the stool, making it more difficult to pass through the lumen. Decreased stool size increases intraluminal pressure, thus promoting diverticula formation.

Clinical Manifestations and Complications

A majority of patients with diverticulosis have no symptoms. Those with symptoms typically have abdominal pain, bloating, flatulence, or changes in bowel habits but no symptoms of inflammation.

The most common symptoms of diverticulitis include acute pain in the left lower quadrant (location of sigmoid colon), a palpable abdominal mass, and systemic symptoms of infection (fever, increased C-reactive protein, and leukocytosis with a shift to the left). Older patients with diverticulitis may be afebrile, with a normal WBC count and little, if any, abdominal tenderness.

The diverticula may bleed, or diverticulitis can develop. Diverticulitis is characterized by inflamed diverticuli and increased luminal pressures that cause erosion of the bowel wall, and thus perforation into the peritoneum. A localized abscess develops when the body is able to wall off the area of perforation. Peritonitis develops if it cannot be contained. Bleeding can be extensive but usually stops spontaneously.

Diagnostic Studies
- History and physical examination
- Abdominal and chest x-rays are used to rule out other causes of acute abdominal pain
- CT scan with oral contrast confirms the diagnosis

Collaborative Care
A high-fiber diet, mainly from fruits and vegetables, and decreased intake of fat and red meat are recommended for preventing diverticular disease. High levels of physical activity may decrease the risk. A high-fiber diet is also recommended once diverticular disease is present. Weight reduction is important for the obese person.

In acute diverticulitis, the goal of treatment is to allow the colon to rest and the inflammation to subside. Some patients can be managed at home with oral antibiotics and a clear liquid diet. Hospitalization is necessary if symptoms are severe, the patient is unable to tolerate oral fluids, or the patient has comorbid diseases.

Surgery is reserved for patients with complications, such as an abscess or obstruction that cannot be managed medically. The usual surgical procedures involve resection of the involved colon with either a primary anastomosis if adequate bowel cleansing is feasible or a temporary diverting colostomy. The colostomy is reanastomosed after the colon is healed.

Nursing Management
Teach patients with diverticular disease to avoid increased intraabdominal pressure because it may precipitate an attack.
- Factors that increase intraabdominal pressure are straining at stool, vomiting, bending, lifting, and wearing tight, restrictive clothing.
- When the acute attack subsides, give oral fluids first and then progress the diet to semisolids. Ambulation is allowed.

- Provide the patient with a full explanation of the condition. Patients who understand the disease process well and adhere to the prescribed regimen are less likely to experience an exacerbation of the disease and its complications.

DYSMENORRHEA

Description

Dysmenorrhea is abdominal cramping pain or discomfort associated with menstrual flow. The degree of pain and discomfort varies with the individual. The two types of dysmenorrhea are *primary* (no pathology exists) and *secondary* (pelvic disease is the underlying cause). Dysmenorrhea is one of the most common gynecologic problems.

Pathophysiology

Primary dysmenorrhea is not a disease. Rather it is caused by either an excess of or an increased sensitivity to prostaglandin $F_2\alpha$ ($PGF_2\alpha$). Primary dysmenorrhea begins in the first few years after menarche, typically with the onset of regular ovulatory cycles.

- With the onset of menses, degeneration of the endometrium releases prostaglandins. Prostaglandins locally increase myometrial contractions and constriction of small endometrial blood vessels, with consequent tissue ischemia and increased sensitization of the pain receptors resulting in menstrual pain.

Secondary dysmenorrhea occurs most commonly in women in their 30s and 40s. Secondary dysmenorrhea is caused by pelvic conditions such as endometriosis, chronic pelvic inflammatory disease (PID), and uterine leiomyomas (fibroids).

Clinical Manifestations

Primary dysmenorrhea starts 12 to 24 hours before the onset of menses. The pain is most severe the first day of menses and rarely lasts more than 2 days.

- Characteristic manifestations include lower abdominal cramping pain that is colicky in nature, frequently radiating to the lower back and upper thighs. The abdominal pain is often accompanied by nausea, diarrhea, loose stools, fatigue, and headache.

Secondary dysmenorrhea usually occurs after the woman has experienced problem-free periods for some time. The pain, which may be unilateral, is generally more constant in nature and continues for a longer time than primary dysmenorrhea.

- Depending on the cause, symptoms such as *dyspareunia* (painful intercourse), painful defecation, or irregular bleeding may occur at times other than menstruation.

Diagnostic Studies

Evaluation begins with distinguishing primary from secondary dysmenorrhea.

- Obtain a health history with special attention to menstrual and gynecologic history. A pelvic examination is also done.
- If the pelvic examination is normal and the history reveals an onset shortly after menarche with symptoms only associated with menses, the probable diagnosis is primary dysmenorrhea.
- If a specific cause is evident, the diagnosis is secondary dysmenorrhea.

Collaborative Care

Treatment for primary dysmenorrhea includes heat applied to the lower abdomen or back, exercise, and drug therapy. Regular exercise is beneficial because it may reduce endometrial hyperplasia and subsequent prostaglandin production.

Drug therapy involves nonsteroidal antiinflammatory drugs (NSAIDs), such as naproxen (Naprosyn), which has antiprostaglandin activity. NSAIDs should be started at the first sign of menses and continued every 4 to 8 hours for the duration of the usual discomfort.

Oral contraceptives may also be used to decrease dysmenorrhea by reducing endometrial hyperplasia. Treatment for secondary dysmenorrhea depends on the cause with some of the same approaches being used that are recommended for primary dysmenorrhea.

Nursing Management

- Advise women that during acute pain, relief may be obtained by applying heat to the abdomen or back and taking NSAIDs for analgesia.
- Suggest noninvasive pain-relieving practices such as relaxation breathing and guided imagery.
- Health care measures that can decrease discomfort include proper nutritional habits, regular exercise, avoidance of constipation, maintaining good body mechanics, and avoidance of stress and fatigue, particularly during the time preceding menstrual periods.
- Staying active and interested in activities may also help.

DYSRHYTHMIAS

Description

Dysrhythmias are abnormal cardiac rhythms. Prompt assessment of abnormal cardiac rhythms and the patient's response to the rhythm is critical. Dysrhythmias result from disorders of impulse formation, conduction of impulses, or both. A pacemaker from a site other than the sinoatrial (SA) node may be fired in two ways.

- If the SA node fires more slowly than a secondary pacemaker, electrical discharges from the secondary pacemaker may passively "escape" and fire automatically at its intrinsic rate. Secondary pacemakers can also originate when they fire more rapidly than the normal pacemaker of the SA node. *Triggered beats* (early or late) may come from an *ectopic focus* (area outside the normal conduction pathway) in the atria, atrioventricular (AV) node, or ventricles. This results in a dysrhythmia, which replaces the normal sinus rhythm.

- Dysrhythmias occur as the result of various abnormalities and disease states. The cause of a dysrhythmia influences the patient's treatment. Common causes of dysrhythmias are presented in Table 34. Table 35 presents a systematic approach to assessing a cardiac rhythm.

D

Table 34	Common Causes of Dysrhythmias*

Cardiac Conditions
- Accessory pathways
- Cardiomyopathy
- Conduction defects
- Heart failure
- Myocardial ischemia, infarction
- Valve disease

Other Conditions
- Acid-base imbalances
- Alcohol
- Caffeine, tobacco
- Connective tissue disorders
- Drug effects (e.g., antidysrhythmia drugs, stimulants, β-adrenergic blockers) or toxicity
- Electric shock
- Electrolyte imbalances (e.g., hyperkalemia, hypocalcemia)
- Emotional crisis
- Herbal supplements (e.g., areca nut, wahoo root bark, yerba maté)
- Hypoxia
- Metabolic conditions (e.g., thyroid dysfunction)
- Near-drowning
- Sepsis, shock
- Toxins

*List is not all-inclusive.

Table 35	Approach to Assessing Heart Rhythm

When assessing a heart rhythm, use a consistent and systematic approach. One such approach includes the following:

1. Look for the P wave. Is it upright or inverted? Is there one for every QRS complex or more than one? Are atrial fibrillatory or flutter waves present?
2. Evaluate the atrial rhythm. Is it regular or irregular?
3. Calculate the atrial rate.
4. Measure the duration of the PR interval. Is it normal duration or prolonged?
5. Evaluate the ventricular rhythm. Is it regular or irregular?
6. Calculate the ventricular rate.
7. Measure the duration of the QRS complex. Is it normal duration or prolonged?
8. Assess the ST segment. Is it isoelectric (flat), elevated, or depressed?
9. Measure the duration of the QT interval. Is it normal duration or prolonged?
10. Note the T wave. Is it upright or inverted?

Additional questions to consider include the following:

1. What is the dominant or underlying rhythm and/or dysrhythmia?
2. What is the clinical significance of your findings?
3. What is the treatment for the particular rhythm?

Types of Dysrhythmias

Examples of ECG tracings of common dysrhythmias are presented in Figs. 36-11 to 36-19, Lewis et al, *Medical-Surgical Nursing,* ed. 9, pp. 793, 795, 797 to 799. The characteristics of common dysrhythmias are described in the Reference Appendix on pp. 760 to 762.

Sinus Bradycardia

This condition occurs when the SA node discharges at a rate less than 60 beats/minute. It may be a normal sinus rhythm in aerobically trained athletes or in some people during sleep. It also occurs in response to carotid sinus massage, Valsalva maneuver, hypothermia, increased intraocular pressure, vagal stimulation, and the administration of certain drugs (e.g., β-adrenergic blockers, calcium channel blockers). Disease states associated with sinus bradycardia are hypothyroidism, increased intracranial pressure, hypoglycemia, and inferior wall myocardial infarction (MI).

- Clinical significance depends on how the patient tolerates it. Signs of symptomatic bradycardia include pale, cool skin; hypotension;

weakness; angina; dizziness or syncope, confusion, or disorientation; and shortness of breath.

■ Treatment consists of administration of atropine for patients with symptoms. Pacemaker therapy may be required. If caused by drugs, these may need to be held or discontinued, or given in reduced dosages.

Sinus Tachycardia

This dysrhythmia involves a heart rate (HR) of 101 to 200 beats per minute from the SA node as a result of vagal inhibition or sympathetic stimulation. Sinus tachycardia is associated with physiologic and psychologic stressors, such as exercise, fever, pain, hypotension, hypovolemia, anemia, hypoglycemia, myocardial ischemia, heart failure (HF), hyperthyroidism, and anxiety. It can also be an effect of drugs such as epinephrine, norepinephrine, caffeine, theophylline, nifedipine (Procardia), or hydralazine (Apresoline). Pseudoephedrine (Sudafed) found in many over-the-counter cold remedies can also cause tachycardia.

■ Clinical significance depends on the patient's tolerance of the increased HR. The patient may experience dizziness, dyspnea, and hypotension. Angina or an increase in infarction size may accompany sinus tachycardia in the patient with an acute MI.

■ Treatment is based on the underlying cause. For example, if the patient is experiencing tachycardia from pain, effective pain management is important to treat the tachycardia. In patients who are clinically stable, vagal maneuvers can be attempted. In addition, IV β-adrenergic blockers (e.g., metoprolol [Lopressor]) can be given to reduce HR and decrease myocardial oxygen consumption.

Premature Atrial Contraction (PAC)

PAC is a contraction starting from an ectopic focus in the atrium (in a location other than the SA node) and coming sooner than the next expected sinus beat. The ectopic focus starts in the left or right atrium and travels across the atria by an abnormal pathway, creating a distorted P wave. At the AV node it may be stopped (nonconducted PAC), delayed (lengthened PR interval), or conducted normally. If the impulse moves through the AV node, in most cases it is conducted normally through the ventricles.

In a normal heart, a PAC can result from emotional stress or physical fatigue or from the use of caffeine, tobacco, or alcohol. A PAC can also result from hypoxia, electrolyte imbalances, and disease states such as hyperthyroidism, chronic obstructive pulmonary disease (COPD), and heart disease, including coronary artery disease (CAD) and valvular disease.

■ HR varies with the underlying rate and frequency of PAC, and the rhythm is irregular.

- Isolated PACs are not significant in people with healthy hearts. In people with heart disease, PACs may warn of or start more serious dysrhythmias (e.g., supraventricular tachycardia).
- Treatment depends on patient symptoms. Withdrawal of sources of stimulation such as caffeine may be warranted. β-Adrenergic blockers may also be used to decrease PACs.

Paroxysmal Supraventricular Tachycardia (PSVT)

PSVT is a dysrhythmia originating in an ectopic focus anywhere above the bifurcation of the bundle of His. Identification of the ectopic focus is often difficult even with a 12-lead ECG, because it requires recording the dysrhythmia as it starts. *Paroxysmal* refers to an abrupt onset and termination. Some degree of AV block may be present. In the normal heart, PSVT is associated with overexertion, emotional stress, deep inspiration, and stimulants such as caffeine and tobacco. PSVT is also associated with rheumatic heart disease, *Wolff-Parkinson-White (WPW) syndrome* (conduction by way of accessory pathways), digitalis intoxication, CAD, and cor pulmonale.

- HR is 150 to 220 beats/minute, and rhythm is regular.
- Clinical significance depends on the associated symptoms. A prolonged episode and HR above 180 beats/minute will cause decreased cardiac output (CO), resulting in hypotension, dyspnea, and angina.
- Treatment includes vagal stimulation and drug therapy. Common vagal maneuvers include Valsalva, carotid massage, and coughing. IV adenosine (Adenocard) is the drug of choice to convert PSVT to a normal sinus rhythm. IV β-adrenergic blockers (e.g., sotalol [Betapace]), calcium channel blockers (e.g., diltiazem [Cardizem]), and amiodarone (Cordarone) can also be used. If vagal stimulation and drug therapy are ineffective and the patient becomes hemodynamically unstable, direct current (DC) cardioversion is used.

Atrial Flutter

This condition is an atrial tachydysrhythmia identified by recurring, regular, sawtooth-shaped flutter waves that originate from a single ectopic focus in the right atrium. Atrial flutter rarely occurs in a normal heart. It is associated with CAD, hypertension, mitral valve disorders, pulmonary embolus, chronic lung disease, cor pulmonale, cardiomyopathy, hyperthyroidism, and the use of drugs such as digoxin, quinidine, and epinephrine.

- The atrial rate is 250 to 350 beats/minute. The ventricular rate varies based on the conduction ratio. In 2:1 conduction, the ventricular rate is typically about 150 beats/minute. Atrial and ventricular rhythms are usually regular.
- High ventricular rates (>100) can decrease CO and cause serious consequences, such as HF.

- The primary treatment goal is to slow ventricular response by increasing AV block. Drugs used to control the ventricular rate include calcium channel blockers and β-adrenergic blockers. Antidysrhythmic drugs used to convert atrial flutter to sinus rhythm or maintain sinus rhythm include amiodarone, ibutilide (Corvert), dronedarone [Multaq]), and flecainide (Tambocor). Electrical cardioversion may be used to convert atrial flutter to sinus rhythm in an emergency situation. Radiofrequency catheter ablation is the treatment of choice for atrial flutter.

Atrial Fibrillation

This condition is a total disorganization of atrial electrical activity because of multiple ectopic foci, resulting in loss of effective atrial contraction. The dysrhythmia may be paroxysmal (i.e., beginning and ending spontaneously) or persistent (lasting >7 days).

Atrial fibrillation is the most common, clinically significant dysrhythmia with respect to morbidity, mortality, and economic impact. It occurs in about 3% of people over age 65, and its prevalence increases with age. Atrial fibrillation usually occurs in the patient with underlying heart disease. It often develops acutely with thyrotoxicosis, alcohol intoxication, caffeine use, electrolyte disturbances, stress, and cardiac surgery.

- The atrial rate may be as high as 350 to 600 beats/minute. The ventricular rate varies, and the rhythm is usually irregular.
- Atrial fibrillation results in a decrease in CO because of ineffective atrial contractions and/or rapid ventricular response. Thrombi form in the atria because of blood stasis. An embolized clot may develop and pass to the brain, causing a stroke.

The goals of treatment include a decrease in ventricular response to <100 beats/minute, prevention of cerebral embolic events, and conversion to sinus rhythm, if possible. Drugs used for rate control include calcium channel blockers (e.g., diltiazem), β-adrenergic blockers (e.g., metoprolol), dronedarone, and digoxin (Lanoxin). The most common antidysrhythmic drugs used for cardioversion to and maintenance of sinus rhythm include amiodarone and ibutilide. Cardioversion may convert atrial fibrillation to normal sinus rhythm.

- If a patient is in atrial fibrillation for longer than 48 hours, anticoagulation therapy with warfarin is needed for 3 to 4 weeks before the cardioversion and for several weeks after successful cardioversion.
- For patients with drug-refractory atrial fibrillation or those who do not respond to electrical conversion, radiofrequency catheter ablation (similar to procedure for atrial flutter) and the Maze procedure (surgical intervention that interrupts ectopic electrical signals) may be used.

First-Degree AV Block
In this type of AV block every impulse from the atria is conducted to the ventricles, but the time of AV conduction is prolonged. After the impulse moves through the AV node, the ventricles usually responded normally. First-degree AV block is associated with MI, CAD, rheumatic fever, hyperthyroidism, vagal stimulation, and drugs such as digoxin, β-adrenergic blockers, calcium channel blockers, and flecainide.

HR is normal, and rhythm is regular.

- First-degree AV block may be a precursor of higher degrees of AV block.
- Patients with first-degree AV block are asymptomatic.
- There is no treatment for first-degree AV block.

Second-Degree AV Block, Type I (Mobitz I, Wenckebach)
A type I, second-degree AV block is characterized by gradual lengthening of the PR interval. It occurs because of an AV conduction time that is prolonged until an atrial impulse is nonconducted and a QRS complex is blocked (missing). Type I AV block may result from use of digoxin or β-adrenergic blockers. It may be associated with CAD. It is usually the result of myocardial ischemia or inferior MI. It is generally transient and well tolerated. However, it may be a warning signal of a more serious AV conduction disturbance (e.g., complete heart block).

- The rhythm appears on the ECG in a pattern of grouped beats.
- If the patient is symptomatic, atropine is used to increase HR, or a temporary pacemaker may be needed, especially if the patient has experienced an MI.

Second-Degree Heart Block, Type II (Mobitz II)
In this type of heart block, the P wave is nonconducted without progressive PR lengthening. This usually occurs when a bundle branch block is present. On conducted beats, the PR interval is constant. In a second-degree heart block a certain number of impulses from the SA node are not conducted to the ventricles. This occurs in ratios of 2:1, 3:1, and so on when there are two P waves to one QRS complex, three P waves to one QRS complex, and so on. It may occur with varying ratios. Type II AV block is associated with rheumatic heart disease, CAD, anterior MI, and drug toxicity.

- The atrial rate is usually normal. The ventricular rate depends on the intrinsic rate and degree of AV block. The atrial rhythm is regular, but the ventricular rhythm may be irregular.
- Type II AV block often progresses to third-degree AV block and is associated with a poor prognosis.
- Reduced HR frequently results in decreased CO with subsequent hypotension and myocardial ischemia.

- Type II AV block is an indication for a permanent pacemaker (see Pacemakers, p. 725).

Third-Degree AV Heart Block (Complete Heart Block)

This condition constitutes one form of AV dissociation in which no impulses from the atria are conducted to the ventricles. The atria are stimulated and contract independently of the ventricles. Ventricular rhythm is an escape rhythm, and focus may be above or below the bifurcation of the bundle of His. This rhythm is associated with severe heart disease, including CAD, MI, myocarditis, cardiomyopathy, and some systemic diseases such as amyloidosis and progressive systemic sclerosis (scleroderma). Some medications can also cause third-degree AV block, such as digoxin, β-adrenergic blockers, and calcium channel blockers.

- Atrial rate is usually a sinus rate of 60 to 100 beats/minute. Ventricular rate depends on the site of the block. If it is in the AV node, the rate is 40 to 60 beats/minute, and if it is in the Purkinje system, it is 20 to 40 beats/minute. Atrial and ventricular rhythms are regular but unrelated to each other.
- Third-degree AV block almost always results in reduced CO with subsequent ischemia and heart failure.
- For symptomatic patients, a temporary transcutaneous pacemaker is used until a permanent pacemaker can be inserted. Use of drugs such as atropine, epinephrine, and dopamine is a temporary measure to increase HR and support blood pressure (BP) before pacemaker insertion (see Pacemakers, p. 725).

Premature Ventricular Contractions (PVCs)

These contractions originate in an ectopic focus in the ventricles. PVCs are a premature occurrence of the QRS complex, which is wide and distorted in shape. PVCs that are initiated from different foci appear different in shape from each other and are termed *multifocal PVCs*. When every other beat is a PVC, it is called *ventricular bigeminy*. When every third beat is a PVC, it is called *ventricular trigeminy*. Two consecutive PVCs are called *couplets*. *Ventricular tachycardia* occurs when there are three or more consecutive PVCs. When a PVC falls on the T wave of a preceding beat, the *R-on-T phenomenon* occurs and is considered to be dangerous because it may precipitate ventricular tachycardia or ventricular fibrillation.

PVCs are associated with stimulants such as caffeine, alcohol, nicotine, epinephrine, isoproterenol, and digoxin. They are also associated with electrolyte imbalances, hypoxia, fever, exercise, and emotional stress. Disease states associated with PVCs include MI, mitral valve prolapse, HF, and CAD.

- HR varies according to the intrinsic rate and the number of PVCs. Rhythm is irregular because of premature beats.

- PVCs are usually not harmful in the patient with a normal heart. In heart disease, PVCs may reduce CO and precipitate angina and HF. PVCs in CAD or acute MI represent ventricular irritability.
- Treatment relates to the cause of the PVCs (e.g., oxygen therapy for hypoxia, electrolyte replacement). Assessing the patient's hemodynamic status is important to determine if drug therapy is indicated. Drug therapy includes β-adrenergic blockers, procainamide, amiodarone, or lidocaine (Xylocaine).

Ventricular Tachycardia (VT)

This dysrhythmia is a run of three or more PVCs that occurs when an ectopic focus or foci fire repetitively and the ventricle takes control as the pacemaker. Different forms of VT exist. The development of VT is an ominous sign. It is a life-threatening dysrhythmia because of decreased CO and the possibility of the development of ventricular fibrillation, which is a lethal dysrhythmia. Ventricular tachycardia is associated with MI, CAD, significant electrolyte imbalances, hypoxemia, cardiomyopathy, mitral valve prolapse, long QT syndrome, digitalis toxicity, and central nervous system disorders. The dysrhythmia can be seen in patients who have no evidence of cardiac disease.

- The ventricular rate is 150 to 250 beats/minute.
- VT can be stable (patient has a pulse) or unstable (patient is pulseless). Sustained VT causes a severe decrease in CO because of decreased ventricular diastolic filling times and loss of atrial contraction. This results in hypotension, pulmonary edema, decreased cerebral blood flow, and cardiopulmonary arrest.
- The dysrhythmia must be treated quickly, even if it occurs only briefly and stops abruptly. Episodes may recur if prophylactic treatment is not started. Ventricular fibrillation may also develop.
- If the patient is hemodynamically stable and has monomorphic VT (QRS complexes have same shape, size, and direction) with preserved left ventricular function, then IV procainamide, sotalol, amiodarone, or lidocaine is used. If the patient is unstable or has poor left ventricular function, amiodarone or lidocaine is given followed by cardioversion.
- If VT is polymorphic (QRS complexes change from one shape, size, or direction over a series of beats) with a normal baseline QT interval, any one of the following medications is used: β-adrenergic blockers, lidocaine, amiodarone, procainamide, or sotalol. Cardioversion is used when drug therapy is ineffective.
- Ventricular tachycardia without a pulse is a lethal dysrhythmia and is treated in the same manner as ventricular fibrillation.

Ventricular Fibrillation (VF)

This condition is a severe derangement of the heart rhythm characterized on the ECG by irregular waveforms of varying shapes and amplitude. This represents the firing of multiple ectopic foci in the ventricle. Mechanically, the ventricle is simply "quivering," and no effective contraction or CO occurs. This dysrhythmia is lethal. VF occurs in acute MI and myocardial ischemia and in chronic diseases such as CAD and cardiomyopathy. It may occur during cardiac pacing or cardiac catheterization procedures because of catheter stimulation of the ventricle. It may also occur with coronary reperfusion after thrombolytic therapy. Other clinical associations are accidental electrical shock, hyperkalemia, hypoxemia, acidosis, and drug toxicity.

- HR is not measurable. Rhythm is irregular and chaotic.
- VF results in an unresponsive, pulseless, and apneic state. If it is not rapidly treated, the patient will die.
- Treatment consists of immediate initiation of cardiopulmonary resuscitation (CPR) and advanced cardiac life support (ACLS) with the use of defibrillation and definitive drug therapy (e.g., epinephrine, vasopressin [Pitressin]). There should be no delay in using a defibrillator once available.

EATING DISORDERS

Description

Eating disorders are primarily psychiatric disorders and occur more often in women. Men are also at risk, but are less likely to seek treatment because eating disorders are perceived to be a women's disease.

Patients with eating disorders may be hospitalized for fluid and electrolyte alterations; cardiac dysrhythmias; nutritional, endocrine, and metabolic disorders; and menstrual problems. A number of nutritional problems associated with these disorders require you to implement a nutritional plan of care.

The three most common types of eating disorders are anorexia nervosa, bulimia nervosa, and binge-eating disorder.

Anorexia Nervosa

Anorexia nervosa is characterized by self-imposed weight loss, endocrine dysfunction, and a distorted psychopathologic attitude toward weight and eating. Anorexia nervosa is a serious mental illness affecting 1.2% to 2.2% of people during their lifetime, and it occurs more frequently in women.

Anorexia nervosa clinically manifests as abnormal weight loss, deliberate self-starvation, intense fear of gaining weight, *lanugo* (soft, downy hair covering the body except the palms and soles), refusal to eat, continuous dieting, hair loss, sensitivity to cold, compulsive exercise, absent or irregular menstruation, dry and yellowish skin, and constipation. Signs of malnutrition are noted during the physical examination.

Diagnostic studies often show iron-deficiency anemia and an elevated blood urea nitrogen level that reflects marked intravascular volume depletion and abnormal renal function.

■ Lack of potassium in the diet and loss of potassium in the urine lead to potassium deficiency. Manifestations of potassium deficiency include muscle weakness, cardiac dysrhythmias, and renal failure.

■ Leukopenia, hypoglycemia, hyponatremia, hypomagnesemia, and hypophosphatemia may also be present.

Interdisciplinary treatment must involve a combination of nutritional support and psychiatric care. Nutritional rehabilitation focuses on reaching and maintaining a healthy weight, normal eating patterns, and perception of hunger and satiety.

Hospitalization may be necessary if the patient has medical complications that cannot be managed in an outpatient therapy program. Nutritional repletion must be closely supervised to ensure consistent and ongoing weight gain. Refeeding syndrome is a rare but serious complication of behavioral refeeding programs. The use of EN or PN may be necessary (see Enteral Nutrition, p. 709, and Parenteral Nutrition, p. 728).

Improved nutrition, however, is not a cure for anorexia nervosa. The underlying psychiatric problem must be addressed by identification of the disturbed patterns of individual and family interactions, followed by individual and family counseling.

Bulimia Nervosa

Bulimia nervosa is a disorder characterized by frequent binge eating and self-induced vomiting associated with loss of control related to eating and a persistent concern with body image. Individuals with bulimia nervosa may have normal weight for height, or their weight may fluctuate with bingeing and purging. They may also abuse laxatives, diuretics, exercise, or diet drugs. They may have signs of frequent vomiting, such as macerated knuckles, swollen salivary glands, broken blood vessels in the eyes, and dental problems.

■ The individual with bulimia nervosa goes to great lengths to conceal abnormal eating habits. Abnormal laboratory parameters, including hypokalemia, metabolic alkalosis, and elevated serum amylase, may occur with frequent vomiting.

The cause of bulimia remains unclear but is thought to be similar to that of anorexia nervosa. Substance abuse, anxiety, affective disorders, and personality disturbances have been reported among people with bulimia.

■ Over time, problems associated with bulimia become increasingly hard to deal with effectively. A treatment combination of psychologic counseling and diet therapy is essential.

- Antidepressants are helpful for some but not all patients with bulimia. Education and emotional support for the patient and the family are vital. Support groups such as the National Association of Anorexia Nervosa and Associated Disorders (ANAD) *(www.anad.org)* are helpful to those affected by these disorders.

Binge-eating disorder is less severe than bulimia nervosa and anorexia nervosa. Individuals with binge-eating disorder do not have a distorted body image and are often overweight or obese.

ENCEPHALITIS

Description

Encephalitis is a serious, sometimes fatal, acute inflammation of the brain. It is usually caused by a virus. Many different viruses have been implicated in encephalitis; some of them are associated with certain seasons of the year and are endemic to certain geographic areas. Ticks and mosquitoes transmit epidemic encephalitis, whereas nonepidemic encephalitis may occur as a complication of measles, chickenpox, or mumps.

- Herpes simplex virus (HSV) encephalitis is the most common form of nonepidemic viral encephalitis.
- Cytomegalovirus encephalitis is one of the common complications in patients with acquired immunodeficiency syndrome (AIDS).

Clinical Manifestations and Diagnostic Studies

The onset of infection is typically nonspecific, with fever, headache, nausea, and vomiting. It can be acute or subacute. Signs of encephalitis appear on day 2 or 3 and may vary from minimal alterations in mental status to coma.

- Almost any central nervous system (CNS) abnormality can occur, including hemiparesis, tremors, seizures, dysphasia, cranial nerve palsies, personality changes, memory impairment, and amnesia.
- Diagnostic findings related to viral encephalitis are shown in Table 36.
- Brain imaging techniques include CT, MRI, and positron emission tomography (PET).
- Polymerase chain reaction (PCR) tests can be used to detect herpes simplex virus (HSV) and West Nile encephalitis.

West Nile virus should be strongly considered in adults older than 50 years who develop encephalitis or meningitis in summer or early fall. The best diagnostic test for West Nile virus is a blood test that detects viral ribonucleic acid (RNA).

Table 36 Comparison of Cerebral Inflammatory Conditions

	Meningitis	Encephalitis	Brain Abscess
Cause	Bacteria (*Streptococcus pneumoniae*, *Neisseria meningitidis*, group B streptococci, viruses, fungi)	Bacteria, fungi, parasites, herpes simplex virus (HSV), other viruses (e.g., West Nile virus)	Streptococci, staphylococci through bloodstream
CSF (Reference Interval)			
▪Pressure (70-150 mm H$_2$O)	Increased	Normal to slight increase	Increased
▪WBC count (0-5 cells/µL)	*Bacterial:* >1000/µL (mainly neutrophils) *Viral:* 25-500/µL (mainly lymphocytes)	500/µL, neutrophils (early), lymphocytes (later)	25-300/µL (neutrophils)
▪Protein (15-45 mg/dL [0.15-0.45 g/L])	*Bacterial:* >500 mg/dL *Viral:* 50-500 mg/dL	Slight increase	Normal
▪Glucose (40-70 mg/dL [2.2-3.9 mmol/L])	*Bacterial:* Decreased *Viral:* Normal or low	Normal	Low or absent
▪Appearance	*Bacterial:* Turbid, cloudy *Viral:* Clear or cloudy	Clear	Clear
Diagnostic studies	CT scan, Gram stain, smear, culture, PCR*	CT scan, EEG, MRI, PET, PCR, IgM antibodies to virus in serum or CSF	CT scan
Treatment	Antibiotics, dexamethasone, supportive care, prevention of ↑ ICP	Supportive care, prevention of ↑ ICP, acyclovir (Zovirax) for HSV	Antibiotics, incision and drainage Supportive care

*PCR is used to detect viral ribonucleic acid (RNA) or deoxyribonucleic acid (DNA).
CSF, Cerebrospinal fluid; *ICP,* intracranial pressure; *PCR,* polymerase chain reaction.

Nursing and Collaborative Management

To prevent encephalitis, mosquito control should be practiced, including cleaning rain gutters, removing old tires, draining bird baths, and removing water where mosquitoes can breed. In addition, insect repellant should be used during mosquito season.

Management of encephalitis, including West Nile virus infection, is symptomatic and supportive. Initially many patients require intensive care. Acyclovir (Zovirax) and vidarabine suspension (Vira-A) are used to treat HSV encephalitis. For maximal benefit, antiviral agents must be started before the onset of coma.

- Prophylactic treatment with antiseizure drugs may be used in severe cases of encephalitis.

ENDOCARDITIS, INFECTIVE

Description

Infective endocarditis (IE) is an infection of the endocardial surface of the heart. The endocardium is the innermost layer of the heart and heart valves. Therefore IE affects the valves. An estimated 10,000 to 15,000 new cases of IE are diagnosed in the United States each year.

Classification

IE can be classified as subacute or acute.

- The *subacute form* typically affects those with preexisting valve disease and has a clinical course that may extend over months.
- The *acute form* typically affects those with healthy valves and presents as a rapidly progressive illness.

IE can also be classified based on the cause (e.g., IV drug abuse, fungal endocarditis) or site of involvement (e.g., prosthetic valve endocarditis).

Pathophysiology

The most common causative agents, *Staphylococcus aureus* and *Streptococcus viridans,* are bacterial. Other pathogens include fungi and viruses.

IE occurs when blood flow turbulence within the heart allows the causative organism to infect previously damaged valves or other endothelial surfaces. This can occur in individuals with a variety of underlying cardiac conditions, including prior endocarditis, prosthetic valves, acquired valve disease, and cardiac lesions. A variety of invasive procedures (e.g., IV drug abuse, renal dialysis) can also allow large numbers of organisms to enter the bloodstream and trigger the infectious process.

Vegetations, the primary lesions of IE, consist of fibrin, leukocytes, platelets, and microbes, which adhere to the valve surface or endocardium. The loss of portions of this vegetation into the circulation results in embolization. Systemic embolization occurs from left-sided heart vegetation, progressing to various organs (e.g., kidney, spleen, brain) and extremities causing limb infarction. Right-sided heart lesions embolize to the lungs, resulting in pulmonary emboli.

The infection may spread locally to cause damage to valves or their supporting structures. This results in dysrhythmias, valve dysfunction, and eventual invasion of the myocardium leading to heart failure (HF), sepsis, and heart block.

At one time rheumatic heart disease was the most common cause of IE. However, now it accounts for less than 20% of cases. The main contributing factors to IE include (1) aging (more than 50% of older people have aortic stenosis), (2) IV drug abuse, (3) use of prosthetic valves, (4) use of intravascular devices resulting in health care–associated infections (e.g., methicillin-resistant *S. aureus* [MRSA]), and (5) renal dialysis.

Clinical Manifestations

The clinical manifestations are nonspecific and can involve multiple organ systems. Low-grade fever occurs in more than 90% of patients.

Nonspecific manifestations include chills, weakness, malaise, fatigue, and anorexia. Arthralgias, myalgias, abdominal discomfort, back pain, weight loss, headache, and clubbing of fingers may occur in subacute forms of endocarditis.

Vascular manifestations include splinter hemorrhages (black longitudinal streaks) that may occur in the nail beds. Petechiae, which may result from fragmentation and microembolization of vegetative lesions, are common in the conjunctivae, lips, buccal mucosa, and palate and over the ankles, feet, and antecubital and popliteal areas. *Osler's nodes* (painful, tender, red or purple, pea-size lesions) may be found on the fingertips or toes. *Janeway lesions* (flat, painless, small, red spots) may be found on the palms and soles. Funduscopic examination may reveal hemorrhagic retinal lesions called *Roth's spots.* Onset of a new or changing murmur is frequently noted, with the aortic and mitral valves most commonly affected.

Clinical manifestations secondary to embolization in various body organs may also be present. These include:

- Embolization to the spleen may result in sharp, left upper quadrant pain and splenomegaly, local tenderness, and abdominal rigidity.
- Embolization to the kidneys may cause pain in the flank, hematuria, and renal failure.

- Emboli may lodge in the small peripheral blood vessels of the arms and legs causing ischemia and gangrene.
- Embolization to the brain may result in hemiplegia, ataxia, aphasia, visual changes, and change in the level of consciousness.
- Pulmonary emboli may occur in right-sided endocarditis.

Diagnostic Studies

A recent health history should be obtained with inquiry made regarding any recent dental, urologic, surgical, or gynecologic procedures including normal or abnormal obstetric delivery. Document any previous history of heart disease, IV drug abuse, recent cardiac catheterization, cardiac surgery, intravascular device placement, renal dialysis, and infections (e.g., skin, respiratory, urinary tract).

- Two blood cultures drawn 30 minutes apart from two different sites will be positive in more than 90% of patients.
- A mild leukocytosis occurs in acute endocarditis.
- Erythrocyte sedimentation rate (ESR) and C-reactive protein (CRP) levels may be elevated.
- Chest x-ray is used to detect an enlarged heart.
- ECG may show first- or second-degree heart block because the valves lie in close proximity to the atrioventricular (AV) node.
- Cardiac catheterization may be used to evaluate valve functioning.

Major criteria to diagnose IE include at least two of the following: positive blood cultures, new or changed cardiac murmur, or intracardiac mass or vegetation noted on echocardiography.

Collaborative Care

Prophylactic Treatment

Antibiotic prophylaxis is recommended for high cardiac risk conditions. These include prosthetic heart valves, history of endocarditis, surgically constructed systemic-pulmonary shunts, and pacemakers.

- Specific antibiotic regimens are recommended for dental, respiratory, GI and genitourinary (GU) procedures (see Table 37-2, Lewis et al, *Medical-Surgical Nursing,* ed. 9, p. 813).

Drug Therapy

Accurate identification of the infecting organism is the key to successful treatment. Complete eradication of the organisms generally takes weeks and relapses are common. Initially patients are hospitalized and IV antibiotic therapy is started.

- Blood cultures are done to evaluate the effectiveness of antibiotic therapy. Blood cultures that remain positive indicate inadequate or inappropriate antibiotic administration, aortic root or myocardial abscess, or the wrong diagnosis (e.g., an infection elsewhere).

- Fever may persist for several days after treatment has been started and is treated with aspirin, acetaminophen, fluids, and rest.
- Complete bed rest is usually not indicated unless the temperature remains elevated or there are signs of heart failure.
- Endocarditis coupled with heart failure responds poorly to antibiotic therapy and valve replacement and is often life threatening.

Nursing Management

Goals

The patient with IE will have normal or baseline cardiac function, perform activities of daily living without fatigue, and know the therapeutic regimen to prevent recurrence of endocarditis.

Nursing Diagnoses

- Decreased cardiac output
- Activity intolerance

Nursing Interventions

The incidence of IE can be decreased by identifying individuals who are at risk for development of the disease. Assessment of the patient's history and an understanding of the disease process are crucial for planning and implementing appropriate health maintenance strategies.

IE generally requires treatment with antibiotics for 4 to 6 weeks. After initial treatment in the hospital, the patient may continue treatment in the home setting if hemodynamically stable and adherent.

- Patients who receive outpatient IV antibiotics require vigilant home nursing care. Instruct the patient or caregiver about the importance of monitoring body temperature because persistent, prolonged temperature elevations may mean that the drug therapy is ineffective. Teach patients and caregivers to recognize signs and symptoms of these complications (e.g., change in mental status, dyspnea, chest pain).
- The patient needs adequate periods of physical and emotional rest. Bed rest may be necessary when fever is present or there are complications (e.g., heart damage). Otherwise the patient may ambulate and perform moderate activity.
- Monitor laboratory data to determine the effectiveness of the antibiotic therapy. Assess IV lines for patency and any signs of complications (e.g., phlebitis). Administer antibiotics as scheduled and monitor the patient for any adverse drug reactions.

- To prevent problems related to decreased mobility, instruct the patient to wear elastic compression gradient stockings, perform range-of-motion (ROM) exercises, and cough and deep breathe every 2 hours.
- The patient may experience anxiety and fear associated with the illness. Recognize this and implement strategies to help the patient cope with the illness.

▼ **Patient and Caregiver Teaching**

- Instruct the patient about symptoms that may indicate recurrent infection, such as fever, fatigue, malaise, and chills, and the importance of notifying the health care provider if they occur.
- Inform the patient about the importance of prophylactic antibiotic therapy before certain invasive procedures.
- Explain to the patient the relationship of follow-up care, good nutrition, and early treatment of common infections (e.g., colds) to maintain good health.

ENDOMETRIAL CANCER

Description

Endometrial cancer is the most common gynecologic malignancy. However, it has a relatively low mortality, because most cases are diagnosed early. The survival rate is 95% if the cancer has not spread at the time of diagnosis.

- The major risk factor for endometrial cancer is estrogen, especially unopposed estrogen. Additional risk factors include increasing age, nulliparity, late menopause, obesity, smoking, and diabetes mellitus (DM), and having a personal or family history of hereditary nonpolyposis colorectal cancer (HNPCC). Pregnancy and oral contraceptives are protective factors.

Pathophysiology

Endometrial cancer arises from the endometrial lining. The precursor may be a hyperplastic state that progresses to invasive carcinoma. Hyperplasia occurs when estrogen is not counteracted by progesterone. The cancer directly extends into the cervix and through the uterine serosa. As invasion of the myometrium occurs, regional lymph nodes, including the paravaginal and paraaortic, become involved. Hematogenous metastases develop concurrently. The usual sites of metastases are the lung, bone, liver, and eventually the brain. Endometrial cancer grows slowly, metastasizes late, and is curable with therapy if diagnosed early.

Clinical Manifestations

- The first sign is abnormal uterine bleeding, usually in postmeno-pausal women. Because perimenopausal women have sporadic periods for a time, it is important that this sign not be ignored or attributed to menopause.
- Pain occurs late in the disease process, and other manifestations that may arise are related to metastasis to other organs.

Diagnostic Studies

Endometrial biopsy is the primary diagnostic procedure for endo-metrial cancer.

- Occurrence of abnormal or unexpected bleeding in a postmeno-pausal woman mandates obtaining a tissue sample to exclude endometrial cancer.
- The Pap test is not a reliable diagnostic tool for endometrial cancer, but it can rule out cervical cancer.

Collaborative Care

Treatment is a total hysterectomy and bilateral salpingo-oophorectomy with lymph node biopsies. Most cases of endome-trial cancer are diagnosed at an early stage when surgery alone may result in cure. Surgery may be followed by radiation, either to the pelvis or abdomen externally or intravaginally, to decrease local recurrence.

Treatment of advanced or recurrent disease is difficult. Proges-terone hormonal therapy (e.g., megestrol [Megace]) is the treat-ment of choice when the progesterone receptor status is positive and the tumor is well differentiated. Tamoxifen (Nolvadex), either alone or in combination with progesterone therapy, is also effec-tive in women with advanced or recurrent endometrial cancer. Chemotherapy is considered when progesterone therapy is unsuc-cessful. Agents used include doxorubicin (Adriamycin), cisplatin (Platinol), 5-fluorouracil (5-FU), carboplatin (Paraplatin), and paclitaxel (Taxol).

Nursing Management: Cancers of the Female Reproductive Tract

See Cervical Cancer, p. 119.

ENDOMETRIOSIS

Description

Endometriosis is the presence of normal endometrial tissue in sites outside the endometrial cavity. The most frequent sites are in or near the ovaries, uterosacral ligaments, and uterovesical peritoneum. Endometrial tissues can also be found in other locations, such as the stomach, lungs, intestines, and spleen. The tissue responds to hormones of the ovarian cycle and undergoes a mini–menstrual cycle similar to that in uterine endometrium. Endometriosis is one of the most common gynecologic problems.

- The typical patient with endometriosis will be in her late twenties or early thirties and has never had a full-term pregnancy.
- Endometriosis is a common cause of infertility and increases the risk of ovarian cancer.

The etiology of endometriosis is unknown. A widely held view is that retrograde menstrual flow passes through the fallopian tubes, carrying viable endometrial tissues into the pelvis and attaching to various sites.

Clinical Manifestations

A wide range of manifestations and severity exists. The magnitude of a woman's symptoms does not necessarily correlate with the clinical extent of her endometriosis.

- The most common symptoms are secondary dysmenorrhea, infertility, pelvic pain, dyspareunia, and irregular bleeding.
- Less common symptoms include backache, painful bowel movements, and dysuria.
- With menopause, estrogen is no longer produced in the ovaries, which may lead to the disappearance of symptoms.

When the ectopic endometrial tissues "menstruate," blood collects in cystlike nodules. When a cyst ruptures, the pain may be acute, and the resulting irritation promotes the formation of adhesions, which attach and fix the affected area to another pelvic structure. The adhesions may become severe enough to cause a bowel obstruction or painful micturition.

Diagnostic Studies

Diagnosis is frequently confirmed by patient history and the palpation of firm nodular lumps in the adnexa on bimanual examination. Laparoscopic examination is necessary for a definitive diagnosis.

Collaborative Care

Treatment is influenced by a patient's age, desire for pregnancy, symptom severity, and the extent and location of the disease. When symptoms are not disruptive, a "watch and wait" approach is used.

Drug Therapy

Drugs are often used to reduce symptoms. Pain may be relieved with nonsteroidal antiinflammatory drugs such as ibuprofen (Advil) and diclofenac (Voltaren). Drugs to inhibit estrogen production by the ovary may be used to shrink the endometrial tissue. These drugs imitate a state of pregnancy or menopause.

- Continuous use (for 9 months) of combined oral contraceptives causes regression of endometrial tissue. Ovulation is suppressed by progestin agents such as medroxyprogesterone (Depo-Provera).
- Another approach to hormonal treatment is danazol (Danocrine), a synthetic androgen that inhibits the anterior pituitary. The drug causes atrophy of ectopic endometrial tissue. Subjective relief of symptoms is noted within 6 weeks of danazol use. Drug expense and side effects of weight gain, acne, hot flashes, and hirsutism restrict its use.
- Another class of drugs used is gonadotropin-releasing hormone (GnRH) agonists, such as leuprolide acetate (Lupron) and na-farelin (Synarel). These drugs result in amenorrhea.

Surgical Therapy

The only cure for endometriosis is surgical removal of all the endometrial implants. Surgical therapy may be conservative or definitive. *Conservative surgery* to confirm the diagnosis or remove implants involves removal or destruction of endometrial implants and lysing or excision of adhesions by means of laparoscopic laser surgery and laparotomy.

- For women wishing to get pregnant, conservative surgical therapy is used to remove implants that may block the fallopian tube. Adhesions are removed from the tubes, ovaries, and pelvic structures.
- *Definitive surgery* involves removal of the uterus, fallopian tubes, ovaries, and as many endometrial implants as possible.

Each woman should be actively involved in making the decision about preserving part or all of her ovaries if surgically possible. Help her to explore her feelings about maintaining her cyclic ovarian function.

Nursing Management

Teach and reassure the patient that a life-threatening situation does not exist, which may permit her to accept a conservative and progressive treatment approach.

- When the symptoms are less severe, teach about nondrug comfort measures that may be helpful.
- Assist the patient to understand the drugs ordered to treat the condition.
- Psychologic support may be needed for the patient experiencing severe disabling pain, sexual difficulties secondary to dyspareunia, and infertility.

- If conservative surgery is the treatment selected, nursing care is similar to general preoperative and postoperative care of a patient undergoing laparotomy (see Abdominal Pain, Acute, pp. 4 to 5).
- If definitive surgery is planned, nursing care is similar to the patient undergoing an abdominal hysterectomy.

ESOPHAGEAL CANCER

Description

Esophageal cancer is uncommon. However, the rates are increasing. Annually in the United States there are approximately 17,500 new cases of esophageal cancer diagnosed and 15,100 deaths from esophageal cancer. The 5-year survival remains low at 35%. Incidence of esophageal cancer increases with age and is higher in men than in women.

Risk factors include Barrett's metaplasia, smoking, excessive alcohol intake, and obesity. Patients with injury to the esophageal mucosa (e.g., from occupational exposure) are at greater risk. *Achalasia,* a condition in which there is delayed emptying of the lower esophagus, is associated with squamous cell cancer.

Pathophysiology

Most esophageal cancers are adenocarcinomas, with the remainder being squamous cell tumors. Adenocarcinomas arise from the glands lining the esophagus and resemble cancers of the stomach and small intestine. The cause of esophageal cancer is unknown.

- Most tumors are located in the middle and lower portions of the esophagus. The tumor may penetrate the muscular layer and extend outside the esophageal wall.
- The malignant tumor usually appears as an ulcerated lesion and has often advanced by the time the patient notices symptoms.
- Obstruction of the esophagus occurs in the later stages.

Clinical Manifestations

The onset of symptoms is usually late relative to tumor growth.

- Progressive dysphagia is the most common symptom and may be expressed as a substernal feeling that food is not passing. Initially dysphagia occurs only with meat, then with soft foods, and eventually with liquids.
- Pain develops late and is described as occurring in the substernal, epigastric, or back areas and usually increases with swallowing. The pain may radiate to the neck, jaw, ears, and shoulders.

E

- If the tumor is in the upper third of the esophagus, symptoms such as sore throat, choking, and hoarseness may occur. Weight loss is fairly common.
- When esophageal stenosis (narrowing) is severe, regurgitation of blood-flecked esophageal contents is common.

Complications may include hemorrhage from cancer eroding through the esophagus and into the aorta. Esophageal perforation into the lung or trachea may also develop. The liver and lung are common metastatic sites.

Diagnostic Studies

- Barium swallow with fluoroscopy may detect esophageal narrowing at the tumor site.
- Endoscopic biopsy is used to make a definitive diagnosis.
- Endoscopic ultrasonography is used for staging.
- Bronchoscopy detects lung involvement.
- CT scan and MRI assess the extent of disease.

Collaborative Care

Treatment depends on tumor location and whether metastasis has occurred. The best results may be obtained with a combination of surgery, endoscopic ablation, chemotherapy, and radiation.

- The surgical approaches may be open (thoracic, abdominal incision) or laparoscopic. Minimally invasive esophagectomy (e.g., laparoscopic vagal nerve–sparing surgery) is also being performed.
- Endoscopic approaches using photodynamic and/or laser therapy are also used.

Concurrent radiation and chemotherapy are used for palliation of symptoms, especially dysphagia, as well as to increase survival. Palliative therapy consists of restoration of the swallowing function and maintenance of nutrition and hydration. Dilation, stent placement, or both can relieve obstruction.

Nutritional Therapy

After esophageal surgery, parenteral fluids are given. A swallowing study is often done before the patient is allowed to have oral fluids. When fluids are permitted, water (30 to 60 mL) is given hourly, with gradual progression to small, frequent, bland meals. The patient should be in an upright position to prevent fluid regurgitation. Observe the patient for signs of intolerance to the feeding or leakage of the feeding into the mediastinum. Symptoms indicating leakage are pain, increased temperature, and dyspnea. A gastrostomy may be performed for the purpose of feeding the patient.

Nursing Management
Goals
The patient with esophageal cancer will have relief of symptoms, including pain and dysphagia, achieve optimal nutritional intake, understand the prognosis of the disease, and experience a quality of life appropriate to disease progression.
Nursing Diagnoses
- Imbalanced nutrition: less than body requirements
- Chronic pain
- Ineffective health maintenance
- Anxiety and grieving
Nursing Interventions
In addition to general preoperative teaching and preparation, pay particular attention to the patient's nutritional needs. Many patients are poorly nourished because of the inability to ingest adequate amounts and fluids. Meticulous oral care is essential. Teaching should include information about chest tubes (if a thoracic approach is used), IV lines, nasogastric (NG) tube, gastrostomy or jejunostomy feeding, turning, coughing, and deep breathing.

Postoperative care should include assessment of drainage; maintenance of the NG tube; oral and nasal care; and prevention of respiratory complications by turning, coughing, and deep breathing, incentive spirometry every 2 hours, and placing the patient in a semi-Fowler's position to prevent gastric reflux and aspiration.

Many patients require long-term follow-up care after surgery for esophageal cancer. The patient may undergo chemotherapy and radiation treatment after surgery. Encourage and assist the patient in maintaining adequate nutrition. A permanent feeding gastrostomy may be needed. The patient usually has fears and anxieties about a diagnosis of cancer.
- Know what the physician has told the patient regarding the prognosis and then provide appropriate counseling.
- Referral to a home health nurse may be needed for continued care of the patient (e.g., gastrostomy teaching and follow-up wound care).

▼ Patient and Caregiver Teaching
- Health promotion includes regular follow-up evaluation for patients diagnosed with gastroesophageal reflux disease (GERD), Barrett's esophagus, and hiatal hernia.
- Health counseling should focus on the elimination of smoking and excessive alcohol intake.
- Encourage patients to seek medical attention for any esophageal problems, especially dysphagia.
- Maintenance of good oral hygiene and dietary habits (intake of fresh fruits and vegetables) are important.

FIBROCYSTIC BREAST CHANGES

Description

Fibrocystic breast changes include the development of excess fibrous tissue, hyperplasia of the epithelial lining of the mammary ducts, proliferation of mammary ducts, and cyst formation. These benign changes are the most frequently occurring breast disorder. Fibrocystic changes occur most frequently in women between 35 and 50 years old, but often begin as early as 20 years old. They are not associated alone with increased breast cancer risk.

Fibrocystic changes most commonly occur in women with premenstrual abnormalities, nulliparous women, women with a history of spontaneous abortion, nonusers of oral contraceptives, and women with early menarche and late menopause.

Pathophysiology

Fibrocystic changes are thought to be heightened responsiveness of breast tissue to circulating estrogen and progesterone. These changes produce pain by nerve irritation from connective tissue edema and fibrosis from nerve pinching.

- Masses or nodularities can appear in both breasts and are often found in the upper, outer quadrants. They usually occur bilaterally.
- Symptoms of fibrocystic changes often worsen in the premenstrual phase and subside after menstruation.

Clinical Manifestations

Manifestations of fibrocystic breast changes include one or more palpable lumps that are usually round, well delineated, and freely movable within the breast. Discomfort ranging from tenderness to pain may also occur.

- The lump usually increases in size and perhaps in tenderness before menstruation. Cysts may enlarge or shrink rapidly.
- Nipple discharge associated with fibrocystic breasts is often milky, watery-milky, yellow, or green.
- Pain and nodularity often increase over time, but tend to subside after menopause unless high doses of estrogen replacement are used.

Mammography may be helpful in distinguishing fibrocystic changes from breast cancer. However, in some women the breast tissue is so dense that it is difficult to obtain a mammogram. In these situations, ultrasound may be more useful in differentiating a cystic mass from a solid mass.

Nursing and Collaborative Management

With the initial discovery of a discrete breast mass, aspiration or surgical biopsy may be indicated. If the nodularity is recurrent, a wait of 7 to 10 days may be planned to note any changes related to the menstrual cycle.

- An excisional biopsy should be done if no fluid is found on aspiration, the fluid that is found is hemorrhagic, or a residual mass remains after fluid aspiration.

Many types of treatment have been suggested for a fibrocystic condition. Some relief may occur if the changes are cyclic with caffeine and coffee and dietary fat reduction; taking vitamins E, A, and B complex and gamma-linolenic acid (evening primrose oil); and the continual wearing of a support bra. Drugs might be recommended, including oral contraceptives and danazol (Danocrine).

Patient and Caregiver Teaching

Your role in the care of the patient with fibrocystic breast changes is primarily one of teaching.

- Teach the patient that she may expect recurrences of the cysts in one or both breasts until menopause, and cysts may enlarge or become painful just before menstruation. In addition, offer reassurance that cysts do not "turn into" cancer.
- Encourage the woman with cystic changes to for regular follow-up care. Also teach her breast self-examination (BSE) to self-monitor changes. Severe fibrocystic changes may make palpation of the breast more difficult. Teach her to report any changes in symptoms or changes found during the BSE so they can be evaluated.

FIBROMYALGIA

Description

Fibromyalgia is a chronic disorder characterized by widespread, nonarticular musculoskeletal pain and fatigue with multiple tender points. People with fibromyalgia may also experience nonrestorative sleep, morning stiffness, irritable bowel syndrome, and anxiety. Fibromyalgia is a commonly diagnosed musculoskeletal disorder and a major cause of disability. It affects an estimated 5 million Americans, 75% to 90% of them women.

Fibromyalgia and chronic fatigue syndrome (CFS) share many commonalities (see Table 25, p. 131).

Pathophysiology

There is general agreement that fibromyalgia is a disorder involving neuroendocrine/neurotransmitter dysregulation. The pain amplification experienced by the affected patient is caused by abnormal sensory processing in the central nervous system.

Multiple physiologic abnormalities have been found, including increased levels of substance P in the spinal fluid, low levels of blood flow to the thalamus, dysfunction of the hypothalamic-pituitary-adrenal (HPA) axis, low levels of serotonin and tryptophan, and abnormalities in cytokine function.

- Serotonin and substance P play a role in mood regulation, sleep, and pain perception. Changes in the HPA axis can lead to depression and a decreased response to stress.
- Genetic factors also contribute to the etiology of fibromyalgia, as a familial tendency exists.
- A recent viral illness or Lyme disease may serve as an infectious trigger in susceptible people.

Clinical Manifestations

The patient complains of a widespread burning pain that worsens and improves through the course of a day. It is often difficult for the patient to discriminate whether pain occurs in the muscles, joints, or soft tissues.

- Head or facial pain often results from stiff or painful neck and shoulder muscles. This pain can accompany temporomandibular joint dysfunction. Physical examination characteristically reveals point tenderness at 11 or more of 18 identified sites (Fig. 5).
- Cognitive effects range from difficulty concentrating to memory lapses and a feeling of being overwhelmed when dealing with multiple tasks. Many individuals report migraine headaches, depression, and anxiety.
- Numbness or tingling in the hands or feet (paresthesia) often accompanies fibromyalgia. Restless legs syndrome is also common.
- Women with fibromyalgia may experience more difficult menstruation, with a worsening of disease symptoms during this time.
- Irritable bowel syndrome with manifestations of diarrhea or constipation, abdominal pain, and bloating can occur. In addition, increased frequency of urination and urinary urgency may occur.

Diagnostic Studies

A definitive diagnosis is often difficult to establish. Laboratory results may serve to rule out other suspected disorders.

- Occasionally a low antinuclear antibody (ANA) titer is found, but it is not considered diagnostic.
- Muscle biopsy may reveal a nonspecific moth-eaten appearance or fiber atrophy.

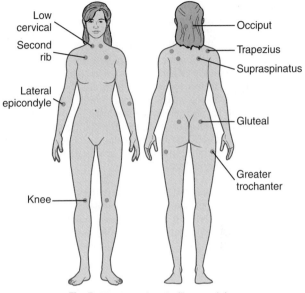

Low cervical
Second rib
Lateral epicondyle
Knee
Occiput
Trapezius
Supraspinatus
Gluteal
Greater trochanter

Fig. 5. Tender points in fibromyalgia.

The American College of Rheumatology classifies an individual as having fibromyalgia if two criteria are met: (1) pain experienced in 11 of the 18 tender points on palpation and (2) a history of widespread pain for at least 3 months.

Collaborative Care

Treatment is symptomatic and requires a high level of patient motivation. You have a key role in teaching the patient to be an active participant in the therapeutic regimen. Rest can help pain, aching, and tenderness.

Drug therapy for the chronic widespread pain associated with fibromyalgia includes pregabalin (Lyrica), duloxetine (Cymbalta), and milnacipran (Savella). Low-dose tricyclic antidepressants, selective serotonin reuptake inhibitors (SSRIs), or benzodiazepines (e.g., diazepam ([Valium]) may also be prescribed. If the tricyclic antidepressant amitriptyline (Elavil) is not well tolerated, other similar drugs can be substituted, such as doxepin (Sinequan), imipramine (Tofranil), or trazodone (Desyrel).

- SSRI antidepressants (e.g., sertraline [Zoloft] or paroxetine [Paxil]) tend to be reserved for fibromyalgia patients who also have depression. Both antidepressants and muscle relaxants (e.g., cyclobenzaprine [Flexeril]) have sedative effects that can help in improving nighttime rest for the patient with fibromyalgia.
- Long-acting opioids generally are not recommended unless fibromyalgia is refractory to other therapies.
- In some patients, pain may be managed with over-the-counter (OTC) analgesics such as acetaminophen (Tylenol), ibuprofen (Motrin, Advil), or naproxen (Aleve). Nonopioids such as tramadol (Ultram) also may be used. In addition, zolpidem (Ambien) is sometimes prescribed for short-term intervention in the patient with severe sleep problems.

Nursing and Collaborative Management

Because of the chronic nature of fibromyalgia and the need to maintain an ongoing rehabilitation program, the patient needs consistent support from you and the other health care team members. Massage is often combined with ultrasound or the application of alternating heat and cold packs to soothe tense, sore muscles and increase blood circulation.

- Gentle stretching can be performed by a physical therapist or practiced by the patient at home to relieve muscle tension and spasm.
- Dietitians often urge fibromyalgia patients to limit their consumption of sugar, caffeine, and alcohol, because these substances have been shown to be muscle irritants.
- Pain and the related symptoms of fibromyalgia can cause significant stress. Patients with fibromyalgia may not deal very effectively with stress. Effective relaxation strategies include biofeedback, guided imagery, and autogenic training. Psychologic counseling (individual or group) may also prove beneficial for the patient.

FLAIL CHEST

Description

Flail chest results from the fracture of several consecutive ribs in two or more separate locations that cause an unstable segment.

Pathophysiology

The affected (flail) area moves in the opposite direction with respect to the intact portion of the chest. During inspiration, the affected portion is sucked in, and during expiration it bulges out. This paradoxic chest movement prevents adequate ventilation of the lung in the injured area and increases the work of breathing.

Clinical Manifestations and Diagnostic Studies

A flail chest is usually apparent on visual examination of the unconscious patient.

- The patient manifests rapid, shallow respirations and tachycardia.
- A flail chest may not be initially apparent in the conscious patient as a result of splinting of the chest wall. The patient moves air poorly, and movement of the thorax is asymmetric and uncoordinated.
- Palpation of abnormal respiratory movements, evaluation for crepitus near the rib fractures, chest x-ray, and arterial blood gases (ABGs) all assist in the diagnosis.

Collaborative Care

Initial therapy consists of airway management, adequate ventilation, supplemental oxygen therapy, careful administration of IV solutions, and pain control. Definitive therapy is to reexpand the lung and ensure adequate oxygenation. Although many patients can be managed without mechanical ventilation, intubation and ventilation may be necessary. Surgical fixation of the flail segment may be done. Lung parenchyma and fractured ribs will heal with time.

F

FRACTURE

Description

A *fracture* is a disruption or break in the continuity of the structure of bone. Traumatic injuries account for the majority of fractures, although some fractures are secondary to a disease process (pathologic fractures from cancer or osteoporosis).

Fractures can be classified as *open* (formerly called compound) or *closed* (formerly called simple) depending on communication or noncommunication with the external environment. In an open fracture, the skin is broken, exposing the bone and causing soft tissue injury. In a closed fracture, the skin has not been ruptured and remains intact.

- Fractures can also be classified as complete or incomplete. Fractures are termed *complete* if the break is completely through the bone and described as *incomplete* if the fracture occurs partly across a bone shaft but the bone is still in one piece. An incomplete fracture is often the result of bending or crushing forces applied to a bone.
- Fractures are also described and classified according to the direction of the fracture line. Types include linear, oblique, transverse, longitudinal, and spiral fractures.

- Fractures can also be classified as *displaced* or *nondisplaced*. In a displaced fracture the two ends of the broken bone are separated from one another and out of their normal positions. Displaced fractures are usually comminuted (more than two fragments) or oblique. In a nondisplaced fracture the periosteum is intact across the fracture and the bone is still in alignment. Nondisplaced fractures are usually transverse, spiral, or greenstick.

Illustrations of the various classifications of fractures can be found in Figs. 63-6 and 63-7 in Lewis et al, *Medical-Surgical Nursing,* ed. 9, p. 1512.

Clinical Manifestations

The clinical manifestations include immediate localized pain, decreased function, and inability to bear weight on or use the affected part.

- The patient guards and protects the extremity against movement. Obvious bone deformity may not be present.
- If a fracture is suspected, the extremity is immobilized in the position in which it is found. Unnecessary movement increases soft tissue damage and may convert a closed fracture to an open fracture or create further injury to adjacent neurovascular structures.

Complications

The majority of fractures heal without complications. If death occurs after a fracture, it is usually the result of damage to underlying organs and vascular structures or from complications of the fracture or immobility.

- Direct complications include problems with bone union, avascular necrosis, and bone infection.
- Indirect complications are associated with blood vessel and nerve damage resulting in conditions such as compartment syndrome, venous thromboembolism, rhabdomyolysis, fat embolism, and traumatic or hypovolemic shock. A discussion of these complications is in Lewis et al, *Medical-Surgical Nursing,* ed. 9, pp. 1522 to 1523. Hypovolemic shock may also occur (see Shock, p. 566).
- Although most musculoskeletal injuries are not life threatening, open fractures or fractures accompanied by severe blood loss and fractures that damage vital organs (e.g., lung, heart) are medical emergencies requiring immediate attention.

Open fractures and soft tissue injuries have a high incidence of infection. Devitalized and contaminated tissue is an ideal medium for many common pathogens, including gas-forming (anaerobic) bacilli.

Diagnostic Studies
- History and physical examination
- X-ray examination
- CT scan and MRI.

Collaborative Care
The goals of treatment are anatomic realignment of bone fragments (reduction), immobilization to maintain realignment, and restoration of function of the injured part.

Fracture Reduction

Closed reduction is a nonsurgical, manual realignment of bones to their previous anatomic position. Traction and countertraction are manually applied to bone fragments to restore position, length, and alignment.
- Closed reduction is usually performed with the patient under local or general anesthesia. After reduction, the injured part is immobilized by casting, traction, external fixation, splints, or orthoses (braces) to maintain alignment until healing occurs.

Open reduction is correction of bone alignment through a surgical incision. It usually includes internal fixation of the fracture with the use of wires, screws, pins, plates, intramedullary rods, or nails.
- Open reduction with internal fixation (ORIF) facilitates early ambulation, which decreases the risk of complications related to prolonged immobility. If ORIF is used for intraarticular fractures, early initiation of range of motion of the joint is indicated. Machines that provide continuous passive motion (CPM) to various joints are used to prevent extraarticular and intraarticular adhesions.

Traction devices apply a pulling force on the fractured extremity while countertraction pulls in the opposite direction. The two most common types of traction are skin traction and skeletal traction.
- *Skin traction* is generally used for short-term treatment (48 to 72 hours) until skeletal traction or surgery is possible. Tape, boots, or slings are applied directly to the skin to maintain alignment, assist in reduction, and help diminish muscle spasms in the injured extremity. A *Buck's traction* boot is a type of skin traction that is used to immobilize a fracture, prevent hip flexion contractures, and reduce muscle spasms.
- *Skeletal traction,* generally in place for longer periods, is used to align injured bones and joints or treat joint contractures and congenital hip dysplasia. It provides a long-term pull that keeps injured bones and joints aligned. Skeletal traction requires the insertion of a pin or wire into the bone to align and immobilize the injured body part. Fracture alignment depends

on correct positioning and alignment of the patient, whereas traction forces remain constant. For extremity traction to be effective, forces must be pulling in the opposite direction *(countertraction)*.

- Countertraction is commonly supplied by the patient's body weight or may be augmented by elevating the end of the bed.

Fracture Immobilization

Casting may occur after closed reduction has been performed. It allows the patient to perform many normal activities of daily living (ADLs) while providing sufficient immobilization to ensure stability.

Immobilization of an acute fracture or soft tissue injury of the upper extremity is often accomplished by use of (1) the sugar-tong splint, (2) the posterior splint, (3) the short arm cast, or (4) the long arm cast. A discussion of these casts is in Lewis et al, *Medical-Surgical Nursing,* ed. 9, p. 1515.

An *external fixator* is a metal device composed of metal pins that are inserted into the bone and attached to external rods to stabilize the fracture while it heals. It can be used to apply traction or to immobilize reduced fragments when the use of a cast or traction is not appropriate. The external fixator is attached directly to the bones by percutaneous pins or wires. Ongoing assessment for pin loosening and infection is critical. Infection signaled by exudate, redness, tenderness, and pain may require removal of the device.

Internal fixation devices (pins, plates, intramedullary rods, and metal and bioabsorbable screws) are surgically inserted to realign and maintain bony fragments. These metal devices are biologically inert and made from stainless steel, vitallium, or titanium. Proper alignment is evaluated by x-ray studies at regular intervals.

Other Therapy

Electrical bone growth stimulation may be used to facilitate the healing process for certain types of fractures, especially when there is nonunion or delayed healing.

Central and peripheral muscle relaxants, such as carisoprodol (Soma), cyclobenzaprine (Flexeril), or methocarbamol (Robaxin), may be prescribed for relief of pain associated with muscle spasms.

In an open fracture, the threat of tetanus can be reduced with tetanus and diphtheria toxoid or tetanus immunoglobulin for the patient who has not been previously immunized. Bone-penetrating antibiotics, such as a cephalosporin (e.g., cefazolin [Kefzol, Ancef]), are used prophylactically before surgery.

Proper nutrition is an essential component of the reparative process in injured tissue. The patient's diet must include ample protein (e.g., 1 g/kg body weight), vitamins (especially B, C, and D), and calcium, phosphorus, and magnesium.

Nursing Management

Goals
The patient with a fracture will have healing with no associated complications, obtain satisfactory pain relief, and achieve maximal rehabilitation potential.

Nursing Diagnoses
- Impaired physical mobility
- Risk for peripheral neurovascular dysfunction
- Acute pain
- Readiness for enhanced self-health management

Nursing Interventions
Patients with fractures may be treated in an emergency department or physician's office and released to home care, or they may require hospitalization. Specific nursing measures depend on the type of treatment used and setting in which patients are placed.

Preoperative Management. If surgical intervention is required to treat the fracture, patients will need preoperative preparation. In addition to the usual preoperative nursing measures, inform patients of the type of immobilization and assistive devices that will be used and the expected activity limitations after surgery.

- Assure patients that their needs will be met by the nursing staff until they can again meet their own needs. Knowing that pain medication will be available if needed is often beneficial.

Postoperative Management. Frequent neurovascular assessments of the affected extremity are necessary to detect early and subtle changes. Closely monitor any limitations of movement or activity related to turning, positioning, and extremity support.

- Pain and discomfort can be minimized through proper alignment and positioning.
- Carefully observe dressings or casts for any overt signs of bleeding or drainage. Report a significant increase in the size of the drainage area.
- If a wound drainage system is in place, regularly assess the patency of the system and the volume of drainage. Whenever the contents of a drainage system are measured or emptied, use sterile technique to avoid contamination.

Plan care to prevent complications of immobility if the patient is immobilized as a result of the fracture. Prevent constipation by increased activity, maintenance of a high fluid intake, and a diet high in bulk and roughage. If these measures are not effective in maintaining the patient's normal bowel pattern, stool softeners, laxatives, or suppositories may be necessary. Maintain a regular time for elimination to promote regularity.

- Renal calculi can develop as a result of bone demineralization. Unless contraindicated, a fluid intake of 2500 mL/day is recommended.
- Rapid deconditioning of the cardiovascular system can occur as a result of prolonged bed rest, resulting in orthostatic hypotension and decreased lung capacity. Unless contraindicated, these effects can be diminished by having the patient sit on the side of the bed, allowing the patient's lower limbs to dangle over the bedside, and having the patient perform standing transfers.
- When the patient is allowed to increase activity, assess for orthostatic hypotension. Also assess patients for deep vein thrombosis (DVT) and pulmonary emboli.

When slings are used with traction, inspect exposed skin areas regularly. Observe skeletal traction pin sites for signs of infection. Pin site care varies but usually includes regular removal of exudate with half-strength hydrogen peroxide, rinsing pin sites with sterile saline, and drying of area with sterile gauze.

▼ **Patient and Caregiver Teaching**

Patient and caregiver teaching are important to prevent complications. In addition to specific instructions for cast care and recognition of complications, encourage the patient to contact the health care provider if questions arise. Validate patient and caregiver understanding of these instructions before discharge.

For further information on rehabilitation management of fractures, including the use of assistive devices such as walkers and crutches, see Lewis et al, *Medical-Surgical Nursing,* ed. 9, p. 1521, and also the specific types of fractures discussed in this *Companion.*

FRACTURE, HIP

Description

Hip fractures are common in older adults, with 90% of these due to a fall. By age 90, approximately 33% of all women and 17% of all men will have sustained a hip fracture. In adults more than 65 years old, hip fracture occurs more frequently in women than in men because of osteoporosis. Many older adults with a hip fracture develop disabilities that require long-term care.

A fracture of the hip refers to a fracture of the proximal (upper) third of the femur, which extends up to 5 cm below the lesser trochanter.

- Fractures that occur within the hip joint capsule are called *intracapsular fractures*. Intracapsular fractures (femoral neck) are further identified by their specific locations: capital, subcapital, and transcervical. These fractures are associated with osteoporosis and minor trauma.

▪ *Extracapsular fractures* occur outside the joint capsule. They are termed intertrochanteric if they occur in a region between the greater and lesser trochanter or subtrochanteric if they occur in the region below the lesser trochanter. Extracapsular fractures are usually caused by severe direct trauma or a fall.

Clinical Manifestations

Manifestations of a hip fracture are external rotation, muscle spasm, shortening of the affected extremity, and severe pain and tenderness in the region of the fracture site. Displaced femoral neck fractures cause serious disruption of the blood supply to the femoral head, which can result in avascular necrosis.

Collaborative Care

Initially the affected extremity may be temporarily immobilized by Buck's traction until the patient's physical condition is stabilized and surgery can be performed. Buck's traction relieves painful muscle spasms and is used for up to a maximum of 24 to 48 hours.

Surgical treatment permits early mobilization of the patient and decreases the risk of major complications. The type of surgery depends on the location of the fracture, the severity of the fracture, and the person's age.

▪ Surgical options include (1) repair with internal fixation devices (e.g., hip compression screw, intramedullary devices), (2) replacement of part of the femur with a prosthesis (partial hip replacement), and (3) total hip replacement (involves both the femur and acetabulum).

These types of surgical repair are shown in Figs. 63-18 and 63-19 in Lewis et al, *Medical-Surgical Nursing,* ed. 9, p. 1525.

Nursing Management

Preoperative Management

Before surgery, severe muscle spasms can increase pain. Appropriate analgesics or muscle relaxants, comfortable positioning unless contraindicated, and properly adjusted traction can help manage spasms.

▪ When possible, teach the patient the method and frequency for exercising the unaffected leg and both arms. Encourage the patient to use the overhead trapeze bar and opposite side rail to assist in changing positions. A physical therapist can begin to teach out-of-bed and chair transfers.

▪ Inform the caregiver about the patient's weight-bearing status after surgery. Plans for discharge begin as the patient enters the hospital, because the length of postoperative stay is only a few days.

Postoperative Management

The principles of patient care for any of the surgical procedures for hip fractures are similar. In the initial postoperative period, assess vital signs and intake and output, monitor respiratory activities such as deep breathing and coughing, administer pain medication, and observe the dressing and incision for signs of bleeding and infection.

In the early postoperative period there is potential for neurovascular impairment. Assess the patient's extremity for motor function, temperature and color, sensation, distal pulses, capillary refill, edema, and pain.

- Edema is alleviated by elevation of the leg whenever the patient is in a chair.
- Pain resulting from poor alignment of the affected extremity can be prevented by keeping pillows (or an abductor splint) between the knees when the patient is turning to either side. Sandbags and pillows are also used to prevent external rotation.
- If the hip fracture has been treated by insertion of a prosthesis with a *posterior approach* (accessing the hip joint from the back), measures to prevent dislocation must be used (Table 37).

Table 37	Patient and Caregiver Teaching Guide *Hip Replacement**

After a hip replacement include the following instructions when teaching a patient and caregiver.

Do	Do Not
▪ Use an elevated toilet seat.	▪ Force hip into greater than 90 degrees of flexion (e.g., sitting in low chairs or toilet seats).
▪ Place chair inside shower or tub and remain seated while washing.	
▪ Use pillow between legs for first 6 wk after surgery when lying on nonoperative side or when supine.	▪ Force hip into adduction.
	▪ Force hip into internal rotation.
▪ Keep hip in neutral, straight position when sitting, walking, or lying.	▪ Cross legs at knees or ankles.
▪ Notify surgeon if severe pain, deformity, or loss of function occurs.	▪ Put on own shoes or stockings without adaptive device (e.g., long-handled shoehorn or stocking-helper) until 4-6 wk after surgery.
▪ Inform dentist of presence of prosthesis before dental work so that prophylactic antibiotics can be given if indicated.	▪ Sit on chairs without arms. They are needed to aid rising to a standing position.

*For patients having surgery by a posterior approach.

- The patient and caregiver must be fully aware of positions and activities that predispose the patient to dislocation (>90 degrees of flexion, abduction, or internal rotation). Many daily activities may reproduce these positions, including putting on shoes and socks, crossing legs or feet while seated, assuming the side-lying position incorrectly, standing up or sitting down while the body is flexed more than 90 degrees relative to the chair, and sitting on low seats, especially low toilet seats.
- Until the soft tissue capsule surrounding the hip has healed sufficiently to stabilize the prosthesis, teach the patient to avoid these activities, usually for at least 6 weeks.

In addition to teaching the patient and caregiver how to prevent prosthesis dislocation, you should also place a large pillow between the patient's legs when turning, avoid extreme hip flexion, and avoid turning the patient on the affected side until it is approved by the surgeon. Some health care providers prefer that patients keep leg abductor splints on except when bathing.

When the hip fracture is accessed during surgery with an *anterior approach* (joint reached from front of body), the hip muscles are left intact. This approach generally results in a more stable hip in the postoperative period with a lower rate of complications. Patient precautions related to motion and weight bearing are few and may include instructions to avoid hyperextension.

The patient is usually out of bed on the first postoperative day. In collaboration with the physical therapist, monitor the patient's ambulation status for proper crutch walking or use of the walker. For the patient to be discharged home, have the patient demonstrate the proper use of crutches or a walker, the ability to transfer into and from a chair and bed, and the ability to ascend and descend stairs.

- Sudden severe pain, a lump in the buttock, limb shortening, and extreme external rotation indicate prosthesis dislocation. This requires a closed reduction or open reduction to realign the femoral head in the acetabulum.

Assist both the patient and caregiver in adjusting to the restrictions and dependence imposed by the hip fracture. Depression can easily occur, but creative nursing care and awareness of the problem can do much to prevent it.

- Inform the patient and caregiver about community referral services that can assist in the postdischarge rehabilitation phase.
- Hospitalization averages 3 or 4 days. Patients frequently require care in a subacute unit, skilled nursing facility, or rehabilitation facility for a few weeks before returning home.

Home care considerations include ongoing assessment of pain management, monitoring for infection, and prevention of deep vein thrombosis (DVT).

FRACTURE, HUMERUS

Fractures involving the shaft of the humerus are a common injury among young and middle-aged adults. Clinical manifestations are an obvious displacement of the humeral shaft, shortened extremity, abnormal mobility, and pain.

- Major complications are radial nerve injury and vascular injury to the brachial artery as a result of laceration, transection, or muscle spasm.

Treatment for a fracture of the humerus depends on the location and displacement of the fracture.

- Nonoperative treatment may include a hanging arm cast, shoulder immobilizer, or the sling and swathe, which is a type of immobilization that prevents glenohumeral movement.

When these devices are used, elevate the head of the bed to assist gravity in reducing the fracture. Allow the arm to hang freely when the patient is sitting and standing.

Include measures in your care to protect the axilla and prevent skin maceration. Carefully place lightly powdered absorption pads in the axilla and change them twice daily or as needed.

- Skin or skeletal traction may be used for purposes of reduction and immobilization.
- During the rehabilitative phase, an exercise program geared toward improving strength and motion of the injured extremity is extremely important. This program should include assisted motion of the hands and fingers. The shoulder can also be exercised to prevent stiffness if the fracture is stable. This helps to prevent stiffness secondary to frozen shoulder or fibrosis of the shoulder capsule.

FRACTURE, PELVIS

Pelvic fractures range from benign to life threatening, depending on the mechanism of injury and associated vascular insult. Although only a small percentage of all fractures are pelvic fractures, this type of injury is associated with a high mortality rate. Preoccupation with more obvious injuries at the time of a traumatic event may result in pelvic injuries being overlooked.

- Pelvic fractures may cause serious intraabdominal injury, such as paralytic ileus, hemorrhage, and laceration of the urethra, bladder, or colon. Patients may survive the initial pelvic injury, only to die from complications such as sepsis, fat embolism syndrome, or thromboembolism.

- Pelvic fractures are diagnosed by x-ray and CT
- Physical examination of the abdomen demonstrates local swelling, tenderness, deformity, unusual pelvic movement, and ecchymosis.

Treatment of pelvic fractures depends on the severity of the injury. Bed rest for stable pelvic fractures is maintained from a few days to 6 weeks. More complex fractures may be treated with pelvic sling traction, skeletal traction, hip spica casts, external fixation, open reduction, or a combination of these methods. Open reduction and internal fixation of a pelvic fracture may be necessary if the fracture is displaced.

- Extreme care in handling or moving the patient is important to prevent serious injury from a displaced fracture fragment. Only turn the patient when ordered by the health care provider. Because a pelvic fracture can damage other organs, assess bowel and urinary tract function, as well as distal neurovascular status.
- Provide back care while the patient is raised from the bed, with either independent use of the trapeze or adequate assistance.

GASTRITIS

Description

Gastritis, an inflammation of the gastric mucosa, is one of the most common problems affecting the stomach. Gastritis may be acute or chronic and diffuse or localized.

Pathophysiology

Gastritis occurs as the result of a breakdown in the normal gastric mucosal barrier. This mucosal barrier normally protects the stomach tissue from the corrosive action of HCl acid and pepsin. When the barrier is broken, HCl acid and pepsin can diffuse back into the mucosa. This back diffusion results in tissue edema, disruption of capillary walls with plasma lost into the gastric lumen, and possible hemorrhage.

Drugs contribute to the development of acute and chronic gastritis. Nonsteroidal antiinflammatory drugs (NSAIDs), including aspirin, and corticosteroids inhibit the synthesis of prostaglandins that are protective to the gastric mucosa, making the mucosa more susceptible to injury. Risk factors for NSAID-induced gastritis include being female; being over age 60; having a history of ulcer disease; taking anticoagulants, other NSAIDs (including low-dose aspirin), or other ulcerogenic drugs (including corticosteroids); and having a chronic debilitating disorder such as cardiovascular disease.

Repeated alcohol abuse results in chronic gastritis. Eating large quantities of spicy, irritating foods and metabolic conditions such as renal failure can also cause acute gastritis.

Another cause of chronic gastritis is *Helicobacter pylori* infection, which is highest in underdeveloped countries and in people of low socioeconomic status.

Autoimmune metaplastic atrophic gastritis (also called autoimmune atrophic gastritis) is an inherited condition in which there is an immune response directed against parietal cells. Atrophic gastritis is associated with an increased risk of stomach cancer.

Clinical Manifestations

- *Acute gastritis* symptoms include anorexia, nausea and vomiting, epigastric tenderness, and a feeling of fullness. Hemorrhage is commonly associated with alcohol abuse and at times may be the only symptom. Acute gastritis is self-limiting, lasting from a few hours to a few days, with complete healing of mucosa expected.
- *Chronic gastritis* symptoms are similar to those of acute gastritis. Some patients are asymptomatic. However, when parietal cells are lost as a result of atrophy, the source of intrinsic factor is lost and cobalamin (vitamin B_{12}) cannot be absorbed in the ileum, ultimately resulting in pernicious anemia and neurologic complications.

Diagnostic Studies

Diagnosis of acute gastritis is most often based on a history of drug and alcohol use.

- Endoscopic examination with biopsy is used to obtain a definitive diagnosis.
- Breath, urine, serum, stool, or gastric tissue biopsy tests are available for determination of *H. pylori* infection.
- CBC may demonstrate anemia from blood loss or lack of intrinsic factor.
- Stools are tested for occult blood.
- Serum tests for antibodies to parietal cells and intrinsic factor are done.

Collaborative Care

Treatment of acute gastritis focuses on eliminating the cause and preventing or avoiding it in the future. The plan of care is supportive and similar to that described for nausea and vomiting.

- If vomiting accompanies acute gastritis, rest, nothing by mouth (NPO) status, and IV fluids may be prescribed. Antiemetics are given for nausea and vomiting. In severe cases, a nasogastric

(NG) tube may be used to monitor for bleeding, lavage the precipitating agent from the stomach, or keep the stomach empty and free of noxious stimuli.

- Clear liquids are resumed when acute symptoms have subsided, with gradual reintroduction of solid, bland foods.
- All of the management strategies discussed in the section on upper GI bleeding apply to the patient with severe gastritis (see Gastrointestinal Bleeding, p. 247).
- Drug therapy focuses on reducing irritation of the gastric mucosa and providing symptomatic relief. Histamine (H_2)-receptor blockers (e.g., ranitidine, cimetidine) or proton pump inhibitors (PPIs; e.g., omeprazole, lansoprazole) reduce gastric HCl acid secretion.

Treatment of chronic gastritis focuses on evaluating and eliminating the specific cause.

- Currently antibiotic combinations are used to eradicate infection with *H. pylori*.
- For the patient with pernicious anemia, lifelong administration of cobalamin is needed.

The patient undergoing treatment for chronic gastritis may have to adapt to lifestyle changes and strictly adhere to a drug regimen. An interdisciplinary team approach in which the physician, nurse, dietitian, and pharmacist provide consistent information and support may increase patient success in making these alterations.

GASTROESOPHAGEAL REFLUX DISEASE

Description

Gastroesophageal reflux disease (GERD) results from mucosal damage caused by reflux of stomach acid into the lower esophagus. GERD is not a disease but a syndrome. GERD is the most common upper GI problem. Approximately 10% to 20% of the U.S. population experience GERD symptoms (heartburn or regurgitation) at least once a week.

Pathophysiology

GERD has no one single cause (Fig. 6). GERD results when the defenses of the esophagus are overwhelmed by the reflux of acidic gastric contents into the esophagus. One of the primary etiologic factors in GERD is an incompetent lower esophageal sphincter (LES). Under normal conditions, the LES acts as an antireflux barrier. An incompetent LES lets gastric contents move from the stomach to the esophagus when the patient is supine or has an increase in intraabdominal pressure.

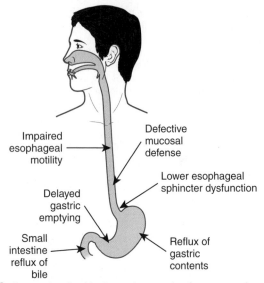

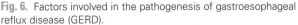

Fig. 6. Factors involved in the pathogenesis of gastroesophageal reflux disease (GERD).

Gastric HCl acid and pepsin secretions that reflux cause esophageal irritation and inflammation *(esophagitis)*. The degree of inflammation depends on the amount and composition of the gastric reflux and on the esophagus's mucosal defense mechanisms.

Clinical Manifestations

Symptoms vary from person to person, with symptoms that persistently occur more than twice a week generally indicative of GERD.

- Heartburn (pyrosis), caused by irritation of the esophagus by secretions, is the most common clinical manifestation. Heartburn is a burning, tight sensation that is felt intermittently beneath the lower sternum and spreads upward to the throat or jaw.
- Patients may complain of dyspepsia, which is pain or discomfort centered in the upper abdomen (mainly in or around the midline as opposed to the right or left hypochondrium).
- Regurgitation is common and often described as a hot, bitter, or sour liquid coming into the throat or mouth.
- GERD-related chest pain can mimic angina. It is described as burning, squeezing or radiating to the back, neck, jaw, or

arms. Unlike angina, GERD-related chest pain is relieved with antacids.

Complications

Complications are related to the effects of gastric acid secretion on the esophageal mucosa. Esophagitis (inflammation of the esophagus) is a common complication of GERD. Repeated esophagitis may cause scar tissue formation, stricture, and ultimately dysphagia. *Barrett's esophagus,* a precancerous lesion, increases the patient's risk for esophageal cancer.

- Respiratory complications due to irritation of the upper airway by gastric secretions include cough, bronchospasm, laryngospasm, asthma, and chronic bronchitis.
- Dental erosion may result from acid reflux into the mouth.

Diagnostic Studies

Diagnostic studies help determine the cause of the GERD.

- Barium swallow determines if there is protrusion of the upper part of the stomach into the esophagus.
- Endoscopy is useful in assessing LES competence and extent of inflammation (if present), potential scarring, and strictures.
- Biopsy and cytologic specimens can be taken to differentiate stomach and esophageal cancer from Barrett's esophagus (see Esophageal Cancer, p. 223).
- Radionuclide tests can also detect reflux of gastric contents and the rate of esophageal clearance.

Collaborative Care

Most patients with GERD can successfully manage this condition through lifestyle modifications and drug therapy. These long-term approaches require patient teaching and adherence to therapies.

Teach the patient to avoid factors that trigger symptoms. Give particular attention to diet and other medications that may affect the LES, acid secretion, or gastric emptying. Encourage patients who smoke to stop.

Food can aggravate symptoms. No specific diet is necessary. Teach patients to avoid foods such as chocolate, peppermint, tomatoes, fatty foods, coffee, and tea that decrease LES pressure and predispose them to reflux. Small, frequent meals help prevent overdistention of the stomach. Late evening meals and nocturnal snacking should be avoided. Weight reduction is recommended if the patient is obese.

Drug Therapy

Drug therapy focuses on improving LES function, increasing esophageal clearance, decreasing volume and acidity of reflux, and protecting esophageal mucosa. Proton-pump inhibitors (PPIs) and H_2-receptor blockers are effective treatments for symptomatic GERD. The goal of HCl acid suppression treatment is to reduce the acidity of the gastric refluxate. Patients who are symptomatic with GERD but do not have evidence of esophagitis achieve symptom relief with PPI and H_2-receptor agents. The PPIs are more effective in healing esophagitis than are H_2-receptor blockers.

- PPIs include omeprazole (Prilosec), esomeprazole (Nexium), lansoprazole (Prevacid), and rabeprazole (AcipHex).
- H_2-receptor blockers such as cimetidine (Tagamet), ranitidine (Zantac), famotidine (Pepcid), and nizatidine (Axid) reduce symptoms and promote esophageal healing in 50% of patients.

Antacids with or without alginic acid (e.g., Gaviscon) may be useful in patients with mild, intermittent heartburn.

Surgical Therapy

Surgical therapy is reserved for patients with complications of reflux, including esophagitis, intolerance of medications, stricture, Barrett's esophagus, and persistence of severe symptoms. Most surgical procedures are performed laparoscopically. The goal of surgery is to reduce reflux by enhancing the integrity of the LES. In these procedures the fundus of the stomach is wrapped around the lower portion of the esophagus to reinforce and repair the defective barrier.

Alternatives to surgical therapy include endoscopic mucosal resection, photodynamic therapy, cryotherapy, and radiofrequency ablation (image-guided technique that kills cells through heating).

Nursing Management

Nursing care for the patient with acute symptoms consists of encouraging the patient to follow the necessary regimen (Table 38).

- The head of the bed is elevated to approximately 30 degrees. This can be done using pillows or with 4- to 6-inch blocks under the bed.
- For 2 to 3 hours after a meal the patient should not be supine. Teach the patient to avoid food and activities that cause reflux (e.g., late-night eating).
- Instruct patients to contact their health care provider if symptoms persist.

Postoperative care focuses on prevention of respiratory complications, maintenance of fluid and electrolyte balance, and prevention of infection. Laparoscopic procedures reduce the risk of respiratory complications. During the postoperative phase, patients require medications to prevent nausea and vomiting and to control pain.

- When peristalsis returns, only fluids are given initially. Measure and record the intake and output. Solids are added gradually with the goal of resuming a normal diet.

| Table 38 | Patient and Caregiver Teaching Guide
Gastroesophageal Reflux Disease (GERD) |

Include the following when teaching the patient and caregiver about management of GERD.

1. Explain the rationale for a low-fat diet.
2. Encourage the patient to eat small, frequent meals to prevent gastric distention.
3. Explain the rationale for avoiding alcohol, smoking (causes an almost immediate, marked decrease in LES pressure), and beverages that contain caffeine.
4. Advise the patient to not lie down for 2-3 hr after eating, wear tight clothing around the waist, or bend over (especially after eating).
5. Have the patient avoid eating within 3 hr of bedtime.
6. Encourage the patient to sleep with head of bed elevated on 4- to 6-in blocks (gravity fosters esophageal emptying).
7. Provide information regarding drugs, including rationale for their use and common side effects.
8. Discuss strategies for weight reduction if appropriate.
9. Encourage patient and caregiver to share concerns about lifestyle changes and living with a chronic problem.

LES, Lower esophageal sphincter.

- In the first month after surgery, the patient may report mild dysphagia caused by edema, but it should resolve. Instruct the patient to report persistent symptoms such as heartburn and regurgitation.

GASTROINTESTINAL BLEEDING, UPPER

Description

In the United States approximately 300,000 hospital admissions occur each year for upper GI bleeding. Approximately 60% of these are adults over age 65. Despite advances in the drug management of predisposing conditions and identification of risk factors, the mortality rate for upper GI bleeding has remained at approximately 6% to 13% for the past 45 years.

Pathophysiology

Although the most serious loss of blood from the upper GI tract is characterized by a sudden onset, insidious occult bleeding can also be a major problem. Bleeding severity depends on whether the origin is venous, capillary, or arterial. Bleeding from an arterial source is profuse, and the blood is bright red. In contrast, "coffee ground" vomitus indicates that the blood has been in the stomach for some time. *Melena* (black, tarry stools) indicates slow bleeding from an upper GI source.

A variety of areas in the GI tract may be involved. Table 39 lists common causes of upper GI bleeding. The most common sites are the esophagus, stomach, and duodenum.

- Bleeding from the esophagus is most likely caused by chronic esophagitis, Mallory-Weiss tear, or esophageal varices. A *Mallory-Weiss tear* occurs in the mucosa near the esophagogastric junction and is often related to severe retching and vomiting. Esophageal varices most often occur secondary to cirrhosis of the liver (see Cirrhosis, p. 144).
- Bleeding peptic ulcers account for 40% of the cases of upper GI bleeding. Drugs, either prescribed by the health care provider or over-the-counter (OTC), are a major cause of upper GI bleeding.
- Stress-related mucosal disease, also called *physiologic stress ulcers,* occurs in patients who have had severe burns or trauma or major surgery.

Complications
Although approximately 80% to 85% of patients who have massive hemorrhage spontaneously stop bleeding, the cause must be identified and treatment initiated immediately.

Table 39	Common Causes of Upper Gastrointestinal Bleeding

Drug Induced
- Corticosteroids
- Nonsteroidal antiinflammatory drugs (NSAIDs)
- Salicylates

Esophagus
- Esophageal varices
- Esophagitis
- Mallory-Weiss tear

Stomach and Duodenum
- Stomach cancer
- Hemorrhagic gastritis
- Peptic ulcer disease
- Polyps
- Stress-related mucosal disease

Systemic Diseases
- Blood dyscrasias (e.g., leukemia, aplastic anemia)
- Renal failure

To facilitate early intervention, the physical examination should focus on early identification of signs and symptoms of shock such as tachycardia, weak pulse, hypotension, cool extremities, prolonged capillary refill, and apprehension. Monitor vital signs every 15 to 30 minutes. The patient is at risk for gut perforation and peritonitis, which may be indicated by a tense, rigid, boardlike abdomen.

- IV lines, preferably two, with a 16- or 18-gauge needle are placed for fluid and blood replacement. An indwelling urinary catheter may also be inserted so that output can be accurately assessed hourly.
- The use of supplemental oxygen delivered by face mask or nasal cannula may help increase blood oxygen saturation.

Diagnostic Studies

- Endoscopy is the primary tool for diagnosing the source (e.g., esophageal or gastric varices, gastritis) of upper GI bleeding.
- Angiography is used in diagnosing upper GI bleeding when endoscopy cannot be done or when bleeding persists after endoscopic therapy.
- Laboratory studies include CBC, blood urea nitrogen (BUN), serum electrolytes, prothrombin time, partial thromboplastin time, liver enzymes, and arterial blood gases (ABGs).

Collaborative Care

Endoscopy performed within the first 24 hours of bleeding is important for diagnosis and the determination of the need for surgical or radiologic intervention. Several techniques are used, including (1) thermal (heat) probe, (2) multipolar and bipolar electrocoagulation probe, (3) argon plasma coagulation (APC), and (4) neodymium:yttrium-aluminum-garnet (Nd:YAG) laser. For variceal bleeding, other strategies include variceal ligation, injection sclerotherapy, and balloon tamponade.

Surgical intervention is indicated when bleeding continues regardless of the therapy provided and when the site of the bleeding has been identified. The site of the hemorrhage determines the choice of operation.

During the acute phase, drugs are used to decrease bleeding, decrease HCl acid secretion, and neutralize the HCl acid that is present. Injection therapy with epinephrine (1:10,000 dilution) during endoscopy is effective for acute hemostasis.

- Efforts are made to reduce acid secretion because the acidic environment can alter platelet function, as well as interfere with clot stabilization. Proton-pump inhibitors (PPIs; e.g., pantoprazole [Protonix]) or H_2-receptor blockers (e.g., cimetidine [Tagamet]) are administered IV to decrease acid secretion (see Table 42-22 Lewis et al, *Medical-Surgical Nursing,* ed. 9, p. 955).

Nursing Management

Goals

The patient with upper GI bleeding will have no further GI bleeding, have the cause of the bleeding identified and treated, experience a return to a normal hemodynamic state, and have minimal or no symptoms of pain or anxiety.

Nursing Diagnoses

- Decreased cardiac output
- Deficient fluid volume
- Ineffective peripheral tissue perfusion
- Anxiety

Nursing Interventions

Consider the patient with a history of chronic gastritis or peptic ulcer disease at high risk for upper GI bleeding. Instruct the at-risk patient to avoid gastric irritants such as alcohol and smoking, prevent or decrease stress-inducing situations at home or at work, and take only prescribed medications.

When working with the patient who has a history of liver cirrhosis with esophageal varices, instructions must be specific regarding the importance of avoiding known irritants, such as alcohol and smoking.

Once an infusion has been started, maintain the IV line for fluid or blood replacement. An accurate intake and output record is essential so that the patient's hydration status can be assessed. If the patient has a central venous pressure line or pulmonary artery catheter in place, record these readings every 1 to 2 hours.

Although room-temperature, cool, or iced gastric lavage is used in some institutions, its effectiveness as a treatment for upper GI bleeding is questionable. When lavage is used, approximately 50 to 100 mL of fluid is instilled at a time into the stomach.

- Monitor vital signs, especially in patients with cardiovascular disease, because dysrhythmias may occur. Keep the head of the bed elevated to provide comfort and prevent aspiration.
- Assess stools for blood. Black, tarry stools are not usually associated with a brisk hemorrhage but are indicative of prolonged bleeding.
- Monitor the patient's laboratory studies to estimate the effectiveness of therapy. The hemoglobin and hematocrit are usually evaluated about every 4 to 6 hours if the patient is actively bleeding.
- When oral nourishment is begun, observe the patient for symptoms of nausea and vomiting and a recurrence of bleeding. Feedings initially consist of clear fluids and are given hourly until tolerance is determined. Gradual introduction of foods follows if the patient exhibits no signs of discomfort.

- When the hemorrhage is the result of chronic alcohol abuse, closely observe the patient for delirium tremens as withdrawal from alcohol takes place.

▼ **Patient and Caregiver Teaching**
- Teach the patient and caregiver how to avoid future bleeding episodes.
- Ulcer disease, drug or alcohol abuse, and liver and respiratory diseases can all result in upper GI bleeding.
- Help the patient and caregiver be aware of the consequences of not adhering to drug therapy.
- Emphasize that no drugs (especially aspirin, NSAIDs) other than those prescribed by the health care provider should be taken.
- Smoking and alcohol should be eliminated because they are sources of irritation and interfere with tissue repair.
- Instruct the patient and the family on what to do if an acute hemorrhage occurs in the future.

GLAUCOMA

Description

Glaucoma is a group of disorders characterized by increased intraocular pressure (IOP) and the consequences of elevated pressure, optic nerve atrophy, and peripheral visual field loss. At least 2 million people have glaucoma. Of these, more than 50% are unaware of their condition.

- Glaucoma is the second leading cause of permanent blindness in the United States and the leading cause of blindness among African Americans.
- Blindness from glaucoma is largely preventable with early detection and appropriate treatment.

Pathophysiology

The etiology of glaucoma is related to the consequences of elevated IOP. Increased IOP results when the rate of aqueous production (inflow) is greater than aqueous reabsorption (outflow). If the pressure remains elevated, permanent visual damage may begin.

- *Primary open-angle glaucoma* (POAG) is the most common type of primary glaucoma. In POAG, the aqueous outflow is decreased in the trabecular meshwork. The drainage channels become clogged, like a clogged kitchen sink. Damage to the optic nerve can then result.
- *Primary angle-closure glaucoma* (PACG) is due to a reduction in the outflow of aqueous humor that results from angle closure.

Usually this is caused by the lens bulging forward as a result of the aging process. Angle closure may also occur as a result of pupil dilation in the patient with anatomically narrow angles. An acute attack may occur because of drug-induced mydriasis, emotional excitement, or darkness. Check the medical record before administering medications to the patient with angle-closure glaucoma and instruct the patient not to take any mydriatic medications.

Clinical Manifestations

- POAG develops slowly without symptoms of pain or pressure. The patient usually does not notice gradual visual field loss until peripheral vision is severely compromised (tunnel vision).
- Acute angle-closure glaucoma causes symptoms of sudden, excruciating pain in or around the eye that is often accompanied by nausea and vomiting. Visual symptoms include seeing colored halos around lights, blurred vision, and ocular redness.
- Manifestations of subacute or chronic angle-closure glaucoma appear gradually. The patient who has had a previous unrecognized episode of subacute angle-closure glaucoma might report a history of blurred vision, colored halos around lights, ocular redness, or eye or brow pain.

Diagnostic Studies

- IOP with tonometry
- Visual acuity measurement and visual field perimetry
- Slit-lamp microscopy
- Ophthalmoscopy (direct and indirect)

Collaborative Care

The primary focus of therapy is to keep the IOP low enough to prevent the patient from developing optic nerve damage. Therapy varies with the type of glaucoma.

- In chronic open-angle glaucoma, initial drug therapy can include β-adrenergic receptor blocking agents, α-adrenergic agents, cholinergic agents (miotics), and carbonic anhydrase inhibitors (hyperosmotic agents).
- When medications are not effective or are not used as recommended, surgical options include argon laser trabeculoplasty (ALT) or trabeculectomy.
- Acute angle-closure glaucoma is an ocular emergency that requires immediate interventions, including miotics and oral or IV hyperosmotic agents. Laser peripheral iridotomy or surgical iridectomy is necessary for long-term treatment and prevention of subsequent episodes.

Nursing Management

Because glaucoma is a chronic condition requiring long-term management, assess the patient's ability to understand and adhere to the rationale and regimen of the prescribed therapy. Also assess the patient's psychologic reaction to the diagnosis of a potentially sight-threatening chronic disorder.

Goals

The patient with glaucoma will have no progression of visual impairment, understand the disease process and rationale for therapy, comply with all aspects of therapy (including medication administration and follow-up care), and have no postoperative complications.

Nursing Diagnoses

- Acute pain
- Self-care deficits
- Noncompliance
- Risk for injury

Nursing Interventions

- The patient with acute angle-closure glaucoma requires immediate medication to lower the IOP. Most surgical procedures for glaucoma are outpatient procedures.
- Encourage the patient to follow therapy recommendations, including information about the disease processes, normal course of the condition, and treatment options that include the rationale underlying each option.

▼ Patient and Caregiver Teaching

See Table 22, Patient and Caregiver Teaching Guide: After Eye Surgery, p. 117.

- Provide accurate information about the disease process and treatment options, including the rationale underlying each option. In addition, the patient needs information about the purpose, frequency, and technique for administration of antiglaucoma drugs.
- Encourage adherence by helping the patient identify the most convenient and appropriate times for medication administration or advocating a change in therapy if the patient reports unacceptable side effects.

GLOMERULONEPHRITIS

Glomerulonephritis is an inflammation of renal glomeruli caused by immunologic processes. It affects both kidneys equally and is the third leading cause of end-stage kidney disease in the United States. Although the glomerulus is the primary site of inflammation, tubular, interstitial, and vascular changes also occur.

- A variety of conditions can cause glomerulonephritis, ranging from kidney infections to systemic diseases. Glomerulonephritis can be acute or chronic. In acute glomerulonephritis symptoms come on suddenly and may be temporary or reversible. In contrast, chronic glomerulonephritis is slowly progressive and generally leads to irreversible renal failure.

Acute Poststreptococcal Glomerulonephritis

Acute poststreptococcal glomerulonephritis (APSGN) is most common in children and young adults. It develops 5 to 21 days after an infection of the tonsils, pharynx, or skin (e.g., streptococcal sore throat, impetigo) by certain nephrotoxic strains of group A β-hemolytic streptococci. Antibodies are produced to the streptococcal antigen, and tissue injury occurs as the antigen-antibody complexes are deposited in the glomeruli and complement is activated.

- More than 95% of patients with APSGN recover completely or improve rapidly with conservative management. Accurate recognition and assessment are critical, because chronic glomerulonephritis develops in 5% to 15% of affected people.

Clinical manifestations of APSGN include generalized body edema, hypertension, oliguria, hematuria with a smoky or rusty appearance, and proteinuria. Fluid retention occurs as a result of decreased glomerular filtration.

- Edema initially appears in low-pressure tissues, such as the eyes (periorbital edema), but later progresses to involve the total body as ascites or peripheral edema in the legs.
- Smoky urine indicates bleeding in the upper urinary tract. The degree of proteinuria varies with the severity of the glomerulonephropathy.
- Hypertension mainly results from increased extracellular fluid volume.
- The patient may have abdominal or flank pain. At times the patient has no symptoms, with the problem found on routine urinalysis.

An immune response to the streptococci is often demonstrated by assessment of antistreptolysin-O (ASO) titers. Decreased complement levels indicate an immune-mediated response. Renal biopsy may be done to confirm the disease. Urinalysis reveals significant numbers of erythrocytes. Erythrocyte casts are highly suggestive of acute glomerulonephritis. Proteinuria may be mild to severe. CBC, blood urea nitrogen (BUN), serum creatinine, and albumin assess the extent of renal impairment.

Nursing and Collaborative Care

Management of APSGN focuses on symptomatic relief. Rest is recommended until the signs of glomerular inflammation (proteinuria, hematuria) and hypertension subside. Edema is treated by restricting sodium and fluid intake and administering diuretics.

- Severe hypertension is treated with antihypertensive drugs.
- Dietary protein intake may be restricted if there is evidence of an increase in nitrogenous wastes (e.g., elevated BUN).
- Antibiotics should be given only if streptococcal infection is still present. Corticosteroids and cytotoxic drugs have not been shown to be of value.

One of the most important ways to prevent APSGN is to encourage early diagnosis and treatment of sore throats and skin lesions. If streptococci are found in the culture, treatment with appropriate antibiotic therapy (usually penicillin) is essential. The patient must be encouraged to take the full course of antibiotics to ensure that the bacteria have been eradicated.

- Good personal hygiene is an important factor in preventing the spread of cutaneous streptococcal infections.

Chronic Glomerulonephritis

Chronic glomerulonephritis is a syndrome that reflects the end stage of glomerular inflammatory disease. Most types of glomerulonephritis and nephrotic syndrome can eventually lead to chronic glomerulonephritis.

- Some people who develop chronic glomerulonephritis have no history of kidney disease. Frequently the cause of chronic glomerulonephritis is not found.
- The syndrome is characterized by proteinuria, hematuria, and the slow development of the uremic syndrome as a result of decreasing renal function.

Chronic glomerulonephritis is often found coincidentally when an abnormality on a urinalysis or elevated BP is detected. It is common to find that the patient has no recollection or history of acute nephritis or any renal problems. A renal biopsy may be performed to determine the exact cause of the glomerulonephritis. Ultrasound and CT scan are preferred diagnostic measures. Treatment is supportive and symptomatic (see Kidney Disease, Chronic, p. 373).

GONORRHEA

Description

Gonorrhea is the second most frequently occurring sexually transmitted infection (STI) in the United States. In 2009 the gonorrhea rates were the lowest since recording of rates began. Since that time there has been a slight increase in the rate of gonorrhea to a total of about 309,000 cases today.

- Gonorrhea rates are highest in adolescents of all racial and ethnic groups and among African Americans.
- Most states have enacted laws that permit examination and treatment of minors without parental consent.

Pathophysiology

Gonorrhea is caused by *Neisseria gonorrhoeae,* a gram-negative diplococcus. Mucosal tissues present in the genitalia (urethra in men, cervix in women), rectum, and oropharynx are especially sensitive to gonococcal infection.

- The infection is spread by direct physical contact with an infected host, usually during sexual activity (vaginal, oral, or anal).
- Neonates can develop a gonococcal infection during delivery from an infected mother.
- Indirect transmission by instruments or linens is rare because the delicate gonococcus is easily killed by drying, heating, or washing with an antiseptic.
- Incubation period is 3 to 8 days. The infection confers no immunity to subsequent reinfection.
- Gonococcal infection elicits an inflammatory response, which, if left untreated, leads to formation of fibrous tissue and adhesions. This fibrous scarring is subsequently responsible for many complications such as strictures and tubal abnormalities, which can lead to tubal pregnancy, chronic pelvic pain, and infertility.

Clinical Manifestations

Men. Initial site of infection in men is usually the urethra.

- Symptoms of urethritis consist of dysuria and profuse, purulent urethral discharge developing 2 to 5 days after infection. Painful or swollen testicles may also occur.
- Men generally seek medical evaluation early in the infection because symptoms are usually obvious and distressing. It is unusual for men with gonorrhea to be asymptomatic.

Women. Many women who contract gonorrhea are asymptomatic or have minor symptoms that are often overlooked, making it possible for them to remain a source of infection.

- A few women may complain of vaginal discharge, dysuria, or frequency of urination. Changes in menstruation may be a symptom, but these changes are often disregarded by the woman.
- After the incubation period, redness and swelling occur at the site of contact, which is usually the cervix or urethra.

A greenish-yellow purulent exudate often develops with a potential for abscess formation.

- The infection may remain local or can spread by direct tissue extension to the uterus, fallopian tubes, and ovaries. Although the vulva and vagina are uncommon sites for a gonorrheal infection, they may become involved when little or no estrogen is present, such as in prepubertal girls and postmenopausal women.

Anorectal gonorrhea may be present and is usually caused by anal intercourse. Symptoms may include mucopurulent anal discharge, bleeding, and tenesmus.

- Most patients with anorectal infections and infections in the throat have few symptoms. A small percentage of individuals develop gonococcal pharyngitis resulting from orogenital sexual contact. When the gonococcus can be demonstrated by culture, individuals of either gender are infectious to their sexual partners.

Complications

Because men often seek treatment early in the course of the infection, they are less likely to develop complications. Complications that do occur in men are prostatitis, urethral strictures, and sterility from orchitis or epididymitis.

Because women who are asymptomatic seldom seek treatment, complications are more common and usually are the reason for seeking medical attention. Pelvic inflammatory disease (PID), Bartholin's abscess, ectopic pregnancy, and infertility are the main complications in women.

- A small percentage of infected people, mainly women, may develop a disseminated gonococcal infection (DGI). In DGI the appearance of skin lesions, fever, arthralgia, arthritis, or endocarditis usually causes the patient to seek medical help.

Diagnostic Studies

- For men, a presumptive diagnosis of gonorrhea is made if there is a history of sexual contact with an infected individual followed within a few days by a urethral discharge. Typical clinical manifestations combined with a positive finding in a Gram-stained smear of discharge from the penis give an almost certain diagnosis.
- A culture of the discharge is indicated for men whose smears are negative in the presence of strong clinical evidence.
- Making a diagnosis in women is difficult because most women are symptom free. A culture must be performed to confirm the diagnosis.

- The nucleic acid amplification test (NAAT) is a nonculture test with sensitivity similar to culture tests for *N. gonorrhoeae*. It can be done on a wide variety of samples, including vaginal, endocervical, urethral, and urine specimens.

Collaborative Care

Because of a short incubation period and high infectivity, treatment is generally instituted without awaiting culture results.

Treatment of gonorrhea in the early stage is curative, with the most common treatment being an intramuscular (IM) dose of ceftriaxone (Rocephin) or cefixime (Suprax) orally. The high frequency (up to 20% in men and 40% in women) of coexisting chlamydial and gonococcal infections has led to the addition of azithromycin (Zithromax) or doxycycline (Vibramycin) to the treatment regimen. Patients with coexisting syphilis are likely to be treated by the same drugs used for gonorrhea.

- All sexual contacts of patients with gonorrhea must be treated to prevent reinfection after resumption of sexual relations. The "Ping-Pong" effect of reexposure, treatment, and reinfection can cease only when infected partners are treated simultaneously.
- Counsel the patient to abstain from sexual intercourse and alcohol during treatment. Sexual intercourse allows the infection to spread and can delay healing as a result of vascular congestion. Alcohol has an irritant effect on the healing urethral walls.
- Caution men against squeezing the penis to look for further discharge.
- Reinfection, rather than treatment failure, is the main cause of infections identified after treatment has ended.

Nursing Management

See Nursing Management: Sexually Transmitted Infections, p. 564.

GOUT

Description

Gout is a type of recurring acute arthritis characterized by the accumulation of uric acid crystals in one or more joints. Characteristic deposits of sodium urate crystals occur in articular, periarticular, and subcutaneous tissues. More than 3 million Americans are affected by gout. The incidence among African American men is nearly twice that of white men.

Gout may be classified as primary or secondary. In *primary gout,* a hereditary error of purine metabolism leads to overproduction or retention of uric acid. Primary gout, which accounts for 90% of cases, occurs predominantly in middle-aged men. *Secondary gout* may be related to another acquired disorder (e.g., atherosclerosis, obesity, malignant disease) or may be the result of medications known to inhibit uric acid excretion (e.g., thiazide, diuretics). Secondary gout may also be caused by drugs that increase the rate of cell death, such as the chemotherapeutic agents used in treating leukemia.

Pathophysiology

Uric acid is the major end product of purine catabolism and is primarily excreted by the kidneys. Gout is caused by an increase in uric acid production, underexcretion of uric acid by the kidneys (the most common cause), or increased intake of foods containing purines, which are metabolized to uric acid by the body.

- A high dietary intake of purine alone has little effect on uric acid levels. Hyperuricemia may result from prolonged fasting or excessive drinking because of increased production of keto-acids, which then inhibit uric acid excretion.

Clinical Manifestations

In the acute phase, gouty arthritis may occur in one or more joints. Affected joints may appear dusky or cyanotic and are extremely tender. Inflammation of the great toe *(podagra)* is the most common initial problem. Other joints affected may include the midtarsal area of the foot, ankle, knee, wrist, and the olecranon bursa.

- Acute gouty arthritis is usually precipitated by events such as trauma, surgery, alcohol ingestion, or systemic infection. Onset of symptoms is usually rapid, with swelling and pain peaking within several hours, often accompanied by a low-grade fever.
- Individual attacks usually subside, treated or untreated, in 2 to 10 days. The affected joint returns entirely to normal, and patients are often free of symptoms between attacks.

Chronic gout is characterized by multiple joint involvement and deposits of sodium urate crystals *(tophi)*. These are typically seen in the synovium, subchondral bone, olecranon bursa, and vertebrae; along tendons; and in the skin and cartilage. Tophi are generally noted many years after the onset of the disease.

Chronic inflammation may result in joint deformity, and cartilage destruction may predispose the joint to secondary osteoarthritis. Large and unsightly tophaceous deposits may perforate overlying skin, producing draining sinuses that often become infected. Excessive uric acid excretion may lead to urinary tract stone formation. Pyelonephritis associated with intrarenal sodium urate deposits and obstruction may contribute to renal disease.

The severity of gouty arthritis is variable. The clinical course may consist of infrequent mild attacks or multiple severe episodes associated with a slowly progressive disability.

Diagnostic Studies

- Serum uric acid levels are usually elevated above 6 mg/dL.
- Specimens for 24-hour urine uric acid levels may be obtained to determine if the disease is caused by decreased renal excretion or overproduction of uric acid.
- X-rays appear normal in the early stages of gout, with tophi, an indicator of chronic disease, appearing as eroded areas in the bone.
- Synovial fluid aspiration helps distinguish gout from septic arthritis and *pseudogout* (calcium phosphate crystals are formed). Affected fluid characteristically contains needlelike crystals of sodium urate.

Collaborative Care

Goals for care include termination of an acute attack through the use of an antiinflammatory agent such as colchicine. Drug therapy is the primary therapy used in treating acute and chronic gout. In addition, weight reduction (as needed) and possible avoidance of alcohol and foods high in purine (red and organ meats) are recommended.

Drug Therapy

Acute gouty arthritis is treated with colchicine and nonsteroidal antiinflammatory drugs (NSAIDs). Future attacks are prevented in part by combining colchicine with a xanthine oxidase inhibitor such as allopurinol or a uricosuric drug such as probenecid (Benemid). Febuxostat (Uloric), a selective inhibitor of xanthine oxidase, is given for long-term management of hyperuricemia in people with chronic gout.

- Aspirin inactivates the effect of uricosurics, resulting in urate retention, and should be avoided while patients are taking uricosuric drugs (e.g., probenecid [Benemid]). Acetaminophen can be used safely if analgesia is required.

Patients who cannot take or do not respond to drugs that lower uric acid in the blood may be given pegloticase (Krystexxa). This drug is an enzyme that metabolizes uric acid into a harmless chemical that is excreted in the urine.

- Corticosteroids, either orally or by intraarticular injection, can be helpful in treating acute attacks.
- Adequate urine volume with normal renal function (2 to 3 L/day) must be maintained to prevent precipitation of uric acid in

the renal tubules. Allopurinol, which blocks production of uric acid, is particularly useful in patients with uric acid stones or renal impairment, in whom uricosuric drugs may be ineffective or dangerous.

Regardless of which drugs are used to treat gout, serum uric acid levels must be checked regularly to monitor treatment effectiveness.

Nutritional Therapy

Dietary restrictions may include limiting the use of alcohol and foods high in purine. However, drugs can generally control gout without necessitating these changes. Instruct obese patients in a carefully planned weight-reduction program.

Nursing Management

Nursing intervention is directed at supportive care of the inflamed joints.

- Bed rest may be appropriate, with affected joints properly immobilized. Involvement of a lower extremity may require use of a cradle or footboard to protect the painful area from the weight of bed clothes.
- Assess the limitation of motion and degree of pain and document treatment effectiveness.

▼ **Patient and Caregiver Teaching**

Help the patient and caregiver to understand that hyperuricemia and gouty arthritis are chronic problems that can be controlled with careful adherence to a treatment program.

- Offer explanations concerning the importance of drug therapy and the need for periodic determination of serum uric acid levels.
- Teach the patient about precipitating factors that may cause an attack, including overindulgence in purine-containing foods and alcohol, starvation (fasting), medication use (e.g., aspirin, diuretics), and major medical events (e.g., surgery, myocardial infarction).

GUILLAIN-BARRÉ SYNDROME

Description

Guillain-Barré syndrome (postinfectious polyneuropathy and ascending polyneuropathic paralysis) is an acute, rapidly progressing, and potentially fatal form of polyneuritis. It is characterized by ascending, symmetric paralysis that usually affects cranial nerves and the peripheral nervous system. The syndrome is rare, affecting an estimated 3000 to 6000 Americans each year.

- Although 85% to 95% of patients recover completely, it is generally a slow process that takes months or years.

Pathophysiology

The etiology is unknown. Both cellular and humoral immune mechanisms play a role in the immune reaction directed at the nerves. The result is a loss of myelin (a segmental demyelination) and edema and inflammation of the affected nerves. As demyelination occurs, the transmission of nerve impulses is stopped or slowed down. The muscles innervated by the damaged peripheral nerves undergo denervation and atrophy. In the recovery phase, remyelination occurs slowly and returns in a proximal-to-distal pattern.

- The syndrome is often preceded by immune system stimulation from a viral infection, trauma, surgery, or viral immunizations. *Campylobacter jejuni* gastroenteritis is thought to precede Guillain-Barré syndrome in approximately 30% of cases.

Clinical Manifestations

Guillain-Barré syndrome is a heterogeneous condition with symptoms ranging from mild to severe.

- Weakness of the lower extremities (evolving more or less symmetrically) occurs over hours to days to weeks, usually peaking about day 14. Paresthesia (numbness and tingling) is frequent, and paralysis usually follows in the extremities. Hypotonia and areflexia are common manifestations.
- Autonomic nervous system dysfunction results, with manifestations of orthostatic hypotension, hypertension, and abnormal vagal responses (bradycardia, heart block, and asystole). Other autonomic dysfunctions include bowel and bladder dysfunction, facial flushing, and diaphoresis.
- Patients may also have the syndrome of inappropriate antidiuretic hormone (SIADH) secretion.
- Pain is a common symptom including paresthesias, muscular aches and cramps, and hyperesthesias. Pain appears to be worse at night. Opioids may be indicated for those experiencing severe pain. Pain may lead to a decrease in appetite and interfere with sleep.

The most serious complication is respiratory failure, which occurs as paralysis progresses to the nerves that innervate the thoracic area. Respiratory infections or urinary tract infections (UTIs) may occur. Immobility from the paralysis can cause problems such as paralytic ileus, muscle atrophy, deep vein thrombosis, pulmonary emboli, skin breakdown, nutritional deficiencies, and orthostatic hypotension.

Diagnostic Studies

Diagnosis is based primarily on patient history and clinical signs.

- Cerebrospinal fluid is normal or has a low protein content initially, but after 7 to 10 days it shows a greatly elevated protein level.
- Electromyographic (EMG) and nerve conduction studies are markedly abnormal (showing reduced nerve conduction velocity) in affected extremities.
- Brain MRI may be done to rule out multiple sclerosis.

Nursing and Collaborative Care

Management is aimed at supportive care, particularly ventilatory support, during the acute phase. Plasmapheresis is used in the first 2 weeks. IV administration of high-dose immunoglobulin (Sandoglobulin) has been as effective as plasma exchange and is more readily available. Beyond 3 weeks after disease onset, plasmapheresis and immunoglobulin therapies have little value. Corticosteroids appear to have little effect on the prognosis or duration of the disease.

Assessment of the patient is the most important aspect of nursing care during the acute phase. During the assessment, monitor the ascending paralysis; assess respiratory function; monitor arterial blood gases (ABGs); and assess the gag, corneal, and swallowing reflexes. Reflexes are usually decreased or absent.

- Monitor BP and cardiac rate and rhythm during the acute phase because dysrhythmias may occur. Autonomic dysfunction is common and usually takes the form of bradycardia and dysrhythmias. Orthostatic hypotension secondary to muscle atony may occur in severe cases. Vasopressor agents and volume expanders may be needed to treat the low BP.
- Monitoring vital capacity and ABGs is essential. A tracheostomy or endotracheal intubation may be done so that the patient can be mechanically ventilated (see Tracheostomy, p. 732, and Artificial Airways: Endotracheal Tubes, p. 679).
- If fever develops, obtain sputum cultures to identify the pathogen. Appropriate antibiotic therapy is then initiated.

Nutritional needs must be met in spite of possible problems associated with gastric dilation, paralytic ileus, and aspiration potential if the gag reflex is lost.

- Note drooling and other difficulties with secretions, which may indicate an inadequate gag reflex.
- Initially enteral feedings or parenteral nutrition may be used to ensure adequate caloric intake. Monitor fluid and electrolyte therapy to prevent electrolyte imbalances.

HEAD AND NECK CANCER

Description

Most head and neck cancers arise from squamous cells that line the mucosal surfaces of the head and neck. Most people present with locally advanced disease. Disability from the disease and treatment is great because of the potential loss of voice, disfigurement, and social consequences.

- Most head and neck cancers are caused by tobacco use. Excessive alcohol consumption is also a major risk factor. Head and neck cancer occurs most frequently in patients 50 to 60 years of age.
- Cancers in patients younger than 50 have been associated with human papillomavirus (HPV) infection. Other risk factors include sun exposure (oral cavity), radiation therapy to the head and neck, exposure to asbestos and other industrial carcinogens, and poor oral hygiene.
- Men are affected twice as often as women.

Clinical Manifestations

Early signs of head and neck cancer vary with tumor location. Cancer of the oral cavity may be initially seen as a red or white patch in the mouth, an ulcer that does not heal, or a change in the fit of dentures.

- Hoarseness that lasts more than 2 weeks may be a symptom of early laryngeal cancer. Some patients experience what feels like a lump in the throat or a change in voice quality.
- Other clinical manifestations include sore throat that does not get better with treatment, unilateral sore throat or otalgia (ear pain), swelling or lumps in the neck, and coughing up blood.
- Difficulty with chewing, swallowing, moving the tongue, and breathing are typically late symptoms.

Diagnostic Studies

- If lesions are suspected, upper airways may be examined using an indirect laryngoscopy or a flexible nasopharyngoscope. The larynx and vocal cords are visually inspected for lesions and tissue mobility.
- A CT scan or MRI may be performed to detect local and regional spread.
- Multiple biopsy specimens are obtained to determine the extent of the disease.

Collaborative Care

The stage of the disease is determined based on tumor size (T), number and location of involved nodes (N), and extent of metastasis (M). TNM classifies disease as stage I to stage IV (see p. 777).

- Stage I and II cancers are potentially curable with single-modality radiation therapy or larynx-sparing surgery.
- Patients with advanced disease (stages III and IV) are treated with various combinations of surgery, radiation, chemotherapy, and targeted therapy. Radiation therapy can be delivered by either external-beam therapy or internal implants (brachytherapy).
- Advanced lesions of the larynx are treated by a total laryngectomy in which the entire larynx and preepiglottic region are removed and a permanent tracheostomy is performed (see Tracheostomy, p. 732). Radical neck dissection frequently accompanies total laryngectomy. Depending on the extent of involvement, extensive dissection and reconstruction may be performed.
- Changes following a total laryngectomy include loss of speech, loss of the ability to taste and smell, inability to produce audible sounds (including laughing and crying), and a permanent tracheal stoma.
- Some patients refuse surgical intervention for advanced lesions because of the extent of the procedure and the potential risk. In this situation, external radiation therapy is used as the sole treatment or in combination with chemotherapy.
- Chemotherapy (e.g., cisplatin [Platinol] and targeted therapy (cetuximab [Erbitux]) are used in combination with radiation therapy for patients with stage III or IV cancers.

Nutritional Therapy

After radical neck surgery, the patient may be unable to take in nutrients through the normal route of ingestion. Parenteral fluids are given for the first 24 to 48 hours.

- Because of swelling and difficulty swallowing postoperatively, tube feedings are usually given through a nasogastric, nasointestinal, or gastrostomy tube that was placed during surgery.

When the patient can swallow, give small amounts of thickened liquids or pureed foods with the patient in high Fowler's position. Close observation for choking is essential. Suctioning may be necessary to prevent aspiration.

Nursing Management

Goals

The patient with head or neck cancer will have a patent airway, no complications related to therapy, adequate nutritional intake, minimal to no pain, the ability to communicate, and an acceptable body image.

Nursing Diagnoses
- Anxiety
- Ineffective airway clearance
- Risk for aspiration
- Impaired verbal communication
- Acute pain

Nursing Interventions

Include information about risk factors in health teaching. Encourage good oral hygiene. Teach patients about safe sex practices to prevent HPV infection. If cancer has been diagnosed, tobacco and alcohol cessation is still important as the likelihood of a cure is diminished if these behaviors continue.

- Interventions to reduce side effects of radiation therapy include measures to reduce dry mouth, teaching oral care to the patient, and encouraging patients to engage in regular exercise to reduce fatigue.

For procedures that involve a laryngectomy, teaching should include information about expected changes in speech. Establish a means of communication for the immediate postoperative period.

After surgery, maintenance of a patent airway is essential and a laryngectomy (tracheostomy) tube will be in place. Keep the patient in semi-Fowler's position to decrease edema and tension on the suture lines. Monitor vital signs frequently because of the risk of hemorrhage and respiratory compromise. Immediately after surgery the postlaryngectomy patient requires frequent suctioning via the tracheostomy tube.

- Encourage deep breathing and coughing and provide tracheostomy care as needed.
- Depression and changes in sexuality patterns because of altered body image are common in the patient who has had radical neck dissection. Help the patient regain an acceptable self-concept.
- A speech therapist should meet with the patient having a total laryngectomy to discuss voice restoration options.

▼ **Patient and Caregiver Teaching**
- Monitor patency of wound drainage tubes (if in place) every 4 hours to ensure proper functioning. After drainage tubes are removed, closely monitor the area to detect any swelling. If fluid continues to accumulate, aspiration may be necessary.
- Instruct the patient and caregiver on how to manage tubes and whom to call if there are problems.
- Provide pictorial instructions for tracheostomy care, suctioning, stoma care, and tube feedings as appropriate.

- Teach the patient to cover the stoma before performing activities such as shaving and applying makeup to avoid inhalation of foreign materials.
- Address measures to provide adequate humidity at home using a bedside humidifier and high oral fluid intake.
- Encourage preparation of food that is colorful, attractive, and nutritious because taste may also be diminished secondary to the loss of smell and radiation therapy.

HEAD INJURY

Description

Head injury includes any trauma to the scalp, skull, or brain. A serious form of head injury is *traumatic brain injury* (TBI). In the United States in hospital emergency departments, an estimated 1.7 million people are treated and released with TBI.

- Motor vehicle crashes and falls are the most common causes of head injury. Other causes of head injury include firearms, assaults, sports-related trauma, recreational injuries, and war-related injuries.
- Males are twice as likely to sustain a TBI as females.

Deaths from head trauma occur at three time points after injury: immediately after injury, within 2 hours of injury, and approximately 3 weeks after injury.

- The majority of deaths occur immediately after the injury, either from the direct head trauma or massive hemorrhage and shock.
- Deaths occurring within a few hours of the trauma are caused by progressive worsening of the head injury or internal bleeding. Immediately recognizing changes in neurologic status and rapid surgical intervention are critical in the prevention of deaths.
- Deaths occurring 3 weeks or more after the injury result from multisystem failure.

Types of Head Injuries

Scalp Laceration

Because the scalp contains many blood vessels with poor constrictive abilities, even relatively small wounds can bleed profusely. The major complications of scalp lesions are blood loss and infection.

Skull Fracture

Fractures frequently occur with head trauma. Fractures may be closed or open, depending on the presence of a scalp laceration or extension of the fracture into the air sinuses or dura.

- The type and severity of a skull fracture depend on the velocity, momentum, and direction of the injuring agent, and the site of impact. Specific manifestations of a skull fracture are generally associated with the location of the injury (see Table 57-7, Lewis et al, *Medical-Surgical Nursing,* ed. 9, p. 1369).

Major potential complications of skull fracture are intracranial infections and hematoma, as well as meningeal and brain tissue damage.

Head Trauma

Brain injuries are categorized as diffuse (generalized) or focal (localized). In *diffuse injury* (i.e., concussion, diffuse axonal), damage to the brain cannot be localized to one particular area of the brain, whereas a *focal injury* (e.g., contusion, hematoma) can be localized to a specific area of the brain.

Diffuse Injury

Concussion is a minor, sudden, transient, and diffuse head injury associated with a disruption in neural activity and a change in the level of consciousness (LOC). The patient may not lose total consciousness. Signs include a brief disruption in LOC, amnesia for the event (retrograde amnesia), and headache. Manifestations are generally of short duration.

- Postconcussion syndrome may develop in some patients and is usually seen anywhere from 2 weeks to 2 months after the injury. Symptoms include persistent headache, lethargy, behavior changes, decreased short-term memory, and changes in intellectual ability.

Although concussion is generally considered benign and usually resolves spontaneously, the symptoms may be the beginning of a more serious, progressive problem. At the time of discharge it is important to give the patient and caregiver instructions for observation and accurate reporting of symptoms or changes in neurologic status.

Diffuse axonal injury (DAI) is widespread axonal damage occurring after a mild, moderate, or severe TBI.

- Clinical signs of DAI include decreased LOC, increased intracranial pressure (ICP), decortication or decerebration, and global cerebral edema. Approximately 90% of patients with DAI remain in a persistent vegetative state.
- Patients who survive the initial event are rapidly triaged to an ICU where they will be vigilantly watched for signs of increased ICP and treated for increased ICP (see Increased Intracranial Pressure, p. 346).

Focal Injury

Focal injury can be minor to severe and can be localized to an area of injury. Focal injury consists of lacerations, contusions, hematomas, and cranial nerve injuries.

Lacerations involve actual tearing of brain tissue and often occur with compound fractures and penetrating injuries. Tissue damage is severe, and surgical repair of the laceration is impossible because of the nature of brain tissue. If bleeding is deep into the brain parenchyma, focal and generalized signs develop. Prognosis is generally poor for the patient with a large intracerebral hemorrhage.

A *contusion* is the bruising of brain tissue within a focal area. It is usually associated with a closed head injury. A contusion may contain areas of hemorrhage, infarction, necrosis, and edema and frequently occurs at a fracture site.

- Contusions or lacerations may occur both at the site of the direct impact of the brain on the skull *(coup)* and at a secondary area of damage on the opposite side away from injury *(contre-coup)*, leading to multiple contused areas.
- Neurologic assessment may demonstrate focal findings as well as generalized findings depending on the size and location of the contusion. Seizures are a common complication.

Complications

Epidural Hematoma

An *epidural hematoma* results from bleeding between the dura and inner surface of the skull. An epidural hematoma is a neurologic emergency and is usually associated with a linear fracture crossing a major artery in the dura, causing a tear. It can have a venous or an arterial origin.

- Venous epidural hematomas are associated with a tear of the dural venous sinus and develop slowly.
- With arterial hematomas, the middle meningeal artery lying under the temporal bone is often torn. Because this is an arterial hemorrhage, the hematoma develops rapidly.

Manifestations typically include an initial period of unconsciousness at the scene, with a brief lucid interval followed by a decrease in LOC. Other symptoms may be headache, nausea and vomiting, or focal findings. Rapid surgical intervention to evacuate the hematoma and prevent cerebral herniation, along with medical management for increasing ICP, can dramatically improve outcomes.

Subdural Hematoma

A *subdural hematoma* occurs from bleeding between the dura mater and the arachnoid layer of the meninges. The hematoma usually results from injury to the brain tissue and its blood vessels. A subdural hematoma is usually venous in origin, with a slow development of the hematoma, but rapid development can occur if the hematoma is of arterial origin. Subdural hematomas may be acute, subacute, or chronic (Table 40).

- An *acute subdural hematoma* manifests within 24 to 48 hours of the injury. Manifestations are similar to those associated with

Table 40 Types of Subdural Hematomas

Occurrence After Injury	Progression of Symptoms	Treatment
Acute 24-48 hr after severe trauma	Immediate deterioration	Craniotomy, evacuation and decompression
Subacute 48 hr–2 wk after severe trauma	Alteration in mental status as hematoma develops Progression dependent on size and location of hematoma	Evacuation and decompression
Chronic Weeks or months, usually >20 days after injury Often injury seemed trivial or was forgotten by patient	Nonspecific, nonlocalizing progression Progressive alteration in LOC	Evacuation and decompression, membranectomy

LOC, Level of consciousness.

brain tissue compression in increased ICP (see Increased Intra-cranial Pressure, p. 346). The patient's appearance may range from drowsy and confused to unconscious. The ipsilateral pupil dilates and becomes fixed if ICP is significantly elevated.

- A *subacute subdural hematoma* usually occurs within 2 to 14 days of the injury. After the initial bleeding, a subdural hematoma may appear to enlarge over time as the breakdown products of the blood draw fluid into the subdural space.
- A *chronic subdural hematoma* develops over weeks or months after a seemingly minor head injury. Chronic subdural hematomas are more common in older adults because of a potentially larger subdural space as a result of brain atrophy. The presenting complaints are focal symptoms, rather than signs of increased ICP.

Intracerebral Hematoma

An *intracerebral hematoma* occurs from bleeding within the brain tissue. It usually occurs within the frontal and temporal lobes, possibly from the rupture of intracerebral vessels at the time of injury.

Diagnostic Studies

- CT scan is the best diagnostic test to evaluate for craniocerebral trauma.
- MRI, positron emission therapy (PET), and evoked potential studies assist in diagnosis and differentiation of head injuries.
- Transcranial Doppler studies are used to measure cerebral blood flow velocity.
- Cervical spine x-ray series, CT scan, or MRI of the spine may be done.

Collaborative Care

Emergency management of the patient with head injury includes measures to prevent secondary injury by treating cerebral edema and managing increased ICP (see Table 57-9, Lewis et al, *Medical-Surgical Nursing,* ed. 9, p. 1372). The principal treatment of head injuries is timely diagnosis and surgery if necessary. For the patient with a concussion or contusion, observation and management of increased ICP are primary management strategies.

- The treatment of skull fractures is usually conservative. For depressed fractures and fractures with loose fragments, a craniotomy is necessary to elevate depressed bone and remove free fragments. If large amounts of bone are destroyed, the bone may be removed (craniectomy) and a cranioplasty will be needed at a later time (see the section on cranial surgery, Lewis et al, *Medical-Surgical Nursing,* ed. 9, pp. 1379 to 1381).

- In cases of large acute subdural and epidural hematomas or those associated with significant neurologic impairment, the blood must be removed. A craniotomy is generally performed to visualize and allow control of the bleeding vessels. Burr-hole openings may be used in an extreme emergency for more rapid decompression, followed by a craniotomy. A drain may be placed postoperatively for several days to prevent reaccumulation of blood.

Nursing Management
Goals
The patient with an acute head injury will maintain adequate cerebral oxygenation and perfusion; remain normothermic; achieve control of pain and discomfort; be free from infection; have adequate nutrition; and attain maximal cognitive, motor, and sensory function.

Nursing Diagnoses/Collaborative Problems
- Risk for ineffective cerebral tissue perfusion
- Hyperthermia
- Impaired physical mobility
- Anxiety
- Potential complication: increased ICP

Nursing Interventions
One of the best ways to prevent head injuries is to prevent car and motorcycle crashes.
- Be active in campaigns that promote driving safety, and speak to driver education classes regarding the dangers of unsafe driving and driving after drinking alcohol and using drugs.
- The use of seat belts in cars and the use of helmets for riding on motorcycles are the most effective measures for increasing survival after crashes.

Acute Intervention. The general goal of nursing management of the head-injured patient is to maintain cerebral oxygenation and perfusion and prevent secondary cerebral ischemia. Surveillance or monitoring for changes in neurologic status is critically important because the patient's condition may deteriorate rapidly, necessitating emergency surgery.
- Explain the need for frequent neurologic assessments to both the patient and caregiver.
- Behavioral manifestations associated with head injury can result in a frightened, disoriented patient who is combative and resists help.

The Glasgow Coma Scale (GCS) is useful in assessing the LOC (see Glasgow Coma Scale, p. 766). Indications of a deteriorating neurologic state, such as a decreasing LOC or lessening of motor strength, should be reported to the health care provider, and the patient's condition should be closely monitored.

The major focus of nursing care for the brain-injured patient relates to increased ICP (see Increased Intracranial Pressure: Nursing Management, p. 346).

- Loss of the corneal reflex may necessitate administering lubricating eye drops or taping the eyes shut to prevent abrasion.
- Periorbital ecchymosis and edema disappear spontaneously, but cold and, later, warm compresses provide comfort and hasten the process.
- Diplopia can be relieved by use of an eye patch.
- Hyperthermia can result in increased metabolism, cerebral blood flow, cerebral blood volume, and ICP. Increased metabolic waste also produces further cerebral vasodilation. Avoid hyperthermia, with a goal of 36° C to 37° C as the standard of care.
- If cerebrospinal fluid (CSF) rhinorrhea or otorrhea occurs, inform the physician immediately. The head of the bed may be elevated to decrease the CSF pressure. A loose collection pad may be placed under the nose or over the ear. Instruct the patient not to sneeze or blow the nose.
- Nausea and vomiting may be a problem and can be alleviated by antiemetic drugs.
- Headache can usually be controlled with acetaminophen or small doses of codeine.

If the patient's condition deteriorates, intracranial surgery may be necessary. A burr-hole opening or craniotomy may be indicated, depending on the underlying injury. The patient is often unconscious before surgery, making it necessary for a family member to sign the consent form for surgery. This is a difficult and frightening time for the patient's caregiver and family and requires sensitive nursing management. The suddenness of the situation makes it especially difficult for the family to cope.

Rehabilitation. Once the condition has stabilized, the patient is usually transferred for acute rehabilitation management. There may be chronic problems related to motor and sensory deficits, communication, memory, and intellectual functioning.

- The patient's outward appearance is not a good indicator of how well the patient will function in the home or work environment given recovery time and rehabilitation.
- The mental and emotional sequelae of brain trauma are often the most incapacitating problems. Many of the patients with head injuries who have been comatose for more than 6 hours undergo some personality change. The patient's behavior may indicate a loss of social restraint, judgment, tact, and emotional control.

Progressive recovery may continue for 6 months or more before a plateau is reached and a prognosis for recovery can be made. Nursing management depends on specific residual deficits. In all cases the family must be given special consideration. They need to understand what is happening and be taught appropriate interaction patterns.

- The family often has unrealistic expectations of the patient as the coma begins to recede. The family expects full return to pretrauma status. In reality, the patient usually experiences a reduced awareness and ability to interpret environmental stimuli.
- Prepare the family for the emergence of the patient from coma and explain that the process of awakening often takes several weeks. Arrange for social work and chaplain consultations for the family in addition to providing open visitation and frequent status updates.
- Family members, particularly spouses, go through role transition as the role changes from one of spouse to that of caregiver.

HEADACHE

Description

Headache is probably the most common type of pain experienced by humans. The majority of people have functional headaches, such as migraine or tension type, whereas others have organic headaches caused by intracranial or extracranial disease.

- *Primary headaches* are those not caused by a disease or another medical condition. They include tension-type, migraine, and cluster headaches. Characteristics of primary headaches are shown in Table 41.
- *Secondary headaches* are caused by another condition or disorder, such as sinus infection, neck injury, and stroke.

Tension-Type Headache

Tension-type headache, also called stress headache, is the most common type of headache and is characterized by its bilateral location and pressing/tightening quality. It is usually of mild or moderate intensity and can last from minutes to days. It is likely that neurovascular factors similar to those involved in migraine headaches play a role in the development of tension-type headaches.

Clinical Manifestations. Patients usually present with a bilateral frontal-occipital headache described as a constant, dull pressure, or bandlike headache associated with neck pain and increased tone in the cervical and neck muscles. There is no prodrome (early manifestation of impending disease) in tension-type headache. The

Table 41 Comparison of Types of Headaches

Pattern	Tension-Type Headache	Migraine Headache	Cluster Headache
Site (see Fig. 59-1, Lewis et al, *Medical-Surgical Nursing*, ed 9, p. 1414)	Bilateral, bandlike pressure at base of skull	Unilateral (in 60%), may switch sides, commonly anterior	Unilateral, radiating up or down from one eye
Quality	Constant, squeezing tightness	Throbbing, synchronous with pulse	Severe, bone-crushing
Frequency	Cycles for many years	Periodic, cycles of several months to years	May have months or years between attacks. Attacks occur in clusters over a period of 2 to 12 wk
Duration	30 min to 7 days	4 to 72 hr	5 min to 3 hr
Time and mode of onset	Not related to time	May be preceded by prodrome. Onset after awakening. Gets better with sleep	Nocturnal, commonly awakens patient from sleep
Associated symptoms	Palpable neck and shoulder muscle tension, stiff neck, tenderness	Nausea, vomiting. Irritability, sweating. Photophobia. Phonophobia. Prodrome of sensory, motor, or psychic phenomena. Family history (in 65%)	Facial flushing or pallor. Unilateral lacrimation, ptosis, and rhinitis

H

headache does not involve nausea or vomiting, but may involve sensitivity to light *(photophobia)* or sound *(phonophobia)*.

- Headaches may occur intermittently for weeks, months, or years. Many patients can have a combination of migraine and tension-type headaches with features of both headaches occurring simultaneously.

Diagnostic Studies. Careful history taking is the most important diagnostic tool. Electromyography (EMG) may reveal sustained contraction of the neck, scalp, or facial muscles. If tension-type headache is present during physical examination, increased resistance to passive movement of the head and tenderness of head and neck may be present.

Migraine Headache

Migraine headache is a recurring headache characterized by unilateral or bilateral throbbing pain, a triggering event or factor, and manifestations associated with neurologic and autonomic nervous system dysfunction. The most common age for migraine onset is between ages 20 and 30 years, with women being affected more than men. Risk factors for migraine include family history, low level of education, low socioeconomic status, high workload, and frequent tension-type headaches.

Pathophysiology. The current theory is that a complex series of neurovascular events initiates a migraine headache. People who have migraines have a state of neuronal hyperexcitability in the cerebral cortex, especially in the occipital cortex. Approximately 70% of those with migraine have a first-degree relative who also had migraine headaches.

Migraines can be preceded by prodrome and aura. The prodrome may precede the headache by several hours or several days.

- The *prodrome* may include neurologic (e.g., photophobia), psychologic (e.g., hyperactivity, irritability), and other (e.g., food craving) manifestations.
- An *aura* is a complex experience of neurologic symptoms characterized by visual (e.g., bright lights, scotomas [patchy blindness], visual distortions [zig-zag lines]) and sensory (hearing voices or sounds that do not exist, strange smells) and/or motor (e.g., weakness, paralysis, feeling that limbs are moving) phenomena.

In many cases, migraine headaches have no known precipitating events. However, for other patients, the headache may be precipitated or triggered by foods, hormonal fluctuation, head trauma, physical exertion, fatigue, stress, and drugs.

Clinical Manifestations. Migraine without aura is the most common type of migraine headache. Migraine with aura occurs in only 10% of migraine headache episodes.

The headache may last 4 to 72 hours. During the headache phase, some patients may tend to "hibernate"; that is, they seek shelter from noise, light, odors, people, and problems. The headache is described as a steady, throbbing pain that is synchronous with the pulse. Although the headache is usually unilateral, it may switch to the opposite side in another episode. In some patients, the symptoms of the migraine headaches may become progressively worse over time.

Diagnostic Studies. There are no specific laboratory or radiologic tests for migraine headache. The diagnosis is usually made from the history. Neurologic and other diagnostic examinations are often normal.

Cluster Headache

Cluster headache, a rare form of headache, involves repeated headaches that typically last 2 weeks to 3 months, and then the patient goes into remission for months to years. The clusters occur with regularity, usually occurring at the same time each day, during the same seasons of the year.

Pathophysiology. Neither the cause nor pathophysiology of cluster headache is fully known. The trigeminal nerve has a role in the production of pain, but cluster headaches also involve dysfunction of intracranial blood vessels, the sympathetic nervous system, and pain modulation systems. Imaging studies show hypothalamic activation at the onset of cluster headache. Alcohol is the only dietary trigger. Strong odors, weather changes, and napping are other triggers.

Clinical Manifestations. The cluster headache is one of the most severe forms of headache, with intense pain lasting from a few minutes to 3 hours.

- The pain is generally located around the eye, radiating to the temple, forehead, cheek, nose, or gums.
- Other manifestations include swelling around the eye, lacrimation (tearing), facial flushing or pallor, rhinitis, and constriction of the pupil.
- During the headache, the patient is often agitated and restless, unable to sit still or relax.

Diagnostic Studies. Diagnosis is primarily based on the history. Asking patients to keep a headache diary can be useful. CT scan, MRI, or magnetic resonance angiography (MRA) may rule out an aneurysm, a tumor, or an infection. A lumbar puncture may rule out other disorders.

Collaborative Care

If no systemic underlying disease is found, the type of headache guides the therapy. Table 59-3, Lewis et al, *Medical-Surgical Nursing,* ed. 9, p. 1417 summarizes current therapies for prophylaxis and symptomatic relief of headaches. These therapies include drugs, meditation, yoga, biofeedback, cognitive-behavioral therapy, and relaxation training.

Drug Therapy

Tension-Type Headache. Drug treatment usually involves aspirin, acetaminophen, or nonsteroidal antiinflammatory drugs (NSAIDs) used alone or in combination with a sedative, muscle relaxant, or tranquilizer. However, many of these drugs have serious side effects.

Migraine Headache. Drug treatment is aimed at terminating or decreasing the symptoms of the acute attack. Many people with mild or moderate migraine can obtain relief with NSAIDs, aspirin, or caffeine-containing combination analgesics. For moderate to severe headaches, the triptans have become the first line of therapy.

- Triptans affect selected serotonin receptors, reducing the neurogenic inflammation of the cerebral blood vessels and producing vasoconstriction. They include sumatriptan (Imitrex), naratriptan (Amerge), rizatriptan (Maxalt), almotriptan (Axert), frovatriptan (Frova), zolmitriptan (Zomig), and eletriptan (Relpax). The combination drug sumatriptan/naproxen (Treximet) combines a triptan with an antiinflammatory drug. Because these drugs cause vasoconstriction, they are avoided in patients with heart disease or stroke. Triptan medications should be taken at the first symptom of migraine headache.
- Topiramate (Topamax), taken daily, has been shown to be an effective therapy for migraine prevention in adults. It must be used for 2 to 3 months to determine its effectiveness. Other preventive drugs for migraine headaches can include β-adrenergic blockers (e.g., propranolol [Inderal], atenolol [Tenormin]), tricyclic antidepressants (e.g., amitriptyline [Elavil]), selective serotonin reuptake inhibitors (e.g., fluoxetine [Prozac]), and calcium channel blockers (e.g., verapamil (Calan), flunarizine (Sibelium).
- Botulinum toxin (Botox) may be an effective prophylactic treatment for patients who have chronic migraines or migraines that do not respond to other medications.

Cluster Headache. Because these headaches occur suddenly, often at night, and are not long lasting, drug therapy is not as useful as it is for other types of headache. Prophylactic medications may include verapamil (Isoptin), lithium, ergotamine, melatonin, or divalproex (Depakote).

- Acute treatment of cluster headache is inhalation of 100% oxygen (O_2) delivered at a rate of 6 to 8 L/min for 10 minutes, which may relieve headache by causing vasoconstriction. The triptans (e.g., sumatriptan) are also effective in treating acute cluster headache. Intranasal administration of lidocaine is useful as an adjunctive therapy.

- Methysergide may be used prophylactically when the cluster headache recurs at a known time.

Nursing Management

Goals

The patient with a headache will have reduced or no pain, experience increased comfort and decreased anxiety, demonstrate understanding of triggering events and treatment strategies, use positive coping strategies to deal with pain, and experience increased quality of life and decreased disability.

Nursing Diagnoses

- Acute pain
- Ineffective self-health management

Nursing Interventions

Headaches may result from an inability to cope with daily stresses. An effective therapy may be to help patients examine their lifestyle, recognize stressful situations, and learn to cope with them more appropriately. Help the patient identify precipitating factors and develop ways to avoid them. Encourage daily exercise, relaxation periods, and socializing because each can help decrease the recurrence of headache.

- Suggest alternative ways of handling the pain of headache through techniques such as relaxation, meditation, yoga, and self-hypnosis. Massage and moist hot packs to the neck and head can help a patient with tension-type headaches.
- The patient should learn about drugs prescribed for prophylactic and symptomatic treatment of headache and should be able to describe the purpose, action, dosage, and side effects.
- For the patient whose headaches are triggered by food, provide dietary counseling. The patient needs to be encouraged to eliminate foods that may provoke headaches (e.g., chocolate, alcohol, excessive caffeine, cheese, fermented foods, monosodium glutamate).
- Cluster headache attacks may occur at high altitudes with low oxygen levels during air travel. Ergotamine, taken before the plane takes off, may decrease the likelihood of these attacks.

▼ **Patient and Caregiver Teaching**

A teaching guide for the patient with a headache is provided in Table 42.

Table 42	Patient and Caregiver Teaching Guide *Headaches*

For the patient with a headache, include the following instructions when teaching the patient and caregiver.

- Keep a diary or calendar of headaches and possible precipitating events.
- Avoid factors that can trigger a headache:
  - Foods containing amines (cheese, chocolate), nitrites (meats such as hot dogs), vinegar, onions, monosodium glutamate
  - Fermented or marinated foods
  - Caffeine
  - Oranges
  - Tomatoes
  - Aspartame
  - Nicotine
  - Ice cream
  - Alcohol (particularly red wine)
  - Emotional stress
  - Fatigue
  - Drugs such as ergot-containing preparations (ergotamine tartrate [Ergomar]) and monoamine oxidase inhibitors (e.g., rasagiline [Azilect])
- Learn the purpose, action, dosage, and side effects of drugs taken.
- Self-administer sumatriptan (Imitrex) subcutaneously if prescribed.
- Use stress management techniques such as relaxation.
- Participate in regular exercise.
- Contact health care provider if any of the following occurs:
  - Symptoms become more severe, last longer than usual, or are resistant to medication.
  - Nausea and vomiting (if severe or not typical), change in vision, or fever occurs with the headache.
  - Problems occur with any drugs.

HEART FAILURE

Description

Heart failure (HF) is an abnormal clinical syndrome involving impaired cardiac pumping and/or filling of the heart. This results in the inability of the heart to provide sufficient blood to meet the oxygen needs of the tissues. In clinical practice, the terms acute and chronic HF have replaced the term congestive HF (CHF) because not all HF involves pulmonary congestion.

HF is associated with numerous types of cardiovascular diseases, particularly long-standing hypertension, coronary artery disease (CAD), and MI.

- HF is a major health problem in the United States. In contrast to other cardiovascular diseases, HF is increasing in incidence and prevalence. This is because of improved survival after cardiovascular events and the increased aging population. HF is the most common reason for hospital admission in older adults.
- CAD and hypertension are the primary risk factors for HF. Other factors, including advanced age, diabetes, cigarette smoking, obesity, and high serum cholesterol, contribute to the development of HF.

Pathophysiology

HF may be caused by any interference with the normal mechanisms regulating cardiac output (CO). CO depends on (1) preload, (2) afterload, (3) myocardial contractility, and (4) heart rate (HR). Any changes in these factors can lead to decreased ventricular function and subsequent HF.

- Major causes of HF may be divided into two subgroups: (1) *primary causes,* consisting of underlying cardiac diseases, such as CAD and cardiomyopathy; and (2) *precipitating causes,* such as anemia, pulmonary disease, and hypervolemia (see the complete listing of causes in Tables 35-1 and 35-2, Lewis et al, *Medical-Surgical Nursing,* ed. 9, p. 767).

Heart failure is classified as systolic or diastolic failure. *Systolic failure* results from an inability of the heart to pump effectively. It is caused by impaired contractile function (e.g., MI), increased afterload (e.g., hypertension), cardiomyopathy, and mechanical abnormalities (e.g., valvular heart disease). The hallmark of systolic dysfunction is a decrease in the left ventricular ejection fraction (EF).

Diastolic failure is the inability of the ventricles to relax and fill during diastole. Decreased filling results in decreased stroke volume and CO and venous engorgement in both the pulmonary and systemic vascular systems. The diagnosis of diastolic failure is based on the presence of HF symptoms with a normal EF. Diastolic failure is usually the result of left ventricular hypertrophy from chronic hypertension, aortic stenosis, or hypertrophic cardiomyopathy.

Mixed systolic and diastolic failure is seen in disease states such as dilated cardiomyopathy, in which poor systolic function (weakened muscle function) is further compromised by dilated left ventricular walls that are unable to relax.

The patient with ventricular failure of any type has low systemic arterial BP, low CO, and poor renal perfusion. Whether a patient arrives at this point acutely (from an MI) or chronically

H

(from worsening cardiomyopathy or hypertension), the body's response to this low CO is to mobilize compensatory mechanisms to maintain CO and BP. The main compensatory mechanisms include (1) sympathetic nervous system activation, (2) neurohormonal responses, (3) ventricular dilation, and (4) ventricular hypertrophy.

HF is usually manifested by biventricular failure, although one ventricle may precede the other in dysfunction.

- *Left-sided failure* is the most common form of initial heart failure. Left-sided failure causes blood to back up into the left atrium and pulmonary veins. The increased pulmonary pressure causes fluid leakage from the pulmonary capillary bed into the interstitium and then the alveoli, which is manifested as pulmonary congestion and edema.
- *Right-sided failure* causes a backup of blood into the right atrium and venous circulation. Venous congestion in the systemic circulation results in peripheral edema, hepatomegaly, and jugular venous distention. The primary cause of right-sided failure is left-sided failure. *Cor pulmonale* (right ventricular dilation and hypertrophy caused by pulmonary pathologic conditions) can also cause right-sided failure (see Cor Pulmonale, p. 159).

The primary cause of right-sided HF is left-sided HF. In this situation, left-sided HF results in pulmonary congestion and increased pressure in the blood vessels of the lung (pulmonary hypertension). Eventually, chronic pulmonary hypertension (increased right ventricular afterload) results in right-sided hypertrophy and HF.

Manifestations

Acute Decompensated Heart Failure

In acute decompensated HF (ADHF), an increase in the pulmonary venous pressure is caused by failure of the left ventricle (LV). This results in engorgement of the pulmonary vascular system. This early stage is clinically associated with a mild increase in the respiratory rate and a decrease in partial pressure of oxygen in arterial blood (PaO_2). ADHF can manifest as *pulmonary edema*. This is an acute, life-threatening situation in which the lung alveoli become filled with serosanguineous fluid. The most common cause of pulmonary edema is acute LV failure secondary to CAD.

- Manifestations of pulmonary edema are distinct: the patient is usually anxious, pale, and possibly cyanotic, with clammy and cold skin.
- The patient has dyspnea, respiratory rate greater than 30 breaths/min, and orthopnea. Wheezing and coughing with production of frothy, blood-tinged sputum may also occur.

- Auscultation of the lungs may reveal bubbling crackles, wheezes, and rhonchi. The patient's HR is rapid, and BP may be elevated or decreased depending on the severity of the HF.

Chronic Heart Failure

Manifestations of chronic HF depend on the patient's age, underlying type and extent of heart disease, and which ventricle is failing to pump effectively. Table 43 lists manifestations of left-sided and right-sided failure. The patient with chronic HF usually has manifestations of biventricular failure.

- Fatigue after usual activities is one of the earliest symptoms.

Table 43	Manifestations of Heart Failure

Right-Sided Heart Failure	Left-Sided Heart Failure
Signs	
■ RV heaves	■ LV heaves
■ Murmurs	■ Pulsus alternans (alternating pulses: strong, weak)
■ Jugular venous distention	■ ↑ HR
■ Edema (e.g., pedal, scrotum, sacrum)	■ PMI displaced inferiorly and posteriorly (LV hypertrophy)
■ Weight gain	■ ↓ PaO_2, slight ↑ $PaCO_2$ (poor O_2 exchange)
■ ↑ HR	■ Crackles (pulmonary edema)
■ Ascites	■ S_3 and S_4 heart sounds
■ Anasarca (massive generalized body edema)	■ Pleural effusion
■ Hepatomegaly (liver enlargement)	■ Changes in mental status
	■ Restlessness, confusion
Symptoms	
■ Fatigue	■ Weakness, fatigue
■ Anxiety, depression	■ Anxiety, depression
■ Dependent, bilateral edema	■ Dyspnea
■ Right upper quadrant pain	■ Shallow respirations up to 32-40/min
■ Anorexia and GI bloating	■ Paroxysmal nocturnal dyspnea
■ Nausea	■ Orthopnea (shortness of breath in recumbent position)
	■ Dry, hacking cough
	■ Nocturia
	■ Frothy, pink-tinged sputum (advanced pulmonary edema)

LV, Left ventricle; *$PaCO_2$,* partial pressure of CO_2 in arterial blood; *PaO_2,* partial pressure of O_2 in arterial blood; *PMI,* point of maximal impulse; *RV,* right ventricle.

- Dyspnea is a common sign. Shortness of breath occurs when the patient is in the recumbent position (orthopnea).
- Paroxysmal nocturnal dyspnea (PND) occurs when the patient is asleep. The patient awakens in a panic, has feelings of suffocation, and has a strong desire to sit or stand up.
- A cough is often associated with HF and may be the first clinical symptom. It begins as a dry, nonproductive cough that is not relieved by position change or over-the-counter cough medicine.
- Other common signs include tachycardia; edema in the legs, liver, abdominal cavity, and lungs; nocturia; dusky skin; restlessness and confusion; angina; and weight changes.

Complications

Pleural effusion results from increasing pressure in the pleural capillaries. Enlargement of the heart chambers in chronic HF can cause atrial fibrillation. Patients also are at risk for ventricular dysrhythmias.

Left ventricular thrombus may occur with ADHF or chronic HF in which the enlarged LV and decreased CO combine to increase the chance of thrombus formation in the LV. This places the patient at risk for stroke.

Hepatomegaly may result as the liver becomes congested with venous blood. Hepatic congestion leads to impaired liver function; eventually liver cells die, and cirrhosis can develop. The decreased CO that accompanies chronic HF also results in decreased perfusion to the kidneys and can lead to renal insufficiency or failure.

Diagnostic Studies

Diagnosing HF is often difficult because neither patient signs nor symptoms are highly specific, and both may mimic many other medical conditions (e.g., anemia, lung disease). Diagnostic tests for acute decompensated and chronic heart failure are presented in Table 44.

A primary diagnostic goal is to determine the underlying etiology. An endomyocardial biopsy (EMB) may be done in patients who develop unexplained, new-onset HF that is unresponsive to usual care. EF is used to differentiate systolic and diastolic HF. In general, b-type natriuretic peptide (BNP) levels correlate positively with the degree of left ventricular dysfunction.

Nursing and Collaborative Management: Acute Decompensated Heart Failure

With the addition of new drugs and device therapies, the management of HF has dramatically changed in the past few years. Table 44 lists collaborative therapy for the patient with ADHF.

Table 44 Collaborative Care
Heart Failure

Both ADHF and Chronic HF	ADHF	Chronic HF
Diagnostic	▪ ABGs	▪ Exercise stress testing
▪ History and physical examination	▪ Endomyocardial biopsy	
▪ Determination of underlying cause		
▪ Serum chemistries, cardiac enzymes, BNP or NT-proBNP level (see Table 32-6, Lewis et al, *Medical-Surgical Nursing*, 9e, p. 699), liver function tests, thyroid function tests, CBC		
▪ Chest x-ray		
▪ 12-lead ECG		
▪ Hemodynamic monitoring		
▪ Echocardiogram		
▪ Nuclear imaging studies (see Table 32-6, Lewis et al, *Medical-Surgical Nursing*, 9e, pp. 701-702)		
▪ Cardiac catheterization		

H

Continued

Table 44 Collaborative Care
Heart Failure—cont'd

Both ADHF and Chronic HF	ADHF	Chronic HF
Collaborative Therapy ■ Treatment of underlying cause ■ Circulatory assist devices (e.g., ventricular assist device) ■ Daily weights ■ Sodium- and, possibly, fluid-restricted diet	■ High Fowler's position ■ O₂ by mask or nasal cannula ■ BiPAP ■ Circulatory assist device: intraaortic balloon pump ■ Endotracheal intubation and mechanical ventilation ■ Vital signs, urine output at least q1hr ■ Continuous ECG and pulse oximetry monitoring ■ Hemodynamic monitoring (e.g., intraarterial BP, PAWP, CO) ■ Drug therapy (see Table 35-7, Lewis et al, *Medical-Surgical Nursing*, 9e, p. 774) ■ Possible cardioversion (e.g., atrial fibrillation) ■ Ultrafiltration	■ O₂ therapy at 2-6 L/min by nasal cannula if indicated ■ Rest-activity periods ■ Cardiac rehabilitation ■ Home health nursing care (e.g., telehealth monitoring) ■ Drug therapy (see Table 35-7, Lewis et al, *Medical-Surgical Nursing*, 9e, p. 774) ■ Cardiac resynchronization therapy with biventricular pacing and internal cardioverter-defibrillator ■ LVAD ■ Cardiac transplantation ■ Palliative and end-of-life care

ABGs, Arterial blood gases; *ADHF,* acute decompensated heart failure; *BiPAP,* bilevel positive airway pressure; *BNP,* b-type natriuretic peptide; *CO,* cardiac output; *HF,* heart failure; *LVAD,* left ventricular assist device; *NT-proBNP,* N-terminal prohormone of BNP; *PAWP,* pulmonary artery wedge pressure.

Patients with ADHF need continuous monitoring and assessment, which may be done in an intensive care unit (ICU) setting. Monitor ECG and oxygen saturation. The patient may have continuous hemodynamic monitoring. Supplemental oxygen helps increase the percentage of oxygen in inspired air. In severe pulmonary edema the patient may need noninvasive ventilatory support or intubation and mechanical ventilation.

- If the patient is dyspneic, place in a high Fowler's position with the feet horizontal in the bed or dangling at the bedside. This position helps decrease venous return because of the pooling of blood in the extremities.
- Ultrafiltration is an option for the patient with volume overload. It can rapidly remove intravascular fluid volume while maintaining hemodynamic stability.
- Circulatory assist devices are used to manage patients with worsening HF. The intraaortic balloon pump (IABP) increases coronary blood flow to the heart muscle and decreases the heart's workload. Ventricular assist devices can be used to maintain the pumping action of the heart.
- Assess patients with HF for depression and anxiety, and treatment plans should be initiated if appropriate.

Drug Therapy

Drug therapy is essential in treating acute heart failure.

- *Diuretics:* Diuretics are the mainstay of treatment in patients with volume overload. They act to decrease sodium reabsorption within the nephrons, thereby enhancing sodium and water loss. Decreasing venous return (preload) reduces the amount of volume returned to the LV during diastole. Decreasing intravascular volume with the use of loop diuretics (e.g., furosemide [Lasix], bumetanide [Bumex]) reduces venous return.
- *Vasodilators:* IV nitroglycerin reduces preload, slightly reduces afterload (in high doses), and increases myocardial oxygen supply. Sodium nitroprusside (Nipride) reduces both preload and afterload, thus improving myocardial contraction, increasing CO, and reducing pulmonary congestion. IV nesiritide (Natrecor), a recombinant form of BNP, causes both arterial and venous dilation.
- *Morphine:* Morphine sulfate reduces preload and afterload and is used in the treatment of ADHF and pulmonary edema. It dilates the pulmonary and systemic blood vessels, thereby decreasing pulmonary pressures and improving gas exchange.
- *Positive inotropics:* Inotropic therapy increases myocardial contractility. Drugs include β-adrenergic agonists (e.g., dopamine [Intropin], dobutamine [Dobutrex], epinephrine, norepinephrine [Levophed]), phosphodiesterase inhibitors (inamrinone [Inocor], milrinone [Primacor]), and digitalis.

Digitalis is a positive inotrope that improves LV function but also increases myocardial oxygen consumption. Inotropic therapy is only recommended for use in the short-term management of patients with ADHF who have not responded to conventional pharmacotherapy (e.g., diuretics, vasodilators, morphine).

Collaborative Care: Chronic Heart Failure

The main goals in the treatment of chronic HF are to treat the underlying cause and contributing factors, maximize CO, reduce symptoms, improve ventricular function, improve quality of life, preserve target organ function, and improve mortality and morbidity. The treatment of causes such as dysrhythmias, hypertension, valvular disorders, and CAD is discussed elsewhere in this book.

Nondrug Therapy

- Administration of O_2 improves O_2 saturation and assists in meeting tissue oxygen needs, thereby helping to relieve dyspnea and fatigue.
- Physical and emotional rest conserves energy and decreases the need for additional O_2. A patient with severe HF may be on bed rest with limited activity. A patient with mild to moderate HF can be ambulatory with a restriction of strenuous activity.

Cardiac resynchronization therapy (CRT), unlike traditional pacing, coordinates right and left ventricular contractility through biventricular pacing. The ability to have normal simultaneous electrical conduction (synchrony) within the right and left ventricles increases left ventricular function and CO.

Mechanical options such as the IABP and ventricular assist devices (VADs) are available for patients with deteriorating conditions, especially those awaiting cardiac transplantation. Limitations of bed rest, infection, and vascular complications preclude long-term use of IABPs. VADs provide highly effective long-term support and have become standard care in many heart transplant centers.

Drug Therapy

- *Diuretics:* Diuretics reduce edema, pulmonary venous pressure, and preload. Thiazide diuretics (e.g., hydrochlorothiazide [Hydrodiuril]) inhibit sodium reabsorption in the distal tubule, thus promoting excretion of sodium and water. Loop diuretics such as furosemide (Lasix), bumetanide (Bumex), and torsemide (Demadex) are potent but can cause hypokalemia and ototoxicity. In chronic HF the lowest effective dose of diuretic should be used.
- *Angiotensin-converting enzyme (ACE) inhibitors:* ACE inhibitors (e.g., captopril [Capoten], enalapril [Vasotec]) are the primary drugs of choice for blocking the renin-angiotensin-aldosterone system in HF patients with systolic failure. A reduction in systemic vascular resistance (SVR) with the use of ACE inhibitors

causes a significant increase in CO. Although BP decreases, tissue perfusion is maintained or increased as a result of improved CO, and diuresis is enhanced by the suppression of aldosterone.

- *Nitrates:* Nitrates (e.g., nitroglycerin) cause vasodilation by acting directly on the smooth muscle of the vessel wall. Nitrates are of particular benefit in the management of myocardial ischemia related to HF because they promote vasodilation of the coronary arteries.
- *BiDil:* A combination drug containing isosorbide dinitrate and hydralazine (BiDil) is used for the treatment of HF in African Americans who are already being treated with standard therapy.
- *β-Adrenergic blockers:* β-Adrenergic blockers including carvedilol (Coreg), metoprolol (Toprol-XL), and bisoprolol (Zebeta) directly block the negative effects of the sympathetic nervous system on the failing heart.
- *Positive inotropes:* Positive inotropes are used to improve cardiac contractility. Digitalis preparations (e.g., digoxin [Lanoxin]) increase the force of cardiac contraction *(inotropic action).* They also decrease conduction speed within the myocardium and slow the HR *(chronotropic action).* This allows for more complete emptying of the ventricles, reducing the volume remaining in the ventricles during diastole. CO increases because of increased stroke volume from improved contractility.

Nutritional Therapy

Diet teaching and weight management are essential to the patient's control of chronic HF. You or a dietitian should obtain a detailed diet history to determine not only what foods the patient eats but also when, where, and how often they dine out.

The edema associated with chronic HF is often treated by dietary restriction of sodium. Teach the patient what foods are low and high in sodium and ways to enhance food flavors without the use of salt (e.g., substituting lemon juice, various spices). The degree of sodium restriction depends on the severity of the HF and the effectiveness of diuretic therapy.

- A commonly prescribed diet for a patient with mild HF is a 2-g sodium diet. All foods high in sodium should be eliminated. (For sample menu plans for sodium-restricted diets see Table 35-8, Lewis et al, *Medical-Surgical Nursing,* ed. 9, p. 778).

Fluid restrictions are not commonly prescribed for mild to moderate HF. However, in moderate to severe HF, fluid restrictions are usually implemented.

- Instruct patients to weigh themselves at the same time each day, preferably before breakfast, while wearing the same type of clothing. For a weight gain of 3 lb (1.4 kg) over 2 days or a 5-lb (2.3-kg) gain over 1 week, the primary health care provider should be called.

Nursing Management: Chronic Heart Failure

Goals

The patient with HF will have a decrease in symptoms (e.g., shortness of breath, fatigue), decreased peripheral edema, increased exercise tolerance, adherence with medical regimen, and no complications related to HF.

See NCP 35-1 for the patient with HF, Lewis et al, *Medical-Surgical Nursing,* ed. 9, pp. 780 to 781.

Nursing Diagnoses

- Activity intolerance
- Excess fluid volume
- Decreased cardiac output
- Impaired gas exchange

Nursing Interventions

Help to aggressively identify and treat risk factors for HF to prevent or slow the progression of the disease. For example, teach a patient with hypertension or hyperlipidemia measures to manage BP or cholesterol with medication, diet, and exercise. Patients with valvular disease should have valve replacement planned before lung congestion develops.

Acute Intervention.   Many people with HF will experience one or more episodes of ADHF. When they do, they are usually managed in an intensive care unit, an intermediate care unit with continuous cardiac monitoring capability, or a specialized HF unit.

- Successful HF management depends on several important principles: (1) HF is a progressive disease, and treatment plans are established along with quality-of-life goals; (2) symptom management is controlled by the patient with self-management tools (e.g., daily weights, drug regimens, diet and exercise plans); (3) salt and, at times, water must be restricted; (4) energy must be conserved; and (5) support systems are essential to the success of the entire treatment plan.
- Reduction of anxiety is an important nursing function, since anxiety may increase the sympathetic nervous system (SNS) response and further increase myocardial workload. Reducing anxiety may be facilitated by a variety of nursing interventions and the use of sedatives (e.g., benzodiazepines, morphine sulfate).

Ambulatory and Home Care.   HF is a chronic illness for most people. Important nursing responsibilities are to (1) teach the patient about physiologic changes that have occurred, (2) help the patient adapt to both physiologic and psychologic changes, and (3) integrate the patient and caregiver in the overall care plan.

A patient and caregiver teaching guide for HF is presented in Table 45.

Table 45	**Patient and Caregiver Teaching Guide** *Heart Failure*

Include the following instructions when teaching the patient and caregiver management of heart failure.

Dietary Therapy

- Consult the written diet plan and list of permitted and restricted foods.
- Examine labels to determine sodium content. Also examine the labels of over-the-counter drugs such as laxatives, cough medicines, and antacids for sodium content.
- Avoid salt when preparing foods or adding salt to foods.
- Weigh yourself at the same time each day, preferably in the morning, using the same scale and wearing the same or similar clothes.
- Eat smaller, more frequent meals.

Activity Program

- Increase walking and other activities gradually, provided they do not cause fatigue or dyspnea. Consider a cardiac rehabilitation program.
- Avoid extremes of heat and cold.

Ongoing Monitoring

- Know the signs and symptoms of worsening heart failure (see eTable 35-1: Who Is the Patient With Heart Failure? Think FACES [Fatigue, limitation of Activities, chest Congestion/cough, Edema, and Shortness of breath], Lewis et al, *Medical-Surgical Nursing*, 9e, on the Evolve website for Chapter 35).
- Recall the symptoms experienced when illness began. Reappearance of previous symptoms may indicate a recurrence.
- Report immediately to health care provider any of the following:
  - Weight gain of 3 lb (1.4 kg) in 2 days, or 3-5 lb (2.3 kg) in a week
  - Difficulty breathing, especially with exertion or when lying flat
  - Waking up breathless at night
  - Frequent dry, hacking cough, especially when lying down
  - Fatigue, weakness
  - Swelling of ankles, feet, or abdomen; swelling of face or difficulty breathing (if taking ACE inhibitors)
  - Nausea with abdominal swelling, pain, and tenderness
  - Dizziness or fainting
- Follow up with health care provider on regular basis.
- Consider joining a local support group with your family members and/or caregiver(s).

H

Continued

| Table 45 | Patient and Caregiver Teaching Guide
Heart Failure—cont'd |

Health Promotion
- Obtain annual flu vaccination.
- Obtain pneumococcal vaccine (e.g., Pneumovax) and revaccination after 5 yr (for people at high risk of infection or serious disease).
- Develop plan to reduce risk factors (e.g., BP control, smoking cessation, weight reduction).

Rest
- Plan a regular daily rest and activity program.
- After exertion, such as exercise and ADLs, plan a rest period.
- Shorten working hours or schedule rest period during working hours.
- Avoid emotional upsets. Verbalize any concerns, fears, feelings of depression, etc., to health care provider.

Drug Therapy
- Take each drug as prescribed.
- Develop a system (e.g., daily chart, weekly pillbox) to ensure medications have been taken.
- Take pulse rate each day before taking medications (if appropriate). Know the parameters that your health care provider wants for your heart rate.
- Take BP at determined intervals (if appropriate). Know your target BP limits.
- Know signs and symptoms of orthostatic hypotension and how to prevent them (see Table 33-12, Lewis et al, *Medical-Surgical Nursing*, ed. 9, p. 724).
- Know signs and symptoms of internal bleeding (bleeding gums, increased bruises, blood in stool or urine) and what to do if taking anticoagulants.
- Know own INR if taking warfarin (Coumadin) and how often to have blood monitored.

ACE, Angiotensin-converting enzyme; *INR,* international normalized ratio.

HEMOPHILIA AND VON WILLEBRAND DISEASE

Description

Hemophilia is an X-linked recessive genetic disorder caused by a defective or deficient coagulation factor. The two major types of hemophilia that can occur in mild to severe forms are *hemophilia A* (classic hemophilia, factor VIII deficiency) and *hemophilia B*

(Christmas disease, factor IX deficiency). *von Willebrand disease* is a related disorder involving a deficiency of the von Willebrand coagulation protein.

Hemophilia A is the most common form of hemophilia, accounting for about 85% of all cases. von Willebrand disease is considered the most common congenital bleeding disorder in humans, with estimates as high as 1 or 2 in 100 people.

Deficiency and inheritance patterns of these three forms of inherited coagulopathies are compared in Table 46.

Clinical Manifestations and Complications

Clinical manifestations and complications related to hemophilia include (1) slow, persistent, prolonged bleeding from minor trauma and small cuts; (2) delayed bleeding after minor injuries (the delay may be several hours or days); (3) uncontrollable hemorrhage after dental extractions or irritation of the gingiva with a hard-bristle toothbrush; (4) epistaxis, especially after a blow to the face; (5) GI bleeding from ulcers and gastritis; (6) hematuria from genitourinary (GU) trauma and splenic rupture resulting from falls or abdominal trauma; (7) ecchymoses and subcutaneous hematomas; (8) neurologic signs, such as pain, anesthesia, and paralysis, that may develop from nerve compression caused

H

| Table 46 | Types of Hemophilia |

Type	Inheritance Pattern
Hemophilia A	
Factor VIII	Recessive sex-linked (transmitted by female carriers, displayed almost exclusively in men)
Hemophilia B	
Factor IX	Recessive sex-linked (transmitted by female carriers, displayed almost exclusively in men)
von Willebrand Disease	
vWF, variable factor VIII deficiencies and platelet dysfunction	Autosomal dominant, seen in both genders
	Recessive (in severe forms of the disease)

vWF, von Willebrand factor.

by hematoma formation; and (9) hemarthrosis (bleeding into the joints), which may lead to joint deformity severe enough to cause crippling (commonly in knees, elbows, shoulders, hips, and ankles).

Diagnostic Studies

Laboratory studies determine the type of hemophilia present. Any factor deficiency within the intrinsic system (factor VIII, IX, XI, or XII or von Willebrand factor [vWF]) will yield the laboratory results presented in Table 31-18, Lewis et al, *Medical-Surgical Nursing,* ed 9, p. 656.

Collaborative Care

The goal of care is to prevent and treat bleeding. People with hemophilia or von Willebrand disease require preventive care, the use of replacement therapy during acute bleeding episodes and as prophylaxis, and treatment of complications of the disease and its therapy.

- Replacement of deficient clotting factors is the primary means of supporting patients with hemophilia. In addition to treating acute crises, replacement therapy may be given before surgery and dental care as a prophylactic measure.
- For mild hemophilia A or certain subtypes of von Willebrand disease, desmopressin acetate (DDAVP), a synthetic analog of vasopressin, may be used to stimulate an increase in factor VIII and vWF.

Complications of treatment of hemophilia include development of inhibitors to factors VIII or IX, transfusion-transmitted infectious disorders, allergic reactions, and thrombotic complications with the use of factor IX because it contains activated coagulation factors.

The most common difficulty with acute management is starting factor replacement therapy too late and stopping it too soon. Generally, minor bleeding episodes should be treated for at least 72 hours. Surgery and traumatic injuries may need more prolonged support. Chronically, the development of inhibitors to the factor products has occurred and requires individualized expert patient management.

Nursing Management

Because of the hereditary nature of hemophilia, referral of affected people for genetic counseling before reproduction is an essential preventive measure. Counseling is especially important because people with hemophilia are living into adulthood.

Acute interventions are related primarily to controlling the bleeding and include the following:

1. Stop the topical bleeding as quickly as possible by applying direct pressure or ice, packing the area with Gelfoam or

fibrin foam, and applying topical hemostatic agents, such as thrombin.

2. Administer the specific coagulation factor concentrate as ordered. Monitor the patient for signs and symptoms such as hypersensitivity.

3. When joint bleeding occurs, it is important to totally rest the involved joint to prevent crippling deformities from hemarthrosis. Pack the joint in ice. Give analgesics (e.g., acetaminophen, codeine) to reduce severe pain. Aspirin and aspirin-containing compounds should never be used. As soon as bleeding ceases, encourage mobilization of the affected area through range-of-motion (ROM) exercises and physical therapy. Weight bearing is avoided until all swelling has resolved and muscle strength has returned.

4. Manage life-threatening complications that may develop as a result of hemorrhage. Examples include prevention or treatment of airway obstruction from hemorrhage into the neck and pharynx, as well as early assessment and treatment of intracranial bleeding.

▼ Patient and Caregiver Teaching

Quality and length of life may be significantly affected by the patient's knowledge of the illness and how to live with it. Provide ongoing assessment of the patient's adaptation to the illness.

- Teach the patient with hemophilia that immediate medical attention is required for severe pain or swelling of a muscle or joint that restricts movement or inhibits sleep and for a head injury, swelling in the neck or mouth, abdominal pain, hematuria, melena, and skin wounds in need of suturing.
- Teach the patient to perform daily oral hygiene without causing trauma.
- Advise the patient to only participate in noncontact sports (e.g., golf) and to wear gloves when doing household chores to prevent cuts or abrasions from knives, hammers, and other tools.
- The patient should wear a Medic Alert tag to ensure that health care providers know about the hemophilia in case of an accident.
- Many patients or their caregivers can be taught to self-administer the factor replacement therapies at home.

HEMORRHOIDS

Description

Hemorrhoids are dilated veins that may be internal (occurring above the internal sphincter) or external (occurring outside the external sphincter).

Pathophysiology

Hemorrhoids develop as a result of increased anal pressure and weakened connective tissue that normally supports the hemorrhoidal veins. When supporting tissues in the anal canal weaken, usually as a result of straining at defecation, venules become dilated. In addition, blood flow through the veins of the hemorrhoidal plexus is impaired. An intravascular clot in the venule results in a thrombosed external hemorrhoid.

Hemorrhoids are the most common reason for bleeding with defecation. Hemorrhoids may be precipitated by many factors, including pregnancy, prolonged constipation, straining in an effort to defecate, heavy lifting, prolonged standing and sitting, and portal hypertension (as found in cirrhosis).

Clinical Manifestations

Classic manifestations of hemorrhoids include bleeding, anal pruritus, prolapse, and pain.

- *Internal hemorrhoids* may be asymptomatic, but when they become constricted, pain occurs. Internal hemorrhoids can bleed, resulting in blood on toilet paper after defecation or blood on the outside of the stool. The patient may report a chronic, dull aching discomfort, particularly when hemorrhoids have prolapsed.
- *External hemorrhoids* are reddish blue and seldom bleed or cause pain unless a vein ruptures. Blood clots in external hemorrhoids cause pain and inflammation and are described as thrombosed. External hemorrhoids cause intermittent pain, pain on palpation, itching, and burning. Patients also report bleeding associated with defecation. Constipation or diarrhea can aggravate these symptoms.

Diagnostic Studies

- *Internal hemorrhoids* are diagnosed by digital examination, anoscopy, and sigmoidoscopy.
- *External hemorrhoids* can be diagnosed by visual inspection and digital examination.

Collaborative Care

Therapy is directed toward the causes of the condition and the patient's symptoms. A high-fiber diet and increased fluid intake prevent constipation and reduce straining. Ointments, creams, suppositories, and impregnated pads that contain antiinflammatory agents (e.g., hydrocortisone) or astringents and anesthetics (e.g., witch hazel, benzocaine, pramoxine) may be used to shrink mucous membranes and relieve discomfort. The use of topical corticosteroids such as hydrocortisone agents should be limited to 1 week or less to prevent side effects such as contact dermatitis and mucosal atrophy. Stool softeners may keep stools soft, and sitz baths help relieve pain.

- External hemorrhoids are usually managed by conservative therapy unless they become thrombosed. For internal hemorrhoids, nonsurgical approaches (band ligation, infrared coagulation, cryotherapy, laser treatment) can be used.
- In general, a hemorrhoidectomy (surgical excision of hemorrhoids) is reserved for patients with severe symptoms related to multiple thrombosed hemorrhoids or marked protrusion. Surgical removal may be done by cautery, clamp, or excision. Hemorrhoids may recur. Occasionally, anal strictures develop and dilation is necessary.

Nursing Management

Nursing care includes teaching measures to prevent constipation, avoidance of prolonged standing or sitting, proper use of over-the-counter medications available for hemorrhoidal symptoms, and instructions on when to seek medical care for symptoms (e.g., excessive pain and bleeding, prolapsed hemorrhoids).

- Pain caused by sphincter spasm is a common problem after a hemorrhoidectomy. Be aware that even though the procedure is minor, the pain is severe. Opioids are usually given initially. Postoperatively, topical nitroglycerin preparations may be used to decrease pain and subsequent opioid use.
- Sitz baths are started 1 or 2 days after surgery. A sponge ring in the sitz bath helps relieve pressure on the area. Initially the patient should not be left alone because of the possibility of weakness or fainting.
- Packing may be inserted into the rectum to absorb drainage with a T-binder used to hold the dressing in place. If packing is inserted, it usually is removed the first or second postoperative day. Assess for rectal bleeding. The patient may be embarrassed when the dressing is changed, and privacy should be provided.
- A stool softener such as docusate sodium (Colace) is usually ordered the first few postoperative days. If the patient does not have a bowel movement within 2 or 3 days, an oil retention enema is given.
- The patient usually dreads the first bowel movement and often resists the urge to defecate. Pain medication may be given before the bowel movement to reduce discomfort.

▼ **Patient and Caregiver Teaching**

After surgery:

- Teach the importance of diet, care of the anal area, symptoms of complications (especially bleeding), and avoidance of constipation and straining.
- Sitz baths are recommended for 1 to 2 weeks.
- The health care provider may order a stool softener to be taken for a time.
- Regular checkups are important in the prevention of any further problems.

HEPATITIS, VIRAL

Description

Hepatitis is an inflammation of the liver. Viral hepatitis is the most common cause of hepatitis. The types of viral hepatitis are A, B, C, D, E, and G. They differ in their modes of transmission and clinical manifestations (Table 47). Other viruses known to damage the liver include cytomegalovirus, Epstein-Barr virus, herpes virus, coxsackievirus, and rubella virus.

Hepatitis A

Hepatitis A viral infection can cause a mild flu-like illness or acute hepatitis with jaundice. It can also cause acute liver failure. It does not result in a chronic (long-term) infection.

Hepatitis A virus (HAV) is a ribonucleic acid (RNA) virus. Foodborne hepatitis A outbreaks are usually due to food contaminated by an infected food handler.

- Anti-HAV (antibody to HAV) immunoglobulin (Ig) M appears in the serum as the stool becomes negative for the virus. Detection of hepatitis A IgM indicates acute hepatitis. Hepatitis A IgG indicates past infection.
- Hepatitis A vaccination and thorough hand washing are the best measures to prevent outbreaks.

Hepatitis B

Hepatitis B virus (HBV) can cause either acute or chronic disease. Transmission occurs when the virus (from infected blood or body fluids) enter the body of an uninfected person who has not received the HBV vaccine. Since the 1990s, the incidence of HBV infection has decreased because of the widespread use of the HBV vaccine. HBV is a deoxyribonucleic acid (DNA) virus.

- About 12 million Americans have been infected with HBV. In the majority of adults with acute hepatitis B, the infection completely resolves. Of the more than 1 million Americans

Table 47   Characteristics of Hepatitis Viruses

Incubation Period and Mode of Transmission	Sources of Infection	Infectivity
Hepatitis A Virus (HAV) 15-50 days (average 28) Fecal-oral (primarily fecal contamination and oral ingestion)	Crowded conditions (e.g., day care, nursing home). Poor personal hygiene. Poor sanitation. Contaminated food, milk, water, shellfish. People with subclinical infections, infected food handlers; sexual contact, IV drug users.	Most infectious during 2 wk before onset of symptoms. Infectious until 1-2 wk after the start of symptoms.
Hepatitis B Virus (HBV) 45-180 days (average 56-96) Percutaneous (parenteral) or permucosal exposure to blood or blood products Sexual contact Perinatal transmission	Contaminated needles, syringes, and blood products. Sexual activity with infected partners. Asymptomatic carriers. Tattoos or body piercing with contaminated needles.	Before and after symptoms appear. Infectious for 4-6 mo. Carriers continue to be infectious for life.
Hepatitis C Virus (HCV) 14-180 days (average 56) Percutaneous (parenteral) or mucosal exposure to blood or blood products High-risk sexual contact Perinatal contact	Blood and blood products. Needles and syringes. Sexual activity with infected partners.	1-2 wk before symptoms appear. Continues during clinical course. 75%-85% go on to develop chronic hepatitis C and remain infectious.

Continued

H

Table 47 Characteristics of Hepatitis Viruses—cont'd

Incubation Period and Mode of Transmission	Sources of Infection	Infectivity
Hepatitis D Virus (HDV) 2-26 wk HBV must precede HDV Chronic carriers of HBV always at risk	Same as HBV. Can cause infection only when HBV is present. Routes of transmission same as for HBV.	Blood infectious at all stages of HDV infection.
Hepatitis E Virus (HEV) 15-64 days (average 26-42 days) Fecal-oral route Outbreaks associated with contaminated water supply in developing countries	Contaminated water, poor sanitation. Found in Asia, Africa, and Mexico. Not common in United States.	Not known. May be similar to HAV.

who develop chronic infections, liver impairment may range from a normal liver to severe liver disease. Approximately 15% to 25% of chronically infected people die from chronic liver disease.

Hepatitis C

Infection with the hepatitis C virus (HCV) can result in both acute and chronic illness. Acute hepatitis C, which is usually asymptomatic, can be difficult to detect unless diagnosed with laboratory testing.

- Chronic HCV results in a potentially progressive liver disease, with 20% to 30% of these patients developing cirrhosis. Hepatitis C is the most common cause of chronic liver disease and the most common indication for liver transplantation in the United States.

Hepatitis D

Hepatitis D virus (HDV), also called *delta virus,* is a defective single-stranded RNA virus that cannot survive on its own. It requires hepatitis B virus to replicate. It can be acquired at the same time as HBV, or a person with HBV can be infected with HDV at a later time. HDV is transmitted percutaneously.

- It can cause a spectrum of illness ranging from an asymptomatic chronic carrier state to acute liver failure. There is no vaccine for HDV. However, vaccination against HBV reduces the risk of HDV co-infection.

Hepatitis E

Hepatitis E virus (HEV) is an RNA virus transmitted by the fecaloral route. The usual mode of transmission is drinking contaminated water. Hepatitis E infection occurs primarily in developing countries, with epidemics reported in India, Asia, Mexico, and Africa.

For a more complete description of each hepatitis virus, see Lewis et al, *Medical-Surgical Nursing,* ed. 9, pp. 1007 to 1015.

Pathophysiology

During acute infection, liver damage is mediated by cytotoxic cytokines and natural killer cells that cause lysis of infected hepatocytes. Inflammation can interrupt bile flow (cholestasis).

- Liver cells can regenerate and, if no complications occur, resume their normal appearance and function.
- Antigen-antibody complexes between the virus and its corresponding antibody may form circulating immune complexes in the early phases of hepatitis. The circulating complexes activate the complement system. Manifestations of this activation are rash, angioedema, arthritis, fever, and malaise.

Clinical Manifestations

A large number of patients with acute hepatitis have no symptoms. Manifestations of viral hepatitis may be classified into acute and chronic phases. The *acute phase* usually lasts 1 to 4 months.

- During the incubation period, symptoms may include malaise, anorexia, fatigue, nausea, occasional vomiting, and right upper quadrant abdominal discomfort. Other symptoms may include headache, low-grade fever, arthralgias, and skin rashes.
- Physical examination may reveal hepatomegaly, lymphadenopathy, and sometimes splenomegaly. This is the period of maximal infectivity for hepatitis A.
- The acute phase may be *icteric* (jaundice) or anicteric. Jaundice, a yellowish discoloration of body tissues, results from an alteration in normal bilirubin metabolism or flow of bile into the hepatic or biliary duct systems. The urine may darken because of excess bilirubin being excreted by the kidneys. If conjugated bilirubin cannot flow out of the liver because of bile duct obstruction, stools will be light or clay colored. Pruritus, caused by bile salts beneath the skin, may result if cholestasis is present.
- The convalescence following the acute phase begins as jaundice is disappearing and lasts weeks to months, with an average of 2 to 4 months. During this period the patient's major complaints are malaise and easy fatigability. Hepatomegaly remains for several weeks.

In the *chronic phase* patients may be asymptomatic. Others, however, may have intermittent or ongoing malaise, fatigue, myalgias, arthralgias, and hepatomegaly.

Complications

Most patients with acute viral hepatitis recover completely with no complications. The overall mortality rate for acute hepatitis is less than 1%. Complications include acute liver failure, chronic hepatitis, cirrhosis of the liver (see Cirrhosis, p. 144), and hepatocellular carcinoma (see Liver Cancer, p. 393).

The disappearance of jaundice does not mean the patient has totally recovered. Some HBV infections and the majority of HCV infections result in chronic (lifelong) viral infection.

- Risk factors for progression of chronic HCV to cirrhosis include male gender, alcohol consumption, and excess iron deposition in the liver.

Diagnostic Studies

The only definitive way to distinguish among the various forms of viral hepatitis is by testing the patient's blood for the specific antigen or antibody. Table 48 presents the serologic tests for the different types of viral hepatitis.

- Many of the liver function tests show significant abnormalities.
- Physical assessment may reveal hepatic tenderness, hepatomegaly, and splenomegaly.
- Liver biopsy allows for histologic examination of liver cells in chronic hepatitis.

Collaborative Care

There is no specific treatment for acute viral hepatitis. Most patients can be managed at home. Emphasis is on measures to rest the body and assist the liver in regenerating. Adequate nutrients and rest seem to be most beneficial for healing and liver cell regeneration. The degree of rest ordered depends on symptom severity; usually alternating periods of activity with rest is adequate.

Drug Therapy

There are no specific drug therapies for the treatment of acute hepatitis A infection. Treatment of acute hepatitis B is indicated only in patients with severe hepatitis and liver failure. In people with acute hepatitis C, treatment with pegylated interferon within the first 12 to 24 weeks of infection has shown a marked reduction in the development of chronic hepatitis C. Supportive drug therapy may include antiemetics for nausea, such as prochlorperazine (Compazine), promethazine (Phenergan), or ondansetron (Zofran).

Drug therapy for chronic HBV is focused on decreasing the viral load and liver enzymes and slowing the rate of disease progression. Current drug therapies for chronic HBV do not eradicate the virus, but work well to suppress viral replication and prevent complications of hepatitis B. First-line therapies include pegylated interferon and nucleoside and nucleotide analogs.

- α-Interferon interferes with viral replication and is available in long-acting preparations (Pegasys, peg Intron). One third of the patients receiving α-interferon will have a significant reduction of serum HBV DNA levels, normalization of alanine aminotransferase (ALT) levels, and loss of HBV e antigen (HBeAg).
- Nucleoside and nucleotide analogs suppress HBV replication by inhibiting viral DNA synthesis. The drugs used in the treatment of chronic HBV when there is evidence of active viral replication include lamivudine (Epivir), adefovir (Hepsera), entecavir (Baraclude), tenofovir (Viread), and telbivudine (Tyzeka). These drugs can reduce viral load and liver damage.

Drug therapy for hepatitis C is directed at eradicating the virus and preventing HCV-related complications.

- Treatment for HCV includes pegylated interferon given with ribavirin (Rebetol, Copegus).

Table 48   Tests for Viral Hepatitis

Virus	Tests	Significance
A	Anti-HAV immunoglobulin M (IgM)	Acute infection.
	Anti-HAV immunoglobulin G (IgG)	Previous infection or immunization. Not routinely done in clinical practice.
B	HBsAg (hepatitis B surface antigen)	Marker of infectivity.
		Present in acute or chronic infection.
		Positive in chronic carriers.
	Anti-HBs (hepatitis B surface antibody)	Indicates previous infection with HBV or immunization.
	HBeAg (hepatitis B e antigen)	Indicates high infectivity.
		Used to determine the clinical management of patients with chronic hepatitis B.
	Anti-HBe (hepatitis B e antibody)	Indicates previous infection.
		In chronic hepatitis B, indicates a low viral load and low degree of infectivity.
	Anti-HBc (antibody to hepatitis B core antigen) IgM	Indicates acute infection.
		Does not appear after vaccination.
	Anti-HBc IgG	Indicates previous infection or ongoing infection with hepatitis B.
		Does not appear after vaccination.

	HBV DNA quantitation	Indicates active ongoing viral replication. Best indicator of viral replication and effectiveness of therapy in patient with chronic hepatitis B.
	HBV genotyping	Indicates the genotype of HBV.
C	Anti-HCV (antibody to HCV)	Marker for acute or chronic infection with HCV.
	HCV RNA quantitation	Indicates active ongoing viral replication.
	HCV genotyping	Indicates the genotype of HCV.
D	Anti-HDV	Present in past or current infection with HDV.
	HDV Ag (hepatitis D antigen)	Present within a few days after infection.
E*	Anti-HEV IgM and IgG	Present 1 wk to 2 mo after illness onset.
	HEV RNA quantitation	Indicates active ongoing viral replication.

*Currently, no serologic tests to diagnose HEV infection are commercially available in the United States. However, diagnostic tests are available in research laboratories to detect IgM and IgG anti-HEV and HEV RNA levels.

A, Hepatitis A virus (HAV); B, hepatitis B virus (HBV); C, hepatitis C virus (HCV); D, hepatitis D virus (HDV); E, hepatitis E virus (HEV).

H

- Patients who have HCV genotype 1 also receive either telaprevir (Incivek) or boceprevir (Victrelis), which are HCV protease inhibitors. Protease is an enzyme that is essential in viral replication.

Prevention

Drug therapy is also used for prevention of HAV and HBV infection. Both hepatitis A vaccine and immune globulin (IG) are used for prevention of hepatitis A.

- The vaccine is used for preexposure prophylaxis, and IG can be used either before or after exposure.
- IG provides temporary (1 to 2 months) passive immunity and is effective for preventing hepatitis A if given within 2 weeks after exposure.
- IG is recommended for people who do not have anti-HAV antibodies and are exposed because of close contact with people who have HAV or foodborne exposure.
- Although IG may not prevent infection in all people, it may modify the illness to a subclinical infection.
- Twinrix, a combined HAV and HBV vaccine, is available for people over the age of 18 years.
- Immunization with hepatitis B vaccine is the best means for preventing HBV infection. The vaccine is given in a series of three intramuscular (IM) injections in the deltoid muscle. The vaccine is more than 95% effective.
- For postexposure prophylaxis, the vaccine and hepatitis B immune globulin (HBIG) are used. HBIG contains antibodies to HBV and confers temporary passive immunity. HBIG is recommended for postexposure prophylaxis in cases of needle stick, mucous membrane contact, or sexual exposure and for infants born to mothers who are positive for HBsAg.

Nutritional Therapy

No special diet is required in the treatment of viral hepatitis. Emphasis is placed on a well-balanced diet that the patient can tolerate. Vitamin supplements, particularly B-complex vitamins and vitamin K, are frequently used. If anorexia, nausea, and vomiting are severe, IV solutions of glucose or supplemental enteral nutrition therapy may be used.

Nursing Management

Goals

The patient with viral hepatitis will have relief of discomfort, be able to resume normal activities, and return to normal liver function without complications.

Nursing Diagnoses

- Imbalanced nutrition: less than body requirements
- Activity intolerance
- Risk for impaired liver function

Nursing Interventions

Viral hepatitis is a community health problem. Your role is important in the prevention and control of this disease (see Lewis et al, *Medical-Surgical Nursing,* ed. 9, pp. 1013 to 1015, for a summary of preventive measures).

Hepatitis A. Vaccination is the best protection against HAV. Preventive measures include personal and environmental hygiene and health education to promote good sanitation. Hand washing is essential and is probably the most important precaution. Teach about careful hand washing after bowel movements and before eating.

Hepatitis B. The best way to reduce HBV infection is to identify those at risk, screen them for HBV, and vaccinate those who are not infected. Teach individuals at high risk of contracting HBV to reduce risks. Good hygienic practices, including hand washing and using gloves when expecting contact with blood, are important.

- A condom is advised for sexual intercourse, and the partner should be vaccinated. Razors, toothbrushes, and other personal items should not be shared. Close contacts of the patient with hepatitis B who are HBsAg negative and antibody negative should be vaccinated.

Hepatitis C. There currently is no vaccine available. Primary measures to prevent HCV transmission are similar to those for HBV, including the screening of blood, organ, and tissue donors; use of infection control measures; and modification of high-risk sexual behavior.

During acute intervention, assess for the presence and degree of jaundice. Comfort measures to relieve pruritus (if present), headache, and arthralgias are helpful.

- Ensuring that the patient receives adequate nutrition is not always easy. Small, frequent meals may be preferable to three large ones and may also help prevent nausea. Measures to stimulate the appetite, such as mouth care, antiemetics, and attractively served meals in pleasant surroundings, should be in your plan of care.
- Assess the patient's response to the rest and activity plan and modify accordingly.
- Psychologic and emotional rest is as essential as physical rest. Bed rest may produce anxiety and extreme restlessness in some patients. Diversional activities, such as reading and hobbies, may help.

▼ Patient and Caregiver Teaching

- Teach the patient and caregiver how to prevent transmission to other family members. Also teach what symptoms need to be reported to the health care provider.
- Caution the patient about overexertion and the need to follow the health care provider's advice about when to return to work.

- Assess the patient for manifestations of complications. Bleeding tendencies with increasing prothrombin time values, symptoms of encephalopathy, or elevated liver function tests indicate problems.
- Instruct the patient to have regular follow-up for at least 1 year after the diagnosis of hepatitis. Because relapses occur with hepatitis B and C, teach the patient the symptoms of recurrence and the need for follow-up evaluations. All patients with chronic HBV or HCV should avoid alcohol, because it can accelerate disease progression.
- The patient who is receiving interferon for the treatment of hepatitis B or C requires teaching regarding this drug.

HERNIA

Description

A *hernia* is a protrusion of the viscus through an abnormal opening or a weakened area in the wall of the cavity in which it is normally contained. A hernia may occur in any part of the body, but it usually occurs within the abdominal cavity.

- Hernias that easily return to the abdominal cavity are called *reducible.* The hernia can be reduced manually or may reduce spontaneously when the person lies down.
- If the hernia cannot be placed back into the abdominal cavity, it is known as *irreducible* or *incarcerated.* In this situation intestinal flow may be obstructed. When the hernia is irreducible and intestinal flow and blood supply are obstructed, the hernia is *strangulated.* The result is an acute intestinal obstruction.

Types

Types of hernias include inguinal, femoral, umbilical, and ventral (incisional).

- *Inguinal hernia* is the most common type of hernia and occurs at the point of weakness in the abdominal wall where the spermatic cord in men or the round ligament in women emerges. An inguinal hernia is more common in men.
- *Femoral hernia* occurs when there is a protrusion through the femoral ring into the femoral canal. It becomes strangulated easily and occurs more frequently in women.
- *Umbilical hernia* occurs when the rectus muscle is weak (as with obesity) or the umbilical opening fails to close after birth.
- *Ventral* or *incisional hernia* is caused by a weakness of the abdominal wall at the site of a previous incision. It occurs most commonly in patients who are obese, who have had multiple surgical procedures in the same area, or who have had inadequate wound healing because of poor nutrition or infection.

Clinical Manifestations

A hernia may be readily visible, especially when the person tenses the abdominal muscles. Discomfort may result from tension.

- If the hernia becomes strangulated, the patient will experience severe pain and symptoms of a bowel obstruction, such as vomiting, cramping abdominal pain, and distention.
- Strangulated hernias or painful, inflamed hernias that cannot be reduced require emergency surgery.

Diagnosis is based on history and physical examination findings.

Collaborative Care

Laparoscopic surgery is the treatment of choice for hernias. The surgical repair of a hernia, known as a *herniorrhaphy,* is usually an outpatient procedure. Reinforcement of the weakened area with wire, fascia, or mesh is known as a *hernioplasty.* Strangulated hernias are treated immediately with resection of the involved area or a temporary colostomy so that necrosis and gangrene do not occur.

Nursing Management

After a hernia repair, the patient may have difficulty voiding. Measure intake and output and observe for a distended bladder.

- Scrotal edema is a painful complication after an inguinal hernia repair. A scrotal support with application of an ice bag may help relieve pain and edema.
- Encourage deep breathing, but not coughing. Teach patients to splint the incision and keep their mouths open when coughing or sneezing when possible.
- The patient may be restricted from heavy lifting for 6 to 8 weeks.

HERPES, GENITAL

Description

Genital herpes is caused by herpes simplex virus (HSV). Its true incidence is difficult to determine, as most people have few to no symptoms. In the United States at least 50 million people are infected with herpes simplex virus type 2. In people ages 14 to 49, approximately one in six have genital herpes.

Pathophysiology

The HSV enters through the mucous membranes or breaks in the skin during contact with an infected person. HSV then reproduces inside the cell and spreads to surrounding cells. The virus next enters the peripheral or autonomic nerve endings and ascends to the sensory or autonomic nerve ganglion, where it often becomes dormant. Viral reactivation (recurrence) may occur when the virus travels down to the initial site of infection.

When a person is infected with HSV, the virus usually persists within the individual for life. Transmission of HSV occurs through direct contact with skin or mucous membranes when an infected individual is symptomatic or through asymptomatic viral shedding.

Two different strains of herpes simplex virus (HSV) cause infection.

- HSV type 1 (HSV-1) generally causes infection above the waist, involving the gingivae, dermis, upper respiratory tract, and central nervous system (CNS).
- HSV type 2 (HSV-2) most frequently involves the genital tract and perineum (i.e., locations below the waist).

Clinical Manifestations

In the *primary (initial) episode* of genital herpes, the patient may complain of burning, itching, or tingling at the site of inoculation. Multiple, small vesicular lesions may occur on the penis, scrotum, vulva, perineum, perianal region, vagina, or cervix and contain large quantities of infectious viral particles. The lesions rupture and form shallow, moist ulcerations. Finally, crusting and epithelialization of the erosions occur.

- Primary infections tend to be associated with local inflammation and pain accompanied by systemic manifestations of fever, headache, malaise, myalgia, and regional lymphadenopathy.
- Urination may be painful from urine touching active lesions. Urinary retention may occur as a result of HSV urethritis or cystitis. A purulent vaginal discharge may develop with HSV cervicitis.
- Primary lesions are generally present for 17 to 20 days, but new lesions sometimes continue to develop for 6 weeks.
- The lesions heal spontaneously unless secondary infection occurs.

Recurrent genital herpes occurs in about 50% to 80% of individuals during the year following the primary episode. Common trigger factors include stress, fatigue, sunburn, general illness, immunosuppression, and menses.

- Many patients can predict a recurrence by noticing early prodromal symptoms of tingling, burning, and itching at the site where lesions will eventually appear. Symptoms of recurrent episodes are less severe, and the lesions usually heal within 8 to 12 days. With time the recurrent lesions will generally occur less frequently.

Complications

- Although most infections are relatively benign, complications of genital herpes may involve the CNS, causing aseptic meningitis and lower motor neuron damage.
- Autoinoculation of the virus to extragenital sites such as the fingers and lips ("cold sores") may occur.
- Neuron damage may result in atonic bladder, impotence, and constipation.
- Immunocompromised patients (e.g., HIV-infected patients) should be monitored closely for treatment failure and a slower healing time of HSV lesions.

Diagnostic Studies

- Diagnosis is usually based on the patient's symptoms and history.
- Highly accurate serologic tests are available for the diagnosis of HSV-1 and HSV-2. These type-specific immunoassays test for the presence of antibodies to HSV.
- A viral culture of the active lesion can also be used to isolate the virus.

Collaborative Care

Encourage symptomatic treatment such as good genital hygiene and the wearing of loose-fitting cotton undergarments. The lesions should be kept clean and dry. To ensure complete drying of the perineal area, women may use a hair dryer set on a cool setting. Drying agents such as colloidal oatmeal (Aveeno) and aluminum salts (Burow's solution) may provide relief from the burning and itching.

- Frequent sitz baths may soothe the area and reduce inflammation. Pain may require a local anesthetic, such as lidocaine (Xylocaine), or systemic analgesics, such as codeine and aspirin.
- Barrier forms of contraception, especially condoms, used during asymptomatic periods, decrease the transmission of the disease. When lesions are present, the patient should avoid sexual activity altogether because even barrier protection is not satisfactory in eliminating disease transmission.

Women with a primary episode of HSV near the time of delivery have the highest risk of transmitting genital herpes to the neonate. An active genital lesion at the time of delivery is usually an indication for cesarean section. Acyclovir may be given to pregnant women who have reached at least 36 weeks of gestation to prevent neonatal transmission.

Drug Therapy

Three antiviral agents are available for the treatment of HSV: acyclovir (Zovirax), valacyclovir (Valtrex), and famciclovir (Famvir).

These drugs inhibit herpetic viral replication and are prescribed for primary and recurrent infections. Although not a cure, these drugs shorten the duration of viral shedding and healing time of genital lesions and reduce outbreaks by 75%. Continued use of oral acyclovir for up to 5 years is safe and effective.

Acyclovir ointment appears to have no clinical benefit in the treatment of recurrent lesions, either in the speed of healing or in resolution of pain. IV acyclovir is reserved for severe or life-threatening infections.

Nursing Management: Genital Herpes
See Sexually Transmitted Infections, p. 564.

HIATAL HERNIA

Description
Hiatal hernia is herniation of a portion of the stomach into the esophagus through an opening or hiatus in the diaphragm. It is also referred to as diaphragmatic hernia or esophageal hernia. Hiatal hernias are common in older adults and occur more frequently in women than men. Hiatal hernias are classified into two types (Fig. 7).

- A *sliding hernia* is the most common type. It occurs at the junction of the stomach and esophagus located above the hiatus of the diaphragm. A part of the stomach "slides" through the hiatal opening in the diaphragm. This occurs when the patient is supine, and it usually goes back into the abdominal cavity when the patient is standing upright.
- A *paraesophageal* or *rolling hernia* occurs at the esophago-gastric junction where the fundus and greater curvature of the stomach roll up through the diaphragm to form a pocket alongside the esophagus.

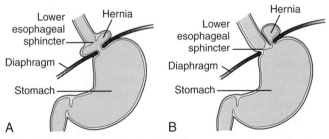

Fig. 7. **A,** Sliding hiatal hernia. **B,** Rolling or paraesophageal hernia.

Pathophysiology

Many factors contribute to the development of hiatal hernia, including structural changes, such as weakening of the muscles in the diaphragm around the esophagogastric opening. Factors that increase intraabdominal pressure including obesity, pregnancy, ascites, intense physical exertion, and heavy lifting on a continual basis may also predispose patients to a hiatal hernia.

Clinical Manifestations

Some individuals are asymptomatic. When present, signs and symptoms of hiatal hernia are similar to those described for gastroesophageal reflux disease (GERD).

- Heartburn, especially after a meal or after lying supine, is a common symptom. Bending over may cause a severe burning pain, which is usually relieved by sitting or standing. Large meals, alcohol, and smoking may precipitate pain.
- Nocturnal attacks are common, especially if the person has eaten before lying down.

Complications may include GERD, esophagitis, hemorrhage from erosion, stenosis, ulcerations of the herniated portion of the stomach, strangulation of the hernia, and regurgitation with tracheal aspiration.

Diagnostic Studies

- Barium swallow (esophagram) may show gastric mucosa protrusion through the esophageal hiatus.
- Upper GI endoscopy with biopsy and cytologic analysis determines if the lower esophageal sphincter (LES) is incompetent and gastric reflux is present.
- Esophageal motility (manometry) studies determine pressure gradients.

Nursing and Collaborative Management

Conservative therapy is similar to that described under GERD, including lifestyle modifications (elimination of constricting garments, avoidance of lifting and straining, elevating the head of the bed, and elimination of alcohol and smoking), reducing body weight if overweight, and the administration of antacids and antisecretory agents (see Gastroesophageal Reflux Disease, p. 243). Teach the patient to reduce intraabdominal pressure by eliminating constricting garments and avoiding lifting and straining.

Surgical approaches include reduction of the herniated stomach into the abdomen, *herniotomy* (excision of the hernia sac), *herniorrhaphy* (closure of the hiatal defect), an antireflux procedure, and *gastropexy* (attachment of the stomach subdiaphragmatically to prevent reherniation).

H

- Laparoscopically performed Nissen and Toupet fundoplication techniques are the standard antireflux surgeries for hiatal hernia.

HODGKIN'S LYMPHOMA

Description

Hodgkin's lymphoma, also called Hodgkin's disease, is a malignant condition characterized by proliferation of abnormal, giant, multinucleated cells called *Reed-Sternberg cells,* which are located in lymph nodes. The disease makes up 11% of all lymphomas and has a bimodal age-specific incidence, occurring most frequently in people from 15 to 35 years old and above 50 years old. In adults it is twice as prevalent in men as in women. Each year, approximately 9060 new cases of Hodgkin's lymphoma are diagnosed and approximately 1200 deaths occur. However, long-term survival exceeds 85% for all stages.

Pathophysiology

Although the cause of Hodgkin's lymphoma remains unknown, several key factors are thought to play a role in its development. The main interacting factors include infection with the Epstein-Barr virus, genetic predisposition, and exposure to occupational toxins.

In Hodgkin's lymphoma the normal structure of the lymph nodes is destroyed by hyperplasia of monocytes and macrophages. The disease is believed to arise in a single location (it originates in the cervical lymph nodes in 70% of patients) and then spreads along adjacent lymphatics. It eventually infiltrates other organs, especially the lungs, spleen, and liver.

Clinical Manifestations

The initial sign is most often an enlargement of the cervical, axillary, or inguinal lymph nodes. The enlarged nodes are not painful unless pressure is exerted on adjacent nerves.

- The patient may note weight loss, fatigue, weakness, fever, chills, tachycardia, or night sweats. A group of initial findings, including fever, night sweats, and weight loss (referred to as *B symptoms*), correlates with a worse prognosis.
- Generalized pruritus without skin lesions may develop. Cough, dyspnea, stridor, and dysphagia may all reflect mediastinal node involvement.
- In more advanced disease there may be hepatomegaly and splenomegaly. Anemia results from increased destruction and decreased production of erythrocytes. Intrathoracic involvement

may lead to superior vena cava syndrome. Enlarged retroperitoneal nodes may cause palpable abdominal masses or interfere with renal function.

- Jaundice may result from liver involvement.
- Spinal cord compression leading to paraplegia may occur with extradural involvement.

Diagnostic Studies

Peripheral blood analysis, excisional lymph node biopsy, bone marrow examination, and radiologic studies are important means of evaluating Hodgkin's lymphoma.

- Microcytic hypochromic anemia, leukopenia, and thrombocytopenia may develop, but they are usually a consequence of treatment, advanced disease, or hypersplenism (related to the disease process).
- Other blood studies may show hypoferremia caused by excessive iron uptake by the liver and spleen, elevated alkaline phosphatase from liver and bone involvement, hypercalcemia from bone involvement, and hypoalbuminemia from liver involvement.
- Positron emission tomography (PET) scans with or without CT is used to stage and then assess response to therapy. The scans may show increased uptake of carbohydrate by cancer cells (by PET) and masses (by CT) such as mediastinal lymphadenopathy, renal displacement caused by retroperitoneal node enlargement, abdominal lymph node enlargement, and liver, spleen, bone, and brain infiltration.

Collaborative Care

Treatment decisions are made based on the clinical stage of the disease. The standard for chemotherapy is the ABVD regimen: doxorubicin (**A**driamycin), **b**leomycin, **v**inblastine, and **d**acarbazine given for two to eight cycles of treatment depending on disease stage and prognosis.

Combination chemotherapy works well because, as in leukemia, the drugs used have an additive antitumor effect without increasing side effects. As with leukemia, therapy must be aggressive. Therefore potentially life-threatening problems are encountered in an attempt to achieve a remission.

A variety of chemotherapy regimens and newer agents, such as brentuximab vedotin (Adcetris), are used to treat patients who have relapsed or refractory disease. Ideally, once remission is obtained, a treatment option with the goal of cure may be intensive chemotherapy with the use of autologous or allogeneic hematopoietic stem cell transplantation.

The role of radiation as a supplement to chemotherapy varies depending on site of disease and the presence of resistant disease after chemotherapy.

Nursing Management

Nursing care for patients with Hodgkin's lymphoma is largely based on managing problems related to the disease, such as pain, and side effects of therapy, such as pancytopenia.

- Because the survival of patients with Hodgkin's lymphoma depends on their response to treatment, supporting the patient through the consequences of treatment is extremely important.
- Psychosocial considerations are as important as they are with leukemia (see Leukemia, p. 387). However, the prognosis for Hodgkin's lymphoma is better than that for many forms of cancer or leukemia. The physical, psychologic, social, and spiritual consequences of the patient's disease must be addressed.
- Evaluation of patients for long-term effects of therapy is important because delayed consequences of the disease and treatment, such as secondary malignancies and long-term endocrine, cardiac, and pulmonary toxicities, may not be apparent for many years.

HUMAN IMMUNODEFICIENCY VIRUS INFECTION

Description

Human immunodeficiency virus (HIV) infection is caused by HIV, a retrovirus that causes immunosuppression. The viral infection causes the person to be susceptible to infections that would normally be controlled through immune responses.

More than 1 million people are living with HIV in the United States, with an estimated 50,000 new infections each year. In North America HIV has been most prevalent among men who have sex with men, but women, people of color, people who live in poverty, and adolescents represent an expanding proportion of new HIV infections. With advances in treatment, HIV is managed as a chronic disease because people are living longer.

Pathophysiology

HIV is a ribonucleic acid (RNA) virus. Like all viruses, HIV cannot replicate unless it is in a living cell. HIV infects human cells that have $CD4^+$ receptors on their surfaces. These include lymphocytes, monocytes/macrophages, astrocytes, and oligodendrocytes. Immune dysfunction in HIV disease is caused predominantly by destruction of $CD4^+$ T cells (also known as T-helper cells or $CD4^+$

lymphocytes). The major concern related to immune suppression is the development of opportunistic diseases (infections and cancers that occur in immunosuppressed patients that can lead to disability, disease, and death).

HIV can be transmitted as a result of contact with infected blood, semen, vaginal secretions, or breast milk. HIV-infected individuals can transmit HIV to others within a few days of becoming infected. The ability to transmit HIV is lifelong.

Clinical Manifestations

The typical course of untreated HIV infection follows the pattern shown in Fig. 8. It is important to remember that disease progression is highly individualized and that treatment can significantly alter the pattern. HIV infections are divided into acute and chronic stages.

Acute Infection

During acute HIV infection, HIV-specific antibodies are produced (seroconversion) and a mononucleosis-like syndrome of fever, lymphadenopathy, pharyngitis, headache, malaise, nausea, and/or a diffuse rash may occur.

- Symptoms generally occur 2 to 4 weeks after initial infection and last for 1 to 3 weeks.

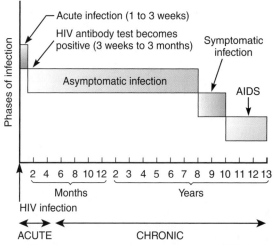

Fig. 8. Timeline for the spectrum of untreated HIV infection. The timeline represents the course of untreated illness from the time of infection to clinical manifestations of disease.

- During this time a high viral load is noted and CD4$^+$ T-cell counts fall temporarily but quickly return to baseline. Many people, including health care providers, mistake acute HIV symptoms for a bad case of the flu.

Chronic Infection

There are three stages of chronic infection: asymptomatic infection, symptomatic infection, and acquired immunodeficiency syndrome (AIDS). The interval between untreated HIV infection and a diagnosis of AIDS is about 10 years.

- *Asymptomatic infection*—during this time CD4$^+$ lymphocyte counts remain above 500 cells/μL (normal or slightly decreased) and the viral load in the blood is low. This phase has been referred to as asymptomatic infection, but fatigue, headache, low-grade fever, night sweats, persistent generalized lymphadenopathy (PGL), and other symptoms often occur.
- *Symptomatic infection* occurs as the CD4$^+$ T-cell count drops to 200 to 500 cells/μL and the viral load increases. Symptoms seen in earlier phases tend to become worse and other problems, including infections, lymphadenopathy, and nervous system manifestations, may occur.
- *AIDS* is characterized by severe immune system suppression and CD4$^+$ T-cell counts below 200 cells/μL. A diagnosis of AIDS is made when an HIV-infected patient meets criteria established by the Centers for Disease Control and Prevention (CDC), which include the development of at least one of these conditions:
  1. CD4$^+$ lymphocyte count less than 200/μL
  2. Development of opportunistic infection (see Tables 15-9 and 15-10, Lewis et al, *Medical-Surgical Nursing,* ed. 9, pp. 235, 236)
  3. Development of opportunistic cancer (e.g., Kaposi sarcoma)
  4. *Wasting syndrome* (defined as a loss of 10% or more of ideal body mass)
  5. Development of AIDS-dementia complex (ADC)

Diagnostic Studies

Screening

The most useful screening tests are those that detect HIV-specific antibodies. A major problem is that there is a delay of several weeks after infection before antibodies can be detected.

- Standard antibody tests can be completed on blood or oral fluid specimens. They are sent to a laboratory with results available from a day to a week later.
- Rapid HIV-antibody tests are done in the office, and results can be shared with patients before they leave. They can also be done at home using a self-administered HIV test kit.

- A positive antibody test should be followed by a confirming test (usually the Western blot).

Progression of HIV Infection

- $CD4^+$ T-cell count and viral load monitor progression of infection.
- WBC count, RBC count, and platelets decrease with progression of HIV.

Collaborative Care

Treatment focuses on (1) monitoring HIV progression and immune function; (2) initiating and monitoring antiretroviral therapy (ART); (3) preventing, detecting, and treating opportunistic diseases; (4) managing symptoms; (5) preventing or decreasing the complications of treatment; and (6) preventing further transmission of HIV.

Drug Therapy

Goals of drug therapy in HIV infection are to decrease the viral load, maintain or increase $CD4^+$ T cell counts, prevent HIV-related symptoms and opportunistic diseases, delay disease progression, and prevent HIV transmission.

Drugs used for treatment work at various points in the HIV replication cycle (Table 49). Stribild (elvitegravir, cobicistat, emtricitabine, tenofovir disoproxil fumarate) is a newer once-a-day combination pill to treat HIV-1 infection in adults who have never been treated for HIV infection.

The major advantage of using drugs from different classes is that combination therapy can inhibit viral replication in several ways, making it difficult for the virus to recover and decreasing the likelihood of drug resistance.

- A major problem with most drugs used in ART is that resistance develops rapidly when drugs are used alone or taken in inadequate doses. The most effective means to suppress HIV replication is using at least three effective antiretroviral drugs from at least two different drug classes in optimum schedules and at full dosages (see Table 49).
- Many ART agents cause dangerous and potentially lethal interactions when used in combination with other commonly used drugs, including over-the-counter drugs and herbal therapies.

Opportunistic diseases associated with HIV can be delayed or prevented through prophylactic interventions, including (1) pneumococcal, influenza, and hepatitis B vaccines; (2) trimethoprim-sulfamethoxazole (TMP-SMX) inhalation for *Pneumocystis jiroveci* and toxoplasma; and (3) rifabutin (Mycobutin) for *Mycobacterium avium* complex. See Table 15-10, Lewis et al, *Medical-Surgical Nursing,* ed. 9, p. 236, for a complete description.

Table 49 Drug Therapy
HIV Infection

Drug Classification	Mechanism of Action	Examples*
Entry Inhibitors	Prevent binding of HIV to cells, thus preventing entry of HIV into cells where replication would occur	enfuvirtide (Fuzeon) maraviroc (Selzentry)
Reverse Transcriptase Inhibitors		
Nucleoside reverse transcriptase inhibitors (NRTIs)	Insert a piece of DNA into the developing HIV DNA chain, blocking further development of the chain and leaving the production of the new strand of HIV DNA incomplete	zidovudine (AZT, ZDV, Retrovir) didanosine (ddI, Videx, Videx-EC [time-released]) stavudine (d4T, Zerit) lamivudine (3TC, Epivir) abacavir (Ziagen) emtricitabine (FTC, Emtriva)
Nonnucleoside reverse transcriptase inhibitors (NNRTIs)	Inhibit the action of reverse transcriptase	nevirapine (Viramune) delavirdine (Rescriptor) efavirenz (Sustiva) etravirine (Intelence) rilpivirine (Edurant)
Nucleotide reverse transcriptase inhibitor (NtRTI)	Combines with reverse transcriptase enzyme to block the process needed to convert HIV RNA into HIV DNA	tenofovir (Viread)

Integrase Inhibitors	Bind with integrase enzyme and prevent HIV from incorporating its genetic material into the host cell	raltegravir (Isentress) elvitegravir
Protease Inhibitors (PIs)	Prevent the protease enzyme from cutting HIV proteins into the proper lengths needed to allow viable virions to assemble and bud out from the cell membrane	saquinavir (Fortovase, Invirase) indinavir (Crixivan) ritonavir (Norvir)‡ nelfinavir (Viracept) atazanavir (Reyataz) fosamprenavir (Lexiva) tipranavir (Aptivus) darunavir (Prezista) lopinavir + ritonavir (Kaletra)
Fixed-Dose Combinations (More than one drug combined into a single tablet. Drugs may be from the same or different classes.)		Atripla (tenofovir DF + emtricitabine + efavirenz) Combivir (lamivudine + zidovudine) Complera (tenofovir + emtricitabine + rilpivirine) Epzicom (abacavir + lamivudine) Trizivir (abacavir + lamivudine + zidovudine) Truvada (tenofovir + emtricitabine) Stribild (tenofovir + emtricitabine + elvitegravir + cobicistat§)

*Side effects of these drugs are listed in eTable 15-3, Lewis, et al. *Medical-Surgical Nursing*, ed. 9 on the website for Chapter 15.
†Part of the combination pill Stribild (see below).
‡Most often used in low doses with other PIs to boost effect.
§Cobicistat is a pharmacologic booster that enhances the potency of some HIV antiretrovirals. It has no direct effects against HIV.
DF, Disoproxil fumarate.

H

Nursing Management

Goals

The patient with HIV infection will adhere to drug regimens; adopt a healthy lifestyle that includes avoiding exposure to other sexual and blood-borne diseases; protect others from HIV; maintain or develop healthy and supportive relationships; maintain activities and productivity; explore spiritual issues; come to terms with issues related to disease, disability, and death; and cope with the frequent symptoms caused by HIV and its treatments.

Nursing Interventions

The complexity of HIV disease is related to its chronic nature. As with most chronic and infectious diseases, primary prevention and health promotion are the most effective health care strategies. See eTable 15-7 on the website for Chapter 15 of Lewis et al, *Medical-Surgical Nursing,* ed. 9, for a synopsis of nursing goals, assessments, and interventions at each stage of HIV infection.

HIV infection is preventable. Avoiding and/or modifying risky behaviors are the most effective prevention tools. Provide culturally sensitive, language-appropriate, and age-specific teaching and behavior change counseling.

- Early intervention after detection of HIV infection can promote health and limit disability. It should focus on early detection of symptoms, opportunistic diseases, and psychosocial problems.

Useful interventions for HIV-infected patients include nutritional support; moderation or elimination of alcohol, tobacco, and drug use; keeping recommended vaccines up to date; adequate rest, exercise, and stress reduction; avoiding exposure to new infectious agents; mental health counseling; and getting involved in support groups and community activities.

- Teach patients to recognize symptoms that may indicate disease progression and/or drug side effects so that prompt medical care can be initiated.
- During acute exacerbations of opportunistic diseases or adverse effects of treatment, symptomatic care may include teaching and treatment for diarrhea, pneumonia, fatigue, wasting syndrome, and ADC.
- The focus of terminal care is patient comfort, facilitation of emotional and spiritual issues, and helping significant others deal with grief and loss.

▼ **Patient and Caregiver Teaching**

HIV education emphasizes prevention and risk-reducing activities. Teach the proper use and placement of male and female condoms and how to access drug-using equipment that promotes risk reduction. For an infected patient, teaching is directed toward health promotion, managing the problems caused by HIV infection, and maximizing the patient's quality of life.

- Teach advantages and disadvantages of new treatments, including drug therapy, dangers of nonadherence to therapeutic regimens, how and when to take each medication, drug interactions to avoid, and side effects that need to be reported to the primary care provider. Tables 15-14, 15-15, and 15-16, Lewis et al, *Medical-Surgical Nursing,* ed. 9, pp. 240 and 242, provide guidance for patient teaching in these areas.
- Teach energy conservation measures and the use of assistive devices to increase safety and decrease fatigue.
- Discuss infection control measures with the patient, caregiver, family, and visitors.
- Provide information about support groups and community resources.

HUNTINGTON'S DISEASE

Description

Huntington's disease (HD) is a genetically transmitted, autosomal dominant disorder that affects both men and women of all races. The onset of HD is usually between 30 and 50 years of age. About 15,000 Americans are symptomatic, and 150,000 are at risk. Offspring of a person with this disease have a 50% risk of inheriting it.

Pathophysiology

Like Parkinson's disease, the pathologic process of HD involves the basal ganglia and the extrapyramidal motor system. However, instead of a deficiency of dopamine (DA), HD involves a deficiency of the neurotransmitters acetylcholine (ACh) and γ-aminobutyric acid (GABA). The net effect is an excess of DA, which leads to symptoms that are the opposite of those of parkinsonism.

Clinical Manifestations

Manifestations are characterized by a movement disorder and cognitive and psychiatric disorders. The movement disorder is characterized by abnormal and excessive involuntary movements *(chorea).* These are writhing, twisting movements of the face, limbs, and body. The movements get worse as the disease progresses.

- Facial movements involving speech, chewing, and swallowing are affected and may cause aspiration and malnutrition. The gait deteriorates, and ambulation eventually becomes impossible.

- Psychiatric symptoms are very frequently present in the early stage of the disease, often before the onset of motor symptoms. Depression is common. Other psychiatric symptoms include anxiety, agitation, impulsivity, apathy, social withdrawal, and obsessiveness.
- Cognitive deterioration is more variable and involves perception, memory, attention, and learning.

Eventually all psychomotor processes, including the ability to eat and talk, are impaired. Death usually occurs 10 to 20 years after the onset of symptoms, most commonly due to pneumonia, followed by suicide.

Diagnosis

The diagnostic process begins with a review of family history and clinical symptoms. Genetic testing confirms the presence of the disease in a person with symptoms.

- People who are asymptomatic but who have a positive family history of HD face the dilemma of whether or not to be genetically tested. If the test is positive, the person will develop HD, but when and to what extent the disease develops cannot be determined.

Collaborative Care

Because there is no cure, collaborative care is palliative. Tetrabenazine (Xenazine) is used to treat the chorea. It works to decrease the amount of dopamine available at synapses in the brain and thus decreases the involuntary movements of chorea.

- Other medications include antipsychotics such as haloperidol [Haldol]) and risperidone (Risperdal), benzodiazepines such as diazepam (Valium) and clonazepam (Klonopin), and dopamine-depleting agents such as reserpine and tetrabenazine.
- Cognitive disorders are treated with nondrug therapies (e.g., counseling). The psychiatric disorders can be treated with selective serotonin uptake inhibitors such as sertraline (Zoloft) and paroxetine (Paxil).

The goal of nursing management is to provide the most comfortable environment possible for the patient and caregiver by maintaining physical safety, treating physical symptoms, and providing emotional and psychologic support.

- Because of the choreic movements, caloric requirements are high. Patients may require as many as 4000 to 5000 cal/day to maintain body weight. As the disease progresses, meeting caloric needs becomes a greater challenge when the patient has difficulty swallowing and holding the head still. Depression and mental deterioration can also compromise nutritional intake.

- End-of-life issues need to be discussed with the patient and caregiver. These include care in the home or long-term care facility, artificial methods of feeding, advance directives and CPR, use of antibiotics to treat infections, and guardianship.

HYPERPARATHYROIDISM

Description

Hyperparathyroidism is a condition involving increased secretion of parathyroid hormone (PTH). PTH helps regulate serum calcium and phosphate levels by stimulating bone resorption, renal tubular reabsorption of calcium, and activation of vitamin D. Thus oversecretion of PTH is associated with increased serum calcium levels. Hyperparathyroidism affects approximately 1% of the U.S. population and is more common in women than in men.

Hyperparathyroidism is classified as primary, secondary, or tertiary.

- *Primary hyperparathyroidism* is caused by an increased secretion of PTH leading to disorders of calcium, phosphate, and bone metabolism. The most common cause is a benign tumor (adenoma) in the parathyroid gland. Previous head and neck radiation may be a predisposing factor for a parathyroid adenoma.
- *Secondary hyperparathyroidism* is a compensatory response to conditions that induce or cause hypocalcemia, the main stimulus of PTH secretion. These conditions include vitamin D deficiencies, malabsorption, chronic kidney disease, and hyperphosphatemia.
- *Tertiary hyperparathyroidism* occurs when there is hyperplasia of the parathyroid glands and a loss of negative feedback from circulating calcium levels. This causes autonomous secretion of PTH even with normal calcium levels. It is observed in the patient who has had a kidney transplant after a long period of dialysis treatment for chronic kidney disease.

Pathophysiology

Excessive levels of circulating PTH usually lead to hypercalcemia and hypophosphatemia, with multiple body systems affected (see Table 50-12, Lewis et al, *Medical-Surgical Nursing,* ed. 9, p. 1205).

- Decreased bone density can occur as a result of the effect of PTH on osteoclastic (bone-resorption) and osteoblastic (bone-formation) activity.
- In the kidneys, excess calcium cannot be reabsorbed, which leads to hypercalciuria. This urinary calcium, along with a large amount of urinary phosphate, can lead to formation of calculi.

Clinical Manifestations

Manifestations range from the asymptomatic individual (diagnosed through testing for unrelated problems) to the patient with overt symptoms. The manifestations are associated with hypercalcemia.

- Muscle weakness, loss of appetite, constipation, fatigue, emotional disorders, and shortened attention span are often noted.
- Other signs of hyperparathyroidism include osteoporosis, fractures, and kidney stones (nephrolithiasis). Neuromuscular abnormalities are characterized by muscle weakness, particularly in the proximal muscles of the lower extremities.

Complications include renal failure; pancreatitis; cardiac changes; and long bone, rib, and vertebral fractures.

Diagnostic Studies

- PTH levels are elevated.
- Serum calcium levels are elevated with decreased phosphorus levels.
- Urine calcium, serum chloride, serum uric acid, and serum creatinine are elevated.
- Serum amylase (if pancreatitis is present) and alkaline phosphatase (if bone disease is present) are both elevated.
- Bone density tests can detect bone loss.
- MRI, CT scanning, and ultrasound can be used to localize adenoma.

Collaborative Care

Treatment objectives are to relieve the symptoms and prevent complications caused by excess PTH. The choice of therapy depends on the urgency of the clinical situation, the degree of hypercalcemia, and the underlying cause of the disorder.

- The most effective treatment of primary and secondary hyperparathyroidism is partial or complete surgical removal of the parathyroid glands. The procedure most commonly used involves endoscopy on an outpatient basis.

A conservative management approach is used in patients who are asymptomatic or have mild symptoms of hyperparathyroidism. This includes an annual examination with tests for serum PTH, calcium, phosphorus, and alkaline phosphatase levels and renal function; x-rays to assess for metabolic bone disease; and measurement of urinary calcium excretion.

- X-rays and dual-energy x-ray absorptiometry (DXA) are done to assess for metabolic bone loss. Dietary measures include high fluid and moderate calcium intake.
- Bisphosphonates (e.g., alendronate [Fosamax]) inhibit osteoclastic bone resorption and improve bone mineral density.

Phosphorus is usually supplemented unless contraindicated in a person with an increased risk for urinary calculi formation. Phosphates should be used only if the patient has normal renal function and low serum phosphate levels.

- Calcimimetic agents (e.g., cinacalcet [Sensipar]) increase the sensitivity of the calcium receptor on the parathyroid gland, resulting in decreased PTH secretion and calcium blood levels.
- Loop diuretics may be given to increase urinary excretion of calcium.

Nursing Management

Nursing care after surgery is similar to that for the patient after thyroidectomy (see Hyperthyroidism, p. 336). The major postoperative complications are hemorrhage and fluid and electrolyte disturbances. Tetany is usually apparent early in the postoperative period but may develop over several days. Mild tetany, characterized by an unpleasant tingling of the hands and around the mouth, may be present but should resolve without problems. IV calcium should be readily available for use if tetany becomes more severe (e.g., muscular spasms or laryngospasms).

- Monitor intake and output to evaluate fluid status.
- Assess calcium, potassium, phosphate, and magnesium levels frequently.
- Encourage mobility to promote bone calcification.
- If surgery is not performed, treatment to relieve symptoms and prevent complications is initiated.

▼ **Patient and Caregiver Teaching**

- Assist the patient with hyperparathyroidism to adapt the meal plan to his or her lifestyle. A referral to a dietitian may be useful.
- Because immobility can aggravate bone loss, stress the importance of an exercise program.
- Encourage the patient to keep annual appointments. Instruct the patient regarding the symptoms of hypocalcemia or hypercalcemia and to report them when they occur.

HYPERTENSION

Description

One in three adults in the United States has *hypertension,* or high BP. An additional 30% of adults have prehypertension, and approximately 8% have undiagnosed hypertension. There is a direct relationship between hypertension and cardiovascular disease (CVD). As BP increases, so does the risk of MI, heart failure, stoke, and renal disease.

Hypertension is defined as a persistent systolic BP (SBP) of 140 mm Hg or greater, diastolic BP (DBP) of 90 mm Hg or greater, or current use of antihypertensive medication. *Prehypertension* is defined as SBP 120 to 139 mm Hg or DBP 80 to 89 mm Hg. Classification of hypertension for adults according to stages is described in Table 50.

- The classification is based on the average of two or more properly measured BP readings on two or more office visits.

Isolated systolic hypertension (ISH) is an average SBP greater than 140 mm Hg coupled with an average DBP less than 90 mm Hg and is associated with loss of elasticity in larger arteries from atherosclerosis in older adults. SBP increases with aging. DBP rises until approximately age 55 and then declines. Control of ISH decreases the incidence of stroke, heart failure, and death.

Hypertension can be classified as primary (essential or idiopathic) or secondary. *Primary hypertension* accounts for 90% to 95% of all cases of hypertension. Although the exact cause of primary hypertension is unknown, several contributing factors have been identified, including greater-than-ideal body weight, diabetes mellitus (DM), increased sympathetic nervous system (SNS) activity, increased sodium intake, and excessive alcohol intake.

Secondary hypertension is elevated BP with a specific cause that often can be identified and corrected. This type of hypertension accounts for 5% to 10% of hypertension in adults. Causes of secondary hypertension include coarctation or congenital narrowing of the aorta, renal artery stenosis, endocrine disorders such as Cushing syndrome, cirrhosis, neurologic disorders such as brain tumors and head injury, sleep apnea, and pregnancy-induced hypertension. Treatment of secondary hypertension is directed at removing or treating the underlying cause.

| Table 50 | Classification of Hypertension |

Category	SBP (mm Hg)		DBP (mm Hg)
Normal	<120	and	<80
Prehypertension	120-139	or	80-89
Hypertension, stage 1	140-159	or	90-99
Hypertension, stage 2	≥160	or	≥100

From the National Heart, Lung, and Blood Institute: Seventh report of the Joint National Committee on Detection, Evaluation, and Treatment of High Blood Pressure (JNC-7), NIH Publication No. 04-5230, Bethesda, Md, 2004, The Institute. Retrieved from *www.nhlbi.nih.gov/guidelines/hypertension/jnc7full.pdf*.
DBP, Diastolic blood pressure; *SBP,* systolic blood pressure.

Pathophysiology of Primary Hypertension

The hemodynamic hallmark of hypertension is persistently increased systemic vascular resistance (SVR). Table 51 presents factors that relate to the development of primary hypertension or contribute to its consequences.

Clinical Manifestations

Hypertension is often called the "silent killer" because it is frequently asymptomatic until it becomes severe and target organ disease has occurred. A patient with severe hypertension may experience a variety of symptoms secondary to effects on blood vessels in the various organs and tissues or to the increased workload of the heart. These secondary symptoms include fatigue, reduced activity tolerance, dizziness, palpitations, angina, and dyspnea.

The most common complications of hypertension are target organ diseases occurring in the heart (hypertensive heart disease), brain (cerebrovascular disease), peripheral vasculature (peripheral vascular disease), kidney (nephrosclerosis), and eyes (retinal damage).

Hypertensive Heart Disease

Hypertension is a major risk factor for coronary artery disease (CAD). The mechanisms by which hypertension contributes to the development of atherosclerosis are not fully known. The "response-to-injury" theory of atherogenesis suggests that hypertension disrupts the coronary artery endothelium. This results in a stiff arterial wall with a narrowed lumen and accounts for a high rate of CAD, angina, and MI. Sustained high BP also increases the cardiac workload and produces left ventricular hypertrophy (LVH). Progressive LVH, especially in association with CAD, is associated with the development of heart failure.

Heart failure occurs when the heart's compensatory adaptations are overwhelmed and the heart can no longer pump enough blood to meet the body's demands.

- The patient may complain of shortness of breath on exertion, paroxysmal nocturnal dyspnea, and fatigue.

Cerebrovascular Disease

Atherosclerosis is the most common cause of cerebrovascular disease. Atherosclerotic plaques are commonly distributed at the bifurcation of the common carotid artery. Portions of the atherosclerotic plaque, or the blood clot that forms on the plaque, may break off and travel to intracerebral vessels, producing a thromboembolism. The patient may experience transient ischemic attacks or a stroke.

H

| Table 51 | Risk Factors for Primary Hypertension |

Risk Factor	Description
Age	SBP rises progressively with increasing age.
	After age 50, SBP >140 mm Hg is a more important cardiovascular risk factor than DBP.
Alcohol	Excessive alcohol intake is strongly associated with hypertension.
	Patients with hypertension should limit their daily intake to 1 oz of alcohol.
Tobacco use	Smoking tobacco greatly ↑ risk of cardiovascular disease.
	People with hypertension who smoke tobacco are at even greater risk for cardiovascular disease.
Diabetes mellitus	Hypertension is more common in diabetics.
	When hypertension and diabetes coexist, complications (e.g., target organ disease) are more severe.
Elevated serum lipids	↑ Levels of cholesterol and triglycerides are primary risk factors in atherosclerosis.
	Hyperlipidemia is more common in people with hypertension.
Excess dietary sodium	High sodium intake can
	▪ Contribute to hypertension in some patients
	▪ Decrease the effectiveness of certain antihypertensive medications
Gender	Hypertension is more prevalent in men in young adulthood and early middle age (<55 yr of age).
	After age 64, hypertension is more prevalent in women. (See Gender Differences box, Lewis et al, *Medical-Surgical Nursing*, ed. 9, p. 710.)
Family history	History of a close blood relative (e.g., parents, sibling) with hypertension is associated with an ↑ risk for developing hypertension.

DBP, Diastolic blood pressure; *SBP,* systolic blood pressure.

Table 51	Risk Factors for Primary Hypertension—cont'd

Risk Factor	Description
Obesity	Weight gain is associated with increased frequency of hypertension. The risk is greatest with central abdominal obesity.
Ethnicity	Incidence of hypertension is two times higher in African Americans than in whites. (See Cultural & Ethnic Health Disparities box, Lewis et al, *Medical-Surgical Nursing*, ed. 9, p. 710.)
Sedentary lifestyle	Regular physical activity can help control weight and reduce cardiovascular risk. Physical activity may ↓ BP.
Socioeconomic status	Hypertension is more prevalent in lower socioeconomic groups and among the less educated.
Stress	People exposed to repeated stress may develop hypertension more frequently than others. People who develop hypertension may respond differently to stress than those who do not develop hypertension.

H

Peripheral Vascular Disease

Hypertension speeds up the process of atherosclerosis in peripheral blood vessels, leading to the development of aortic aneurysm, aortic dissection, and peripheral vascular disease. *Intermittent claudication* (ischemic muscle pain precipitated by activity and relieved with rest) is a classic symptom of peripheral vascular disease.

Nephrosclerosis. Hypertension is one of the leading risk factors for chronic kidney disease, especially among African Americans. Some degree of renal disease is usually present in the hypertensive patient, even one with a minimally elevated BP. This disorder is the result of ischemia caused by the narrowing of renal blood vessels. This leads to the destruction of glomeruli, atrophy of tubules, and eventual death of nephrons. These changes may eventually lead to renal failure. The earliest symptom of renal disease is usually nocturia.

Retinal Damage. The appearance of the retina provides important information about the severity and duration of hypertension. The blood vessels of the retina can be directly visualized with an ophthalmoscope. Damage to the retinal vessels provides an indication of related vessel damage in the heart, brain, and kidneys. Symptoms of severe retinal damage include blurring of vision, retinal hemorrhage, and loss of vision.

Diagnostic Studies

Basic laboratory studies are performed to evaluate target organ disease, determine overall cardiovascular risk, or establish baseline levels before initiating therapy.

- Routine urinalysis, blood urea nitrogen (BUN), and serum creatinine levels to screen for renal involvement.
- Serum electrolytes, especially potassium levels, to detect hyperaldosteronism.
- Blood glucose level to assess for diabetes mellitus.
- Lipid profile to assess for risk factors for atherosclerosis.
- ECG for baseline cardiac status.

Collaborative Care

Treatment goals include achieving and maintaining goal BP and reducing cardiovascular risk and target organ disease. Lifestyle modifications are indicated for all patients with prehypertension and hypertension. These modification measures include weight reduction, Dietary Approaches to Stop Hypertension (DASH) eating plan, dietary sodium reduction, regular physical activity, moderation of alcohol consumption, management of psychosocial risk factors, and avoidance of tobacco use.

- Dietary therapy consists of restricting sodium intake to less than 2300 mg/day and following the DASH eating plan, which emphasizes fruits, vegetables, fat-free or low-fat milk and milk products, whole grains, fish, poultry, beans, seeds, and nuts. Compared with the typical American diet, the plan contains less red meat, salt, sweets, added sugars, and sugar-containing beverages and is rich in vegetables, fruit, and nonfat dairy products. Men should limit their intake of alcohol to no more than two drinks per day and women and lighter men to no more than one drink per day.
- Adults should perform moderate-intensity aerobic physical activity for at least 30 minutes most days (i.e., more than 5 days per week) or vigorous-intensity aerobic activity for at least 20 minutes 3 days a week.
- Muscle-strengthening activities should also be performed using the major muscles of the body at least twice a week. Flexibility

and balance exercises are recommended at least twice a week for older adults, especially for those at risk for falls. Advise sedentary people to increase activity levels gradually.

- Psychosocial risk factors (e.g., depression, social isolation, low socioeconomic status) can contribute to the risk of developing CVD and to a poorer prognosis and clinical course in patients with CVD. Screening for these factors is important. Make appropriate referrals (e.g., counseling) when indicated.
- Nicotine contained in tobacco causes vasoconstriction and increases BP in hypertensive people. Strongly encourage everyone, especially a hypertensive patient, to avoid tobacco use.

Drug Therapy

The goal for treating primary hypertension is for the patient to have a BP less than 140/90 mm Hg. A lower goal of 130/80 mm Hg is recommended for patients at high risk of CAD (e.g., patients with diabetes mellitus and chronic kidney disease), as well as for patients with preexisting CAD (e.g., stable angina, heart failure, MI). The drugs currently available for treating hypertension have two main actions: reducing SVR and decreasing the volume of circulating blood.

- Drugs used in treatment of hypertension include diuretics, adrenergic (SNS) inhibitors, direct vasodilators, angiotensin inhibitors, and calcium channel blockers. (See Table 33-7, Lewis et al, *Medical-Surgical Nursing,* ed. 9, pp. 717 to 719, for a description of antihypertensive drug therapy.)
- Most patients who are hypertensive require two or more antihypertensive medications to achieve their goal BP (Table 52).
- Once antihypertensive therapy is started, most patients should return for follow-up and adjustment of medications at monthly intervals until the goal BP is reached.

Nursing Management

Goals

The patient with hypertension will achieve and maintain goal BP; understand and follow the therapeutic plan; experience minimal or no unpleasant side effects of therapy; and be confident of ability to manage and cope with this condition.

Nursing Diagnoses/Collaborative Problems

- Ineffective self-health management
- Anxiety
- Sexual dysfunction
- Risk for decreased cardiac perfusion
- Risk for ineffective renal perfusion
- Potential complication: stroke
- Potential complication: hypertensive crisis

Table 52	Patient and Caregiver Teaching Guide
	Hypertension

When teaching the patient and/or caregiver about hypertension, include the following information.

General Instructions

1. Provide the patient's BP reading and explain what it means (e.g., high, low, normal, borderline). Encourage the patient to monitor BP at home and instruct the patient to call health care provider if BP exceeds high or low limits set by health care provider.
2. Hypertension is usually asymptomatic, and symptoms (e.g., nosebleeds) do not reliably indicate BP levels.
3. Hypertension means high BP and does not relate to a "hyper" personality.
4. Long-term therapy and follow-up care are necessary to treat hypertension. Therapy involves lifestyle changes (e.g., weight management, sodium reduction, smoking cessation, regular physical activity) and, in most cases, medications.
5. Therapy will not cure hypertension, but should control it.
6. Controlled hypertension usually results in an excellent prognosis and a normal lifestyle.
7. Explain the potential dangers of uncontrolled hypertension (e.g., target organ disease).

Instructions Related to Medications

1. Be specific about the names, actions, dosages, and side effects of prescribed medications.
2. Help the patient plan regular and convenient times for taking medications and measuring BP.
3. Do not stop drugs abruptly because withdrawal may cause a severe hypertensive reaction.
4. Do not double up on doses when a dose is missed.
5. If BP increases, the patient should not take an increased medication dosage before consulting with the health care provider.
6. Do not take a medication belonging to someone else.
7. Supplement diet with foods high in potassium (e.g., citrus fruits, green leafy vegetables) if taking potassium-wasting diuretics.
8. Avoid hot baths, excessive amounts of alcohol, and strenuous exercise within 3 hr of taking medications that promote vasodilation.

Table 52	Patient and Caregiver Teaching Guide
	Hypertension—cont'd

9. Many medications cause orthostatic hypotension. The effects of orthostatic hypotension can be reduced by rising slowly from bed, sitting on the side of the bed for a few minutes, standing slowly, and beginning to move if no symptoms develop (e.g., dizziness, light-headedness). Do not stand still for prolonged periods, do leg exercises to increase venous return, or sleep with the head of the bed raised. Do lie or sit down when dizziness occurs.

10. Many medications cause sexual problems (e.g., erectile dysfunction, decreased libido). Consult with the health care provider about changing drugs or dosages if sexual problems develop.

11. The side effects of medication(s) may decrease with time.

12. Be careful about taking potentially high-risk, over-the-counter medications, such as high-sodium antacids, appetite suppressants, and cold and sinus medications. Read warning labels and consult with a pharmacist.

Nursing Interventions

You are in an ideal position to assess for the presence of hypertension, identify risk factors for hypertension and CAD, and teach the patient about these conditions.

Initially, take the BP in both arms to note any differences. Atherosclerosis in the subclavian artery can cause a falsely low reading on the side where the narrowing occurs. Use the arm with the highest BP and take at least two readings, at least 1 minute apart.

Assess for orthostatic (or postural) changes in BP and pulse in older adults, in people taking antihypertensive drugs, and in patients who report symptoms consistent with reduced BP on standing (e.g., light-headedness, dizziness, syncope).

Your primary nursing responsibilities for long-term management of hypertension are to assist the patient in reducing BP and adhering to the treatment plan. Your nursing actions include evaluating therapeutic effectiveness, detecting and reporting any adverse treatment effects, assessing and enhancing adherence, and patient and caregiver teaching.

▼ **Patient and Caregiver Teaching**

Help the patient and caregiver understand that hypertension is a chronic illness that cannot be cured. Emphasize that it can be controlled with drug therapy, diet changes, physical activity, periodic follow-up, and other relevant lifestyle modifications (Table 52).

H

HYPERTHYROIDISM

Description

Hyperthyroidism is hyperactivity of the thyroid gland with a sustained increase in synthesis and release of thyroid hormones. The most common form of hyperthyroidism is Graves' disease. Other causes include toxic nodular goiter, thyroiditis, pituitary tumors, and thyroid cancer. *Thyrotoxicosis* is hypermetabolism that results from excess circulating levels of thyroxine (T_4), triiodothyronine (T_3), or both. Hyperthyroidism and thyrotoxicosis usually occur together as in Graves' disease. Graves' disease accounts for up to 80% of the cases of hyperthyroidism. Hyperthyroidism occurs in more women than men, with the highest frequency in people 20 to 40 years old.

Pathophysiology

Graves' disease is an autoimmune disease of unknown etiology marked by diffuse thyroid enlargement and excessive thyroid hormone secretion. The patient develops antibodies to the thyroid-stimulating hormone (TSH) receptor. These antibodies attach to receptors and stimulate the thyroid gland to release T_3, T_4, or both. The excessive release of thyroid hormones leads to the clinical manifestations associated with thyrotoxicosis.

- The disease is characterized by remissions and exacerbations, with or without treatment. It may progress to destruction of thyroid tissue, causing hypothyroidism.
- Precipitating factors, such as insufficient iodine supply, infection, and stressful life events, may interact with genetic factors to cause Graves' disease. Cigarette smoking increases the risk of Graves' disease and the development of eye problems associated with the disease.

Clinical Manifestations

Manifestations of hyperthyroidism are related to the effect of excess thyroid hormones.

- Palpation of the thyroid gland may reveal a goiter. When the thyroid gland is excessively large, a goiter may be noted on inspection. Auscultation of the thyroid gland may reveal bruits, a reflection of increased blood supply.
- *Exophthalmos,* a protrusion of the eyeballs from the orbits, is caused by impaired venous drainage from the orbit leading to increased deposits of fat and fluid (edema) in the orbital tissues.

This sign is a classic finding in Graves' disease. When the eyelids do not close completely, exposed corneal surfaces become dry and irritated. Serious consequences, such as corneal ulcers and eventual loss of vision, can occur. Ocular muscle changes result in muscle weakness, causing diplopia.

- A patient with advanced disease may exhibit many symptoms, whereas a patient in the early stages of hyperthyroidism may only exhibit weight loss and increased nervousness.

Other manifestations of hyperthyroidism are summarized in Table 50-5, Lewis et al, *Medical-Surgical Nursing,* ed. 9, p. 1197.

Complications

Thyrotoxicosis (also called thyrotoxic crisis, thyroid storm) is an acute, severe, and rare condition that occurs when excessive amounts of thyroid hormones are released into the circulation. Although this is considered a life-threatening emergency, death is rare when treatment is initiated early. Thyrotoxicosis is thought to result from stressors (e.g., infection, trauma, surgery) in a patient with preexisting hyperthyroidism, either diagnosed or undiagnosed.

All the symptoms of hyperthyroidism are prominent and severe, including severe tachycardia, heart failure, shock, hyperthermia (up to 105.3° F [40.7° C]), restlessness, agitation, abdominal pain, nausea, vomiting, diarrhea, delirium, and coma.

- Treatment is aimed at reducing circulating thyroid hormone levels by appropriate drug therapy, fever reduction, fluid replacement, and elimination or management of the initiating stressor or stressors.

Diagnostic Studies

- Diagnosis is confirmed with findings of decreased serum TSH levels and elevated free thyroxine (T_4) levels.
- Total T_3 and T_4 may be assessed, but they are not definitive.
- Radioactive iodine uptake (RAIU) differentiates Graves' disease from other forms of thyroiditis.

Collaborative Care

The goal of management is to block the adverse effects of thyroid hormones, suppress oversecretion of thyroid hormone, and prevent complications. There are several treatment options, including antithyroid medications, radioactive iodine therapy, and surgical intervention. The choice of treatment is influenced by the patient's age and preferences, coexistence of other diseases, and pregnancy status.

H

Drug Therapy
Drugs used in the treatment of hyperthyroidism are useful in controlling symptoms in thyrotoxic states, but they are not curative.

Antithyroid Drugs. The first-line antithyroid drugs commonly used are propylthiouracil (PTU) and methimazole (Tapazole). These drugs inhibit the synthesis of thyroid hormones. Indications for their use include Graves' disease in the young patient, hyperthyroidism during pregnancy, and the need to achieve a euthyroid state before surgery or radiation therapy. PTU, which blocks the peripheral conversion of T_4 to T_3, is first-line treatment for thyrotoxic crisis.

Iodine. In large doses, iodine (e.g., Lugol's solution, saturated solution of potassium iodide [SSKI]) inhibits the synthesis of T_3 and T_4 and blocks the release of these hormones into circulation. Iodine decreases thyroid vascularity, making surgery safer and easier. The maximal effect is usually seen within 1 to 2 weeks.

β-Adrenergic Blockers. β-Adrenergic blockers (e.g., propranolol [Inderal]) are used for symptomatic relief of thyrotoxicosis. These drugs block the effects of sympathetic nervous stimulation, thereby decreasing tachycardia, nervousness, irritability, and tremors.

Radioactive Iodine. Radioactive iodine (RAI) limits thyroid hormone secretion by damaging or destroying thyroid tissue. RAI has a delayed response, and the maximum effect may not be seen for up to 3 months. For this reason, other drug therapy may be used until the effects of radiation become apparent. This treatment is usually effective but often results in hypothyroidism.

Surgical Therapy
Thyroidectomy is indicated for individuals who (1) have a large goiter causing tracheal compression, (2) have been unresponsive to antithyroid therapy, or (3) have thyroid cancer unresponsive to antithyroid therapy. A subtotal thyroidectomy is often the preferred surgical procedure and involves the removal of a significant portion (90%) of the thyroid gland. An endoscopic thyroidectomy is a minimally invasive procedure. It is performed for patients with small nodules (less than 3 cm) and no evidence of malignancy.

Nutritional Therapy
There is a high potential for nutritional deficits when an increased metabolic rate is present. A high-calorie diet (4000 to 5000 cal/day) may be ordered to satisfy hunger and prevent tissue breakdown. This can be accomplished with six full meals each day and snacks high in protein, carbohydrates, minerals, and vitamins.

- ▪ Teach the patient to avoid highly seasoned and high-fiber foods because these foods can further stimulate the already hyperactive GI tract. Provide substitutes for caffeine-containing liquids such as coffee, tea, and cola because the stimulating effects of these fluids increase restlessness and sleep disturbances.

- Refer the patient to a dietitian for help in meeting individual nutritional needs.

Nursing Management

Goals

The patient with hyperthyroidism will experience relief of symptoms, have no serious complications related to the disease or treatment, maintain nutritional balance, and cooperate with the therapeutic plan.

Nursing Diagnoses

- Activity intolerance
- Imbalanced nutrition: less than body requirements

Nursing Interventions

Acute thyrotoxicosis requires aggressive treatment, often in an intensive care unit. Administer medications (previously discussed) that block thyroid hormone production and the sympathetic nervous system.

Provide supportive therapy to the patient, including monitoring for cardiac dysrhythmias and decompensation, ensuring adequate oxygenation, and administering IV fluids to replace fluid and electrolyte losses. This is especially important in the patient who experiences fluid losses because of vomiting and diarrhea.

Provision of adequate rest may be a challenge because of the patient's irritability and restlessness. Provide a calm, quiet room because increased metabolism and sensitivity of the sympathetic nervous system cause sleep disturbances.

- Interventions may include placing the patient in a cool room away from very ill patients and noisy, high-traffic areas; using light bed coverings and changing the linen frequently if the patient is diaphoretic; encouraging and assisting with exercise involving large muscle groups (tremors can interfere with small-muscle coordination) to allow the release of nervous tension and restlessness; and establishing a supportive, trusting relationship to help the patient cope with aggravating events and lessen anxiety.

If exophthalmos is present, there is a potential for corneal injury. The patient may also have orbital pain. Interventions to relieve eye discomfort and prevent corneal ulceration include applying artificial tears to soothe and moisten conjunctival membranes, elevating the patient's head to reduce periorbital edema, and providing dark glasses to reduce glare and prevent irritation from smoke, air currents, dust, and dirt. If the eyelids cannot be closed, lightly tape them shut for sleep. To maintain flexibility, teach the patient to exercise intraocular muscles several times each day by turning the eyes in the complete range of motion.

Nursing Management: Patient Having Thyroid Surgery

When a subtotal thyroidectomy is the treatment of choice, the patient must be adequately prepared to avoid postoperative complications.

- Preoperative teaching should include comfort and safety measures and teaching the patient the importance of leg exercises. The patient should also be taught how to support the head manually while turning in bed to minimize stress on the surgery suture line. Range-of-motion (ROM) exercises of the neck should be practiced, and the patient should be told that talking is likely to be difficult for a short time after surgery.
- Recurrent laryngeal nerve damage leads to vocal cord paralysis. If both cords are paralyzed, spastic airway obstruction will occur, requiring an immediate tracheostomy.
- Respiration may become difficult because of excess swelling of the neck tissue, hemorrhage, and hematoma formation.
- Laryngeal stridor (harsh, vibratory sound) may occur during respiration as a result of edema of the laryngeal nerve or because of tetany, which occurs if the parathyroid glands are removed or damaged during surgery. To treat tetany, IV calcium salts such as calcium gluconate or gluceptate should be available.

Important nursing interventions after a thyroidectomy include the following:

- Assess the patient every 2 hours for 24 hours for signs of hemorrhage or tracheal compression, such as irregular breathing, neck swelling, frequent swallowing, sensation of fullness at the incision site, choking, and blood on dressings.
- Place the patient in a semi-Fowler's position and support the head with pillows. Avoid flexion of the neck and any tension on the suture lines.
- Monitor vital signs and calcium levels. Check for signs of tetany secondary to hypoparathyroidism (e.g., tingling of toes, fingers, or around the mouth; muscular twitching; apprehension) and by evaluating any difficulty in speaking and hoarseness.
- Control postoperative pain by giving medication.

▼ **Patient and Caregiver Teaching**

Follow-up care is important for the patient who has undergone thyroid surgery.

- Hormone balance should be monitored periodically to ensure that normal function has returned.
- Caloric intake must be reduced substantially below the amount that was required before surgery to prevent weight gain.
- Adequate iodine is necessary to promote thyroid function, but excesses inhibit the thyroid. Seafood once or twice per week or the normal use of iodized salt should provide sufficient intake.
- Encourage regular exercise to help stimulate the thyroid.

- Teach the patient to avoid high environmental temperatures because they inhibit thyroid regeneration.

If a complete thyroidectomy has been performed, instruct the patient about the need for lifelong thyroid replacement therapy. Teach the patient the signs and symptoms of progressive thyroid failure and instruct him or her to seek medical care if these develop. Hypothyroidism is relatively easy to manage with oral administration of thyroid replacement.

HYPOPARATHYROIDISM

Description

Hypoparathyroidism is an uncommon condition characterized by inadequate circulating parathyroid hormone (PTH) that results in hypocalcemia. PTH resistance at the cellular level may also occur. This is caused by a genetic defect resulting in hypocalcemia in spite of normal or high PTH levels and is often associated with hypothyroidism and hypogonadism.

Pathophysiology

The most common cause of hypoparathyroidism is the accidental removal of parathyroids or damage to the vascular supply of the glands during neck surgery (e.g., thyroidectomy).

- Idiopathic hypoparathyroidism resulting from absence, fatty replacement, or atrophy of the glands is a rare disease that usually occurs early in life and may be associated with other endocrine disorders. Affected patients may have antiparathyroid antibodies.
- Severe hypomagnesemia (e.g., malnutrition, renal failure) also leads to suppression of PTH secretion.

Clinical Manifestations

Clinical features of acute hypoparathyroidism are caused by hypocalcemia (see Table 50-12, Lewis et al, *Medical-Surgical Nursing*, ed. 9, p. 1205).

Sudden decreases in calcium concentration cause tetany, characterized by lip tingling and extremity stiffness. Painful tonic spasms of smooth and skeletal muscles can cause dysphagia and laryngospasms that compromise breathing.

Abnormal laboratory findings include decreased serum calcium and PTH levels and increased serum phosphate levels.

Nursing and Collaborative Management

Treatment goals for the patient with hypoparathyroidism are to treat acute complications such as tetany, maintain normal serum calcium levels, and prevent long-term complications. Emergency treatment of tetany after surgery requires the administration of IV calcium.

- Give IV calcium chloride, calcium gluconate, or calcium glucep-tate slowly. Use ECG monitoring during calcium administration because high serum calcium blood levels can cause hypotension, serious cardiac dysrhythmias, or cardiac arrest.
- Rebreathing may partially alleviate acute neuromuscular symptoms associated with hypocalcemia such as generalized muscle cramps or mild tetany. Instruct the patients (if cooperative) to breathe in and out of a paper bag or breathing mask.

▼ **Patient and Caregiver Teaching**

The patient with hypoparathyroidism needs instruction in the management of long-term nutrition and drug therapy.

- Oral calcium supplements of at least 1.5 to 3 g/day in divided doses are usually prescribed.
- A high-calcium meal plan includes foods such as dark green vegetables, soybeans, and tofu. Tell the patient that foods containing oxalic acid (e.g., spinach, rhubarb), phytic acid (e.g., bran, whole grains), and phosphorus reduce calcium absorption.
- Instruct the patient about the need for lifelong treatment and follow-up care including monitoring of calcium levels three or four times a year.

HYPOTHYROIDISM

Description

Hypothyroidism is a deficiency of thyroid hormone that causes a general slowing of the metabolic rate. About 4% of the U.S. population has mild hypothyroidism, with about 0.3% having more severe disease. Hypothyroidism is more common in American women than men.

Pathophysiology

Hypothyroidism can be *primary* (related to destruction of thyroid tissue or defective hormone synthesis) or *secondary* (related to pituitary disease with decreased thyroid-stimulating hormone [TSH] secretion or hypothalamic dysfunction with decreased thyrotropin-releasing hormone [TRH] secretion). It may also be transient, related to a thyroiditis or discontinuance of thyroid hormone therapy.

- Iodine deficiency is the most common cause of hypothyroidism worldwide. In the United States, the most common cause of primary hypothyroidism is atrophy of the thyroid gland. This atrophy is the end result of Hashimoto's thyroiditis or Graves' disease. These autoimmune diseases destroy the thyroid gland.

- Hypothyroidism may also develop as a result of treatment for hyperthyroidism, specifically the surgical removal of the thyroid gland or radioactive iodine (RAI) therapy. Drugs such as amiodarone (Cordarone) (contains iodine) and lithium (blocks hormone production) can cause hypothyroidism.
- Hypothyroidism that develops in infancy *(cretinism)* is caused by thyroid hormone deficiencies during fetal or early neonatal life.

Clinical Manifestations

Regardless of the cause, hypothyroidism has common features. Manifestations vary depending on severity and duration of thyroid deficiency, as well as the patient's age at onset of the deficiency.

Hypothyroidism has systemic effects characterized by a slowing of body processes. The patient is often fatigued and lethargic and experiences personality and mental changes including impaired memory, slowed speech, decreased initiative, and somnolence. Many individuals with hypothyroidism appear depressed, and weight gain is most likely a result of decreased metabolic rate.

- Hypothyroidism is associated with decreased cardiac output and decreased cardiac contractility. Anemia is a common feature. Increased serum cholesterol and triglyceride levels and the accumulation of mucopolysaccharides in the intima of small blood vessels can result in coronary atherosclerosis.
- GI motility is decreased in hypothyroidism, and *achlorhydria* (absence or decreased secretion of hydrochloric acid) is common. Constipation, which is a common complaint, may progress to obstipation and, rarely, to intestinal obstruction.
- In the older adult, typical manifestations include fatigue, cold and dry skin, hair loss, constipation, hoarseness, and cold intolerance.
- Individuals with hypothyroidism may describe an altered self-image related to their disabilities and altered appearance.

Those with severe long-standing hypothyroidism may display *myxedema,* which alters the physical appearance of the skin and subcutaneous tissues with puffiness, facial and periorbital edema, and a masklike affect. Myxedema occurs because of the accumulation of hydrophilic mucopolysaccharides in the dermis and other tissues.

Other manifestations of hypothyroidism are summarized in Table 50-5, Lewis et al, *Medical-Surgical Nursing,* ed. 9, p. 1197.

Complications

The mental sluggishness, drowsiness, and lethargy of hypothyroidism may progress gradually or suddenly to a notable impairment of consciousness or coma. This situation, termed *myxedema coma,* constitutes a medical emergency.

- Myxedema coma can be precipitated by infection, drugs (especially opioids, tranquilizers, and barbiturates), exposure to cold, and trauma. It is characterized by subnormal temperature, hypotension, and hypoventilation.
- For the patient to survive, vital functions must be supported, and IV thyroid hormone replacement administered.

Diagnostic Studies

- Serum TSH and free thyroxine (FT_4) are the most reliable indicators of thyroid function.
- Serum TSH levels help determine the cause of hypothyroidism. If high, the defect is in the thyroid; if low, it is in the pituitary or hypothalamus.
- The presence of thyroid antibodies suggests an autoimmune origin of the hypothyroidism.
- Elevated cholesterol and triglycerides, anemia, and increased creatine kinase can occur.

Collaborative Care

The treatment goal is the restoration of the euthyroid state as safely and rapidly as possible with hormone therapy. A low-calorie diet is also indicated to promote weight loss or prevent weight gain.

Levothyroxine (Synthroid) is the drug of choice to treat hypothyroidism. In the young, otherwise healthy patient, the maintenance replacement dosage is adjusted according to the patient's response and laboratory findings. The initial dosages are low to avoid increases in resting heart rate and BP. In the patient with compromised cardiac status, careful monitoring is needed when starting and adjusting the dosage because the usual dose may increase myocardial oxygen demand. The increased oxygen demand may cause angina and cardiac dysrhythmias. In the patient without side effects, the dose is increased at 4- to 6-week intervals.

Liotrix is a synthetic mix of levothyroxine (T_4) and liothyronine (T_3) in a 4:1 combination. Levothyroxine has a peak of action of 1 to 3 weeks. In contrast, liotrix has a faster onset of action with a peak of 2 to 3 days. Liotrix can be used in acutely ill individuals with hypothyroidism.

It is important that the patient take replacement medication regularly. Lifelong thyroid therapy is usually required.

Nursing Management

Goals

The patient with hypothyroidism will experience relief of symptoms, maintain a euthyroid state, maintain a positive self-image, and comply with lifelong thyroid therapy.

Nursing Diagnoses
- Imbalanced nutrition: more than body requirements
- Constipation
- Impaired memory

Nursing Interventions

Most individuals with hypothyroidism are treated on an outpatient basis. The patient who develops myxedema coma requires acute nursing care, often in an intensive care setting. Mechanical respiratory support and cardiac monitoring are frequently necessary. Administer thyroid hormone therapy and all other medications IV because paralytic ileus may be present in the patient with myxedema coma. Monitor core temperature because the patient with myxedema coma is often hypothermic.

- Use soap gently and moisturize frequently to prevent skin breakdown. Frequent changes in patient positioning and a low-pressure mattress can also assist in maintaining skin integrity.
- Monitor the patient's progress, vital signs, body weight, fluid intake and output, and visible edema. Cardiac assessment is especially important because the cardiovascular response to hormone therapy determines the medication regimen.
- Note energy level and mental alertness, which should increase within 2 to 14 days and continue to rise steadily to normal levels.

▼ **Patient and Caregiver Teaching**

Initially the hypothyroid patient may have difficulty processing complex instructions. It is important to provide written instructions, repeat the information often, and assess the patient's comprehension level.

- Stress the need for receiving lifelong drug therapy and avoiding abrupt discontinuation of drugs. Instruct the patient in expected and unexpected side effects. In the teaching plan, include the signs and symptoms of hypothyroidism or hyperthyroidism that indicate hormone imbalance.
- Teach the patient to immediately contact a health care provider if signs of overdose appear, such as orthopnea, dyspnea, rapid pulse, palpitations, nervousness, or insomnia.
- The patient with diabetes mellitus should test his or her capillary blood glucose at least daily because a return to the euthyroid state frequently increases insulin requirements.
- In addition, thyroid preparations potentiate the effects of other common drugs, such as anticoagulants, antidepressants, and digitalis compounds. Instruct the patient on the toxic signs and symptoms of these medications and the need to remain under close medical observation until stable.

INCREASED INTRACRANIAL PRESSURE

Description

Increased intracranial pressure (ICP) is a potentially life-threatening situation that results from an increase in any or all of the three components within the skull: brain tissue, blood, and cerebrospinal fluid (CSF).

Pathophysiology

Common causes of increased ICP include a mass lesion (e.g., hematoma, contusion, abscess, tumor) and cerebral edema (associated with brain tumors, hydrocephalus, head injury, or brain inflammation). These cerebral insults, which may result in hypercapnia, cerebral acidosis, impaired autoregulation, and systemic hypertension, increase the formation and spread of cerebral edema. This edema distorts brain tissue, further increasing the ICP, and leads to even more tissue hypoxia and acidosis.

Regardless of the cause, cerebral edema results in an increase in tissue volume that has the potential to increase ICP. The extent and severity of the original insult are factors that determine the degree of cerebral edema. Figure 9 illustrates the progression of increased ICP.

There are three types of cerebral edema, including vasogenic, cytotoxic, and interstitial. More than one type may occur in the same patient.

- *Vasogenic cerebral edema,* the most common type of edema, occurs mainly in the white matter and is characterized by leakage of macromolecules from the capillaries into the surrounding extracellular space. This edema may produce a continuum of symptoms ranging from headache to disturbances in consciousness, including coma and focal neurologic deficits.
- *Cytotoxic cerebral edema* results from disruption of the integrity of the cell membranes. This type of edema develops from destructive lesions or trauma to brain tissue resulting in cerebral hypoxia or anoxia and syndrome of inappropriate antidiuretic hormone (SIADH) secretion.
- *Interstitial cerebral edema* is usually a result of hydrocephalus. It can be due to excess CSF production, obstruction of flow, or an inability to reabsorb the CSF.

Clinical Manifestations

Manifestations of increased ICP can take many forms, depending on the cause, location, and rate of increase of ICP.

- *Change in level of consciousness (LOC).* LOC is a sensitive and reliable indicator of the patient's neurologic status. Changes in LOC may be dramatic, as in coma, or subtle, such as a change in orientation or a decrease in the level of attention.

PATHOPHYSIOLOGY MAP

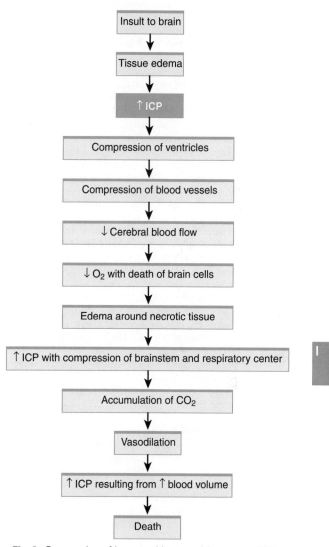

Fig. 9. Progression of increased intracranial pressure (ICP).

- *Changes in vital signs.* Manifestations such as *Cushing's triad* (systolic hypertension with widening pulse pressure, bradycardia with a full and bounding pulse, and irregular respirations) may be present but often do not appear until ICP has been increased for some time or markedly increased (e.g., head trauma). The effect of increased ICP on the hypothalamus can cause a change in body temperature.
- *Ocular signs.* Compression of the oculomotor nerve (CN III) results in dilation of the pupil on the same side (ipsilateral) as the mass lesion, sluggish or no response to light, an inability to move the eye upward, and ptosis of the eyelid. A fixed, unilaterally dilated pupil is a neurologic emergency that indicates brain herniation. Other cranial nerves may also be affected, with signs of blurred vision, diplopia, and changes in extraocular eye movements. Papilledema, a nonspecific sign associated with persistent increases in ICP, is also seen.
- *Decrease in motor function.* As ICP continues to rise, the patient manifests changes in motor ability. A contralateral (opposite side of the mass lesion) hemiparesis or hemiplegia may develop. If a painful stimulus is used to elicit a motor response, the patient may localize to the stimulus or withdraw from it. *Decorticate* (flexor) and *decerebrate* (extensor) posturing may also be elicited by noxious stimuli (see Fig. 57-5, Lewis et al, *Medical-Surgical Nursing,* ed 9, p. 1360).
- *Headache.* Although the brain itself is insensitive to pain, compression of other intracranial structures, such as the walls of arteries and veins and the cranial nerves, can produce headache. The headache is often continuous but is worse in the morning. Straining or movement may accentuate the pain.
- *Vomiting.* Vomiting, usually not preceded by nausea, is often a nonspecific sign of increased ICP.

The major complications of uncontrolled increased ICP are inadequate cerebral perfusion and cerebral herniation.

Diagnostic Studies

- MRI, CT scan, and positron emission tomography (PET) are used to diagnose the cause of increased ICP.
- Other tests may include cerebral angiography, electroencephalography (EEG), ICP measurement, brain tissue oxygenation measurement via the LICOX catheter, transcranial Doppler studies, and evoked potential studies.

Collaborative Care

The goals of management of increased ICP are to identify and treat the underlying cause of increased ICP and to support brain function.

The earlier the condition is recognized and treated, the better the patient outcome. A careful history is an important diagnostic aid that can direct the search for the underlying cause.

Ensuring adequate oxygenation to support brain function is important. Arterial blood gas (ABG) analysis guides the oxygen therapy. To meet the goal of maintaining the partial pressure of oxygen in arterial blood (PaO_2) at 100 mm Hg or greater and to keep $PaCO_2$ in normal range at 35 to 45 mm Hg, an endotracheal tube or tracheostomy and mechanical ventilation may be necessary.

- If the condition is caused by a mass lesion, such as a tumor or hematoma, surgical removal of the mass is the best management (see Brain Tumors, p. 85).
- Nonsurgical intervention for the reduction of tissue volume related to cerebral tissue swelling and edema includes the use of diuretics and corticosteroids.

Drug Therapy

Drug therapy plays an important part in the management of increased ICP.

- IV mannitol (Osmitrol) (25%) is an osmotic diuretic that decreases ICP in two ways: plasma expansion and osmotic effect. The immediate plasma-expanding effect reduces the hematocrit and blood viscosity, thereby increasing cerebral blood flow and cerebral oxygenation. The osmotic effect causes fluid to move from the tissue into the blood vessels, resulting in a decrease in total brain fluid content.
- Hypertonic saline is another drug treatment used to manage increased ICP. It produces massive movement of water out of edematous swollen brain cells and into the blood vessels.
- Corticosteroids (e.g., dexamethasone [Decadron]) are used to treat vasogenic edema surrounding tumors and abscesses, but are not recommended for head-injured patients. Corticosteroids stabilize the cell membrane and inhibit the synthesis of prostaglandins. These drugs also improve cerebral blood flow and restore autoregulation.
- Metabolic demands such as fever (above 38° C), agitation/shivering, pain, and seizures can also increase ICP. The health care team should plan to reduce these metabolic demands in order to lower the ICP in the at-risk patient.
- High-dose barbiturates (e.g., pentobarbital [Nembutal] and thiopental [Pentothal]) are used in patients with an increased ICP refractory to other treatments. These drugs lower cerebral metabolism, which causes a decrease in ICP.

Nutritional Therapy

The patient with increased ICP is in a hypermetabolic and hypercatabolic state that increases the need for glucose to provide the necessary fuel for metabolism of the injured brain. If the patient cannot maintain an adequate oral intake, other means of meeting the nutritional requirements, such as enteral or parenteral nutrition, should be started. Current fluid therapy is directed at keeping patients normovolemic.

Nursing Management

Goals
The overall goals are that the patient with increased ICP will have ICP within normal limits, maintain a patent airway, demonstrate normal fluid and electrolyte balance, and have no complications secondary to immobility and decreased LOC.

Nursing Diagnoses
- Risk for ineffective cerebral tissue perfusion
- Decreased intracranial adaptive capacity
- Risk for disuse syndrome

Nursing Interventions
Respiratory Function. Maintenance of a patent airway is critical in patients with increased ICP and is a primary nursing responsibility. As the LOC decreases, the patient is at increased risk of airway obstruction.

- Be alert to altered breathing patterns. Snoring sounds indicate obstruction and require immediate intervention. An oral airway facilitates breathing and provides an easier suctioning route in the comatose patient.
- In general, any patient with a Glasgow Coma Scale score of 8 or less (see Glasgow Coma scale, p. 766) or an altered LOC who is unable to maintain a patent airway or effective ventilation needs intubation and mechanical ventilation.
- Prevent hypoxia and hypercapnia. Proper positioning of the head is important.
- Elevation of the head of the bed by 30 degrees enhances respiratory exchange and aids in decreasing cerebral edema.
- Suctioning and coughing can cause transient increases in ICP and decreases in PaO_2. Suctioning should be kept to a minimum.
- Try to prevent abdominal distention, as it can interfere with respiratory function. Insertion of a nasogastric tube to aspirate the stomach contents can prevent distention, vomiting, and possible aspiration. In patients with facial and skull fractures, a nasogastric tube is contraindicated, and oral insertion of a gastric tube is preferred.
- ABGs should be measured and evaluated regularly. The appropriate ventilatory support can be ordered on the basis of the PaO_2 and $PaCO_2$ values.

Fluid and Electrolyte Balance. Fluid and electrolyte disturbances can have an adverse effect on ICP. Closely monitor IV fluids. Intake and output, with insensible losses and daily weights taken into account, are important parameters in the assessment of fluid balance.

- Electrolyte determinations should be made daily. It is especially important to monitor serum glucose, sodium, potassium, magnesium, and osmolality. Monitor urinary output for problems related to syndrome of inappropriate antidiuretic hormone (SIADH) and diabetes insipidus (DI) (see Diabetes Insipidus, p. 173).

Monitoring Intracranial Pressure. ICP monitoring is used in combination with other physiologic parameters to guide the care of the patient and assess the patient's response to routine care. Valsalva maneuver, coughing, sneezing, hypoxemia, and arousal from sleep are factors that can increase ICP. Methods of monitoring ICP are discussed in detail in Chapter 57, Lewis et al, *Medical-Surgical Nursing,* ed 9. Also see Intracranial Pressure Monitoring, p. 770.

Body Position. Maintain the patient with increased ICP in the head-up position. Take care to prevent extreme neck flexion, which can cause venous obstruction and contribute to elevated ICP. Adjust the body position to decrease the ICP maximally and to improve cerebral perfusion pressure (CPP).

- Take care to turn the patient with slow, gentle movements because rapid changes in position may increase ICP. Prevent discomfort in turning and positioning the patient because pain or agitation also increases pressure. Increased intrathoracic pressure contributes to increased ICP by impeding venous return. Thus coughing, straining, and the Valsalva maneuver should be avoided. Avoid extreme hip flexion to decrease the risk of raising the intraabdominal pressure, which increases ICP.

Protection From Injury. The patient with increased ICP and a decreased LOC needs protection from self-injury. Confusion, agitation, and the possibility of seizures increase the risk of injury. Use restraints judiciously in the agitated patient. The patient can benefit from a quiet, nonstimulating environment. Touch and talk to the patient, even one who is in a coma.

Psychologic Considerations. Anxiety over the diagnosis and prognosis for the patient with neurologic problems can be distressing to the patient, caregiver, family, and nursing staff. Short, simple explanations are appropriate and allow the patient and family to acquire the amount of information they desire. There is a need for support, information, and education of both patients and families.

Assess the family members' desire and need to assist in providing care for the patient and allow for their participation as appropriate.

INFLAMMATORY BOWEL DISEASE

Description

Inflammatory bowel disease (IBD) is a chronic inflammation of the GI tract. It is characterized by periods of remission interspersed with periods of exacerbation. The cause is unknown, and there is no cure. IBD is classified as either Crohn's disease or ulcerative colitis based on clinical manifestations (Table 53). Ulcerative colitis is usually limited to the colon. Crohn's disease can involve any segment of the GI tract from the mouth to the anus.

Both ulcerative colitis and Crohn's disease commonly occur during the teenage years and early adulthood, and both have a second peak in the sixth decade. IBD is more prevalent in industrialized countries and in the Ashkenazi Jewish population. Many people with IBD have a family member with the disorder.

Pathophysiology

IBD is an autoimmune disease involving an immune reaction to a person's own intestinal tract. Some agent or a combination of agents triggers an overactive, inappropriate, sustained immune response. The resulting inflammation causes widespread tissue destruction.

Evidence suggests that IBD is caused by a combination of factors, including environmental factors, genetic predisposition, and alterations in the function of the immune system. The pattern of inflammation differs between Crohn's disease and ulcerative colitis.

Crohn's Disease

The inflammation in *Crohn's disease* involves all layers of the bowel wall and can occur anywhere in the GI tract from the mouth to the anus. It most commonly occurs in the terminal ileum and colon. Segments of normal bowel can occur between diseased portions, the so-called *skip lesions*.

- Typically, ulcerations are deep and longitudinal and penetrate between islands of inflamed edematous mucosa, causing the classic cobblestone appearance.
- Strictures at the areas of inflammation may cause bowel obstruction.
- Because the inflammation goes through the entire wall, microscopic leaks can allow bowel contents to enter the peritoneal cavity and form abscesses or produce peritonitis.
- Fistulas can develop between adjacent areas of bowel, between the bowel and bladder, and between the bowel and vagina.

Table 53	Comparison of Ulcerative Colitis and Crohn's Disease	
Characteristic	**Ulcerative Colitis**	**Crohn's Disease**
Clinical		
Usual age at onset	Teens to mid-30s*	Teens to mid-30s*
Diarrhea	Common	Common
Abdominal cramping pain	Common	Common
Fever (intermittent)	During acute attacks	Common
Weight loss	Rare	Common, may be severe
Rectal bleeding	Common	Infrequent
Tenesmus	Common	Rare
Malabsorption and nutritional deficiencies	Minimal incidence	Common
Pathologic		
Location	Usually starts in rectum and spreads in a continuous pattern up the colon	Occurs anywhere along GI tract in characteristic skip lesions; most frequent site is terminal ileum
Distribution	Continuous areas of inflammation	Healthy tissue interspersed with areas of inflammation (skip lesions)
Depth of involvement	Mucosa and submucosa	Entire thickness of bowel wall (transmural)
Granulomas (noted on biopsy)	Occasional	Common
Cobblestoning of mucosa	Rare	Common
Pseudopolyps	Common	Rare
Small bowel involvement	Minimal	Common

Continued

Table 53	Comparison of Ulcerative Colitis and Crohn's Disease—cont'd	
Characteristic	**Ulcerative Colitis**	**Crohn's Disease**
Complications		
Fistulas	Rare	Common
Strictures	Occasional	Common
Anal abscesses	Rare	Common
Perforation	Common (because of toxic megacolon)	Common (because inflammation involves entire bowel wall)
Toxic megacolon	Relatively more common	Rare
Carcinoma	Increased incidence of colorectal cancer after 10 yr of disease	Increased incidence of small intestinal cancer Increased incidence of colorectal cancer but not as much as with ulcerative colitis
Recurrence after surgery	Cure with colectomy	Common at site of anastomosis

*Second peak in incidence after age 60.

Ulcerative Colitis

Ulcerative colitis usually starts in the rectum and moves in a continual fashion toward the cecum. Although mild inflammation sometimes occurs in the terminal ileum, ulcerative colitis is a disease of the colon and rectum.

- Inflammation and ulcerations occur in the mucosal layer, the innermost layer of the bowel wall. Because inflammation does not extend through all the bowel layers, fistulas and abscesses are rare.
- Areas of inflamed mucosa form pseudopolyps, tonguelike projections into the bowel lumen.

Clinical Manifestations

Symptoms are often the same (diarrhea, bloody stools, weight loss, abdominal pain, fever, and fatigue) in both conditions. Bloody stools are more common with ulcerative colitis, and weight loss is more common in Crohn's disease because inflammation of the small intestine impairs nutrient absorption. Both forms of IBD are chronic disorders with mild to severe acute exacerbations that occur at unpredictable intervals over many years.

Crohn's Disease

Diarrhea and colicky abdominal pain are common symptoms of Crohn's disease.

- If the small intestine is involved, weight loss occurs from malabsorption.
- Rectal bleeding sometimes occurs with Crohn's disease, although not as often as with ulcerative colitis.

Ulcerative Colitis

The primary symptoms of ulcerative colitis are bloody diarrhea and abdominal pain. Pain may vary from the mild, lower abdominal cramping associated with diarrhea to the severe, constant abdominal pain associated with acute perforations.

- With *mild disease,* diarrhea may consist of one or two semi-formed stools daily that contain small amounts of blood. The patient may have no other manifestations.
- In *moderate disease,* there is increased stool output (up to 10 stools/day), increased bleeding, and systemic symptoms (fever, malaise, mild anemia, anorexia).
- In *severe disease,* diarrhea is bloody, contains mucus, and occurs 10 to 20 times a day. In addition, fever, weight loss (more than 10% of total body weight), anemia, tachycardia, and dehydration are present.

Complications

Patients with IBD experience both local (confined to the GI tract) and systemic complications.

- GI tract complications include hemorrhage, strictures, perforation, fistulas, and colonic dilation (toxic megacolon).
- Toxic megacolon is more common with ulcerative colitis, whereas abscesses and perianal fistulas occur more often with Crohn's disease.
- Hemorrhage may lead to anemia and is corrected with blood transfusions and iron supplements.
- People with a history of IBD are at high risk for colorectal cancer, whereas those with Crohn's disease are at increased risk for small intestine cancer.

Some people with IBD suffer from systemic complications, including joint, eye, mouth, kidney, bone, vascular, and skin problems. Circulating factors such as cytokines trigger inflammation in these areas. Routine liver function tests are important because primary sclerosing cholangitis, a complication of IBD, can lead to liver failure.

Diagnostic Studies

Diagnosis of IBD includes ruling out other diseases with similar symptoms and then determining whether the patient has Crohn's disease or ulcerative colitis.

- Laboratory studies may indicate electrolyte disturbances, anemia, leukocytosis, hypoalbuminemia, and an elevated erythrocyte sedimentation rate.
- Stool is examined for blood, pus, and mucus and cultured to rule out infectious diarrhea.
- Double-contrast barium enema, small bowel series, transabdominal ultrasound, CT, and MRI are useful for IBD diagnosis.
- Colonoscopy allows for examination of the entire large intestine.

Collaborative Care

The goals of treatment are to rest the bowel, control inflammation, combat infection, correct malnutrition, alleviate any stress, provide symptomatic relief, and improve quality of life.

A variety of drugs are available to treat IBD. Hospitalization is indicated if the patient does not respond to drug therapy, if the disease is severe, or if complications are suspected.

Drug Therapy

Drugs are used to induce and maintain a remission of IBD. Drugs are chosen based on the location and severity of inflammation. Five major classes of medications used to treat IBD are aminosalicylates, antimicrobials, corticosteroids, immunosuppressants, and biologic and targeted therapy (Table 54).

- *Aminosalicylates* are combination drugs that contain 5-aminosalicylic acid (5-ASA) and an agent that delivers 5-ASA to the colon when it is taken orally. 5-ASA suppresses proinflammatory cytokines and other inflammatory mediators. Sulfasalazine (Azulfidine) contains sulfapyridine, which helps 5-ASA reach the colon. Because many people cannot tolerate sulfapyridine, preparations such as olsalazine (Dipentum), mesalamine (Pentasa), and balsalazide (Colazal) deliver 5-ASA to the terminal ileum and the colon. These drugs are as effective as sulfasalazine and better tolerated when administered orally. *Aminosalicylates* are first-line therapies for mild to moderate Crohn's disease, especially when the colon is involved, but are more effective for ulcerative colitis.
- *Antimicrobials* (e.g., ciprofloxacin [Cipro]), are used to treat IBD, although no specific infectious agent has been identified.
- *Corticosteroids* such as prednisolone and budesonide (Entocort) are used to achieve remission in IBD. Corticosteroids are given for the shortest possible time because of side effects associated with

Table 54

Drug Therapy
Inflammatory Bowel Disease

Class	Action	Examples
5-Aminosalicylates (5-ASA)	Decrease GI inflammation through direct contact with bowel mucosa	*Systemic:* sulfasalazine (Azulfidine), mesalamine (Asacol, Pentasa), olsalazine (Dipentum), balsalazide (Colazal) *Topical:* 5-ASA enema (Rowasa), mesalamine suppositories (Canasa)
Antimicrobials	Prevent or treat secondary infection	metronidazole (Flagyl), ciprofloxacin (Cipro), clarithromycin (Biaxin)
Corticosteroids	Decrease inflammation	*Systemic:* corticosteroids (prednisone, budesonide [Entocort]) (oral); hydrocortisone or methylprednisolone (IV for severe IBD) *Topical:* hydrocortisone suppository or foam (Cortifoam) or enema (Cortenema)
Immunosuppressants	Suppress immune response	azathioprine (Imuran), 6-mercaptopurine (6-MP), methotrexate, cyclosporine
Biologic and targeted therapy (immunomodulators)	Inhibit the cytokine tumor necrosis factor (TNF) Prevent migration of leukocytes from bloodstream to inflamed tissue	infliximab (Remicade), adalimumab (Humira), certolizumab pegol (Cimzia), golimumab (Simponi) natalizumab (Tysabri)
Antidiarrheals	Decrease GI motility*	diphenoxylate with atropine (Lomotil), loperamide (Imodium)
Hematinics and vitamins	Correct iron-deficiency anemia and promote healing	oral ferrous sulfate or gluconate, iron dextran injection (Imferon), cobalamin, zinc, folate

*Used with caution during severe disease because of potential to produce toxic megacolon.
IBD, Inflammatory bowel disease.

long-term use. When the disease affects the left colon, sigmoid, and rectum, corticosteroid suppositories, enemas, and foams can be used to deliver the drug directly to inflamed tissue with minimal systemic effects. Oral prednisone is given to patients who do not respond to either 5-ASA or topical corticosteroids. IV corticosteroids are reserved for those with severe inflammation.

- *Immunosuppressants* (azathioprine [Imuran] and 6-mercaptopurine [Purinethol]) are given to maintain remission after corticosteroid induction therapy. Methotrexate has also been found to be effective for Crohn's disease.
- *Biologic and targeted drug therapy* includes anti–tumor necrosis factor (TNF) agents (infliximab [Remicade], adalimumab [Humira], certolizumab pegol [Cimzia]), and golimumab (Simponi). Natalizumab [Tysabri] inhibits leukocyte adhesion and movement into inflamed tissue.

Surgical Therapy

Many patients with Crohn's disease will eventually require surgery for complications, such as strictures, bleeding, obstructions, or fistulas.

- When segments of the intestine are removed, the remaining intestine is reanastomosed. Unfortunately, the disease often recurs at the anastomosis site.
- The main surgical treatment for Crohn's disease is strictureplasty to widen areas of narrowed bowel.

In the patient with ulcerative colitis, surgery is indicated if the patient fails to respond to conservative treatment; if exacerbations are frequent and debilitating; or if massive hemorrhage, perforation, strictures, intestinal obstruction, dysplasia, or carcinoma develops. Because ulcerative colitis affects only the colon, a total proctocolectomy is curative.

- Surgical procedures include total colectomy with rectal mucosal stripping and ileoanal reservoir, total proctocolectomy with permanent ileostomy, and total proctocolectomy with continent ileostomy.

For descriptions of these procedures, see Lewis et al, *Medical-Surgical Nursing,* ed 9, pp. 979 to 980.

Nutritional Therapy

Diet is an important component in the treatment of IBD. Consult a dietitian regarding dietary recommendations. The goals of diet management are to provide adequate nutrition without exacerbating symptoms, correct and prevent malnutrition, replace fluid and electrolyte losses, and prevent weight loss.

- Nutritional deficiencies are due to decreased oral intake, blood loss, and, depending on the location of the inflammation, malabsorption of nutrients.

- During an acute exacerbation, patients with IBD may not be able to tolerate a regular diet. Liquid enteral feedings are preferred over parenteral nutrition because atrophy of the gut and bacterial overgrowth occur when the GI tract is not used.
- There are no universal food triggers for IBD, but individuals may find that certain foods initiate diarrhea. A food diary helps to identify problem foods to avoid.

Nursing Management
Goals
The patient with IBD will experience a decrease in the number and severity of acute exacerbations, maintain normal fluid and electrolyte balance, be free from pain or discomfort, adhere to medical regimens, maintain nutritional balance, and have an improved quality of life.

Nursing Diagnoses
- Diarrhea
- Imbalanced nutrition: less than body requirements
- Ineffective coping

Nursing Interventions
During the acute phase, focus your attention on hemodynamic stability, pain control, fluid and electrolyte balance, and nutritional support. Maintain accurate intake and output records and monitor the number and appearance of stools.

- It is important that you establish rapport and encourage the patient to talk about self-care strategies. An explanation of all procedures and treatment will help to build trust and allay apprehension.
- Psychotherapy and behavioral therapies may help the patient experiencing psychologic distress in managing his or her symptoms. Assist the patient in accepting the chronicity of IBD and learning strategies to cope with its recurrent, unpredictable nature.
- Severe fatigue limits the patient's energy for physical activity. Nutritional deficiencies and anemia may leave the patient feeling weak and listless. Rest is important because patients may lose sleep because of frequent episodes of diarrhea and abdominal pain. Schedule activities around rest periods.
- Until diarrhea is controlled, help the patient stay clean, dry, and free of odor. Place a deodorizer in the room. Meticulous perianal skin care using plain water (no harsh soap) together with a skin barrier prevents skin breakdown. Dibucaine (Nupercainal), witch hazel, or other soothing compresses or prescribed ointments may reduce irritation and anal discomfort.

▼ **Patient and Caregiver Teaching**

The patient and caregiver may need help in setting realistic short- and long-term goals.

- Your teaching should include (1) the importance of rest and diet management, (2) perianal care, (3) drug action and side effects, (4) symptoms of disease recurrence, (5) when to seek medical care, and (6) use of diversional activities to reduce stress.
- Excellent teaching resources are available from the Crohn's and Colitis Foundation of America *(www.ccfa.org)*.

INTERSTITIAL CYSTITIS/PAINFUL BLADDER SYNDROME

Description

Interstitial cystitis (IC) is a chronic, painful inflammatory disease of the bladder characterized by symptoms of urgency/frequency and pain in the bladder and/or pelvis. *Painful bladder syndrome* (PBS) is suprapubic pain related to bladder filling.

- The term *IC/PBS* refers to cases of urinary pain that cannot be attributed to other causes such as infection or urinary calculi.
- The average age at onset is 40 years, and the ratio of women to men with IC/PBS is 10:1 to 12:1.

The etiology of IC/PBS remains unknown, with possible causes including neurogenic hypersensitivity of the lower urinary tract, alterations in mast cells in the muscle and/or mucosal layers of the bladder, infection with an unusual organism (e.g., slow-growing virus), or production of a toxic substance in the urine. The bladder wall may be irritated and inflamed and can become scarred.

Clinical Manifestations

Two primary clinical manifestations of IC include pain and bothersome lower urinary tract symptoms (e.g., frequency, urgency).

- The pain is usually located in the suprapubic area but may involve the vagina, labia, or entire perineal region. It varies from moderate to severe and is exacerbated by bladder filling, postponed urination, physical exertion, pressure against the suprapubic area, certain foods, or emotional distress. The pain is transiently relieved by urination.
- Bothersome lower urinary tract symptoms are similar to a urinary tract infection (UTI), and the condition is frequently misdiagnosed as a recurring or chronic UTI or, in men, chronic prostatitis.
- Women report that pain occurs premenstrually and is aggravated by sexual intercourse or emotional stress. Some patients

experience symptoms that disappear altogether after a period of weeks to months, whereas others have persistent symptoms for months to years.

Diagnostic Studies

IC/PBS is a diagnosis of exclusion.

- History and physical examination are necessary to rule out other disorders that produce somewhat similar symptoms, such as UTI or endometriosis.
- Cystoscopic examination may reveal a small bladder capacity and superficial ulceration with bladder filling.

Collaborative Care

No single treatment consistently reverses or relieves symptoms. Elimination of foods and beverages that are likely to irritate the bladder may provide some relief from symptoms. Typical bladder irritants include caffeine; alcohol; citrus products; aged cheeses; nuts; foods containing vinegar or hot peppers; and foods or beverages, including fruits (cranberries), likely to lower urinary pH.

- Advise patients that an over-the-counter (OTC) dietary supplement, calcium glycerophosphate (Prelief), alkalinizes the urine and can provide relief from the irritating effects of certain foods.
- Because stress can exacerbate IC/PBS, relaxation techniques (e.g., sitz baths, application of heat or cold to perineum or bladder, relaxation breathing, imagery) may be helpful.
- Using lubrication or altering positions may decrease pain associated with sexual intercourse.

Two tricyclic antidepressants, amitriptyline (Elavil) and nortriptyline (Aventyl), are used to reduce the burning pain and urinary frequency. In IC, pentosan (Elmiron) is used to enhance the protective effects of the glycosaminoglycan layer of the bladder. These drugs are used to provide relief over weeks to months, but they do not provide the immediate relief that may be needed with an acute exacerbation of symptoms. In this case, a short course of opioid analgesics may be given.

Several agents may be instilled directly into the bladder through a small catheter.

- Dimethyl sulfoxide (DMSO) acts by desensitizing pain receptors in the bladder wall.
- Heparin and hyaluronic acid also may be instilled into the bladder to enhance the protective properties of the glycosaminoglycan layer of the bladder and relieve symptoms.

Several surgical procedures, such as urinary diversion, can be used in an attempt to relieve severe, debilitating pain.

Nursing Management

Assess characteristics of the pain associated with IC/PBS. Ask the patient about specific dietary or lifestyle factors that exacerbate or alleviate pain. Instruct the patient to keep a bladder log or voiding diary over a period of at least 3 days to determine voiding frequency and patterns of nocturia.

Instruct the patient to maintain good nutrition, particularly in light of the dietary restrictions often necessary to control IC-related pain.

- Advise the patient to take a multivitamin containing no more than the recommended dietary allowance for essential vitamins and to avoid high-potency vitamins because they may irritate the bladder.
- Advise the patient to avoid clothing that creates suprapubic pressure, including pants with tight belts or restrictive waistlines.
- Written educational materials concerning diet, ways to cope with the need for frequent urination, and strategies for coping with the emotional burden of IC/PBS are available from the Interstitial Cystitis Association *(www.ichelp.com)*.

INTERVERTEBRAL DISC DISEASE

Description

Intervertebral disc disease is a condition that involves the deterioration, herniation, or other dysfunction of the intervertebral discs. Disc disorders can involve the cervical, thoracic, and lumbar spine.

Pathophysiology

Intervertebral discs separate the vertebrae of the spinal column and provide shock absorption for the spine. Structural degeneration of discs is often caused by *degenerative disc disease* (DDD) (Fig. 10). This progressive degeneration is a normal process of aging and results in the intervertebral discs losing their elasticity, flexibility, and shock-absorbing capabilities.

Thinning of the discs occurs as the *nucleus pulposus* (gelatinous center of the disc) starts to dry out and shrink. These changes limit the ability of the discs to distribute pressure loads between the vertebrae, which can cause progressive, structural deterioration.

- When there is structural damage to the disc, the nucleus pulposus may seep through a torn or stretched annulus. This is called a *herniated disc* (slipped disc), a condition in which a spinal disc herniates and bulges outward between the vertebrae.

A *herniated disc* can be the result of natural degeneration with age or repeated stress and trauma to the spine. The nucleus pulposus

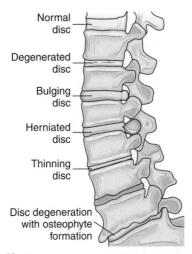

Normal disc

Degenerated disc

Bulging disc

Herniated disc

Thinning disc

Disc degeneration with osteophyte formation

Fig. 10. Common causes of degenerative disc damage.

may first bulge and then it can herniate, placing pressure on nearby nerves. The most common sites of rupture are the lumbosacral discs, specifically L4-5 and L5-S1.

- Disc herniation may be the result of spinal stenosis, in which narrowing of the spinal canal creates a bulging of the intervertebral disc.

Clinical Manifestations

Lumbar Disc Disease

The most common manifestation is low back pain. Radicular pain that radiates down the buttock and below the knee along the distribution of the sciatic nerve generally indicates disc herniation. The straight-leg raise test may be positive indicating nerve root irritation. Back or leg pain may be reproduced by raising the leg and flexing the foot at 90 degrees.

- Reflexes may be depressed or absent, depending on the spinal nerve root involved. Paresthesia or muscle weakness in the legs, feet, or toes may occur.
- Multiple nerve root (cauda equina) compression may be manifested as bowel or bladder incontinence or impotence. This condition is a medical emergency.

Cervical Disc Disease

Pain often radiates into the arms and hands, following the pattern of the nerve involved. Similar to lumbar disc disease, reflexes may or may not be present, and there is often weakness of the handgrip.

Diagnostic Studies

- X-rays are done to detect any structural defects.
- A myelogram, MRI, or CT scan is helpful in localizing the damaged site.
- An epidural venogram or diskogram may be necessary if other methods of diagnosis are unsuccessful.
- An electromyogram (EMG) of the extremities can be performed to determine the severity of nerve irritation or to rule out other pathologic conditions such as peripheral neuropathy.

Collaborative Care

Conservative Therapy

The patient with suspected disc damage is usually managed first with conservative therapy. This includes limitation of extremes of spinal movement (brace/corset/belt), local heat or ice, ultrasound and massage, traction, and transcutaneous electrical nerve stimulation (TENS). Drug therapy includes nonsteroidal antiinflammatory drugs (NSAIDs), short-term opioids, antidepressants, and muscle relaxants. Epidural corticosteroid injections may be effective in reducing inflammation and relieving acute pain.

- Once symptoms subside, back-strengthening exercises are begun twice per day and are encouraged for a lifetime. Teach the patient the principles of good body mechanics. Extremes of flexion and torsion are strongly discouraged.
- Most patients heal with a conservative treatment plan after 6 months.

Surgical Therapy

Surgery for a damaged disc is generally indicated when diagnostic tests indicate that the problem is not responding to conservative treatment and the patient is in consistent pain and/or has a persistent neurologic deficit.

- An *intradiscal electrothermoplasty* (IDET) is a minimally invasive outpatient procedure that may help in treating back and sciatica pain. It involves the insertion of a needle into the affected disc with the guidance of an x-ray. The wire is heated, which denervates the small nerve fibers that have grown into the cracks and invaded the degenerating disc.
- A similar outpatient technique is *radiofrequency discal nucleoplasty,* in which a special radiofrequency probe is inserted into the disc and generates energy that breaks up the molecular bonds of the gel in the nucleus.
- A third procedure is the use of an *interspinous process decompression system* (X Stop). This device is made of titanium and fits onto a mount that is placed on vertebrae in the lower

back. The device works by lifting the vertebrae off the pinched nerve. The X Stop is used in patients with pain due to lumbar spinal stenosis.

- A *diskectomy* is another common type of surgical procedure that may be performed to decompress the nerve root. Microsurgical diskectomy is a version of the standard diskectomy in which the surgeon uses a microscope to allow better visualization of the disc to aid in the removal of the damaged portion.

- A *percutaneous laser diskectomy* is an outpatient surgical procedure that is done by using fluoroscopy and passing a tube through retroperitoneal soft tissues to the lateral border of the disc. A laser is then used on the damaged portion of the disc.

- A traditional and common procedure for lumbar disc disease is a *laminectomy*. It involves the surgical excision of part of the posterior arch of the vertebra (referred to as the lamina) to gain access to part or all of the protruding disc to remove it. A minimal hospital stay is usually required.

- A *spinal fusion* may be performed if the spine is unstable. The spine is stabilized by creating an ankylosis (fusion) of contiguous vertebrae with a bone graft from the patient's fibula or iliac crest or from donated cadaver bone. Metal fixation with rods, plates, or screws may be implanted. A posterior lumbar interbody fusion may be performed to provide extra support for bone grafting or a prosthetic device. Bone morphogenetic protein (BMP), a genetically engineered protein, may be used to stimulate bone growth of the graft in spinal fusions.

- Artificial disc replacement surgery for patients with DDD includes the use of the Charité disc for lower disc damage and the Prestige cervical disc system.

Nursing Management: Vertebral Disc Surgery

Following vertebral disc surgery, postoperative nursing interventions mainly focus on maintaining proper alignment of the spine until healing has occurred. Depending on the type and extent of surgery and the surgeon's preference, the patient may be able to dangle the legs at the side of the bed, stand, or even ambulate the same day of surgery.

When a patient has had a lumbar fusion, place pillows under the thighs of each leg when supine and between the legs when in the side-lying position to provide comfort and ensure alignment.

- The patient often fears turning or any movement that increases pain. Offer reassurance to the patient that the proper technique is being used to maintain body alignment.

- Postoperatively, most patients will require opioids, such as morphine, IV for 24 to 48 hours. Patient-controlled analgesia (PCA) allows for optimal analgesic levels and is the preferred method of continued pain management during this time.
- Once fluids are being taken, the patient may be switched to oral drugs such as acetaminophen with codeine, hydrocodone (Vicodin), or oxycodone (Percocet). Diazepam (Valium) may be prescribed for muscle relaxation.

Because the spinal canal may be entered during the surgical procedure, there is potential for cerebrospinal fluid (CSF) leakage. Immediately report a severe headache or leakage of CSF on the dressing.

- Frequently monitor the peripheral neurologic signs of the patient after spinal surgery. Movement of arms and legs and assessment of sensation should be unchanged when compared with preoperative status. Paresthesias, such as numbness and tingling, may not be relieved immediately after surgery. Document any new muscle weakness or paresthesias and report them to the surgeon.

Paralytic ileus and interference with bowel function may occur for several days and may manifest as nausea, abdominal distention, and constipation. Assess whether the patient is passing flatus, has bowel sounds in all quadrants, and has a flat, soft abdomen. Stool softeners (e.g., docusate sodium [Colace]) may aid in relieving and preventing constipation.

- Adequate bladder emptying may be altered because of activity restrictions, opioids, or anesthesia. Patients should use the commode or ambulate to the bathroom when allowed to promote adequate emptying of the bladder. Intermittent catheterization or an indwelling catheter may be necessary for patients who have difficulty urinating.

Additional nursing responsibilities are required if the patient has also had a spinal fusion. Because a bone graft is usually involved, the postoperative healing time is prolonged compared with that for a laminectomy. Limited activity over an extended time may be necessary. A rigid orthosis (thoracic-lumbar-sacral orthosis or chair-back brace) is often used during this period.

If surgery is done on the cervical spine, be alert for symptoms of spinal cord edema such as respiratory distress and a worsening neurologic status of the upper extremities. After surgery, the patient's neck may be immobilized in either a soft or hard cervical collar.

In addition to the primary surgical site, regularly assess the donor site for the bone graft. The donor site usually causes greater postoperative pain than the fused area. A pressure dressing is applied to the donor site to prevent excessive bleeding. If the donor site is the fibula, neurovascular extremity assessments are a postoperative nursing responsibility.

- Instruct the patient to avoid sitting or standing for prolonged periods. Encourage activities that include walking, lying down, and shifting weight from one foot to the other when standing.
- The patient should learn to think through an activity before starting any potentially injurious task, such as bending or stooping. Any twisting movement of the spine is contraindicated. The thighs and knees, rather than the back, should be used to absorb the shock of activity and movement.
- A firm mattress or bed board is essential.

INTESTINAL OBSTRUCTION

Description

Intestinal obstruction occurs when intestinal contents cannot pass through the GI tract. The obstruction may occur in the small intestine or colon and can be partial or complete, simple or strangulated.

A partial obstruction usually resolves with conservative treatment, whereas a complete obstruction usually requires surgery. A simple obstruction has an intact blood supply, and a strangulated one does not.

Causes of intestinal obstruction can be classified as mechanical or nonmechanical.

- *Mechanical obstruction* is a detectable occlusion of the intestinal lumen that mainly occurs in the small intestine. Surgical adhesion is the most common cause of small bowel obstructions and can occur within days of surgery or several years later. Other causes of intestinal obstruction are hernia, strictures from Crohn's disease, and intussusception following bariatric abdominal surgery. The most common cause of colon obstruction is cancer, followed by diverticular disease.
- *Nonmechanical obstruction* may result from a neuromuscular or vascular disorder. *Paralytic (adynamic) ileus* (lack of intestinal peristalsis and bowel sounds) is the most common form of nonmechanical obstruction. It occurs to some degree after any abdominal surgery. Other causes of paralytic ileus include inflammatory reactions (e.g., acute pancreatitis, acute appendicitis), electrolyte abnormalities (especially hypokalemia), and thoracic or lumbar spinal fractures. Vascular obstructions are rare and are caused by an interference with the blood supply to a portion of the bowel. The most common causes are emboli and atherosclerosis of the mesenteric arteries.

Pathophysiology

When fluid, gas, and intestinal contents accumulate proximal to the obstruction, distention occurs, and the distal bowel collapses. As the proximal bowel becomes increasingly distended, the intraluminal bowel pressure rises. The increased pressure leads to an increase in capillary permeability and extravasation of fluids and electrolytes into the peritoneal cavity. Retention of fluid in the intestine and peritoneal cavity leads to a severe reduction in circulating blood volume and results in hypotension and hypovolemic shock.

- In the most dangerous situation, the bowel becomes so distended that the blood flow is arrested, causing edema, cyanosis, and gangrene of bowel segment. This is called intestinal strangulation. If it is not corrected quickly, the bowel will become necrotic and rupture, leading to infection, septic shock, and death.
- Location of the obstruction determines the extent of fluid, electrolyte, and acid-base imbalances. With a high obstruction (e.g., upper duodenum), metabolic alkalosis may result from the loss of gastric HCl acid through vomiting or nasogastric (NG) intubation and suction. When the obstruction is in the small intestine, dehydration occurs rapidly. If the obstruction is below the proximal colon, solid fecal material accumulates until symptoms of discomfort appear.

Clinical Manifestations

- Manifestations vary, depending on the location of the obstruction. The most important early manifestations of a small bowel obstruction are colicky abdominal pain, nausea, vomiting, and abdominal distention. Constipation and decreased flatus occur later.
- Patients with obstructions in the proximal small intestine rapidly develop nausea and vomiting, which is sometimes projectile and contains bile. Vomiting from more distal obstructions of the small intestine is more gradual in onset. Foul-smelling vomitus that looks like stool indicates a long-standing obstruction requiring immediate surgery. Signs of colonic obstruction include abdominal distention, constipation (new onset), and lack of flatus.
- Vomiting usually relieves abdominal pain in higher intestinal obstructions. Persistent, colicky abdominal pain is seen with lower intestinal obstruction. With mechanical obstruction, pain comes and goes in waves. In contrast, paralytic ileus produces a more constant, generalized discomfort. Strangulation causes severe, constant pain that is rapid in onset.

- Abdominal distention is usually absent or minimally noticeable in proximal small intestine obstructions and markedly increased in lower intestinal obstructions. Abdominal tenderness and rigidity are usually absent unless strangulation or peritonitis has occurred.
- Auscultation of bowel sounds reveals high-pitched sounds above the area of obstruction. Bowel sounds may also be absent. *Borborygmi* (audible abdominal sounds caused by hyperactive intestinal motility) are often noted by the patient. The patient's temperature rarely rises above 100° F (37.8° C) unless strangulation or peritonitis has occurred.

Diagnostic Studies
- CT scans and abdominal x-rays are used.
- Sigmoidoscopy or colonoscopy may provide direct visualization of an obstruction in the colon.
- An elevated WBC count may indicate strangulation or perforation.
- Elevated hematocrit (Hct) values may reflect hemoconcentration.
- Decreased hemoglobin (Hgb) and Hct values may indicate bleeding from a neoplasm or strangulation with necrosis.
- Serum electrolytes, blood urea nitrogen (BUN), and creatinine are monitored frequently to assess the degree of dehydration.

Collaborative Care
Emergency surgery is indicated if the bowel is strangulated, but many obstructions resolve with conservative treatment. Initial treatment of bowel obstruction caused by adhesions includes placing the patient on NPO status, inserting an NG tube, IV fluid therapy, adding potassium to IV fluids after verifying renal function, and analgesics for pain control.

- The treatment goal for the patient with a malignant bowel obstruction is to regain patency and resolve the obstruction. Stents can be placed via endoscopic or fluoroscopic procedures for palliative purposes or until surgery can be performed.
- If the obstruction does not improve within 24 hours or if the patient's condition deteriorates, surgery is performed to relieve the obstruction.
- Surgery may involve simply resecting the obstructed segment of bowel and anastomosing the remaining healthy bowel back together. Partial or total colectomy, colostomy, or ileostomy may be required when extensive obstruction or necrosis is present.
- Occasionally obstructions can be removed nonsurgically. A colonoscope can be used to remove polyps, dilate strictures, and remove and destroy tumors with a laser.

Nursing Management

Goals

The patient with an intestinal obstruction will have relief from the obstruction and a return to normal bowel function, minimal to no discomfort, and normal fluid and electrolyte and acid-base status.

Nursing Diagnoses

- Acute pain
- Deficient fluid volume

Nursing Interventions

If the surgeon decides to wait and see if the obstruction resolves on its own, assess the patient regularly and notify the surgeon of changes in vital signs, changes in bowel sounds, decreased urine output, increased abdominal distention, and pain.

- Maintain a strict intake and output record including emesis and tube drainage.
- Monitor the patient closely for signs of dehydration and electrolyte imbalances. A patient with a high intestinal obstruction is more likely to have metabolic alkalosis. A patient with a low obstruction is at greater risk for metabolic acidosis.
- The patient is often restless and constantly changes position to relieve the pain. Provide comfort measures and promote a restful environment.
- Nursing care of the patient after surgery for an intestinal obstruction is similar to the care of the patient after a laparotomy (see Abdominal Pain, Acute, pp. 4 to 5).

IRRITABLE BOWEL SYNDROME

Description

Irritable bowel syndrome (IBS) is a chronic functional disorder of the colon with an unknown cause. Symptoms of IBS, including abdominal pain or discomfort and alterations in bowel patterns, are intermittent and may occur for years. IBS is more frequently diagnosed in women than in men.

Patients often report a history of GI infections and food intolerances. However, the role of food allergies in IBS is unclear.

- Psychologic stressors (e.g., depression, anxiety, sexual abuse, posttraumatic stress disorder) are associated with the development and exacerbation of IBS.
- In addition to abdominal pain and diarrhea or constipation, patients commonly experience abdominal distention, excessive flatulence, bloating, urgency, and sensation of incomplete

evacuation. Non-GI symptoms may include fatigue and sleep disturbances.

There are no specific physical findings with IBS. The key to accurate diagnosis is a thorough history and physical examination. Diagnostic tests are selectively used to rule out other disorders including colorectal cancer, inflammatory bowel disease, endometriosis, and malabsorption disorders (e.g., celiac disease).

Symptom-based criteria for IBS are referred to as the Rome criteria, which include the following: abdominal discomfort or pain for at least 3 months, with onset at least 6 months before that and has at least two of the following characteristics: (1) relieved with defecation; (2) onset associated with a change in stool frequency; and (3) onset associated with a change in stool appearance.

Treatment is directed at psychologic and dietary factors and drugs to regulate stool output. Patients are more likely to improve with treatment if they have a trusting relationship with their health care provider. Encourage the patient to verbalize concerns.

- Because treatment is often focused on symptoms, patients may benefit from keeping a diary of symptoms, diet, and episodes of stress to help identify factors that seem to trigger the IBS symptoms.
- If tolerated, encourage the patient to increase dietary intake of fiber to at least 20 g/day or use a bulking agent such as Metamucil. Increases in dietary fiber should be instituted gradually to avoid bloating and abdominal discomfort from gas.
- Advise the patient whose primary symptoms are abdominal distention and flatulence to avoid common gas-producing foods such as broccoli or cabbage. Yogurt may be better tolerated than milk products. Probiotics may be used because alterations in intestinal bacteria are believed to exacerbate the condition.

Loperamide (Imodium), a synthetic opioid that slows intestinal transit, may be used to treat diarrhea when it occurs. Alosetron (Lotronex), a serotonergic antagonist, is used for IBS patients with severe symptoms of pain and diarrhea. Lubiprostone (Amitiza) is approved for the treatment of women with IBS-constipation. Linaclotide (Linzess) is approved for the treatment of IBS with constipation in men and women.

Psychologic therapies include cognitive-behavioral therapy, stress management techniques, acupuncture, and hypnosis. Low doses of tricyclic antidepressants seem to provide benefit, possibly because they decrease peripheral nerve sensitivity. No single therapy has been found to be effective for all patients with IBS.

KIDNEY CANCER

Kidney cancer arises from the cortex or pelvis (and calyces). Adenocarcinoma (renal cell carcinoma) is the most common type and is twice as frequent in men as in women. It is typically discovered when the person is 50 to 70 years old. The most significant risk factor is cigarette smoking. Other risk factors include family history (first-degree relatives), obesity, hypertension, and exposure to cadmium, asbestos, and gasoline.

Kidney cancer has no characteristic early symptoms; thus many patients go undiagnosed until the disease has significantly progressed. The most common manifestations are hematuria, flank pain, and a palpable mass in the flank or abdomen. Other symptoms include weight loss, fever, hypertension, and anemia. Local extension of kidney cancer into the renal vein and vena cava is common. The most common sites of metastases include lungs, liver, and long bones.

- Diagnosis is based on CT scan and ultrasound, which differentiates between a solid mass tumor and a cyst. Angiography, biopsy, and MRI are also used in diagnosis. Radionuclide isotope scanning is used to detect metastases.

Nursing and Collaborative Management

Preventive measures, such as quitting smoking, maintaining a healthy weight, controlling BP, and reducing or avoiding exposure to toxins, can help reduce the incidence of kidney cancer. Patients in high-risk groups should be aware of their increased risk for kidney cancer. Teach them about early symptoms (e.g., hematuria, hypertension).

- Partial nephrectomy (for smaller tumors) or a radical nephrectomy (for larger tumors) is the treatment for some renal cancers. Radical nephrectomy involves removal of the kidney, adrenal gland, surrounding fascia, part of the ureter, and draining lymph nodes. Nephrectomy can be performed by a conventional (open) approach or laparoscopically.
- Radiation therapy is used palliatively in inoperable cases and when there is metastasis to bone or lungs.
- Chemotherapy is used for metastatic disease, including 5-fluorouracil (5-FU), floxuridine (FUDR), and gemcitabine (Gemzar). However, renal cell carcinoma is refractory to most chemotherapy drugs.
- Biologic therapy, including α-interferon and interleukin-2 (IL-2), is another treatment in metastatic disease.
- Targeted therapy is the preferred treatment for metastatic kidney cancer. Kinase inhibitors, which block certain proteins

(kinases) that play a role in tumor growth and cancer progression, include sunitinib (Sutent), sorafenib (Nexavar), and axitinib (Inlyta). Bevacizumab (Avastin) and pazopanib (Votrient) inhibit the formation of new blood vessel growth to the tumor. Temsirolimus (Torisel) and everolimus (Afinitor) inhibit a specific protein known as the mammalian target of rapamycin (mTOR).

KIDNEY DISEASE, CHRONIC

Description

Chronic kidney disease (CKD) involves progressive, irreversible loss of kidney function. CKD can be defined as either the presence of kidney damage or a decreased glomerular filtration rate (GFR), less than 60 mL/min/1.73 m^2, for more than 3 months. The classification of CKD is presented in Table 55. The last stage of kidney failure *(end-stage kidney [renal] disease [ESKD])* occurs when the GFR is less than 15 mL/min. At this point, renal replacement therapy (dialysis or transplantation) is required.

Although CKD has many causes, the leading causes of CKD are diabetes mellitus (about 50%) and hypertension (about 25%). One of every nine Americans has CKD. Over half a million Americans are receiving treatment (dialysis, transplant).

Because the kidneys are highly adaptive, kidney disease is often not recognized until there is considerable nephron loss. CKD is often underdiagnosed and undertreated because patients are often asymptomatic. It has been estimated that about 70% of people with CKD are unaware that they have the disease.

Prognosis and course of CKD are highly variable depending on the etiology, patient's condition and age, and adequacy of health care. Some individuals live normal, active lives with compensated renal failure, whereas others may rapidly progress to ESKD.

Clinical Manifestations

As kidney function deteriorates, every body system becomes affected. Manifestations are a result of retained substances including urea, creatinine, phenols, hormones, water, and electrolytes. *Uremia* is a syndrome in which kidney function declines to the point that symptoms develop in multiple body systems. It often occurs when the GFR is less than 10 mL/min (see Fig. 47-2 in Lewis et al., *Medical-Surgical Nursing,* ed. 9, p. 1109). Manifestations of uremia vary among patients according to the etiology of kidney disease, comorbid conditions, age, and degree of adherence to the prescribed medical regimen.

K

Table 55	Stages of Chronic Kidney Disease

Description	GFR (mL/min/1.73 m^2)	Clinical Action Plan
Stage 1 Kidney damage with normal or ↑ GFR	≥90	Diagnosis and treatment CVD risk reduction Slow progression
Stage 2 Kidney damage with mild ↓ GFR	60-89	Estimation of progression
Stage 3 Moderate ↓ GFR	30-59	Evaluation and treatment of complications
Stage 4 Severe ↓ GFR	15-29	Preparation for renal replacement therapy (dialysis, kidney transplant)
Stage 5 Kidney failure	<15 (or dialysis)	Renal replacement therapy (if uremia present and patient desires treatment)

Source: National Kidney Foundation. *www.kidney.org/kidneydisease/aboutckd.cfm.*
CVD, Cardiovascular disease; *GFR,* glomerular filtration rate.

- *Urinary system.* Because most people continue to have good urine output, it is often difficult to convince them they have kidney disease. As CKD progresses, patients have increasing difficulty with fluid retention and require diuretic therapy. After a period on dialysis, patients develop anuria.
- *Metabolic disturbances.* As GFR decreases, blood urea nitrogen (BUN) and serum creatinine levels increase. Serum creatinine and creatinine clearance determinations (calculated GFR) are considered more accurate indicators of kidney function. As BUN increases, nausea, vomiting, lethargy, fatigue, impaired thought processes, and headaches become common.

- *Electrolyte and acid-base imbalances.* Hyperkalemia results from decreased renal excretion, breakdown of cellular protein, bleeding, and metabolic acidosis. Sodium may be elevated, normal, or low in kidney failure. Sodium retention can contribute to edema, hypertension, and heart failure. Sodium intake must be individually determined but is generally restricted to 2 g/day.
- *Altered carbohydrate metabolism and elevated triglycerides.* Mild to moderate hyperglycemia and hyperinsulinemia occur. Insulin and glucose metabolism may improve (but not to normal values) after the initiation of dialysis. Patients with diabetes who develop uremia may require less insulin than before the onset of CKD. This is because insulin, which depends on the kidneys for excretion, remains in circulation longer.
- *Hematologic system.* Anemia results from a lack of erythropoietin. Bleeding tendencies occur because of a defect in platelet function. Cellular and humoral immune responses are suppressed (increased susceptibility to infection results).
- *Cardiovascular system.* The most common cause of death in patients with CKD is cardiovascular disease. Vascular calcification and arterial stiffness are major contributors to cardiovascular disease in CKD. Hypertension is highly prevalent in patients with CKD because hypertension is both a cause and a consequence of CKD. Hypertension is aggravated by sodium retention and increased extracellular fluid volume.

Additional systemic signs include pulmonary edema, constipation, peripheral neuropathy, osteomalacia, pruritus, infertility, and personality and behavior changes.

Diagnostic Studies

- Dipstick evaluation of urine is used to detect protein or micro-albuminuria.
- Urinalysis detects RBCs, WBCs, casts, and glucose.
- BUN and serum creatinine are elevated.
- GFR, obtained from 24-hour urine creatinine clearance measures, is decreased.
- Hematocrit (Hct) and hemoglobin (Hgb) levels are decreased.
- Ultrasound can be used to detect obstructions and the size of kidneys.
- Kidney biopsy provides a definitive diagnosis.

Collaborative Care

The focus in CKD is to preserve existing kidney function, reduce the risks of cardiovascular disease (CVD), prevent complications,

and provide for the patient's comfort. It is important that patients
with CKD receive appropriate follow-up and referral to a nephrol-
ogist early in the course of the disease. A focus on stages 1 through 4
(see Table 55) before the need for dialysis (stage 5) includes the
control of hypertension, hyperparathyroid disease, anemia, hyperglycemia, and dyslipidemia. The following section focuses primarily on the drug and nutritional aspects of care.

- Acute hyperkalemia may require treatment with IV glucose and
  insulin to move potassium into the cells, or IV 10% calcium
  gluconate. Sodium polystyrene sulfonate, a cation-exchange
  resin, is used to lower potassium levels in stage 4 CKD. Dialysis may be required to decrease potassium if dysrhythmias are
  present.
- Control and treatment of hypertension is discussed in Hypertension, pp. 332 to 333. It is recommended that the target BP be less
  than 130/80 mm Hg for patients with CKD and 125/75 for patients with significant proteinuria. Treatment of hypertension includes weight loss (if obese), therapeutic lifestyle changes (e.g.,
  exercise, avoidance of alcohol, smoking cessation), diet recommendations, and administration of antihypertensive drugs. Drugs
  most commonly used include diuretics, β-adrenergic blockers,
  calcium channel blockers, angiotensin-converting enzyme (ACE)
  inhibitors, and angiotensin receptor blockers.
- Phosphate binders such as calcium carbonate (e.g., Caltrate) and
  calcium acetate (e.g., PhosLo) are used to bind phosphate in the
  bowel, which is then excreted in the stool. Phosphate binders
  that do not contain calcium include sevelamer (Renagel) and
  lanthanum (Fosrenol).
- Exogenous erythropoietin (epoetin alfa [Epogen, Procrit]) is
  available to treat the anemia of CKD.

Many drugs are partially or totally excreted by the kidneys. Delayed and decreased elimination lead to an accumulation of drugs
and the potential for drug toxicity. Drugs of particular concern include digoxin, diabetic agents (metformin, glyburide), antibiotics
(e.g., vancomycin, gentamicin), and opioid medication.

Nutritional Therapy

The current diet is designed to be as normal as possible to maintain
good nutrition (see Table 47-10 for specific recommended restrictions in Lewis et al., *Medical-Surgical Nursing,* ed. 9, p. 1114). All
patients with CKD should be referred to a dietitian for nutritional
education and guidance. For CKD stages 1 to 4, many clinicians
encourage a diet with normal protein intake. However, teach patients to avoid high-protein diets and supplements as they may
overstress the diseased kidneys. For patients with malnutrition
or inadequate caloric or protein intake, commercially prepared

products that are high in protein but low in sodium and potassium are available (e.g., Nepro, Amin-Aid).

In addition to protein, nutritional therapy also includes the restriction of water, sodium, potassium, and phosphate (see Table 47-10 for specific recommended restrictions in Lewis et al., *Medical-Surgical Nursing,* ed. 9, p. 1114).

Nursing Management

Goals
The patient with chronic kidney disease will demonstrate the knowledge and ability to comply with the therapeutic regimen, participate in decision making for the plan of care and future treatment modality, demonstrate effective coping strategies, and continue with activities of daily living (ADLs) within physiologic limitations.

Nursing Diagnoses
- Excess fluid volume
- Imbalanced nutrition: less than body requirements
- Risk for electrolyte imbalance

Nursing Interventions
Identify individuals at risk for CKD. These include people who have been diagnosed with diabetes or hypertension and people with a history (or a family history) of kidney disease and repeated urinary tract infections. These individuals should have regular check-ups along with calculation of the estimated GFR and a routine urinalysis.

- Individuals at risk need to take measures to prevent or delay the progression of CKD including glycemic control for patients with diabetes; BP control; and lifestyle modifications, including smoking cessation.
- When potentially nephrotoxic drugs are prescribed, monitor the patient's renal function with serum creatinine and BUN.
- Advise patients with diabetes to report any changes in urine appearance (color, odor), frequency, or volume to the health care provider.
- Inform the patient that if dialysis is chosen, the option of transplantation still remains, and if a transplanted organ fails, the patient can return to dialysis.

Even though transplantation offers the best therapeutic management for patients with kidney failure, the critical shortage of donor organs has limited this treatment option.

It is important to respect the patient's choice to not receive treatment. Many times, patients themselves initiate the conversation about palliative care. Focus the discussion on moving from the curative approach to promotion of comfort care and consideration of hospice care. Listen to the patient and caregiver, allowing them

K

to do most of the talking, and pay special attention to their hopes and fears.

▼ **Patient and Caregiver Teaching**

Teach the patient and family about the diet, drugs, and follow-up medical care (Table 56).

- Teach the patient to take daily BPs and identify the signs and symptoms of fluid overload, hyperkalemia, and other electrolyte imbalances.
- A dietitian should meet with the patient and caregiver on a regular basis for nutritional planning. A diet history and a consideration of cultural variations will facilitate diet planning and adherence.
- The patient needs to understand the drugs, dosages, and common side effects. Because patients with CKD take many medications,

Table 56	Patient and Caregiver Teaching Guide *Chronic Kidney Disease*

Include the following information in the teaching plan for the patient and caregiver.

1. Necessary dietary (protein, sodium, potassium, phosphate) and fluid restrictions.
2. Difficulties in modifying diet and fluid intake.
3. Signs and symptoms of electrolyte imbalance, especially high potassium.
4. Alternative ways of reducing thirst, such as sucking on ice cubes, lemon, or hard candy.
5. Rationales for prescribed drugs and common side effects. Examples:
   - Phosphate binders (including calcium supplements used as phosphate barriers) should be taken with meals.
   - Calcium supplements prescribed to treat hypocalcemia directly should be taken on an empty stomach (but not at the same time as iron supplements).
   - Iron supplements should be taken between meals.
6. The importance of reporting any of the following:
   - Weight gain >4 lb (2 kg)
   - Increasing BP
   - Shortness of breath
   - Edema
   - Increasing fatigue or weakness
   - Confusion or lethargy
7. Need for support and encouragement. Share concerns about lifestyle changes, living with a chronic illness, and decisions about type of dialysis or transplantation.

a pillbox organizer or a list of the drugs and the times of administration that can be posted in the home may be helpful. Instruct the patient to avoid certain over-the-counter drugs, such as nonsteroidal antiinflammatory drugs (NSAIDs) and magnesium-based laxatives and antacids.

KIDNEY INJURY, ACUTE

Description

Acute kidney injury (AKI), previously known as acute kidney failure, is the term used to encompass the entire range of the syndrome ranging from a slight deterioration in kidney function to severe impairment.

AKI is characterized by a rapid loss of kidney function demonstrated by a rise in serum creatinine and/or a reduction in urine output. Severity can range from a small increase in serum creatinine or reduction in urine output to the development of azotemia (an accumulation of nitrogenous waste products [urea nitrogen, creatinine] in the blood).

Although AKI is potentially reversible, it has a high mortality rate. AKI usually affects people with other life-threatening conditions. Most commonly AKI follows severe, prolonged hypotension or hypovolemia or exposure to a nephrotoxic agent.

Pathophysiology

The causes of AKI are categorized as prerenal, intrarenal (or intrinsic), and postrenal causes.

- *Prerenal* AKI is caused by factors external to the kidneys that reduce renal blood flow and lead to decreased glomerular perfusion and filtration. In prerenal oliguria there is no damage to the kidney tissue (parenchyma). The oliguria is caused by a decrease in circulating blood volume (e.g., severe dehydration, decreased cardiac output) and is readily reversible with appropriate treatment. Prerenal conditions can lead to intrarenal disease if renal ischemia is prolonged.
- *Intrarenal* causes include conditions that cause direct damage to the kidney tissue resulting in impaired nephron function. Intrarenal AKI is usually caused by prolonged ischemia, nephrotoxins (e.g., antibiotics), myoglobin released from necrotic muscle cells, or hemoglobin released from hemolyzed RBCs. Primary renal diseases such as systemic lupus erythematosus and glomerulonephritis may also cause AKI. *Acute tubular necrosis* (ATN) is the most common cause of intrarenal AKI and is primarily the result of ischemia, nephrotoxins, or sepsis.

K

- *Postrenal* causes involve mechanical obstruction of urinary outflow. As the flow of urine is obstructed, urine refluxes into the renal pelvis, impairing kidney function. The most common causes are prostate cancer, benign prostatic hyperplasia (BPH), urinary tract calculi, trauma, and extrarenal tumors. Bilateral ureteral obstruction leads to *hydronephrosis* (kidney dilation), increase in hydrostatic pressure, and tubular blockage, resulting in a progressive decline in kidney function. If bilateral obstruction is relieved within 48 hours of onset, complete recovery is likely. After 12 weeks, recovery is unlikely. Prolonged obstruction can lead to tubular atrophy and irreversible kidney fibrosis.

Clinical Manifestations

Clinically, AKI may progress through three phases: oliguric, diuretic, and recovery. In some situations the patient does not recover from AKI, and chronic kidney disease (CKD) results (see Kidney Disease, Chronic, p. 373).

The diagnosis and staging of AKI are standardized with the mnemonic RIFLE (Table 57): *R*isk, the first stage of AKI, is followed by *I*njury, the second stage; AKI then increases in severity to the final or third stage, *F*ailure. The two outcome variables are *L*oss and *E*nd-stage kidney disease.

Oliguric Phase

The most common initial manifestation of AKI is oliguria, a reduction in urine output to less than 400 mL/day. Nonoliguria AKI indicates a urine output greater than 400 mL/day. Oliguria usually occurs within 1 to 7 days of injury to the kidneys. If the cause is ischemia, oliguria often occurs within 24 hours. In contrast, when nephrotoxic drugs are involved, onset may be delayed for up to a week. The oliguric phase lasts on average about 10 to 14 days but can last for months. The longer this phase lasts, the poorer the prognosis for recovery of complete renal function.

About 50% of patients will not be oliguric, making the initial diagnosis more difficult. Changes in urine output generally do not correspond to changes in glomerular filtration rate (GFR).

- A urinalysis may show casts, RBCs, WBCs, a specific gravity fixed at around 1.010, and urine osmolality around 300 mOsm/kg (300 mmol/kg). This is the same specific gravity and osmolality as plasma.
- Fluid retention occurs as urinary output decreases. Neck veins may become distended with a bounding pulse, and edema and hypertension may develop. Fluid overload can lead to heart failure (HF), pulmonary edema, and pericardial and pleural effusions.
- Metabolic acidosis results when the kidneys cannot synthesize ammonia (needed for hydrogen ion excretion) or excrete acid

| Table 57 | RIFLE Classification for Staging Acute Kidney Injury |

Stage	GFR Criteria	Urine Output Criteria
Risk	Serum creatinine increased × 1.5 or GFR decreased by 25%	Urine output <0.5 mL/kg/hr for 6 hr
Injury	Serum creatinine increased × 2 or GFR decreased by 50%	Urine output <0.5 mL/kg/hr for 12 hr
Failure	Serum creatinine increased × 3 or GFR decreased by 75% or Serum creatinine >4 mg/dL with acute rise ≥0.5 mg/dL	Urine output <0.3 mL/kg/hr for 24 hr (oliguria) or Anuria for 12 hr
Loss	Persistent acute kidney failure. Complete loss of kidney function >4 wk	—
End-stage kidney disease	Complete loss of kidney function >3 mo	—

GFR, Glomerular filtration rate.

products of metabolism. The serum bicarbonate level decreases because bicarbonate is depleted in buffering hydrogen ions. The patient may develop Kussmaul (rapid, deep) respirations to increase the excretion of carbon dioxide.

- Serum sodium and potassium levels are altered. Damaged tubules cannot conserve sodium. Urinary excretion of sodium may increase, resulting in normal or below-normal levels of serum sodium. In AKI the serum potassium level increases because the kidney's normal ability to excrete potassium is impaired. Because cardiac muscle is intolerant of acute increases in potassium, treatment is essential whenever hyperkalemia develops.
- Leukocytosis is often present. The most common cause of death in AKI is infection.
- Blood urea nitrogen (BUN) and serum creatinine levels are elevated in kidney failure.

- Neurologic changes can occur as nitrogenous waste products accumulate in the brain and other nervous tissue. Symptoms can be as mild as fatigue and difficulty concentrating and can escalate to seizures, stupor, and coma.

Diuretic Phase

During the diuretic phase, daily urine output of 1 to 3 L/day occurs but may reach 5 L/day or more. The kidneys have recovered their ability to excrete wastes but not to concentrate urine.

- The diuretic phase may last 1 to 3 weeks, with the patient's acid-base, electrolyte, and waste product values beginning to normalize. Because of large losses of fluid and electrolytes, monitor the patient for hyponatremia, hypokalemia, and dehydration.

Recovery Phase

The recovery phase begins when the GFR increases, allowing the BUN and serum creatinine levels to plateau and then decrease. Although major improvements occur in the first 1 to 2 weeks of this phase, kidney function may take up to 12 months to stabilize.

- The outcome of AKI is influenced by the patient's overall health, the severity of renal failure, and the number and type of complications. Some patients do not recover and progress to end-stage kidney disease. Most patients who recover achieve clinically normal kidney function with no complications (e.g., hypertension).

Diagnostic Studies

- History is essential to determine the etiology.
- Urine output and serum creatinine help in making the diagnosis.
- Urinalysis is done to assess sediment, casts, hematuria, pyuria, and crystals.
- Urine osmolality, sodium content, and specific gravity help in differentiating the cause.
- Ultrasound and renal scan are used to assess renal blood flow, tubular function, and the collecting system.
- CT scan can identify lesions, masses, obstructions, and vascular abnormalities.

Collaborative Care

Because AKI is potentially reversible, the primary goals of treatment are to eliminate the cause, manage the signs and symptoms, and prevent complications while the kidneys recover. The first step is to determine if there is adequate intravascular volume and cardiac output (CO) to ensure adequate perfusion of the kidneys. Diuretic therapy is often administered but not in high doses. If AKI is already established, forcing fluids and diuretics will not be effective. Conservative therapy may be all that is necessary until renal function improves.

- Closely monitor fluid intake during the oliguric phase.
- Hyperkalemia is one of the most serious complications because it can cause cardiac dysrhythmias. Both insulin and sodium bicarbonate temporarily shift potassium into the cells, but it eventually shifts back out. Calcium gluconate raises the threshold at which dysrhythmias occur. Only sodium polystyrene sulfonate (Kayexalate) and dialysis actually remove potassium from the body.

Controversy exists about the timing of renal replacement therapy. Common indications for renal replacement therapy in AKI include (1) volume overload, resulting in compromised cardiac and/or pulmonary status; (2) elevated serum potassium level; (3) metabolic acidosis (serum bicarbonate level less than 15 mEq/L [15 mmol/L]); (4) BUN level greater than 120 mg/dL (43 mmol/L); (5) significant change in mental status; and (6) pericarditis, pericardial effusion, or cardiac tamponade.

- If renal replacement therapy is required, there is no consensus regarding the best approach.
- Peritoneal dialysis is considered a viable option for renal replacement, although it is infrequently used.
- Intermittent hemodialysis (HD) (e.g., at intervals of 4 hours either daily, every other day, or three or four times per week) and continuous renal replacement therapy (CRRT) have both been used effectively. CRRT is provided continuously over approximately 24 hours' duration through cannulation of an artery and vein or cannulation of two veins.

Nutritional Therapy

The challenge of nutritional management is to provide adequate calories to prevent catabolism despite the restrictions required to prevent electrolyte and fluid disorders and azotemia. Adequate energy should be primarily from carbohydrate and fat sources to prevent ketosis from endogenous fat breakdown and gluconeogenesis from muscle protein breakdown.

- To maintain adequate caloric intake, 30 to 35 kcal/kg and 0.8 to 1.0 gram protein/kg is recommended to prevent the further breakdown of body protein for energy purposes. Essential amino acid supplements can be given for amino acid and caloric supplementation.
- Potassium and sodium are regulated in accordance with plasma levels. Sodium is restricted as needed to prevent edema, hypertension, and heart failure.
- Fat emulsion IV infusions given as a nutritional supplement provide a good source of nonprotein calories.

K

If a patient cannot maintain adequate oral intake, enteral nutrition is the preferred route for nutritional support (see Enteral Nutrition, p. 709). When the gastrointestinal tract is not functional, parenteral nutrition is necessary for the provision of adequate nutrition (see Parenteral Nutrition, p. 728).

Nursing Management

Goals
The patient with AKI will recover without any loss of kidney function, maintain normal fluid and electrolyte balance, have decreased anxiety, and adhere and understand the need for careful follow-up care.

Nursing Diagnoses/Collaborative Problem
- Excess fluid volume
- Risk for infection
- Fatigue
- Anxiety
- Potential complication: dysrhythmias

Nursing Interventions
Prevention and early recognition of AKI are essential because of the high mortality rate and are primarily directed toward (1) identifying and monitoring high-risk populations, (2) controlling exposure to industrial chemicals and nephrotoxic drugs, and (3) preventing prolonged episodes of hypotension and hypovolemia. In the hospital the factors that increase the risk for developing AKI are advanced age, massive trauma, extensive burns, cardiac failure, obstetric complications, or preexisting chronic kidney disease.

- Carefully monitoring of intake and output and electrolyte balance is essential. Assess and record extrarenal losses of fluid from vomiting, diarrhea, and hemorrhage.
- Prompt replacement of significant fluid losses helps prevent ischemic tubular damage associated with trauma, burns, and extensive surgery. Intake and output records and the patient's weight provide valuable indicators of fluid volume status.
- The individual who is taking drugs that are potentially nephrotoxic must have his or her renal function monitored. Angiotensin-converting enzyme (ACE) inhibitors can also decrease perfusion pressure and cause hyperkalemia. If other measures such as diet modification, diuretics, and sodium bicarbonate cannot control hyperkalemia, the ACE inhibitor may need to be reduced or eliminated.

During acute intervention you have an important role in managing fluid and electrolyte balance during the oliguric and diuretic phases. Observing and recording accurate intake and output is essential.

- Assess for the common signs and symptoms of hypervolemia (in the oliguric phase) or hypovolemia (in the diuretic phase), potassium and sodium disturbances, and other electrolyte imbalances that may occur in AKI.

- Because infection is the leading cause of death in AKI, meticulous aseptic technique is critical. If antibiotics are used to treat infection, the type, frequency, and dosage must be carefully considered because the kidneys are the primary route of excretion for many antibiotics.
- Perform skin care and take measures to prevent pressure ulcers because the patient usually develops edema and decreased muscle tone. Mouth care is important to prevent stomatitis.

▼ **Patient and Caregiver Teaching**

- Once kidney function has returned, follow-up care and regular evaluation of renal function are necessary.
- Teach the patient the signs and symptoms of recurrent renal disease. Emphasize measures to prevent recurrence of AKI.
- The long-term convalescence of 3 to 12 months may cause psychosocial and financial hardships for both the patient and the family. Make appropriate referrals for counseling.
- If the kidneys do not recover, the patient will need to transition to life on chronic dialysis or possible future transplantation.

LACTASE DEFICIENCY

Description

Lactase deficiency is a condition in which the lactase enzyme that breaks down lactose into two simple sugars (glucose and galactose) is deficient or absent.

Primary lactase insufficiency is most commonly caused by genetic factors. Certain ethnic or racial groups, especially those with Asian or African ancestry, develop low lactase levels in childhood. Less common causes include low lactase levels resulting from premature birth and congenital lactase deficiency, a rare genetic disorder. Lactose malabsorption can also occur when conditions leading to bacterial overgrowth promote lactose fermentation in the small bowel, and when intestinal mucosal damage interferes with absorption (e.g., inflammatory bowel disease, celiac disease).

Clinical Manifestations

Symptoms of lactose intolerance include bloating, flatulence, crampy abdominal pain, and diarrhea. They may occur within one-half hour to several hours after drinking a glass of milk or ingesting a milk product. Undigested lactose creates an osmotic action, pulling fluid into the small intestines, resulting in diarrhea.

Diagnostic Studies

Many lactose-intolerant people are aware of their milk intolerance and avoid milk and milk products. Lactose intolerance is diagnosed by a lactose tolerance test, lactose hydrogen breath test, or genetic testing.

Nursing and Collaborative Management

Treatment consists of eliminating lactose from the diet by avoiding milk and milk products and/or replacing lactase with commercially available preparations. Teach the patient the importance of adherence to the diet.

- A lactose-free diet is given initially and may be gradually advanced to a low-lactose diet.
- Many lactose-intolerant people may not exhibit symptoms if lactose is taken in small amounts.
- Because avoidance of milk and milk products can lead to calcium deficiency, supplements may be necessary to prevent osteoporosis.
- Lactase enzyme (Lactaid) is available as an over-the-counter product. It is mixed with milk and breaks down lactose before the milk is ingested.

LEIOMYOMAS

Leiomyomas (uterine fibroids) are benign smooth muscle tumors within the uterus. They are the most common benign tumors of the female genital tract. By 50 years of age, 60% of all women will have had at least one uterine leiomyoma.

The cause of leiomyomas is unknown. They appear to depend on ovarian hormones because they grow slowly during the woman's reproductive years and undergo atrophy after menopause.

A majority of women with leiomyomas do not have symptoms. Of the women who develop symptoms, the most common include abnormal uterine bleeding, pain, and symptoms associated with pelvic pressure. Pain is associated with an infection or twisting of the pedicle from which the tumor is growing.

Pressure on surrounding organs may result in rectal, bladder, and lower abdominal discomfort. Large tumors may cause a general enlargement of the lower abdomen. These tumors are sometimes associated with miscarriage and infertility.

Diagnosis is based on the characteristic pelvic findings of an enlarged uterus distorted by nodular masses.

Treatment depends on the symptoms, age of the patient, her desire to bear children, and the location and size of the tumor or tumors. If the symptoms are minimal, the provider may elect to monitor the patient closely for a time.

- Persistent heavy menstrual bleeding causing anemia and large or rapidly growing tumors are indications for surgery. Leiomyomas are removed by hysterectomy or myomectomy. A myomectomy is performed for women who wish to have children. In this case, only the fibroids are removed to preserve the uterus. Small tumors may be removed using a hysteroscope and laser resection instruments.
- Uterine artery embolization is an alternative treatment for uterine fibroids. In the procedure, embolic material (small plastic or gelatin beads) is injected into the uterine artery and carried to the fibroid branches.
- Cryosurgery and MRI–guided focused ultrasound may also be used to destroy tumors.

LEUKEMIA

Description

Leukemia is a general term used to describe a group of malignant disorders affecting the blood and blood-forming tissues of the bone marrow, lymph system, and spleen. It results in an accumulation of dysfunctional cells because of a loss of regulation in cell division. Although leukemia is often thought of as a disease of children, the number of adults affected is 10 times that of children.

Regardless of the specific type, leukemia has no single cause. Most types of leukemia result from a combination of factors including genetic and environmental influences.

Classification

Leukemia can be classified based on acute versus chronic disease and on the type of WBC involved. By combining the acute and chronic categories with the cell type involved, four major types of leukemia can be identified. Table 58 summarizes the relative incidence and features of the four types of leukemia.

Acute myelogenous leukemia (AML) represents only one fourth of all leukemias, but it makes up approximately 80% of the acute leukemias in adults. Its onset is often abrupt and dramatic. A patient may have serious infections and abnormal bleeding from the onset of the disease. AML is characterized by uncontrolled proliferation of myeloblasts, the precursors of granulocytes. There is hyperplasia of the bone marrow. Clinical manifestations are usually related to replacement of normal hematopoietic cells in the

Table 58   Types of Leukemia

Age of Onset	Clinical Manifestations	Diagnostic Findings
Acute Myelogenous Leukemia (AML)		
Most common cancer in children ages 0-7 yr. Increase in incidence with advancing age after 55 yr.	Fatigue and weakness, headache, mouth sores, anemia, bleeding, fever, infection, sternal tenderness, gingival hyperplasia, mild hepatosplenomegaly (⅓ of patients).	Low RBC count, Hgb, Hct, platelet count. Low to high WBC count with myeloblasts. High LDH. Hypercellular bone marrow with myeloblasts.
Acute Lymphocytic Leukemia (ALL)		
In children median age at diagnosis is 13 yr. Increases in incidence with advancing age after 60 yr.	Fever, pallor, bleeding, anorexia, fatigue and weakness. Bone, joint, and abdominal pain. Generalized lymphadenopathy, infections, weight loss, hepatosplenomegaly, headache, mouth sores, neurologic manifestations: CNS involvement, increased intracranial pressure (nausea, vomiting, lethargy, cranial nerve dysfunction) secondary to meningeal infiltration.	Low RBC count, Hgb, Hct, platelet count. Low, normal, or high WBC count. High LDH. Transverse lines of rarefaction at ends of metaphysis of long bones on x-ray. Hypercellular bone marrow with lymphoblasts. Lymphoblasts also possible in cerebrospinal fluid. Presence of Philadelphia chromosome (20%-25% of patients).

Chronic Myelogenous Leukemia (CML)
Increase in incidence with advancing age after 55 yr.

No symptoms early in disease. Fatigue and weakness, fever, sternal tenderness, weight loss, joint pain, bone pain, massive splenomegaly, increase in sweating.

Low RBC count, Hgb, Hct. High platelet count early, lower count later. ↑ Neutrophils, normal number of lymphocytes, and normal or low number of monocytes. Low leukocyte alkaline phosphatase. Presence of Philadelphia chromosome in 90% of patients.

Chronic Lymphocytic Leukemia (CLL)
Increase in incidence with advancing age after 50 yr, with predominance in men.

Frequently no symptoms. Detection of disease often during examination for unrelated condition, chronic fatigue, anorexia, splenomegaly and lymphadenopathy, hepatomegaly. May progress to fever, night sweats, weight loss, fatigue, and frequent infections.

Mild anemia and thrombocytopenia with disease progression. Total WBC count >100,000/μL. Increase in peripheral lymphocytes and lymphocytes in bone marrow. Hypogammaglobulinemia. May have autoimmune hemolytic anemia, idiopathic thrombocytopenic purpura.

CNS, Central nervous system; *LDH,* lactate dehydrogenase

L

marrow by leukemic myeloblasts and, to a lesser extent, to infiltration of other organs and tissue.

Acute lymphocytic leukemia (ALL) is the most common type of leukemia in children and accounts for about 20% of acute leukemia cases in adults. In ALL, immature lymphocytes proliferate in the bone marrow; most are of B cell origin. Fever is present in the majority of patients at time of diagnosis. Signs and symptoms may appear abruptly with bleeding or fever, or they may be insidious with progressive weakness, fatigue, and bleeding tendencies.

Chronic myelogenous leukemia (CML) is caused by excessive development of mature neoplastic granulocytes in the bone marrow. CML usually has a chronic stable phase that lasts for several years, followed by the development of an acute aggressive phase (blastic phase).

- The Philadelphia chromosome, which is present in 90% to 95% of patients with CML, is a diagnostic hallmark of CML. In addition, its presence is an important indicator of residual disease or relapse after treatment.

Chronic lymphocytic leukemia (CLL) is the most common leukemia in adults and is characterized by the production and accumulation of functionally inactive but long-lived, small, mature-appearing lymphocytes. The B lymphocyte is usually involved. Lymph node enlargement (lymphadenopathy) is present throughout the body. Because CLL is usually a disease of older adults, treatment decisions must be made by considering disease progression and treatment of side effects. Many individuals in the early stages of CLL require no treatment. Others may be followed closely and receive treatment only when the disease progresses; approximately 30% will require immediate intervention at time of diagnosis.

Clinical Manifestations

Although the manifestations of leukemia are varied, they relate to problems caused by bone marrow failure and the formation of leukemic infiltrates (see Table 58). The patient is predisposed to anemia, thrombocytopenia, and decreased number and function of WBCs.

- WBC infiltration into the patient's organs leads to problems such as splenomegaly, hepatomegaly, lymphadenopathy, bone pain, meningeal irritation, and oral lesions.

Diagnostic Studies

- Peripheral blood evaluation and bone marrow examination are the primary methods of diagnosing and classifying the types of leukemia.

- Morphologic, histochemical, immunologic, and cytogenetic methods are all used to identify leukemic cell types and stage of development.
- Studies such as lumbar puncture and CT scan can detect leukemic cells outside the blood and bone marrow.
- The malignant cells in most patients with leukemia have specific cytogenetic abnormalities that are associated with distinct subsets of the disease. These cytogenetic abnormalities have diagnostic, prognostic, and therapeutic importance.

Collaborative Care

Collaborative care first focuses on the initial goal of attaining remission.

- In some cases, such as nonsymptomatic patients with CLL, watchful waiting with active supportive care may be appropriate.
- Because cytotoxic chemotherapy is the mainstay of treatment for some patients, you must understand the principles of cancer chemotherapy, including cellular kinetics, the use of multiple drugs rather than single agents, and the cell cycle (see Chemotherapy, p. 694).
- Corticosteroids and radiation therapy may have a role in therapy for the patient with leukemia. Total body radiation may be used to prepare a patient for bone marrow transplantation, or radiation may be restricted to certain areas (fields), such as the liver, spleen, or other organs affected by infiltrates.
- In ALL, prophylactic intrathecal methotrexate or cytarabine is given to decrease central nervous system (CNS) involvement, which is common in this type of leukemia. When CNS leukemia does occur, cranial radiation may be given. Biologic and targeted therapy may be indicated for specific types of leukemia (see Lewis et al., *Medical-Surgical Nursing,* ed. 9, p. 667).

Chemotherapeutic agents used to treat leukemia vary. Combination chemotherapy is the mainstay of treatment for leukemia. The three purposes for using multiple drugs are to (1) decrease drug resistance, (2) minimize drug toxicity to the patient by using multiple drugs with varying toxicities, and (3) interrupt cell growth at multiple points in the cell cycle.

Hematopoietic stem cell transplantation (HSCT) is another type of therapy used for patients with different forms of leukemia. The goal of HSCT is to totally eliminate leukemia cells from the body using combinations of chemotherapy with or without total body radiation. This treatment also eradicates the patient's hematopoietic stem cells, which are then replaced with those of a human leukocyte antigen (HLA)-matched sibling, with those of a volunteer donor (allogeneic) or an identical twin (syngeneic), or with the patient's own (autologous) stem cells that were removed (harvested) before the intensive therapy. (See content on HSCT in Lewis et al., *Medical-Surgical Nursing,* ed. 9, pp. 667 to 668.)

The primary complications of patients with allogeneic HSCT are graft-versus-host disease (GVHD), relapse of leukemia (especially ALL), and infection (especially interstitial pneumonia). Because HSCT has serious associated risks, the patient must weigh the significant risks of treatment-related death or treatment failure (relapse) with the hope of cure.

Nursing Management

Goals

The patient with leukemia will understand and cooperate with the treatment plan, experience minimal side effects and complications associated with both the disease and its treatment, and feel hopeful and supported during periods of treatment, relapse, or remission.

See nursing care plans for anemia (NCP 31-1, pp. 635 to 636, Lewis et al., *Medical-Surgical Nursing,* ed. 9), thrombocytopenia (eNCP 31-1, available on the website), and neutropenia (eNCP 31-2, available on the website).

Nursing Diagnoses

Nursing diagnoses related to leukemia include those appropriate for anemia (see Anemia, pp. 635 to 636), thrombocytopenia (see Thrombocytopenic Purpura, pp. 653 to 654), and neutropenia (see content on neutropenia in Lewis et al., *Medical-Surgical Nursing,* ed. 9, pp. 660 to 663).

Nursing Interventions

The nursing role during acute phases of leukemia is extremely challenging because the patient has many physical and psychosocial needs. As with other forms of cancer, the diagnosis of leukemia can evoke great fear and be equated with death.

Help the patient realize that although the future may be uncertain, one can have a meaningful quality of life while in remission or with disease control.

Families also need help in adjusting to the stress of the abrupt onset of serious illness and the losses imposed by the sick role. The diagnosis of leukemia often brings with it the need to make difficult decisions at a time of profound stress for the patient and family.

You are an important advocate in helping the patient and family understand the complexities of treatment decisions and manage the side effects and toxicities. A patient may require isolation or may need to temporarily geographically relocate to an appropriate treatment center. This situation can lead a patient to feel deserted and isolated at a time when support is most needed.

From a physical care perspective, you are challenged to make assessments and plan care to help the patient deal with the severe side effects of chemotherapy. The life-threatening results of bone marrow suppression (anemia, thrombocytopenia, neutropenia) require aggressive nursing interventions.

Review all drugs being administered. Assess laboratory data reflecting the effects of the drugs. Patient survival and comfort during aggressive chemotherapy are significantly affected by the quality of nursing care.

▼ **Patient and Caregiver Teaching**

Teach the patient and caregiver to understand the importance of continued diligence in disease management and the need for follow-up care.

Assistance may be needed to reestablish various relationships that are a part of the patient's life.

Involving the patient in survivor networks, support groups, or services may help the patient to adapt to living with a life-threatening illness. Exploring community resources (e.g., American Cancer Society, Leukemia Society) may reduce the financial burden and feelings of dependence. Also provide the resources for spiritual support.

LIVER CANCER

Description

Primary liver cancer (hepatocellular carcinoma [HCC] or malignant hepatoma) is the fifth most common cancer in the world and the second most common cause of cancer death worldwide. It is the most common cause of death in patients with cirrhosis.

The incidence of HCC is rising in the United States because of the large number of patients infected with chronic hepatitis C. Cirrhosis caused by hepatitis C is the most common cause of HCC in the United States, followed by alcoholic cirrhosis. Other primary liver tumors are cholangiomas or bile duct cancers.

Metastatic carcinoma of the liver is more common than primary carcinoma. The liver is a common site of metastatic cancer growth because of its high rate of blood flow and extensive capillary network. Primary liver tumors commonly metastasize to the lung.

- The prognosis for patients with liver cancer is poor. The cancer grows rapidly, and death may occur within 6 to 12 months as a result of hepatic encephalopathy or massive blood loss from GI bleeding.

Clinical Manifestations

Liver cancer can be difficult to diagnose and differentiate from cirrhosis because of similar clinical manifestations (e.g., hepatomegaly,

splenomegaly, jaundice, weight loss, peripheral edema, ascites, portal hypertension).
- Other common manifestations include dull abdominal pain in the epigastric or right upper quadrant region, anorexia, nausea and vomiting, and increased abdominal girth.
- Patients with advanced HCC can have pulmonary emboli and portal vein thrombosis.

Diagnostic Studies
- Ultrasound, CT, and MRI are used to screen and diagnose liver cancer.
- A percutaneous biopsy is performed when the results of diagnostic imaging studies are inconclusive.
- Serum α-fetoprotein (AFP) is often elevated.

Nursing and Collaborative Management
Treatment depends on the size and number of tumors, metastasis beyond the liver, and the patient's age and overall health. In general, management is similar to that for cirrhosis (see Cirrhosis, pp. 148 to 149). Surgical excision (partial hepatectomy) is performed when there is no evidence of portal hypertension, normal liver function, and no evidence of invasion of hepatic blood vessels. Only about 15% of patients have surgically resectable disease, but surgical interventions offer the best chance for cure. Liver transplantation is performed when the tumor is localized. Other treatment options are radiofrequency ablation, chemoembolization, and alcohol injection.

Nursing interventions focus on keeping the patient as comfortable as possible. Because the patient with liver cancer manifests the same problems as the patient with advanced liver disease, the nursing interventions discussed for cirrhosis of the liver apply (see Cirrhosis, pp. 148 to 149).

LOW BACK PAIN, ACUTE

Description
Low back pain is common and has affected 80% of adults in the United States at least once during their lifetime. Risk factors associated with low back pain include cigarette smoking, stress, poor posture, lack of muscle tone, and excess weight. Jobs that require repetitive heavy lifting, vibration (e.g., jackhammer operator), and prolonged periods of sitting are also associated with low back pain. Low back pain is most often caused by a musculoskeletal problem.
- Health care personnel who engage in patient care–related tasks are at high risk for low back pain. Lifting and moving patients,

excessive time in a stooped-over or forward-leaning position, and frequent twisting can result in low back pain.

Pathophysiology

Low back pain is a common problem because the lumbar region (1) bears most of the weight of the body, (2) is the most flexible region of the spinal column, (3) has nerve roots that are vulnerable to injury or disease, and (4) has an inherently poor biomechanical structure. The causes of low back pain of musculoskeletal origin include acute lumbosacral strain, instability of lumbosacral bony mechanism, osteoarthritis of the lumbosacral vertebrae, degenerative disc disease, and herniation of the intervertebral disc.

Acute low back pain lasts 4 weeks or less. It is caused by trauma or activity that causes undue stress (often hyperflexion) on tissues of the lower back. Often symptoms do not appear at the time of injury but develop later because of a gradual increase in pressure on the nerve by an intervertebral disc.

- Symptoms may range from muscle ache to shooting or stabbing pain, limited flexibility and/or range of motion, or inability to stand straight.
- Few definitive diagnostic abnormalities are present with nerve irritation and muscle strain. One test is the straight-leg raise. MRI and CT scans are generally not done unless trauma or systemic disease (e.g., cancer, spinal infection) is suspected.

Collaborative Care

If the acute muscle spasms and accompanying pain are not severe and debilitating, the patient may be treated on an outpatient basis with nonsteroidal antiinflammatory drugs (NSAIDs), muscle relaxants, massage and back manipulation, acupuncture, and alternating use of heat and cold compresses. Severe pain may require a brief course of opioid analgesics.

A brief period (1 to 2 days) of rest at home may be necessary for some individuals, with most people doing better with a continuation of regular activities.

- Patients should refrain from activities that aggravate the pain, including lifting, bending, twisting, and prolonged sitting. Most cases improve within 2 weeks and often resolve with treatment.

L

Nursing Management

As a role model, you need to use proper body mechanics at all times. This includes increasing the patient's bed height, bending at the knees, asking for help in lifting and moving patients, and using lifting devices.

Primary nursing responsibilities in acute low back pain are to assist the patient to maintain activity limitations, promote comfort, and teach the patient about the health problem and appropriate exercises.

- Muscle-strengthening and stretching exercises may be part of the management plan. Although the actual exercises are often taught by the physical therapist, it is your responsibility to ensure that the patient understands the type and frequency of exercise prescribed, as well as the rationale for the program.

▼ **Patient and Caregiver Teaching**

Assess the patient's use of body mechanics and offer advice when the person does activities that could produce back strain (Table 59).

- Advise patients to maintain an appropriate weight. Excess body weight places extra stress on the lower back and weakens abdominal muscles that support the lower back.

Table 59	**Patient and Caregiver Teaching Guide** *Low Back Problems*

Include the following instructions when teaching the patient and caregiver how to manage low back problems.

Do
- Avoid straining the lower back by placing a foot on a step or stool during prolonged standing.
- Sleep in a side-lying position with knees and hips bent.
- Sleep on back with a lift under knees and legs or on back with 10-in-high pillow under knees to flex hips and knees.
- Regularly exercise 15 min in the morning and evening; begin exercises with 2- or 3-min warm-up period by moving arms and legs, alternately relaxing and tightening muscles; exercise slowly with smooth movements.
- Carry light items close to body.
- Maintain appropriate body weight.
- Use local heat and cold application.
- Use a lumbar roll or pillow for sitting.

Do Not
- Lean forward without bending knees.
- Lift anything above level of elbows.
- Stand in one position for prolonged time.
- Sleep on abdomen or on back or side with legs out straight.
- Exercise without consulting health care provider if having severe pain.
- Exceed prescribed amount and type of exercises without consulting health care provider.

■ The position assumed while sleeping is also important in preventing low back pain. Advise patients to avoid sleeping in a prone position because it produces excessive lumbar lordosis, placing excessive stress on the lower back. A firm mattress is recommended. The patient should sleep in either a supine or side-lying position, with the knees and hips flexed to prevent unnecessary pressure on support muscles, ligamentous structures, and lumbosacral joints.

LOW BACK PAIN, CHRONIC

Description

Chronic low back pain lasts more than 3 months or is a repeated incapacitating episode. It is often progressive, and the cause can be difficult to determine.

Causes include (1) degenerative conditions such as arthritis or disc disease; (2) osteoporosis or other metabolic bone diseases; (3) prior injury (scar tissue weakens the back); (4) chronic strain on the lower back muscles from obesity, pregnancy, or job-related stooping, bending, or other stressful postures; and (5) congenital abnormalities in the spine.

Spinal stenosis is a narrowing of the spinal canal. When it occurs in the lumbar area of the spine, it is a common cause of chronic low back pain. Spinal stenosis can be caused by both acquired and/or inherited conditions.

■ A common acquired cause is osteoarthritis in the spine. Arthritic changes (bone spurs, calcification of spinal ligaments, degeneration of discs) narrow the space around the spinal canal and nerve roots, eventually leading to compression. Inflammation caused by the compression results in pain, weakness, and numbness.
■ Inherited conditions that lead to spinal stenosis include congenital spinal stenosis and scoliosis.

The pain associated with lumbar spinal stenosis often starts in the low back and then radiates to the buttock and leg. It worsens with walking and standing without walking. Numbness, tingling, weakness, and heaviness in the legs and buttocks may also be present. A history of the pain lessening when the patient bends forward or sits down is often a sign of spinal stenosis.

■ In most cases the stenosis progresses slowly and does not cause paralysis.

Collaborative Care

Treatment regimens are similar to those recommended for acute low back pain. Relief of pain and stiffness with mild analgesics, such as nonsteroidal antiinflammatory drugs (NSAIDs), is integral to the daily comfort of the individual with chronic low back pain. Antidepressants may help with pain relief and sleep problems. The antiseizure drug gabapentin (Neurontin) may improve walking and relieve leg symptoms. Duloxetine (Cymbalta) may also be used for the treatment of chronic low back pain.

- Weight reduction, sufficient rest periods, local heat/cold application, and exercise and activity throughout the day help keep the muscles and joints mobilized.
- Complementary and alternative therapies such as biofeedback, acupuncture, and yoga may help to reduce the pain.
- Minimally invasive treatments, such as epidural corticosteroid injections and implanted devices that deliver pain medication, may be used for patients with chronic low back pain that is refractory to the usual therapeutic options.
- Surgery may be indicated in patients with severe chronic low back pain who do not respond to conservative care and/or have continued neurologic deficits. (See Surgical Therapy, Intervertebral Disc Disease, p. 364.)

LUNG CANCER

Description

Lung cancer is the leading cause of cancer-related deaths in the United States and accounts for 28% of all cancer deaths. Female smokers have a higher risk of developing lung cancers than male smokers.

- Smoking is the greatest risk factor for lung cancer. Smoking is responsible for approximately 80% to 90% of all lung cancers. Tobacco smoke contains 60 carcinogens and causes a change in the bronchial epithelium, which usually returns to normal when smoking is discontinued.

Assessment of lung cancer risk is divided into three categories: (1) smokers, people who are currently smoking; (2) nonsmokers, people who formerly smoked; and (3) never smokers. The risk of developing lung cancer is directly related to total exposure to tobacco smoke, measured by total number of cigarettes smoked in a lifetime, age of smoking onset, depth of inhalation, tar and nicotine content, and the use of unfiltered cigarettes. Sidestream smoke (smoke from burning cigarettes, cigars) contains the same carcinogens found in mainstream smoke (smoke inhaled and exhaled from the smoker).

- Other causes of lung cancer include high levels of pollution, radiation (especially radon exposure), and asbestos. Heavy or prolonged exposure to industrial agents such as ionizing radiation, coal dust, uranium, formaldehyde, and arsenic can also increase the risk of lung cancer.

- It is also theorized that people have different genetic carcinogen-metabolizing pathways. This may explain why some smokers develop lung cancer and others do not.

Pathophysiology

Most primary lung tumors are believed to arise from mutated epithelial cells. The development of mutations that are caused by carcinogens is influenced by various genetic factors. Once started, tumor development is promoted by epidermal growth factor. These cells grow slowly, taking 8 to 10 years for a tumor to reach 1 cm in size, the smallest lesion detectable on an x-ray. Lung cancers occur primarily in the segmental bronchi or beyond and have a preference for the upper lobes of the lungs.

Primary lung cancers are categorized into two broad types: *non–small cell lung cancer* (NSCLC) (80%) and *small cell lung cancer* (SCLC) (20%). Lung cancer metastasizes primarily by direct extension and by way of the blood and lymph system. Common sites for metastasis are the liver, brain, bones, lymph nodes, and adrenal glands.

Clinical Manifestations

Manifestations are usually nonspecific, appear late in the disease process, and depend on the type of primary lung cancer, its location, and metastatic spread.

- One of the most common first symptoms reported is a persistent cough. Blood-tinged sputum may be produced because of bleeding caused by the malignancy.
- The patient may complain of dyspnea or wheezing. Chest pain, if present, may be localized or unilateral, ranging from mild to severe.

Later manifestations include nonspecific symptoms such as anorexia, fatigue, weight loss, and nausea and vomiting. Hoarseness may be present as a result of laryngeal nerve involvement. Unilateral paralysis of the diaphragm, dysphagia, and superior vena cava obstruction may occur because of intrathoracic spread of malignancy. There may be palpable lymph nodes in the neck or axillae. Mediastinal involvement may lead to pericardial effusion, cardiac tamponade, and dysrhythmias.

Paraneoplastic syndrome is caused by humoral factors (hormones, cytokines) excreted by tumor cells or by an immune response against the tumor. SCLCs are most often associated with the paraneoplastic syndrome. Symptoms of paraneoplastic syndrome may manifest before the diagnosis of a malignancy.

- Examples of paraneoplastic syndrome include hypercalcemia, syndrome of inappropriate antidiuretic hormone (SIADH) secretion, hematologic disorders, and neurologic syndromes. These conditions may stabilize with treatment of the underlying neoplasm.

Diagnostic Studies

- Chest x-ray is used for diagnosis and assessing for metastasis.
- Biopsy is necessary for a definitive diagnosis. If thoracentesis is performed to relieve a pleural effusion, the fluid is also analyzed for malignant cells.
- Additional diagnostic tests include bone scans, CT scans, MRI, positron emission tomography (PET), blood tests, renal function tests, and pulmonary function tests.

Staging of NSCLC is performed according to the TNM staging system (see TNM Classification System, p. 777).

Collaborative Care

Surgical resection is the treatment of choice in NSCLC stages I and IIIA without mediastinal involvement because the disease is potentially curable with resection. The 5-year survival in stage I and II disease ranges from 30% to 50%. For other NSCLC stages, patients may require surgery in conjunction with radiation therapy and/or chemotherapy. Fifty percent of NSCLCs are not resectable at the time of diagnosis. Surgical procedures that may be performed include pneumonectomy (removal of one entire lung), lobectomy (removal of one or more lung lobes), or segmental or wedge resection procedures.

Radiation therapy may be used as treatment for both NSCLC and SCLC (see Radiation Therapy, p. 730).

- Radiation relieves symptoms of dyspnea and hemoptysis from bronchial obstruction tumors and treats superior vena cava syndrome.
- Radiation can be used to treat the pain of metastatic bone lesions or cerebral metastasis, to reduce tumor mass preoperatively, or as an adjuvant measure postoperatively.

A newer type of radiation therapy is stereotactic radiotherapy (SRT), which uses high doses of radiation delivered accurately to the tumor. SRT provides an option for patients with early-stage lung cancers who are not surgical candidates for other medical reasons.

Chemotherapy is the primary treatment for SCLC. It may be used for nonresectable tumors or as an adjuvant therapy to surgery in NSCLC. A variety of chemotherapy drugs and multidrug regimens (i.e., protocols) have been used (see Chemotherapy, p. 694).

One type of targeted therapy for patients with NSCLC is erlotinib (Tarceva), which blocks signals for growth in cancer cells. Other drugs, such as bevacizumab (Avastin), inhibit new blood vessel growth (angiogenesis).

Nursing Management

Goals

The patient with lung cancer will have effective breathing patterns, adequate airway clearance, adequate oxygenation of tissues, minimal to no pain, and a realistic attitude toward treatment and prognosis.

Nursing Diagnoses

- Ineffective airway clearance
- Anxiety
- Ineffective self-health management
- Ineffective breathing pattern
- Impaired gas exchange

Nursing Interventions

Care of the patient with lung cancer initially involves support and reassurance during the diagnostic evaluation. Individualized care will depend on the plan for treatment.

- Assessment and intervention in symptom management are pivotal.
- For many individuals who have lung cancer, little can be done to significantly prolong their lives. Radiation therapy and chemotherapy can provide palliative relief from distressing symptoms. Constant pain may become a major problem.
- Provide patient comfort, monitor for side effects of prescribed medications, foster appropriate coping strategies for patient and caregiver, assess smoking cessation readiness, and help patients access resources to deal with the illness.

▼ **Patient and Caregiver Teaching**

- A wealth of material is available to the smoker who is interested in smoking cessation. The Centers for Disease Control and Prevention (CDC) provides an index of tools *(www.cdc.gov/ tobacco/quit_smoking/cessation/index.htm)*. Also see Chapter 11 in Lewis et al., *Medical-Surgical Nursing,* ed. 9.
- The patient and family should be encouraged to provide a smoke-free environment. This may include smoking cessation for multiple family members. If the treatment plan includes the use of home oxygen, instruct the patient and family on the safe use of oxygen.
- Teach the patient to recognize signs and symptoms that may indicate progression or recurrence of disease.

L

LYME DISEASE

Description

Lyme disease is a spirochetal infection caused by *Borrelia burgdorferi* and transmitted by the bite of an infected deer tick. The tick typically feeds on mice, dogs, cats, cows, horses, deer, and humans. Wild animals do not exhibit the illness, but clinical Lyme disease does occur in domestic animals. Person-to-person transmission does not occur.

The peak season for human infection is during the summer months. Most cases occur in three U.S. endemic areas: along the northeastern coast from Maryland to Massachusetts, in Wisconsin and Minnesota, and along the northwestern coast of northern California and Oregon. Reinfection is not uncommon.

Clinical Manifestations

The most characteristic sign is erythema migrans (EM), a skin lesion that occurs at the site of the tick bite within 3 to 30 days after exposure.

- The lesion begins as a red macule or papule that slowly expands to form a large round lesion of up to 12 inches with a bright red border and central clearing. The EM lesion is often accompanied by acute viral-like symptoms, such as fever, headache, fatigue, stiff neck, swollen lymph nodes, and migratory joint and muscle pain. Loss of tone in facial muscles can manifest as Bell's palsy.
- Symptoms generally resolve over a period of weeks or months, even if untreated.
- If not treated, the spirochete can disseminate within several weeks or months to the heart, joints, and CNS. Carditis may occur with chronic arthritic pain and swelling in the large joints. Nervous system problems may include severe headaches or poor motor coordination.

Diagnostic Studies

Diagnosis is often based on clinical manifestations, in particular the EM lesion, and a history of exposure in an endemic area.

- CBC and erythrocyte sedimentation rate (ESR) results are usually normal.
- A two-step laboratory testing process is recommended to confirm diagnosis. The first step is the enzyme immunoassay (EIA), a test that will have positive results for most people with Lyme disease. If the EIA is positive or inconclusive, a

Western blot test should be done, which will confirm the infection.
- In individuals with neurologic involvement, cerebrospinal fluid should also be examined.

Nursing and Collaborative Management

Active lesions can be treated with oral antibiotics. Doxycycline (Vibramycin), cefuroxime (Ceftin), and amoxicillin are often effective in early-stage infection and in prevention of later stages of the disease. Doxycycline is effective in preventing Lyme disease when given within 3 days after the bite of a deer tick.
- Approximately 10% to 20% of people treated with antibiotics for Lyme disease may experience lingering fatigue or joint and muscle pain.
- Patient and caregiver teaching for the prevention of Lyme disease in endemic areas is outlined in Table 65-13, Lewis et al., *Medical-Surgical Nursing,* ed. 9, p. 1579.

MACULAR DEGENERATION

Description

Age-related *macular degeneration* (AMD) is a degeneration of the retina involving the macula that results in varying degrees of central vision loss. It is the most common cause of irreversible central vision loss in people over 60 years old in the United States. AMD is divided into two classic forms: *dry* (atrophic), which is more common, and *wet* (exudative), which is more severe. Wet AMD accounts for 90% of the cases of AMD-related blindness.

Pathophysiology

AMD is related to retinal aging. Family history is a major risk factor, and a gene responsible for some cases of AMD has been identified. In addition, long-term exposure to ultraviolet light, hyperopia, cigarette smoking, and light-colored eyes may be additional risk factors. Nutritional factors such as vitamins C, E, beta-carotene, and zinc may play a role in the progression of AMD.
- In *dry AMD,* people notice that reading and other close-vision tasks become more difficult. This form starts with the abnormal accumulation of yellowish extracellular deposits called *drusen* in the retinal pigment epithelium. Atrophy and degeneration of macular cells then result, leading to a slowly progressive and painless vision loss.

M

- *Wet AMD* is characterized by the growth of new blood vessels from their normal location in the choroids to an abnormal location in the retinal epithelium. As the new blood vessels leak, scar tissue gradually forms. Acute vision loss may occur in some cases from bleeding.

Clinical Manifestations

The patient may experience blurred and darkened vision, *scotomas* (blind spots in the visual fields), and *metamorphopsia* (distortion of vision).

Diagnostic Studies

- Visual acuity measurement
- Ophthalmoscopic examination to look for drusen and other changes in the fundus
- Amsler grid test to define the involved area and provide a baseline for future comparison
- Fundus photography and IV fluorescein angiography to further define the extent and type of AMD

Nursing and Collaborative Management

Vision does not improve for most people with AMD. Limited treatment options for patients with wet AMD include several medications (i.e., ranibizumab [Lucentis], bevacizumab [Avastin], and pegaptanib [Macugen]) injected directly into the vitreous cavity. These drugs are selective inhibitors of endothelial growth factor and help to slow vision loss.

- Photodynamic therapy is used in wet AMD to destroy abnormal blood vessels without permanent damage to the retinal pigment epithelium and photoreceptor cells.
- Patients at risk for AMD (in consultation with their health care provider) should consider supplements of vitamins and minerals.
- Many patients with low-vision assistive devices can continue reading and retain a license to drive during the daytime and at lowered speeds.

The permanent loss of central vision associated with AMD has significant psychosocial implications for nursing care. Nursing management of the patient with uncorrectable visual impairment is discussed in Lewis et al.: *Medical-Surgical Nursing,* ed. 9, pp. 388 to 389, and is appropriate for the patient with AMD. It is especially important when caring for patients to avoid giving them the impression that "nothing can be done" about their problem. Although therapy will not recover lost vision, much can be done to augment the remaining vision.

MALIGNANT MELANOMA

Description

Malignant melanoma is a tumor arising in cells producing melanin, which are usually the melanocytes of the skin. Melanoma has the ability to metastasize to any organ, including the brain and heart. This is the deadliest form of skin cancer.

The exact cause of melanoma is unknown. Risk factors include long-term UV exposure or overexposure to artificial light, such as a tanning booth. People with fair skin and eyes and those with a prior diagnosis of melanoma or having a first-degree relative diagnosed with melanoma have an increased risk. Immunosuppression and dysplastic nevi also increase a person's risk.

Clinical Manifestations

About 25% of melanomas occur in existing nevi or moles; about 20% occur in dysplastic nevi. Melanoma frequently occurs on the lower legs in women and on the trunk, head, and neck in men. Because most melanoma cells continue to produce melanin, melanoma tumors are often brown or black.

- Individuals should consult their health care provider immediately if their moles or lesions show any of the clinical signs (ABCDEs) of melanoma (see Fig. 24-4, Lewis et al.: *Medical-Surgical Nursing,* ed. 9, p. 433). These signs include **A**symmetry, **B**order irregularity, **C**olor varied from one area of the lesion to another, **D**iameter greater than 6 mm, and **E**volving, changing appearance.
- Any sudden or progressive increase in the size, color, or shape of a mole should be checked. When melanoma begins in the skin, it is called *cutaneous melanoma.* Melanoma can also occur in the eyes, meninges, lymph nodes, digestive tract, and anywhere else in the body where melanocytes are found.

Collaborative Care

All suspicious pigmented lesions should be biopsied using an excisional biopsy technique. The most important prognostic factor is tumor thickness at the time of diagnosis.

- Two methods are used to determine tumor thickness: the *Breslow measurement,* which indicates tumor depth in millimeters, and the *Clark level,* which indicates the depth of invasion of the tumor. The higher the number, the deeper the melanoma.

Treatment depends on the site of the original tumor, stage of the cancer, and patient's age and general health. Initial treatment of

M

malignant melanoma is surgical excision. Melanoma that has spread to the lymph nodes or nearby sites usually requires additional therapy, such as chemotherapy, biologic therapy (e.g., α-interferon, interleukin-2), and/or radiation therapy. Chemotherapy may include dacarbazine (DTIC), temozolomide (TMZ), procarbazine (Matulane), carmustine (BCNU), and lomustine (CCNU). Two newer options for patients with metastatic melanoma are ipilimumab (Yervoy) and vemurafenib (Zelboraf).

Cutaneous melanoma is nearly 100% curable by excision if diagnosed at stage 0. The 5-year survival rate depends on sentinel node biopsy results, which indicate if metastasis has occurred. If metastasis to other organs is found (stage IV), treatment then becomes palliative.

▼ **Patient and Caregiver Teaching**

Emphasize the importance of protection from the damaging effects of the sun, such as wearing a large-brimmed hat, sunglasses, and a long-sleeved shirt of a lightly woven fabric.

- Inform patients that the rays of the sun are most dangerous between 10 AM and 2 PM standard time and 11 AM and 3 PM daylight savings time. Recommend patients use a sunscreen with a minimum SPF of 15 on a daily basis. Sunscreen should be reapplied every 2 hours.
- Teach patients to self-examine their skin at least monthly to detect new or persistent skin lesions.

MALNUTRITION

Description

Malnutrition is an excess, deficit, or imbalance of the essential components of a balanced diet. Malnutrition is also described as undernutrition or overnutrition. *Undernutrition* describes a state of poor nourishment as a result of inadequate diet or diseases that interfere with normal appetite and assimilation of ingested food. *Overnutrition* refers to the ingestion of more food than is required for body needs, as in obesity.

- The incidence of hospitalized patients who are malnourished or at nutritional risk is 20% to 70%. The prevalence of malnutrition in older adults ranges from 6% (community-dwelling older adults) to 50% (rehabilitation settings).

The following etiology-based terminology indicates the interaction and importance of inflammation on nutritional status:

- Starvation-related malnutrition, or primary protein-calorie malnutrition (PCM), occurs when nutritional needs are not met.

It is a clinical state in which there is chronic starvation without inflammation (e.g., anorexia nervosa).

- Chronic disease–related malnutrition, or secondary PCM, is associated with conditions that impose sustained inflammation of a mild to moderate degree. This occurs when tissue needs are not met even though the dietary intake would be satisfactory under normal conditions. Conditions associated with this type of malnutrition include organ failure, cancer, rheumatoid arthritis, obesity, and metabolic syndrome.
- Acute disease- or injury-related malnutrition is associated with acute disease or injury states with marked inflammatory response (e.g., major infection, burns, trauma, closed head injury).

Many factors contribute to the development of malnutrition, including socioeconomic factors, physical illnesses, incomplete diets, and food-drug interactions.

Pathophysiology of Starvation

Initially, the body selectively uses carbohydrates (glycogen) rather than fat and protein to meet metabolic needs. This depletes glycogen stores in the liver and muscles within 18 hours.

- When carbohydrate stores are depleted, skeletal protein begins to be converted to glucose for energy, resulting in a negative nitrogen balance. Within 5 to 9 days, body fat is fully mobilized to supply much of the needed energy.
- In prolonged starvation up to 97% of calories are provided by fat, and protein is conserved. Depletion of fat stores depends on the amount available, but fat stores are generally used up in 4 to 6 weeks. Once fat stores are used, body proteins, including those in internal organs and plasma, can no longer be spared and rapidly decrease because they are the only remaining body source of available energy.
- When the diet is extremely deficient in calories and essential proteins, the sodium-potassium exchange pump fails, leaving sodium inside the cell (along with water, causing cell expansion), and potassium levels in extracellular fluid rise.

The liver is the body organ that loses the most mass during protein deprivation. It gradually becomes infiltrated with fat secondary to decreased synthesis of lipoproteins. If dietary protein and other necessary constituents are not given, death will rapidly ensue.

Clinical Manifestations

Manifestations of malnutrition range from mild to emaciation and death. The most obvious clinical manifestations on physical

M

examination are apparent in the skin (dry and scaly skin, brittle nails, rashes, hair loss), mouth (crusting and ulceration, changes in tongue), muscles (decreased mass and weakness), and CNS (mental changes such as confusion, irritability).

- The person is susceptible to infection. Both humoral and cell-mediated immunity are deficient. There is a decrease in leukocytes in the peripheral blood. Phagocytosis is altered as a result of the lack of energy necessary to drive the process. Many malnourished people are also anemic.

Diagnostic Studies

- Serum albumin, prealbumin, and transferrin levels are decreased.
- C-reactive protein (CRP) and serum potassium are often elevated.
- RBC count and hemoglobin (Hgb) levels indicate the presence and degree of anemia.
- WBC count and total lymphocyte count are decreased.
- Liver enzyme studies may be elevated.
- Waist circumference and hip-to-waist ratio help evaluate the response to therapy.

Nursing and Collaborative Care

Nutritional screening identifies individuals who are malnourished or at risk for malnutrition and to determine if a more detailed nutritional assessment is necessary. Hospital-specific screening tools based on common admission assessment criteria include history of weight loss, prior intake before admission, use of nutritional support, chewing or swallowing issues, and skin breakdown.

Across all care settings, be aware of the patient's nutritional status. Obtaining an accurate measure of body weight and height and recording this information are critical components of this assessment. *Body mass index* (BMI) is a measure of weight for height (see Fig. 41-2, Lewis et al.: *Medical-Surgical Nursing*, ed. 9, p. 907). BMIs outside the normal weight range are associated with increased morbidity and mortality.

Goals

The patient with malnutrition will gain weight (particularly muscle mass), consume a specified number of calories per day (with a diet individualized for the patient), and have no adverse consequences related to malnutrition or nutritional therapies.

Nursing Diagnoses

- Imbalanced nutrition: less than body requirements
- Feeding self-care deficit
- Deficient fluid volume

- Risk for impaired skin integrity
- Noncompliance

Nursing Interventions

Identify patients who are at risk, and determine why they are at risk and how to intervene appropriately. Identify nutritional risk factors and why they might exist. In states of increased stress, such as surgery, severe trauma, and sepsis, more calories and protein are needed.

- Daily weights can give an ongoing record of body weight gain or loss. To obtain an accurate weight, weigh the patient at the same time each day, on the same scale, with the same type or amount of clothing.
- You and the dietitian can assist the patient and caregiver in the selection of high-calorie and high-protein foods.
- If the patient is unable to consume enough nutrition with a high-calorie, high-protein diet, oral liquid nutritional supplements can be added.
- Encourage the family to bring the patient's favorite food while the patient is hospitalized.

Some patients may benefit from appetite stimulants, such as megestrol acetate (Megace) or dronabinol (Marinol), to improve nutritional intake. If the patient is still unable to take in enough calories, enteral feedings may be considered (see Enteral Nutrition, p. 709). Parenteral nutrition (PN) might need to be initiated if enteral feedings are not feasible (see Parenteral Nutrition, p. 728).

▼ **Patient and Caregiver Teaching**

- Teach the patient and caregiver the importance of good nutrition and the rationale for recording the daily weight, intake, and output.
- Assess the patient and caregiver's ability to comply with the dietary instructions related to past eating habits, religious and ethnic preferences, age, income, other resources, and state of health.
- In discharge planning, ensure proper follow-up such as visits by the home health nurse and outpatient dietitian referrals.

MÉNIÈRE'S DISEASE

Description

Ménière's disease is an inner ear disease characterized by episodic vertigo, tinnitus, aural fullness, and fluctuating sensorineural hearing loss. Symptoms are incapacitating as a result of sudden, severe

M

attacks of vertigo with nausea and vomiting. Symptoms usually begin between ages 30 and 60 years.

Pathophysiology

The cause of the disease is unknown, but it results in an excessive accumulation of endolymph in the membranous labyrinth. The volume of endolymph increases until the membranous labyrinth ruptures, mixing high-potassium endolymph with low-potassium perilymph.

Clinical Manifestations

- Attacks may occur without warning or be preceded by an aura consisting of a sense of fullness in the ear, increasing tinnitus, and muffled hearing.
- The patient may report a whirling sensation and experience the feeling of being pulled to the ground ("drop attack").
- Autonomic symptoms include pallor, sweating, nausea, and vomiting.
- Duration of an attack may be hours or days, and attacks may occur several times per year. The clinical course is highly variable.
- Low-pitched tinnitus may be present continuously in the affected ear or it may be intensified during an attack.
- Hearing loss fluctuates, decreasing with each vertigo attack and eventually leading to permanent hearing loss.

Diagnostic Studies

- Audiogram results demonstrate mild, low-frequency hearing loss.
- Vestibular tests
- Glycerol test supports the diagnosis if hearing improvement occurs.

Nursing and Collaborative Care

During an acute attack, antihistamines, anticholinergics, and benzodiazepines can be used to decrease the abnormal sensation and lessen symptoms such as nausea and vomiting. Acute vertigo is treated symptomatically with bed rest, sedation, and antiemetics or antivertigo drugs for motion sickness. Diazepam (Valium), meclizine (Antivert), and fentanyl with droperidol (Innovar) may be used to reduce the vertigo. Most patients respond to the prescribed medications but must learn to live with the unpredictability of the attacks and the loss of hearing.

- During an acute attack, a patient needs reassurance that the condition is not life threatening.

- Focus on providing only essential care because movement aggravates vertigo.
- Side rails should be up and the bed in low position if the patient is in bed. Avoid the use of lights and television, which exacerbate symptoms. Have an emesis basin available because vomiting is common. Assist with ambulation because unsteadiness remains after an attack.

Management between attacks may include calcium channel blockers, diuretics, antihistamines, and a low-sodium diet.

With frequent incapacitating attacks and reduced quality of life, surgical therapy is indicated. Surgical options include endolymphatic shunt, vestibular nerve resection, and labyrinth ablation. Careful management can decrease the possibility of progressive sensorineural loss in many patients.

MENINGITIS, BACTERIAL

Description
Meningitis is an acute inflammation of the meningeal tissues surrounding the brain and spinal cord. Older adults and people who are debilitated are more often affected than is the general population. College students living in dormitories and individuals living in institutions (e.g., prisoners) are also at a high risk for contracting meningitis.

Bacterial meningitis is considered a medical emergency. If it is left untreated, the mortality rate approaches 100%. See Table 36, p. 214, for a comparison of meningitis and encephalitis.

Pathophysiology
Meningitis usually occurs in the fall, winter, or early spring and is often secondary to viral respiratory disease. *Streptococcus pneumoniae* and *Neisseria meningitidis* are the leading causes of bacterial meningitis. Organisms usually gain entry to the central nervous system (CNS) through the upper respiratory tract or bloodstream, but they may enter by direct extension from penetrating wounds of the skull or through fractured sinuses in basal skull fractures.

The inflammatory response to the infection tends to increase cerebrospinal fluid (CSF) production with a moderate increase in intracranial pressure (ICP). The purulent secretion produced by bacteria quickly spreads to other areas of the brain through the CSF.

M

- All patients with meningitis must be observed closely for manifestations of increased ICP, which is thought to be a result of swelling around the dura and increased CSF volume. (See Increased Intracranial Pressure, p. 770.)

Clinical Manifestations

Fever, severe headache, nausea, vomiting, and *nuchal rigidity* (resistance to flexion of the neck) are key signs.

- Photophobia, a decreased level of consciousness (LOC), and signs of increased ICP may also be present.
- If the infecting organism is a meningococcus, a skin rash is common and petechiae may be seen.
- Seizures occur in one third of all cases of meningitis.
- Coma is associated with a poor prognosis and occurs in 5% to 10% of patients with bacterial meningitis.

Complications

The most common acute complication of bacterial meningitis is increased ICP. Another complication is residual neurologic dysfunction. The neurologic dysfunction frequently involves the many cranial nerves.

- The optic nerve (CN II) is compressed by increased ICP. Papilledema is often present, and blindness may occur.
- When the oculomotor (CN III), trochlear (CN IV), and abducens (CN VI) nerves are irritated, ocular movements are affected. Ptosis, unequal pupils, and diplopia are common.
- Irritation of the trigeminal nerve (CN V) results in sensory losses and loss of the corneal reflex. Irritation of the facial nerve (CN VII) may produce facial paresis. Irritation of the vestibulocochlear nerve (CN VIII) causes tinnitus, vertigo, and deafness.
- Hemiparesis, dysphasia, and hemianopsia may also occur, with these signs usually resolving over time.
- Acute cerebral edema may cause seizures, optic nerve palsy, bradycardia, hypertensive coma, and death.
- Headaches may occur for months after the diagnosis of meningitis until the irritation and inflammation have completely resolved.
- A noncommunicating hydrocephalus may occur if the exudate causes adhesions that prevent the normal flow of the CSF from the ventricles. CSF reabsorption by the arachnoid villi may also be obstructed by the exudate. Surgical implantation of a shunt is the only treatment.
- A complication of meningococcal meningitis is the *Waterhouse-Friderichsen syndrome*. The syndrome is manifested by petechiae, disseminated intravascular coagulation (DIC), and adrenal hemorrhage.

Diagnostic Studies

When a patient has manifestations suggestive of bacterial meningitis, a blood culture and CT scan should be done. Diagnosis is usually verified by doing a lumbar puncture with analysis of the CSF.

- CSF protein levels are usually elevated and higher in bacterial than in viral meningitis. CSF glucose concentration is commonly decreased in bacterial meningitis but may be normal in viral meningitis. CSF is purulent and turbid in bacterial meningitis. It may be the same or clear in viral meningitis.
- CSF, sputum, and nasopharyngeal secretions are used to identify the causative organism.
- Skull x-rays may detect infected sinuses.
- CT scans may reveal increased ICP or hydrocephalus.

Collaborative Care

Rapid diagnosis based on a history and physical examination is crucial because the patient is usually in a critical state when health care is sought. When meningitis is suspected, antibiotic therapy is instituted after the collection of specimens for cultures, even before the diagnosis is confirmed. Penicillin, ampicillin, vancomycin, ceftriaxone (Rocephin), or cefotaxime (Claforan) are some commonly prescribed drugs for treating bacterial meningitis. Dexamethasone (Decadron) may also be prescribed before or with the first dose of antibiotics.

Nursing Management

Goals

The patient with meningitis will have a return to maximal neurologic functioning, resolution of infection, and control of pain and discomfort.

Nursing Diagnoses

- Decreased intracranial adaptive capacity
- Risk for ineffective cerebral tissue perfusion
- Acute pain
- Hyperthermia

Nursing Interventions

Prevention of respiratory infections through vaccination programs for pneumococcal pneumonia and influenza is very important. Early and vigorous treatment of respiratory and ear infections is important. People who have close contact with anyone who has meningitis should be given prophylactic antibiotics.

The patient with meningitis is acutely ill. The fever is high, and head pain is severe. Irritation of the cerebral cortex may result in seizures with changes in mental status and LOC dependent on the level of ICP.

M

- Assess and record vital signs, neurologic status, fluid intake and output, skin, and lung fields at regular intervals based on the patient's condition.
- Head and neck pain secondary to movement require attention. Codeine provides some pain relief without undue sedation for most patients. A darkened room and cool cloth over the eyes relieve the discomfort of photophobia. For the delirious patient, additional low lighting may be necessary to decrease hallucinations.
- All patients suffer some degree of mental distortion and hypersensitivity and may be frightened and misinterpret the environment. Make every attempt to minimize environmental stimuli and prevent injury.

If seizures occur, take protective measures. Administer antiseizure medications as ordered. Problems associated with increased ICP need to be managed (see Increased Intracranial Pressure, p. 770).

Fever must be vigorously treated because it increases cerebral edema and the frequency of seizures. Aspirin or acetaminophen may be used to reduce fever. If the fever is resistant to aspirin or acetaminophen, more vigorous means are necessary, such as a cooling blanket. If a cooling blanket is not available, tepid sponge baths with water may be effective. Because high fever greatly increases the metabolic rate, the patient should be assessed for dehydration and adequacy of intake. Supplemental feeding (e.g., enteral nutrition) to maintain adequate nutritional intake may be necessary.

- Meningitis generally requires respiratory isolation until the cultures are negative. Meningococcal meningitis is highly contagious, whereas other causes of meningitis may pose minimal to no infection risk with patient contact.
- After the acute period has passed, stress the importance of good nutrition with an emphasis on a high-protein, high-caloric diet in small, frequent feedings.
- Muscle rigidity may persist in the neck and backs of the legs. Progressive range-of-motion (ROM) exercises and warm baths are useful. Have the patient gradually increase activity as tolerated, but encourage adequate rest and sleep.
- Residual effects can result in sequelae such as dementia, seizures, deafness, hemiplegia, and hydrocephalus. Assess vision, hearing, cognitive skills, and motor and sensory abilities after recovery with appropriate referrals as indicated.
- Throughout the acute and convalescent periods, be aware of the anxiety and stress experienced by the caregiver and other family members.

METABOLIC SYNDROME

Description

Metabolic syndrome is a collection of risk factors that increase an individual's chance of developing cardiovascular disease and diabetes mellitus. It is estimated that about 25% of Americans have metabolic syndrome.

Metabolic syndrome is characterized by a cluster of health problems, including obesity, hypertension, abnormal lipid levels, and high blood glucose. Metabolic syndrome is diagnosed if an individual has three or more of the conditions listed in Table 60.

Pathophysiology

The main underlying risk factor for metabolic syndrome is insulin resistance related to excessive visceral fat (Fig. 11). Insulin resistance

Table 60 Criteria for Metabolic Syndrome*

Measure	Criteria
Waist circumference	≥40 in (102 cm) in men
	≥35 in (89 cm) in women
Triglycerides	>150 mg/dL (1.7 mmol/L)
	or
	Drug treatment for elevated triglycerides
High-density lipoprotein (HDL) cholesterol	<40 mg/dL (0.9 mmol/L) in men
	<50 mg/dL (1.1 mmol/L) in women
	or
	Drug treatment for reduced HDL cholesterol
BP	≥130 mm Hg systolic BP
	or
	≥85 mm Hg diastolic BP
	or
	Drug treatment for hypertension
Fasting blood glucose	≥110 mg/dL
	or
	Drug treatment for elevated glucose

Source: National Heart, Lung, and Blood Institute: *How is metabolic syndrome diagnosed?* Retrieved from *www.nhlbi.nih.gov/health/dci/Diseases/ms/ms_diagnosis.html*.
*Any three of the five measures are needed for a diagnosis of metabolic syndrome.

M

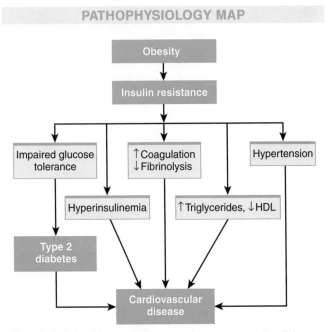

Fig. 11. Relationship among insulin resistance, obesity, diabetes mellitus, and cardiovascular disease. *HDL,* High-density lipoprotein.

is diminished ability of the body's cells to respond to the action of insulin. The pancreas compensates by secreting more insulin, resulting in hyperinsulinemia.

Other characteristics of metabolic syndrome include hypertension, increased risk for clotting, and abnormalities in cholesterol levels. The net effect of these conditions is an increased prevalence of coronary artery disease.
- African Americans, Hispanics, Native Americans, and Asians are at an increased risk for metabolic syndrome.
- Environmental factors that influence the chances of having the syndrome are the same as those involved in the development of obesity.
- Metabolic syndrome is also associated with aging.

Clinical Manifestations

Manifestations include impaired fasting blood glucose, hypertension, abnormal cholesterol levels, and obesity. Patients with this syndrome are at a higher risk of heart disease, stroke, diabetes, renal disease, and polycystic ovary syndrome.

Nursing and Collaborative Management

Lifestyle modifications are the first-line interventions to reduce the risk factors for metabolic syndrome. Management or reversal of metabolic syndrome can be achieved by reducing the major risk factors of cardiovascular disease: reducing low-density lipoprotein (LDL) cholesterol, stopping smoking, lowering BP, and reducing glucose levels. For long-term risk reduction, weight should be decreased, physical activity increased, and healthy dietary habits established.

You can assist patients by providing information on healthy diets, exercise, and positive lifestyle changes. Although there is no specific medication for metabolic syndrome, cholesterol-lowering medication and antihypertensives can be used. Metformin (Glucophage) has also been used to prevent diabetes by lowering glucose levels and enhancing the cells' sensitivity to insulin.

MULTIPLE MYELOMA

Description

Multiple myeloma, or plasma cell myeloma, is a condition in which neoplastic plasma cells infiltrate the bone marrow and destroy bone. The disease is twice as common in men as in women and usually develops after age 40 years. Although it was previously not considered curable, many patients are living 7 or more years because of the variety of treatments that can be provided throughout the course of the disease.

Pathophysiology

The cause of multiple myeloma is unknown. Exposure to radiation, organic chemicals (e.g., benzene), herbicides, and insecticides may play a role. Genetic factors and viral infection may also influence the risk of developing multiple myeloma.

Instead of a variety of plasma cells producing antibodies to fight different infections, myeloma tumors produce monoclonal antibodies (immunoglobulins). *Monoclonal* means they are all of one kind, making them ineffective and even harmful. Not only do they not fight infections, but they also infiltrate the bone marrow. These monoclonal proteins (called M proteins) are made up of two light chains and two heavy chains. *Bence Jones proteins* are the light chain part of these monoclonal antibodies. They show up in the urine in many patients with multiple myeloma.

M

Production of excessive and abnormal amounts of interleukins (IL-4, IL-5, IL-6) also contributes to the pathologic process of bone destruction. The body's normal immune response is compromised by the reduction of normal plasma cells.

- Ultimately the end-organ effects of myeloma are seen in the bones and kidneys and possibly the spleen, lymph nodes, and liver.

Clinical Manifestations

Multiple myeloma develops slowly and insidiously.

- The patient often does not manifest symptoms until the disease is advanced, at which time skeletal pain is the major symptom. Pain in the pelvis, spine, and ribs is common.
- Diffuse osteoporosis develops as the myeloma protein destroys bone. Osteolytic lesions are seen in the skull, vertebrae, and ribs. Vertebral destruction can lead to vertebral collapse with compression of the spinal cord.
- Loss of bone integrity can lead to the development of pathologic fractures. Bony degeneration causes calcium loss from bones, resulting in hypercalcemia. Hypercalcemia may cause renal, GI, or neurologic changes, such as polyuria, anorexia, confusion, and ultimately seizures, coma, and cardiac problems.
- High protein levels caused by the myeloma protein can result in renal failure from renal tubular obstruction and interstitial nephritis.
- The patient may display symptoms of anemia, thrombocytopenia, and granulocytopenia, all of which are related to the replacement of normal bone marrow with plasma cells.

Diagnostic Studies

- Pancytopenia, hyperuricemia, hypercalcemia, and elevated creatinine may be found.
- Excessive production and secretion of monoclonal (M) protein is found in blood and urine.
- The light-chain part of the M protein (called Bence Jones protein) can be detected in the urine.
- Bone marrow examination shows significantly increased numbers of plasma cells.
- Skeletal bone surveys, MRI, and/or PET and CT scans show distinct lytic areas of bone erosions; generalized thinning of the bones; or fractures, especially in the vertebrae, ribs, pelvis, and bones of the thigh and upper arms.
- The simplest measure of prognosis in multiple myeloma is based on blood levels of two markers: β_2-microglobulin and albumin. In general, higher levels of these two markers are associated with a poorer prognosis.

Collaborative Care

The therapeutic approach involves managing both the disease and its symptoms. Multiple myeloma is seldom cured, but treatment can relieve symptoms, produce remission, and prolong life. Current treatment options include "watchful waiting" (for early multiple myeloma), chemotherapy, biologic and targeted therapy, and hematopoietic stem cell transplantation (HSCT).

Ambulation and adequate hydration are used to treat hypercalcemia, dehydration, and potential renal damage. Weight bearing helps the bones reabsorb some calcium, and fluids dilute calcium and prevent protein precipitates from causing renal tubular obstruction.

Control of pain and prevention of pathologic fractures are other goals of collaborative care. Analgesics, orthopedic supports, and localized radiation help reduce skeletal pain. Surgical procedures, such as vertebroplasty, may be done to support degenerative vertebrae.

Chemotherapy with corticosteroids is usually the first treatment recommended and is used to reduce the number of plasma cells (see Chemotherapy, p. 694). High-dose chemotherapy followed by autologous HSCT has evolved as the standard of care in eligible patients. Radiation therapy is another component of treatment, primarily because of its effect on localized lesions.

Biologic and targeted therapy for multiple myeloma may include bortezomib (Velcade) and carfilzomib (Kyprolis). Drugs may be used to treat the complications of multiple myeloma. For example, allopurinol (Zyloprim) may be given to reduce hyperuricemia, and IV furosemide (Lasix) promotes renal excretion of calcium.

Nursing Management

Maintaining adequate hydration is a primary nursing consideration to minimize problems from hypercalcemia. Fluids are administered to attain a urine output of 1.5 to 2 L/day. Because of the myeloma proteins, the patient is at additional risk of renal dysfunction. You need to monitor electrolytes and fluid balance.

Because of the potential for pathologic fractures, use caution when moving and ambulating the patient. A slight twist or strain in the wrong area (e.g., weak area in patient's bones) may be sufficient to cause a fracture.

Pain management requires innovative and knowledgeable nursing interventions. Analgesics, such as nonsteroidal antiinflammatory drugs (NSAIDs), acetaminophen, or acetaminophen with codeine, may be more effective than opioids alone in

M

diminishing bone pain. Braces, especially for the spine, may also help control pain.

- Assessment and prompt treatment of infection are important.
- The patient's psychosocial needs require sensitive, skilled management. Help the patient and significant others adapt to changes fostered by chronic sickness and adjust to the losses related to the disease process, while helping to maximize functioning and quality of life.

MULTIPLE SCLEROSIS

Description

Multiple sclerosis (MS) is a chronic, progressive, degenerative disorder of the central nervous system (CNS) characterized by demyelination of the nerve fibers of the brain and spinal cord. The onset of MS is usually between 20 and 50 years of age, although it can occur in young teens and much older adults. Women are affected more often than men.

- Incidence of MS is five times higher in temperate climates (between 45 and 65 degrees of latitude), such as those found in Europe, Canada, and the northern United States, as compared with tropical regions.

Pathophysiology

The cause of MS is unknown, although research suggests that it is unlikely MS is related to a single cause. Researchers believe the disease develops in a genetically susceptible person as a result of environmental exposure, such as an infection. Multiple genes are believed to be involved in the inherited susceptibility to MS, and first-, second-, and third-degree relatives of patients with MS are at an increased risk.

Possible precipitating factors include infection, smoking, physical injury, emotional stress, excessive fatigue, pregnancy, and a poorer state of health.

MS is characterized by chronic inflammation, demyelination, and gliosis (scarring) in the CNS. The primary neuropathologic condition is an autoimmune disease caused by autoreactive T cells (lymphocytes). An environmental factor or virus in genetically susceptible individuals may initially trigger this process. The activated T cells migrate to the CNS, causing blood-brain disruption. This is likely the initial event in the development of MS. Subsequent antigen-antibody reaction within the CNS results in an inflammatory response and leads to axon demyelination.

- Initially, attacks on the neuron myelin sheaths in the brain and spinal cord result in damage to the myelin sheath. However, the nerve fiber is not affected. Transmission of nerve impulses still occurs, though transmission is slowed. The patient may complain of a noticeable impairment of function (e.g., weakness). However, the myelin can regenerate, and when it does, symptoms disappear. At that point, the patient experiences a remission.
- As ongoing inflammation occurs, the nearby oligodendrocytes are affected, and the myelin loses the ability to regenerate. Eventually damage occurs to the underlying axon. Nerve impulse transmission is disrupted, resulting in the permanent loss of nerve function.
- As inflammation subsides, glial scar tissue replaces the damaged tissue, leading to the formation of hard, sclerotic plaques. These plaques are found throughout the CNS white matter.

Clinical Manifestations

The onset is often insidious and gradual, with vague symptoms that occur intermittently over months or years. The disease may not be diagnosed until long after the onset of the first symptom.

- The disease is characterized by chronic progressive deterioration in some patients and remissions and exacerbations in others. With repeated exacerbations, the overall trend is progressive deterioration in neurologic function. Clinical manifestations vary according to areas of the CNS involved. A classification scheme with four primary patterns of MS has been developed (Table 61).
- Common manifestations include motor, sensory, cerebellar, and emotional problems.
- Motor symptoms include weakness or paralysis of the limbs, trunk, or head; diplopia; and spasticity of muscles.
- Sensory symptoms include numbness and tingling, patchy blindness (scotomas), blurred vision, vertigo, tinnitus, decreased hearing, and chronic neuropathic pain.
- Cerebellar signs include nystagmus, ataxia, dysarthria, and dysphagia.
- Severe fatigue is present in many MS patients and is aggravated by heat, humidity, deconditioning, and drug side effects.
- Bowel and bladder function can be affected if the sclerotic plaque is located in the areas of the CNS that control elimination. Problems usually include constipation and a spastic (uninhibited) bladder.
- Sexual dysfunction occurs in many people. Physiologic erectile dysfunction may result from spinal cord involvement in men. Women may experience decreased libido, difficulty with

M

Table 61	Patterns of Multiple Sclerosis
Category	**Characteristics**
Relapsing-remitting	▪ Clearly defined relapses with full recovery or sequelae and residual deficit on recovery. ▪ Approximately 85% of people are initially diagnosed with this type of multiple sclerosis (MS).
Primary-progressive	▪ Slowly worsening neurologic function from the beginning with no distinct relapses or remissions. ▪ About 10% of people are diagnosed with this type of MS.
Secondary-progressive	▪ A relapsing-remitting initial course, followed by progression with or without occasional relapses, minor remissions, and plateaus. ▪ New treatments may slow progression. ▪ About 50% of people with relapsing-remitting MS develop this type within 10 yr.
Progressive-relapsing	▪ Progressive disease from onset, with clear acute relapses, with or without full recovery. Periods between relapses are characterized by continuing progression. ▪ Only 5% of people experience this type of MS.

orgasmic response, painful intercourse, and decreased vaginal lubrication.
▪ About half of people with MS will experience some problems with cognitive function, including difficulties with short-term memory, attention, information processing, and word finding. General intellect remains unchanged and intact, including long-term memory, conversational skills, and reading comprehension.

The average life expectancy after the onset of symptoms is more than 25 years. Death usually occurs because of the infectious complications (e.g., pneumonia) of immobility or because of unrelated disease.

Diagnostic Studies

Because there is no definitive diagnostic test for MS, factors considered are history, clinical manifestations, and results of diagnostic testing.

- MRI of the brain and spinal cord may show the presence of plaques, inflammation, atrophy, and tissue breakdown and destruction.
- Cerebrospinal fluid (CSF) analysis may show an increase in immunoglobulin G (IgG) or the presence of oligoclonal banding.
- Evoked potential response testing results are often delayed as a result of decreased nerve conduction from the eye and ear to the brain.

In order to make a diagnosis of multiple sclerosis, there must be evidence of at least two inflammatory demyelinating lesions in at least two different locations within the CNS, along with evidence of damage or an attack occurring at different times (usually 1 month or more apart); in addition, all other possible diagnoses must have been ruled out.

Collaborative Care

Because there is currently no cure for MS, collaborative care is aimed at treating the disease process and providing symptomatic relief.

Drug Therapy

The initial treatment of MS is the use of immunomodulator drugs to modify the disease progression and prevent relapses. These drugs include interferon β-1b (Betaseron), interferon β-1a (Avonex, Rebif), and glatiramer acetate (Copaxone).

- Fingolimod (Gilenya) reduces MS disease activity by preventing lymphocytes from reaching the CNS and causing damage.
- Teriflunomide (Aubagio) is an immunomodulatory agent with antiinflammatory properties.
- Dimethyl fumarate (Tecfidera) provides a new approach to treating MS by activating the Nrf2 pathway. This pathway provides a way for cells in the body to defend themselves against inflammation and oxidative stress caused by MS. Dimethyl fumarate is used to treat relapsing-remitting MS.
- For more active and aggressive forms of MS, IV natalizumab (Tysabri) and mitoxantrone (Novantrone) may be used. Natalizumab increases the risk of progressive multifocal leukoencephalopathy, a potentially fatal viral infection of the brain. Mitoxantrone, an antineoplastic medication, has serious effects, including cardiotoxicity, leukemia, and infertility.
- Corticosteroids (e.g., methylprednisolone, prednisone) are the most helpful in treating acute exacerbations of the disease. They reduce edema and acute inflammation at the site of demyelination. However, these drugs do not affect the ultimate

M

outcome or degree of residual neurologic impairment from the exacerbation.

Many other medications are used to treat the symptoms of MS. Antispasmodics are used for spasticity. Amantadine (Symmetrel) and CNS stimulants (pemoline [Cylert], methylphenidate [Ritalin], and modafinil [Provigil]) are used to alleviate fatigue. Anticholinergics are used to treat bladder symptoms. Donepezil (Aricept), an acetylcholinesterase inhibitor, is used to treat cognitive impairment. Tricyclic antidepressants and antiseizure medications are used for chronic pain. Table 59-15, Lewis et al.: *Medical-Surgical Nursing,* ed. 9, p. 1430 lists drugs used for symptomatic treatment of MS.

Other Therapy

Surgical intervention (e.g., neurectomy, rhizotomy, cordotomy), dorsal-column electrical stimulation, or intrathecal baclofen (Lioresal) delivered by pump may be required if spasticity is not controlled with antispasmodics. Tremors that become unmanageable with medication are sometimes treated by thalamotomy or deep brain stimulation.

Neurologic dysfunction sometimes improves with physical therapy and speech therapy. Exercise decreases spasticity, increases coordination, and retrains unaffected muscles to substitute for impaired ones. An especially beneficial type of physical therapy is water exercise.

Nursing Management

Goals

The patient with MS will maximize neuromuscular function, maintain independence in activities of daily living for as long as possible, manage disabling fatigue, optimize psychosocial well-being, adjust to the illness, and reduce factors that precipitate exacerbations.

Nursing Diagnoses

- Impaired physical mobility
- Impaired urinary elimination
- Ineffective self-health management

Nursing Interventions

The patient with MS should be aware of triggers that may cause exacerbations or worsening of the disease. Exacerbations of MS are triggered by infection (especially upper respiratory and urinary tract infections), trauma, childbirth, stress, fatigue, and climatic changes. Assist the patient to identify particular triggers and develop ways to avoid them or minimize their effects.

- During the diagnostic phase, the patient needs reassurance that even though there is a tentative diagnosis of MS, certain diagnostic studies must be made to rule out other neurologic disorders.

The patient with recently diagnosed MS may need assistance with the grieving process.

- During an acute exacerbation the patient may be immobile and confined to bed. The focus of nursing intervention at this phase is to prevent the hazards of immobility, such as respiratory and urinary tract infections and pressure ulcers.

▼ **Patient and Caregiver Teaching**

- Focus teaching on building a general resistance to illness. This includes avoiding fatigue, extremes of heat and cold, and exposure to infection.
- Teach the patient to achieve a good balance of exercise and rest, eat nutritious and well-balanced meals, and minimize caffeine intake.
- Patients should know their treatment regimens, the side effects of drugs, and drug interactions with over-the-counter medications.
- Bladder control is a major problem for many patients with MS. Although anticholinergics may be beneficial for some patients to decrease spasticity, you may need to teach others self-catheterization.
- Increasing dietary fiber may help some patients achieve regularity in bowel habits.

The National Multiple Sclerosis Society and its local chapters can offer a variety of services to meet the needs of MS patients and their families.

MYASTHENIA GRAVIS

Description
Myasthenia gravis (MG) is an autoimmune disease of the neuromuscular junction characterized by fluctuating weakness of certain skeletal muscle groups. The peak age at onset in women is during the childbearing years. In men the peak onset of MG is between the ages of 50 and 70 years.

Pathophysiology
MG is caused by an autoimmune process in which antibodies are produced that attack acetylcholine (ACh) receptors. A reduction in the number of ACh receptor sites at the neuromuscular junction prevents ACh molecules from attaching to the receptors and stimulating muscle contraction. Anti-ACh receptor antibodies are detectable in the serum of most patients with MG. Thymic tumors are found in about 15% of all patients with MG, and abnormal thymus tissue is found in most others.

M

Clinical Manifestations

The primary feature is fluctuating weakness of skeletal muscle. Strength is usually restored after a period of rest. The muscles most often involved are those used for moving the eyes and eyelids, chewing, swallowing, speaking, and breathing. The muscles are generally the strongest in the morning and become exhausted with continued activity. By the end of the day, muscle weakness is prominent.

- In 90% of cases, the eyelid muscles or extraocular muscles are involved. Facial mobility and expression can be impaired. There may be difficulty in chewing and swallowing food. Speech is affected, and the voice often fades during long conversations.
- No other signs of neural disorder accompany MG. There is no sensory loss, reflexes are normal, and muscle atrophy is rare.
- The course of the disease is highly variable. Some patients may have short-term remissions, others may stabilize, and still others may have severe progressive involvement.
- Exacerbations of MG can be precipitated by emotional stress, pregnancy, menses, secondary illness, trauma, temperature extremes, and hypokalemia. Ingestion of drugs, including β-adrenergic blockers and psychotropic drugs, can aggravate MG.

The major complications of MG result from muscle weakness in areas that affect swallowing and breathing. An acute exacerbation of MG that results in aspiration, respiratory infection, and respiratory insufficiency is known as a *myasthenic crisis*.

Diagnostic Studies

The diagnosis of MG can be made on the basis of history and physical examination.

- Electromyogram (EMG) may show a decremental response to repeated stimulation of the hand muscles, indicative of muscle fatigue.
- The Tensilon test reveals improved muscle contractility after an IV injection of the anticholinesterase agent edrophonium chloride (Tensilon).
- If a confirmed diagnosis of MG has been made, a chest CT scan may be done to evaluate the thymus.

Collaborative Care

Drug Therapy

Drug therapy for MG includes anticholinesterase drugs, alternate-day corticosteroids, and immunosuppressants.

- Acetylcholinesterase is the enzyme that breaks down ACh in the synaptic cleft. Acetylcholinesterase inhibitors prolong the action of ACh and facilitate transmission of impulses at the neuromuscular junction. Pyridostigmine (Mestinon) is the most successful drug in this group.
- Corticosteroids (prednisone) are used to suppress the immune response. Drugs such as azathioprine (Imuran), mycophenolate (CellCept), and cyclosporine (Sandimmune) may also be used for immunosuppression.

Other Therapies

Because the presence of the thymus gland in the patient with MG appears to enhance the production of ACh receptor antibodies, removal of the thymus gland results in improvement in a majority of patients.

- Plasmapheresis and IV immunoglobulin G can yield a short-term improvement in symptoms and is indicated for patients in crisis or in preparation for surgery when corticosteroids must be avoided.

Nursing Management

Goals

The patient with MG will have a return of normal muscle endurance, manage fatigue, avoid complications, and maintain a quality of life appropriate to disease course.

Nursing Diagnoses

- Ineffective airway clearance
- Impaired verbal communication
- Activity intolerance
- Disturbed body image

Nursing Interventions

The patient with MG who is admitted to the hospital usually has a respiratory tract infection or is in acute myasthenic crisis. Nursing care is aimed at maintaining adequate ventilation, continuing drug therapy, and watching for side effects of therapy. Be able to distinguish cholinergic from myasthenic crisis because the causes and treatment of the two differ greatly (Table 62).

- As with other chronic illnesses, care focuses on the neurologic deficits and their impact on daily living.
- Teach the patient about a balanced diet that can be chewed and swallowed. Semisolid foods may be easier to eat than solids or liquids. Scheduling doses of medication so that peak action is reached at mealtime may make eating less difficult.
- Arrange diversional activities that require little physical effort and match the interests of the patient. Help the patient plan activities of daily living to avoid fatigue.

M

Table 62	Comparison of Myasthenic and Cholinergic Crises
Myasthenic Crisis	**Cholinergic Crisis**
Causes	
Exacerbation of myasthenia following precipitating factors or failure to take drug as prescribed or drug dose too low	Overdose of anticholinesterase drugs resulting in increased ACh at the receptor sites, remission (spontaneous or after thymectomy)
Differential Diagnosis	
Improved strength after IV administration of anticholinesterase drugs	Weakness within 1 hr after ingestion of anticholinesterase
Increased weakness of skeletal muscles manifesting as ptosis, bulbar signs (e.g., difficulty swallowing, difficulty articulating words), or dyspnea	Increased weakness of skeletal muscles manifesting as ptosis, bulbar signs, dyspnea; effects on smooth muscle include pupillary miosis, salivation, diarrhea, nausea or vomiting, abdominal cramps, increased bronchial secretions, sweating, or lacrimation

ACh, Acetylcholine.

▼ **Patient and Caregiver Teaching**

Teaching should focus on the importance of following the medical regimen, potential adverse reactions to specific drugs, planning activities of daily living to avoid fatigue, availability of community resources, and complications of the disease and therapy (crisis conditions) and what to do about them.

- Explore community resources such as the Myasthenia Gravis Society and MG support groups.

MYOCARDIAL INFARCTION

Myocardial infarction is part of the spectrum referred to as acute coronary syndrome. See Acute Coronary Syndrome, p. 5, for the discussion of this disorder.

MYOCARDITIS

Description

Myocarditis is a focal or diffuse inflammation of the myocardium that has been associated with viruses, bacteria, fungi, radiation therapy, pharmacologic and chemical factors, and autoimmune disorders. Coxsackie A and B viruses are the most common etiologic agents. Myocarditis is frequently associated with acute pericarditis, particularly when it is caused by coxsackievirus B strains.

Pathophysiology

When the myocardium becomes infected, the causative agent invades the myocytes and causes cellular damage and necrosis. The immune response is activated, cytokines and oxygen free radicals are released, and an autoimmune response occurs, resulting in further destruction of myocytes. Myocarditis results in cardiac dysfunction and possibly dilated cardiomyopathy (see Cardiomyopathy, p. 108).

Clinical Manifestations

Clinical manifestations of myocarditis are variable, ranging from a benign course without overt manifestations to severe heart involvement or sudden cardiac death. Fever, fatigue, malaise, myalgias, pharyngitis, dyspnea, lymphadenopathy, and nausea and vomiting are early systemic manifestations of the viral illness.

- *Early:* Cardiac manifestations appear 7 to 10 days after viral infection and include pericardial chest pain with a pericardial friction rub and effusion.
- *Late:* Cardiac signs relate to the development of heart failure and may include S_3, crackles, jugular venous distention, syncope, peripheral edema, and angina.

Diagnostic Studies

- ECG changes are often nonspecific and reflect associated pericardial involvement, including diffuse ST segment abnormalities. Dysrhythmias and conduction disturbances may be present.
- Laboratory findings are often inconclusive, with mild to moderate leukocytosis and atypical lymphocytes, increased erythrocyte sedimentation rate (ESR) and C-reactive protein (CRP) levels, elevated levels of myocardial markers such as troponin, and elevated viral titers. (Virus is generally present in tissue and fluid samples only during the initial 8 to 10 days of illness.)

M

- Histologic confirmation is through an endomyocardial biopsy. A biopsy done during the initial 6 weeks of acute illness is most diagnostic because this is the period in which lymphocytic infiltration and myocyte damage indicative of myocarditis are present.
- Echocardiography, nuclear scans, and MRI are used to evaluate cardiac function.

Collaborative Care

The treatment for myocarditis consists of managing associated cardiac symptoms.

- Digoxin improves myocardial contractility and reduces ventricular rate but is used cautiously in patients with myocarditis because of the heart's increased sensitivity to the adverse effects of this drug (e.g., dysrhythmias, potential toxicity).
- Angiotensin-converting enzyme (ACE) inhibitors and β-blockers are used if the heart is enlarged or to treat heart failure.
- Diuretics reduce fluid volume and decrease preload. If hypertension is not present, nitroprusside (Nitropress), inamrinone (Inocor), and milrinone (Primacor) may be used to reduce afterload and improve cardiac output by decreasing systemic vascular resistance.

Immunosuppressive agents may reduce myocardial inflammation and prevent irreversible myocardial damage. However, the use of these agents for the treatment of myocarditis remains controversial.

General supportive measures for the management of myocarditis include oxygen therapy, bed rest, and restricted activity. In cases of severe heart failure, intraaortic balloon pump therapy and ventricular assist devices may be required.

Nursing Management

Focus your interventions on managing the signs and symptoms of heart failure and instituting measures to decrease cardiac workload (e.g., use of semi-Fowler's position, spaced activity and rest periods, provisions for a quiet environment). Carefully monitor medications that increase the heart's contractility and decrease the preload, afterload, or both.

The patient may be anxious about the diagnosis of myocarditis and recovery. Assess the level of anxiety, institute measures to decrease anxiety, and keep the patient and caregiver informed about the therapeutic plan.

The patient who receives immunosuppressive therapy is at an increased risk for infection. Monitor for complications and provide the patient with proper infection control standards.

NARCOLEPSY

Description

Narcolepsy is a chronic neurologic disorder caused by the brain's inability to regulate sleep-wake cycles normally. During the day, people with narcolepsy experience uncontrollable urges to sleep. As the urge to sleep becomes overwhelming, individuals fall asleep for a few seconds to several minutes.

- Patients often go directly into rapid-eye-movement (REM) sleep from wakefulness, which is a unique feature of narcolepsy.
- Narcolepsy typically occurs in adolescence or early in the third decade.
- Head trauma, sudden change in sleep-wake habits, and infection may trigger symptom onset.

Narcolepsy can occur with *cataplexy,* which is a brief and sudden loss of skeletal muscle tone or muscle weakness.

Pathophysiology

The cause of narcolepsy remains unknown. It is associated with a deficiency of orexin (hypocretin), a neuropeptide linked to waking, from the destruction of orexin neurons. An autoimmune process is suspected for the neuron loss.

Clinical Manifestations

Manifestations in some patients include brief episodes of sleep paralysis, hallucinations, cataplexy, and fragmented nighttime sleep.

- Sleep paralysis is a temporary paralysis of skeletal muscles (except respiratory and extraocular muscles) that occurs in the transition from REM sleep to waking. The loss of muscle tone usually lasts less than 2 minutes.
- Unwanted episodes of REM sleep occur throughout the day. These episodes are usually of short duration, but can last for more than 1 hour, and patients feel refreshed afterward.

Diagnostic Studies

Diagnosis is based on a history of sleepiness, polysomnography (PSG), and daytime multiple sleep latency tests (MSLTs). For MSLT, patients undergo an overnight PSG evaluation followed by four or five naps scheduled every 2 hours during the next day. Short sleep latencies and onset of REM sleep in more than two MSLTs are diagnostic signs of narcolepsy.

Nursing and Collaborative Management

Management of narcolepsy is focused on symptom management. Narcolepsy cannot be cured.

- Drug treatment is combined with behavioral strategies such as cognitive behavioral therapy for patients to maintain a full, normal state of alertness.
- Provide teaching about sleep and sleep hygiene. Advise the patient with narcolepsy to take three or more short (15 minute) naps throughout the day and to avoid large or heavy meals and alcohol.
- You can play a key role in ensuring patient safety by teaching safety behaviors and encouraging adherence to the prescribed medication regimen.

Excessive daytime sleepiness and cataplexy can be controlled with drug treatment (see Table 8-8, Lewis et al.: *Medical-Surgical Nursing,* ed. 9, p. 107).

- A nonamphetamine wake-promotion drug, modafinil (Provigil), is considered first-line drug therapy.
- Other agents, including amphetamine drugs such as dextroamphetamine (Dexedrine), and methylphenidate (Concerta), are used for daytime sleepiness.
- Tricyclic antidepressant drugs such as atomoxetine (Strattera) and desipramine (Norpramin) are effective in managing cataplexy.
- Selective serotonin reuptake inhibitors (SSRIs) such as fluoxetine (Prozac) and venlafaxine (Effexor) may be prescribed for cataplexy.
- Sodium oxybate, or γ-hydroxybutyrate (Xyrem), a metabolite of γ-aminobutyric acid (GABA), may also be used.

NAUSEA AND VOMITING

Description

Nausea and vomiting are the most common manifestations of GI diseases. Although each symptom can occur independently, they are closely related and usually treated as one problem. They occur in a wide variety of GI disorders and in conditions unrelated to GI disease, including pregnancy, infection, central nervous system (CNS) disorders (e.g., meningitis), cardiovascular problems (e.g., myocardial infarction [MI], heart failure [HF]), metabolic disorders (e.g., diabetes mellitus), side effects of drugs (e.g., chemotherapy, digitalis), and psychologic factors (e.g., stress, fear).

Nausea is a feeling of discomfort in the epigastrium with a conscious desire to vomit. Anorexia usually accompanies nausea.

Vomiting is a complex act that results in the forceful ejection of partially digested food and secretions *(emesis)* from the upper GI tract.

Pathophysiology

A vomiting center in the brainstem coordinates the multiple components involved in vomiting. Neural impulses reach the vomiting center by way of afferent pathways through branches of the autonomic nervous system. Receptors for these afferent fibers are located in the GI tract, kidneys, heart, and uterus. When stimulated, these receptors relay information to the vomiting center, which initiates the vomiting reflex. The simultaneous closure of the glottis, deep inspiration with contraction of the diaphragm in the inspiratory position, closure of the pylorus, relaxation of the stomach and lower esophageal sphincter, and contraction of the abdominal muscles with increasing intraabdominal pressure force stomach contents up and out of the mouth.

In addition, the chemoreceptor trigger zone (CTZ) located in the brain responds to chemical stimuli of drugs and toxins. Once stimulated (e.g., motion sickness), the CTZ transmits impulses directly to the vomiting center.

Clinical Manifestations

When nausea and vomiting occur over a long period, dehydration can develop rapidly. Water and essential electrolytes (e.g., potassium, sodium, chloride, hydrogen) are lost. As vomiting persists, the patient may have severe electrolyte imbalances, loss of extracellular fluid volume, decreased plasma volume, and eventually circulatory failure.

- Metabolic alkalosis may result from loss of gastric HCl acid. Less frequently metabolic acidosis can occur when the contents of the small intestine are vomited.
- Weight loss may occur in a short time when vomiting is severe.

The threat of pulmonary aspiration is a concern when vomiting occurs in older or unconscious patients or those with other conditions that impair the gag reflex. To prevent aspiration, put the patient who cannot adequately manage self-care in a semi-Fowler's or side-lying position.

Collaborative Care

The goals of management are to determine and treat the underlying cause of nausea and vomiting and provide symptomatic relief. Assess the patient for precipitating factors, and describe the contents of the emesis.

It is important to differentiate among vomiting, regurgitation, and projectile vomiting. *Regurgitation* is an effortless process in which partially digested food slowly comes up from the stomach. Retching or vomiting rarely occurs before it. *Projectile vomiting* is a forceful expulsion of stomach contents without nausea and is characteristic of CNS (brain and spinal cord) tumors.

The use of drugs in the treatment of nausea and vomiting depends on the cause of the problem. Because the cause cannot always be readily determined, use drugs with caution. Using antiemetics before determining the cause can mask the underlying disease process and delay diagnosis and treatment. Many antiemetic drugs act in the CNS via the CTZ to block the neurochemicals that trigger nausea and vomiting.

▪ Drugs may include anticholinergics (e.g., scopolamine), antihistamines (e.g., promethazine [Phenergan]), phenothiazines (e.g., prochlorperazine [Compazine]), and butyrophenones (e.g., droperidol [Inapsine]). Other drugs with antiemetic effects include benzamides (metoclopramide [Reglan]) and 5-HT (serotonin) receptor antagonists (e.g., ondansetron [Zofran]). A comprehensive list of drugs used for nausea and vomiting is included in Table 42-1, Lewis et al.: *Medical-Surgical Nursing,* ed. 9, p. 926.

The patient with severe vomiting requires IV fluid therapy with electrolyte and glucose replacement until able to tolerate oral intake. In some cases a nasogastric (NG) tube and suction are used to decompress the stomach. Once symptoms have subsided, oral nutrition beginning with clear liquids is started. Water is the initial fluid of choice for rehydration by mouth. As the patient's condition improves, provide a diet high in carbohydrates and low in fat.

Alternative therapies such as acupressure or acupuncture have been shown to be effective in reducing postoperative nausea and vomiting, and herbs such as ginger and peppermint oil may be used by patients. Relaxation breathing exercises, changes in body position, or exercise may be helpful for some patients.

Nursing Management
Goals
The patient with nausea and vomiting will experience minimal or no nausea and vomiting, have normal electrolyte levels and hydration status, and return to a normal pattern of fluid balance and nutrient intake.
Nursing Diagnoses
▪ Nausea
▪ Deficient fluid volume
▪ Imbalanced nutrition: less than body requirements
Nursing Interventions
Until a diagnosis is confirmed, the patient is kept NPO and given IV fluids. An NG tube connected to suction may be necessary for

persistent vomiting or when a bowel obstruction or paralytic ileus is suspected. Secure the NG tube to prevent its movement in the nose and back of the throat because this can stimulate nausea and vomiting.

- Record intake and output, position the patient to prevent aspiration, and monitor vital signs.
- Assess for signs of dehydration, and observe for changes in the patient's physical comfort and mentation. Provide physical and emotional support, and maintain a quiet, odor-free environment.

▼ **Patient and Caregiver Teaching**
- Provide explanations for diagnostic tests and procedures.
- Instruct the patient and caregiver how to manage the unpleasant sensations of nausea, methods to prevent nausea and vomiting, and strategies to maintain fluid and nutritional intake.
- Use of relaxation techniques, frequent rest periods, effective pain management strategies, and diversional tactics can prevent or reduce nausea and vomiting.
- Cleansing the face and the hands with a cool washcloth and providing mouth care between episodes increase the person's comfort level.
- When food is identified as the precipitating cause of nausea and vomiting, help the patient identify the specific food and when it was eaten, prior history with that food, and whether anyone else in the family is sick.

A patient may be reluctant to resume fluid intake because of fear of nausea recurring. Suggest that he or she begin with clear liquids or cola beverages, Gatorade, tea or broth, dry crackers or toast, and then plain gelatin. Bland foods, such as pasta, rice, and cooked chicken, are generally well tolerated in small amounts.

NEPHROTIC SYNDROME

Description

Nephrotic syndrome results when the glomerulus of the kidney is excessively permeable to plasma protein, causing proteinuria and leading to low plasma albumin and tissue edema. Common causes include primary glomerular disease (e.g., focal glomerulonephritis), infections (e.g., hepatitis, streptococcal), neoplasms (e.g., Hodgkin's lymphoma), allergens (e.g., bee sting), drugs (e.g., nonsteroidal antiinflammatory drugs [NSAIDs]), and multisystem diseases (e.g., diabetes mellitus, systemic lupus erythematosus [SLE]).

Pathophysiology and Clinical Manifestations

The increased glomerular membrane permeability found in nephrotic syndrome is responsible for massive excretion of protein in the urine. This results in decreased serum protein and subsequent edema formation, including ascites and anasarca.

- Diminished plasma oncotic pressure from the decrease in serum proteins stimulates hepatic lipoprotein synthesis, which results in hyperlipidemia. Fat bodies (fatty casts) commonly appear in the urine.
- Immune responses, both humoral and cellular, are altered in nephrotic syndrome. As a result, infection is a major cause of morbidity and mortality.
- Calcium and skeletal abnormalities may occur, including hypocalcemia, blunted calcemic response to parathyroid hormone, hyperparathyroidism, and osteomalacia.
- With nephrotic proteinuria, loss of clotting factors can result in a relative hypercoagulable state. Hypercoagulability with thromboembolism is potentially the most serious complication of nephrotic syndrome. The renal vein is the most commonly involved site for thrombus formation. Pulmonary emboli occur in about 40% of nephrotic patients with thrombosis.

Characteristic manifestations include peripheral edema, massive proteinuria, hypertension, hyperlipidemia, and hypoalbuminemia. Laboratory findings include decreased serum albumin, decreased total serum protein, and elevated serum cholesterol.

Collaborative Care

The goals are to relieve the symptoms and cure or control the primary disease. Corticosteroids and cyclophosphamide may be used. Prednisone has been effective to varying degrees for some causes of nephrotic syndrome (e.g., membranous glomerulonephritis, lupus nephritis). Management of diabetes and treatment of edema are also important.

Management of edema includes the cautious use of angiotensin-converting enzyme (ACE) inhibitors, NSAIDs, low sodium intake (2 to 3 g/day), and a low to moderate protein diet (1 to 2 g/kg/day). Some patients may need thiazide or loop diuretics. The treatment of hyperlipidemia includes lipid-lowering agents, such as colestipol (Colestid) and lovastatin (Mevacor).

Nursing Management

The major focus of care is related to edema. Assess the edema by weighing the patient daily, accurately recording intake and output, and measuring abdominal girth or extremity size. Compare this information on a daily basis to assess the effectiveness of treatment.

Clean edematous skin carefully. Avoid trauma to the skin. Monitor effectiveness of diuretic therapy.

Patients have the potential to become malnourished from anorexia and the excessive loss of protein in the urine. Serve small, frequent meals in a pleasant setting to encourage better dietary intake.

- Because the patient is susceptible to infection, teach the patient to avoid exposure to people with known infections.
- Support for the patient, in terms of coping with an altered body image, is essential because of the embarrassment often associated with the edematous appearance.

NON-HODGKIN'S LYMPHOMAS

Description

Non-Hodgkin's lymphomas (NHLs) are a heterogeneous group of malignant neoplasms of B, T, or natural killer (NK) cell origin. NHLs affect all ages. B cell lymphomas constitute about 90% of all NHLs.

NHLs are categorized by the level of differentiation, cell of origin, and rate of cellular proliferation. A variety of clinical presentations and courses are recognized, from indolent (slowly developing) to rapidly progressive disease. NHL is the most commonly occurring hematologic cancer and the fifth leading cause of cancer death.

Pathophysiology

The cause of NHL is usually unknown. NHLs may result from chromosomal translocations, infections, environmental factors, and immunodeficiency states. Chromosomal translocations have an important role in the pathogenesis of many NHLs. Some viruses and bacteria are implicated in the pathogenesis of NHL, including Epstein-Barr virus, hepatitis B and C, *Helicobacter pylori, Campylobacter jejuni,* and *Borrelia burgdorferi.*

Environmental factors linked to the development of NHL include chemicals (e.g., pesticides, herbicides, solvents, organic chemicals, wood preservatives). NHL is also more common in individuals who have inherited immunodeficiency syndromes and who have used immunosuppressive medications (e.g., to prevent rejection after an organ transplant or to treat autoimmune disorders) or received chemotherapy or radiation therapy.

Although there is no hallmark feature in NHL, all NHLs involve lymphocytes arrested in various stages of development. *Diffuse large B cell lymphoma,* the most common aggressive lymphoma, is a neoplasm that originates in the lymph nodes, usually in the neck or the abdomen. *Burkitt's lymphoma* is the most highly aggressive type of NHL and is thought to originate from B cell blasts in the lymph nodes.

Clinical Manifestations

NHLs can originate outside the lymph nodes, and the method of spread can be unpredictable. The majority of patients have widely disseminated disease at the time of diagnosis.

- The primary manifestation is painless lymph node enlargement. Because the disease is usually disseminated when diagnosed, other symptoms are present depending on where the disease has spread (e.g., hepatomegaly with liver involvement, neurologic symptoms with central nervous system disease). NHL can also manifest nonspecifically with airway obstruction, renal failure, pericardial tamponade, and gastrointestinal complaints.
- Patients with high-grade (very aggressive) lymphomas may have lymphadenopathy and constitutional ("B") symptoms, such as fever, night sweats, and weight loss.
- An overlap exists between leukemia and NHL because both involve proliferation of lymphocytes or their precursors. A leukemia-like picture with peripheral lymphocytosis and bone marrow involvement may be present in about 20% of adults with some types of NHL.

Diagnostic Studies

Diagnostic studies for NHL resemble those used for Hodgkin's lymphoma. However, because NHL is more often in extranodal sites, more diagnostic studies may be done, such as MRI to rule out central nervous system (CNS) or bone marrow infiltration, or a barium enema, upper endoscopy, or CT to visualize suspected GI involvement.

Lymph node biopsy establishes cell type and pattern. Prognosis is based on the histopathology.

Nursing and Collaborative Management

Treatment for NHL involves chemotherapy and sometimes radiation therapy (see Chemotherapy, p. 694, Radiation Therapy, p. 730). Ironically, aggressive lymphomas are more responsive to treatment and more likely to be cured. Indolent lymphomas have a naturally long course but are more difficult to treat effectively.

- Hematopoietic stem cell transplants in NHL may have benefit in certain subtypes with aggressive or refractory lymphoma
- Rituximab (Rituxan), a monoclonal antibody against the CD20 antigen on the surface of normal and malignant B lymphocytes, is used to treat NHL.

- Numerous chemotherapy combinations have been used to try to overcome the resistant nature of this disease (see Table 31-30, Lewis et al.: *Medical-Surgical Nursing,* ed. 9, p. 673).
- Complete remissions are uncommon, but the majority of patients respond with improvement in symptoms.
- Other therapies for some types of NHL include the monoclonal antibodies ibritumomab tiuxetan (Zevalin) and tositumomab (Bexxar).
- For more diffuse disease, treatment may include phototherapy, α-interferon, oral bexarotene (Targretin), vorinostat (Zolinza), or denileukin diftitox (Ontak).

Nursing care for patients with NHL is similar to that for Hodgkin's lymphoma. It is largely based on managing problems related to the disease (pain, spinal cord compression, tumor lysis syndrome), pancytopenia, and other effects of therapy.

- The patient undergoing external beam radiation therapy has special nursing needs. The skin in the radiation field requires attention. Concepts related to safety issues regarding radiation therapy are important in the plan of care (see Chapter 16, Lewis et al.: *Medical-Surgical Nursing,* ed. 9).
- Psychosocial considerations are important. Help the patient and family understand the disease, treatment, and expected and potential side effects.
- As in Hodgkin's lymphoma, evaluation of patients with NHL for long-term effects of therapy is important because the delayed consequences of disease and treatment may not become apparent for many years.

OBESITY

Description

Obesity is an excessively high amount of body fat or adipose tissue. Obesity is a major health problem because it increases the risk of numerous other diseases such as diabetes and cancer.

Currently, more than 35% of adults in the United States are obese. The highest prevalence of obesity occurs between ages 40 and 59 for women and after 60 years of age for men.

Obesity in adulthood is often a problem that begins in childhood or adolescence. Nearly one third of children and teens are currently obese or overweight.

- It is estimated that almost 50% of overweight adults were overweight in childhood, and two thirds of obese children remained obese into adulthood. Reversing the childhood obesity crisis is key to addressing the overall obesity epidemic.

The most common measure of obesity is the *body mass index* (BMI). BMI is calculated by dividing a person's weight (in kilograms) by the square of the height in meters.

- Individuals with a BMI less than 18.5 kg/m^2 are considered underweight, whereas those with a BMI between 18.5 and 24.9 kg/m^2 reflect a normal body weight. A BMI of 25 to 29.9 kg/m^2 is classified as being *overweight,* and those with values at 30 kg/m^2 or above are considered *obese.* The term *severely* (morbid, extreme) *obese* is used for those with a BMI greater than 40 kg/m^2.
  - The incidence of the adult American population with a BMI greater than 25 kg/m^2 is over 68%.
- The waist-to-hip ratio (WHR) is another tool used to assess obesity. This ratio is a method of describing the distribution of both subcutaneous and visceral adipose tissue and is calculated by using the waist measurement divided by the hip measurement. A WHR less than 0.8 is optimal, and a WHR greater than 0.8 indicates more truncal fat, which puts the individual at a greater risk for health complications.
- Individuals with fat located primarily in the abdominal area *(apple-shaped body)* are at a greater risk for obesity-related complications than those whose fat is primarily located in the upper legs *(pear-shaped body).*

Pathophysiology

The cause of obesity involves significant genetic/biologic susceptibility factors that are highly influenced by environmental and psychosocial factors.

Most obese people have *primary obesity,* which is excess calorie intake over energy expenditure for the body's metabolic demands. Others have *secondary obesity,* which can result from various congenital anomalies, chromosomal anomalies, metabolic problems, or central nervous system lesions and disorders.

- Neuropeptide Y, produced in the hypothalamus, is a powerful appetite stimulant. When it is imbalanced, it leads to overeating and obesity. Hormones and peptides produced in the gut and adipocyte cells affect the hypothalamus and have a critical role in appetite and energy balance.

The two major consequences of obesity are due to the sheer increase in fat mass and the production of adipokines produced by fat cells. Adipocytes produce at least 100 different proteins. These proteins, secreted as enzymes, adipokines, growth factors, and hormones, contribute to the development of insulin resistance and atherosclerosis.

Environmental factors include greater access to prepackaged and fast foods, larger portion sizes, lack of physical activity and sedentary recreation, and high-calorie foods that may be more accessible to those of low socioeconomic status.

- The association of food with comfort, reward, pleasure, and fun is a powerful incentive for overeating.

There is a 20% to 40% increase in mortality for both men and women who are overweight in midlife. Many problems occur in obese people at higher rates than people of normal weight, including cardiovascular disease, respiratory problems, cancer, diabetes mellitus, and musculoskeletal, gastrointestinal, and liver problems.

Diagnostic Studies

- History and physical examination are done to assess the extent and duration of obesity.
- Laboratory tests of liver function, fasting glucose level, triglyceride level, and low- and high-density lipoprotein cholesterol levels assist in evaluating the cause and effects of obesity.
- Classifications of body weight and obesity are defined by BMI, standardized height-weight charts, or hip/waist ratio.

Collaborative Care

A multifaceted approach needs to be taken, with attention to nutritional therapy, exercise, behavior modification, and for some, medication or surgical intervention. Stress healthy eating habits and adequate physical activity as lifestyle patterns to develop and maintain.

- Restricting dietary intake so that it is below energy requirements is a cornerstone for any weight loss or maintenance program. A good weight loss plan should contain foods from the basic food groups (see Table 40-1, Lewis et al.: *Medical-Surgical Nursing,* ed. 9, p. 887).
- Setting a realistic and healthy goal, such as losing 1 to 2 lb/wk, should be mutually agreed on at the beginning of counseling.
- During normal plateau periods, when no weight is lost for several days to several weeks, patients need encouragement and support to prevent giving up on the weight loss plan.
- Exercise is an essential part of a weight control program. Patients should exercise daily, preferably 30 minutes to an hour. Exercise is especially important in maintaining weight loss.
- People who participate in a behavioral therapy program are more successful in maintaining their losses over an extended time than those who do not participate in such training.
- The person who is on a weight control program may be encouraged to join a support or self-help group if the support of others having the same experiences is helpful.

Drug Therapy

Medications should be part of a comprehensive weight-reduction program that includes reduced-calorie diet, exercise, and behavior modification. Drugs that increase energy expenditure (e.g., ephedrine) are not recommended or approved by the Food and Drug Administration for weight loss.

- Nutrient absorption-blocking drugs such as orlistat (Xenical) work by blocking fat breakdown and absorption in the intestine. Alli, a low-dose form of orlistat, is available for over-the-counter use.
- Lorcaserin (Belviq) is a selective serotonin (5-HT) agonist that suppresses appetite and creates a sense of satiety. Lorcaserin works by activating the serotonin receptor in the brain.
- Qsymia is a combination of two drugs, phentermine and topiramate. In overweight patients, phentermine suppresses appetite, and topiramate induces a sense of satiety.

Drugs will not cure obesity, and individuals must understand that without substantial changes in food intake and increased physical activity, they will gain weight when drug therapy is stopped. Teach patients about administration, and how the drugs fit into the overall weight loss plan. Discourage the purchase of over-the-counter diet aids except for Alli.

Surgical Therapy

Bariatric surgery is a surgical procedure that is used to treat obesity. Criteria for bariatric surgery include having a BMI of 40 kg/m^2 or a BMI of 35 kg/m^2 with one or more severe obesity-related medical complications (e.g., hypertension, type 2 diabetes mellitus, heart failure, sleep apnea).

- Bariatric surgeries are categorized as restrictive, malabsorptive, or a combination of restrictive and malabsorptive. In restrictive procedures the stomach is reduced in size (less food eaten), and in malabsorptive procedures the length of the small intestine is decreased (less food absorbed). The majority of procedures are performed laparoscopically.
- Common restrictive surgeries include adjustable gastric banding and vertical sleeve gastrectomy. These surgeries are discussed further on pp. 916 to 920 in Lewis et al.: *Medical-Surgical Nursing,* ed. 9.

The Roux-en-Y gastric bypass (RYGB) procedure is a combination of restrictive and malabsorptive surgery. This surgical procedure is the most common bariatric procedure performed in the United States and is considered the gold standard among bariatric procedures.

- This procedure, which is irreversible, involves creating a small gastric pouch and attaching it directly to the small intestine using a Y-shaped limb of the small bowel. After the procedure, food bypasses 90% of the stomach, the duodenum, and a small segment of jejunum.

- A complication of the RYGB is *dumping syndrome,* in which gastric contents empty too rapidly into the small intestine, overwhelming its ability to digest nutrients. Symptoms can include vomiting, nausea, weakness, sweating, faintness, and diarrhea.

Cosmetic surgeries may be used to reduce fatty tissue and skinfolds. These procedures include a *lipectomy* (adipectomy) to remove unsightly adipose folds and liposuction for cosmetic purposes.

Nursing Management

Goals

The overall goals are that the patient with obesity will modify eating patterns, participate in a regular physical activity program, achieve weight loss to a specified level, maintain weight loss at a specified level, and minimize or prevent health problems related to obesity.

Nursing Interventions

Together with other members of the health care team, you have a major role in planning for and managing the care of an obese patient. It is essential that you have a nonjudgmental approach in helping patients manage their problems related to obesity.

- Exploring an individual's motivation for weight loss is essential for overall success.
- Focusing on the reasons for wanting to lose weight may help patients develop strategies for a weight loss program. The supervised plan of care must be directed at two different processes: (1) successful weight loss, which requires a short-term energy deficit; and (2) successful weight control, which requires long-term behavior changes.

Preoperative care for gastric surgery includes planning for special needs of an obese patient, such as the availability of a larger sized BP cuff, hospital gown, bed, and chair. Consider how the patient will be weighed, transported through the hospital, and turned. Instruct the patient in the proper coughing technique, deep breathing, use of an incentive spirometer, and methods of turning and positioning to prevent pulmonary complications after surgery.

Postoperative care focuses on careful assessment and immediate intervention for cardiopulmonary complications, deep vein thrombosis, anastomosis leaks, and electrolyte imbalances. Facilitate patient respiratory efforts (elevating the head of the bed, turning, coughing, deep breathing); monitor for wound infection, dehiscence, and delayed healing; promote early ambulation; and monitor nasogastric

(NG) tube patency. The transfer from surgery may require many trained staff members.

- Patients experience considerable abdominal pain after surgery. Give pain medications as necessary during the immediate post-operative period.
- Several potential psychologic problems may arise after surgery. Some patients express guilt feelings concerning the fact that the only way they could lose weight was by surgical means rather than by the "sheer willpower" of reduced dietary intake. Be ready to provide support so that the patient does not dwell on negative feelings.
- Emphasize the importance of long-term follow-up care, in part because of potential complications late in the recovery period. Encourage patients to adhere strictly to the prescribed diet and to inform the health care provider of any changes in their physical or emotional condition.

OBSTRUCTIVE SLEEP APNEA

Description

Obstructive sleep apnea (OSA), also called *obstructive sleep apnea–hypopnea syndrome,* is characterized by partial or complete upper airway obstruction during sleep. *Apnea* is the cessation of spontaneous respirations lasting longer than 10 seconds. *Hypopnea* is a condition characterized by shallow respirations (30% to 50% reduction in airflow).

- Sleep apnea occurs in 2% to 10% of Americans. Risk increases with obesity, age greater than 65 years, craniofacial abnormalities that affect the upper airway, and acromegaly. Smokers are more likely to have OSA. OSA patients with excessive daytime sleepiness have increased mortality.

Pathophysiology

- Airflow obstruction occurs because (1) narrowing of the air passages with relaxation of muscle tone during sleep leads to apnea and hypopnea and (2) the tongue and soft palate fall backward and partially or completely obstruct the pharynx.
- Each obstruction may last 10 to 90 seconds. During the apneic period, hypoxemia and hypercapnia may occur, causing a brief arousal, but the patient may not fully awaken. The patient has a generalized startle response, snorts, and gasps, which causes the tongue and soft palate to move forward and the airway to open.
- Apnea and arousal cycles occur repeatedly, as many as 200 to 400 times during 6 to 8 hours of sleep.

Clinical Manifestations

Manifestations of sleep apnea include frequent arousals during sleep, insomnia, excessive daytime sleepiness, and witnessed apneic episodes. The patient's bed partner may complain about the patient's loud snoring. Other symptoms include morning headaches, personality changes, and irritability.

- Untreated sleep apnea may cause hypertension, right-sided heart failure from pulmonary hypertension, and cardiac dysrhythmias. Chronic sleep loss can lead to decreased ability to concentrate, impaired memory, failure to accomplish daily tasks, and interpersonal difficulties.

Diagnostic Studies

- Sleep and medical history
- Polysomnography. OSA is defined as more than five apnea/hypopnea events per hour accompanied by a 3% to 4% decrease in oxygen saturation.

Nursing and Collaborative Management

Conservative Treatment

Conservative home treatment for mild sleep apnea (5 to 10 apnea/hypopnea events per hour) includes sleeping on one's side rather than the back, elevating head of the bed, and avoiding sedatives or alcoholic beverages 3 to 4 hours before sleep. Because excessive weight worsens sleep apnea, refer patient to a weight loss program if indicated.

- Using a special mouth guard during sleep to prevent airflow obstruction may reduce symptoms.

Continuous positive airway pressure (CPAP) by mask is often used for patients with severe symptoms (more than 15 apnea/hypopnea events per hour). With CPAP, the patient applies a nasal mask attached to a high-flow blower (see Fig. 8-5, Lewis et al.: *Medical-Surgical Nursing,* ed. 9, p. 109). CPAP reduces apnea episodes, daytime sleepiness, and fatigue.

Surgery

If conservative measures fail, surgery may be done. Two common procedures are uvulopalatopharyngoplasty and genioglossal advancement and hyoid myotomy. Radiofrequency ablation may also be used.

- Postoperative complications include airway obstruction or hemorrhage. Patients are usually discharged within 1 day after surgery. Tell patients their throat will be sore and they may have a foul breath odor that can be reduced by rinsing with diluted mouthwash and then salt water after several days. Snoring may persist until inflammation has subsided. Follow-up of patients after surgery is important.

ORAL CANCER

Description

There are two types of *oral cancer:* oral cavity cancer, which starts in the mouth, and oropharyngeal cancer, which develops in the part of the throat just behind the mouth (called the oropharynx). *Head and neck squamous cell carcinoma* (HNSCC) is a term for cancers of the oral cavity, pharynx, and larynx and accounts for 90% of malignant oral tumors. Carcinoma of the lip has the most favorable prognosis of any oral tumor because these cancers are usually diagnosed earlier.

- The 5-year survival rate for all stages of cancer of the oral cavity and pharynx is 61%.

Pathophysiology

Although the definitive cause of oral cancer is unknown, it has a number of predisposing factors, including a diet low in fruits and vegetables, prolonged exposure to sunlight, tobacco use (cigar, cigarette, pipe, snuff), and frequent alcohol consumption. Human papillomavirus (HPV) contributes to 25% of oral cancer cases. HPV-associated oropharyngeal cancer is associated with multiple sexual partners, especially multiple oral sex partners.

Clinical Manifestations

Common manifestations include:

- *Leukoplakia,* called "smoker's patch," is a whitish precancerous lesion on the mucosa of the mouth or tongue that results from chronic irritation, especially from smoking. The patch becomes keratinized (hard and leathery) and is sometimes described as hyperkeratosis.
- *Erythroplakia,* which is a red velvety patch on the mouth or tongue, is also a precancerous lesion. More than 50% of cases of erythroplakia progress to squamous cell carcinoma.

Patients may also report nonspecific symptoms such as chronic sore throat, sore mouth, and voice changes. Some patients with oral cancer have an asymptomatic neck mass. Later symptoms of oral cancer are pain, dysphagia (difficulty swallowing), and difficulty in moving the jaw (e.g., chewing and speaking).

Cancer of the lip usually appears as an indurated, painless lip ulcer. The first sign of tongue cancer is an ulcer or area of thickening. Soreness or pain of the tongue may occur, especially on eating hot or highly seasoned foods.

- Later symptoms of tongue cancer include increased salivation, slurred speech, dysphagia, toothache, and earache.

Diagnostic Studies
- Biopsy of suspected lesion
- Oral exfoliative cytology and toluidine blue test are used to screen for oral cancer.
- Once cancer is diagnosed, CT scan, MRI, and positron emission tomography (PET) are used in staging.

Collaborative Care
Management usually consists of surgery, radiation, and/or chemotherapy. Surgery remains the most effective treatment. Many surgeries are radical procedures involving extensive resections. Some examples are hemiglossectomy (removal of one half of the tongue), glossectomy (removal of the entire tongue), and radical neck dissection (wide excision of the lymph nodes and their lymphatic channels). A tracheostomy (see Tracheostomy, p. 732) is commonly done with radical neck dissection.

Chemotherapy and radiation are used together when there are positive margins, bone erosion, or positive lymph nodes (see Chemotherapy, p. 694, and Radiation Therapy, p. 730). Chemotherapeutic agents used include 5-fluorouracil (5-FU), methotrexate, cisplatin (Platinol), carboplatin (Paraplatin), paclitaxel (Taxol), docetaxel (Taxotere), cetuximab (Erbitux), and bleomycin (Blenoxane).
- Brachytherapy with implantations of radioactive seeds may be used to treat early-stage oral cancer.

Palliative treatment may be the best management when the prognosis is poor, the cancer is inoperable, or the patient decides against surgery. If it becomes difficult for the patient to swallow, a gastrostomy may be performed to provide adequate nutritional intake, and frequent suctioning will be necessary when swallowing becomes difficult.

Nursing Management
Goals
The patient with carcinoma of the oral cavity will have a patent airway, be able to communicate, have adequate nutritional intake to promote wound healing, and have relief of pain and discomfort.
Nursing Diagnoses
- Imbalanced nutrition: less than body requirements
- Chronic pain
- Anxiety
- Ineffective health maintenance
Nursing Interventions
You have a significant role in early detection and treatment of oral cancer. Identify patients at risk (users of tobacco products,

alcoholism, poor dental care, pipe smokers) and provide information regarding predisposing factors.

- Refer any individual with an ulcerative lesion that does not heal within 2 to 3 weeks to a health care provider.
- Teach the patient to report unexplained pain or soreness of the mouth, unusual bleeding, dysphagia, sore throat, voice changes, or swelling or lump in the neck.

Preoperative care for the patient who is having radical neck dissection involves consideration of the patient's physical and psychosocial needs with a special emphasis on oral hygiene. Explanations and emotional support are of special significance and should include postoperative measures relating to communication and feeding.

Postoperative care for a radical neck dissection focuses on the maintenance of a patent airway, including tracheostomy care and observing for signs of respiratory distress. See Head and Neck Cancer, p. 264, for further discussion and teaching.

OSTEOARTHRITIS

Osteoarthritis (OA), the most common form of joint (articular) disease in North America, is a slowly progressive noninflammatory disorder of the diarthrodial (synovial) joints. Currently 27 million Americans are affected by OA, with the numbers expected to greatly increase as the population ages.

OA is not considered to be a normal part of the aging process, but aging is one risk factor for disease development. Cartilage destruction can actually begin between the ages of 20 and 30 years, and the majority of adults are affected by age 40. Few patients experience symptoms until after age 50 or 60 years, but more than half of those older than 65 years of age have x-ray evidence of the disease in at least one joint. After 55 years of age, women are more often affected than men.

- Modifiable risk factors include obesity, which contributes to hip and knee OA. Regular moderate exercise decreases the likelihood of disease development and progression. Anterior cruciate ligament injury, which is associated with quick stops and pivoting as in football and soccer, has been linked to an increased risk of knee OA. Occupations that require frequent kneeling and stooping are also linked to a higher risk of knee OA.

Pathophysiology

The pathogenesis of OA is complex and is due to genetic, metabolic, and local factors that interact and cause a process of deterioration of the cartilage. OA results from cartilage damage at the level of the chondrocytes. Progression of OA causes the normally smooth, white, translucent articular cartilage to become dull, yellow, and granular. Affected cartilage gradually becomes softer, less elastic, and less able to resist wear with heavy use.

Continued changes in the cartilage collagen lead to fissuring and erosion of the articular surfaces. Incongruity in joint surfaces creates an uneven distribution of stress across the joint and contributes to a reduction in motion.

Although inflammation is not characteristic of OA, a secondary synovitis may result when phagocytic cells try to rid the joint of small pieces of cartilage torn from the joint surface. These inflammatory changes contribute to the early pain and stiffness of OA. The pain of later disease results from contact between exposed bony joint surfaces after the articular cartilage has deteriorated completely.

Clinical Manifestations

Systemic manifestations such as fatigue or fever are not present in OA. This is an important differentiation between OA and inflammatory joint disorders, such as rheumatoid arthritis (Table 63). Manifestations of OA range from mild discomfort to significant disability.

Joints. Joint pain is the predominant symptom of OA. Pain generally worsens with joint use. In the early stages of OA, joint pain is relieved by rest. In advanced disease, however, the patient may complain of pain with rest or experience sleep disruptions resulting from increasing joint discomfort. The pain of OA may be referred to the groin, buttock, or medial side of the thigh or knee. Sitting down becomes difficult, as does rising from a chair when the hips are lower than the knees. As OA develops in intervertebral (apophyseal) joints of the spine, localized pain and stiffness are common.

Unlike pain, which is typically provoked by activity, joint stiffness occurs after periods of rest or static position. Early-morning stiffness is common but generally resolves within 30 minutes, a factor distinguishing OA from inflammatory arthritic disorders such as rheumatoid arthritis.

- Overactivity can temporarily increase stiffness. *Crepitation,* a grating sensation caused by loose particles of cartilage in the joint cavity, can also contribute to stiffness.
- OA usually affects joints asymmetrically. The most commonly involved joints are shown in Fig. 65-2, Lewis et al.: *Medical-Surgical Nursing,* ed. 9, p. 1564.

Deformity. Deformity or instability associated with OA is specific to the involved joint. For example, *Heberden's nodes* occur on the distal interphalangeal joints as an indication of osteophyte

Table 63   Comparison of Rheumatoid Arthritis and Osteoarthritis

Parameter	Rheumatoid Arthritis	Osteoarthritis
Age at onset	Young to middle age.	Usually >40 yr.
Gender	Female/male ratio is 2:1 or 3:1. Less marked sex difference after age 60.	Before age 50, more men than women. After age 50, more women than men.
Weight	Lost or maintained weight.	Often overweight.
Disease	Systemic disease with exacerbations and remissions.	Localized disease with variable, progressive course.
Affected joints	Small joints typically first (PIPs, MCPs, MTPs), wrists, elbows, shoulders, knees. Usually bilateral, symmetric joint involvement.	Weight-bearing joints of knees and hips, small joints (MCPs, DIPs, PIPs), cervical and lumbar spine. Often asymmetric.
Pain characteristics	Stiffness lasts 1 hr to all day and may decrease with use. Pain is variable, may disrupt sleep.	Stiffness occurs on arising but usually subsides after 30 min. Pain gradually worsens with joint use and disease progression, relieved with rest.
Effusions	Common.	Uncommon.
Nodules	Present, especially on extensor surfaces.	Heberden's (DIPs) and Bouchard's (PIPs) nodes.
Synovial fluid	WBC count >20,000/μL with mostly neutrophils.	WBC count <2000/μL (mild leukocytosis).
X-rays	Joint space narrowing and erosion with bony overgrowths, subluxation with advanced disease. Osteoporosis related to corticosteroid use.	Joint space narrowing, osteophytes, subchondral cysts, sclerosis.
Laboratory findings	RF positive in 80% of patients. Elevated ESR, CRP indicative of active inflammation.	RF negative. Transient elevation in ESR related to synovitis.

CRP, C-reactive protein; *DIPs,* distal interphalangeal; *ESR,* erythrocyte sedimentation rate; *MCPs,* metacarpophalangeals; *MTPs,* metatarsophalangeals; *PIPs,* proximal interphalangeals; *RF,* rheumatoid factor.

formation and loss of joint space. *Bouchard's nodes* on the proximal interphalangeal joints indicate similar disease involvement. Heberden's and Bouchard's nodes are often red, swollen, and tender. These bony enlargements do not usually cause significant loss of function.

Knee OA often leads to joint malalignment as a result of cartilage loss in the medial compartment. The patient has a characteristic bow-legged appearance and may develop an altered gait. In advanced hip OA, one of the patient's legs may become shorter because of loss of joint space.

Diagnostic Studies

- A bone scan, CT scan, or MRI may be useful to diagnose OA. X-rays also confirm disease and monitor the progression of joint damage.
- No laboratory abnormalities or biomarkers are specific diagnostic indicators. The erythrocyte sedimentation rate (ESR) is normal except in instances of acute synovitis, when minimal elevations may be noted.
- Synovial fluid analysis allows differentiation between OA and other forms of inflammatory arthritis. In OA, fluid remains clear yellow with little or no sign of inflammation.

Collaborative Care

Collaborative care focuses on managing pain and inflammation, preventing disability, and maintaining and improving joint function. Nondrug interventions are the foundation of management and should be maintained throughout the patient's treatment period. Drug therapy serves as an adjunct to nondrug treatments.

The affected joint should be rested during any periods of acute inflammation and maintained in a functional position with splints or braces if necessary. Immobilization should not exceed 1 week because joint stiffness increases with inactivity. The patient may need to modify usual activities or use an assistive device to decrease stress on affected joints. Teach the patient with knee OA to avoid prolonged periods of standing, kneeling, or squatting.

- Applications of heat and cold may help reduce complaints of pain and stiffness. Heat therapy is helpful for stiffness, including hot packs, whirlpool, ultrasound, and paraffin wax baths.
- If the patient is overweight, a weight reduction program is a critical part of the treatment plan. Help the patient evaluate the current diet to make appropriate changes. Aerobic conditioning, range-of-motion exercises, and specific programs for strengthening the quadriceps have been beneficial for many patients with knee OA.

Complementary and alternative therapies for symptom management of arthritis have become increasingly popular with patients who have failed to find relief through traditional medical care. Therapies include yoga, acupuncture, massage, guided imagery, and therapeutic touch. Nutritional supplements such as glucosamine and chondroitin may be helpful in some patients for relieving moderate to severe arthritis and improving joint mobility.

Drug Therapy

Drug therapy is based on the severity of the patient's symptoms (see Table 65-3, Lewis et al.: *Medical-Surgical Nursing,* ed. 9, pp. 1565 to 1567). The patient with mild to moderate joint pain may receive relief from acetaminophen (Tylenol). The patient may receive up to 1000 mg every 6 hours, with a daily dose not to exceed 4 g. A topical agent such as capsaicin cream (Zostrix) may also be beneficial. It blocks pain by locally interfering with substance P, which is responsible for pain impulse transmission. Other topical over-the-counter products that contain salicylates, camphor, eucalyptus oil, and menthol may also provide temporary pain relief.

For the patient who fails to obtain adequate pain management with acetaminophen, or for the patient with moderate to severe OA pain, a nonsteroidal antiinflammatory drug (NSAID) may provide greater relief.

- NSAID therapy is typically initiated in low-dose, over-the-counter strengths (e.g., ibuprofen [Motrin], 200 mg up to four times per day), with the dose increased as the patient's symptoms indicate. If the patient is at risk for or experiences GI side effects with NSAID use, supplemental treatment with a protective agent such as misoprostol (Cytotec) may be indicated.
- As an alternative to traditional NSAIDs, treatment with the COX-2 inhibitor celecoxib (Celebrex) may be considered in selected patients.

Intraarticular injections of corticosteroids may be appropriate for the patient with local inflammation and effusion. Systemic use of corticosteroids is not indicated and may actually accelerate the disease process.

- Another treatment for mild to moderate knee OA is intraarticular injections of hyaluronic acid (HA). HA is found in normal joint fluid and articular cartilage. Synthetic and naturally occurring HA derivatives (Orthovisc, Synvisc, Supartz, Euflexxa, Hyalgan) are administered in three weekly injections directly into the joint space.

Symptoms are often managed conservatively for many years, but the patient's loss of joint function, unrelieved pain, and diminished ability to independently perform self-care may prompt a need for surgery. In patients younger than 55 years of age, arthroscopic surgery for knee OA may delay the need for more serious surgery, such as a knee replacement. The main indication for arthroscopic surgery for OA is to remove debris (e.g., bits of cartilage known as loose bodies) that may be causing problems with joint motion.

Nursing Management

Goals

The patient with OA will maintain or improve joint function through a balance of rest and activity, use joint protection measures to improve activity tolerance, achieve independence in self-care and maintain optimal role function, and use drug and nondrug strategies to manage pain satisfactorily.

Nursing Diagnoses

- Acute and chronic pain
- Impaired physical mobility
- Imbalanced nutrition: more than body requirements
- Depression

Nursing Interventions

Community education should focus on decreasing modifiable risk factors for OA through weight loss and the reduction of occupational and recreational hazards. Athletic instruction and physical fitness programs should include safety measures that protect and reduce trauma to the joint structures.

The patient with OA is usually treated on an outpatient basis, often by an interdisciplinary team of health care providers that includes a rheumatologist, a nurse, an occupational therapist, and a physical therapist.

- Drugs are administered for the treatment of pain and inflammation. Nondrug pain management strategies may include massage, the application of heat (thermal packs) or cold (ice packs), relaxation, and guided imagery.
- Home and work environment modification is essential for patient safety, accessibility, and self-care. Measures include removing scatter rugs, providing rails at the stairs and bathtub, using night-lights, and wearing well-fitting supportive shoes. Assistive devices such as canes, walkers, elevated toilet seats, and grab bars reduce joint load and promote safety.
- Sexual counseling may help the patient and significant other to enjoy physical closeness by introducing the idea of alternate positions and timing for intercourse.

▼ Patient and Caregiver Teaching

Patient and caregiver teaching related to OA is an important nursing responsibility.

- Provide information about the nature and treatment of the disease, pain management, correct posture and body mechanics, and correct use of assistive devices such as a cane or walker, principles of joint protection and energy conservation, and an exercise program.

- Individualize home management goals to meet the patient's needs. Include the caregiver, family, and significant others in goal setting and teaching.
- Assure the patient that OA is a localized disease and that severe deforming arthritis is not the usual course. The patient can also gain support and understanding of the disease process through community resources such as the Arthritis Foundation's Self-Help Course *(www.arthritis.org)*.

OSTEOMALACIA

Osteomalacia is caused by a vitamin D deficiency, resulting in decalcification and softening of bones. It is an uncommon disease in the United States. This disease is the same as rickets in children except that the epiphyseal growth plates are closed in the adult.

- Vitamin D is required for absorption of calcium from the intestine. Insufficient vitamin D intake can interfere with the normal bone mineralization, causing failure or insufficient calcification of bone, which results in bone softening.
- Causes include lack of exposure to UV rays (which is needed for vitamin D synthesis), GI malabsorption, extensive burns, chronic diarrhea, pregnancy, kidney disease, and drugs such as phenytoin (Dilantin).
- Severely obese people are at higher risk for developing osteomalacia due to inadequate calcium intake, decreased physical activity, vitamin D deficiency, coexisting chronic diseases (e.g., hyperlipidemia), and the use of medications associated with these diseases (cholestyramine [Questran]).

Common clinical features are localized bone pain, difficulty rising from a chair, and difficulty walking. Other manifestations include low back and bone pain, progressive muscular weakness especially in the pelvic girdle, weight loss, and progressive deformities of the spine (kyphosis) or extremities. Fractures are common and demonstrate delayed healing.

Laboratory findings often include decreased serum calcium or phosphorus levels, decreased serum 25-hydroxyvitamin D, and elevated serum alkaline phosphatase. X-rays may demonstrate the effects of generalized bone demineralization, especially a loss of calcium in the bones of the pelvis, and the presence of associated bone deformity.

- *Looser's transformation zones* (ribbons of decalcification in bone found on x-ray) are diagnostic of osteomalacia. Significant osteomalacia may exist without demonstrable x-ray changes.

Collaborative care is directed toward the correction of the vitamin D deficiency. When vitamin D_3 (cholecalciferol) and vitamin D_2 (ergocalciferol) are used as supplements, the patient often shows a dramatic response. Calcium or phosphorus supplements may also be prescribed. Dietary ingestion of eggs, meat, oily fish, and milk and breakfast cereals fortified with calcium and vitamin D is encouraged. Exposure to sunlight (and UV rays) is also valuable, along with weight-bearing exercise.

OSTEOMYELITIS

Description

Osteomyelitis is a severe infection of the bone, bone marrow, and surrounding soft tissue. Although *Staphylococcus aureus* is a common cause of infection, a variety of microorganisms may cause osteomyelitis (Table 64).

Pathophysiology

Infecting microorganisms can invade by indirect or direct entry. The *indirect entry* (hematogenous) of microorganisms most frequently

| Table 64 | Organisms Causing Osteomyelitis |

Organism	Predisposing Problem
Staphylococcus aureus	Pressure ulcer, penetrating wound, open fracture, orthopedic surgery, vascular insufficiency disorders (e.g., diabetes, atherosclerosis)
Staphylococcus epidermidis	Indwelling prosthetic devices (e.g., joint replacements, fracture fixation devices)
Streptococcus viridans	Abscessed tooth, gingival disease
Escherichia coli	Urinary tract infection
Mycobacterium tuberculosis	Tuberculosis
Neisseria gonorrhoeae	Gonorrhea
Pseudomonas	Puncture wounds, IV drug use
Salmonella	Sickle cell disease
Fungi, mycobacteria	Immunocompromised host

affects growing bone in boys younger than 12 years old and is associated with their higher incidence of blunt trauma. Adults with vascular insufficiency disorders (e.g., diabetes mellitus) and genitourinary and respiratory infections are at higher risk for a primary infection to spread by way of the blood to the bone. The pelvis, tibia, and vertebrae, which are vascular-rich sites of bone, are the most common sites of infection.

Direct-entry osteomyelitis can occur at any age when there is an open wound (e.g., penetrating wounds, fractures) and microorganisms gain entry to the body. Osteomyelitis may also occur in the presence of a foreign body, such as an implant or an orthopedic prosthetic device (e.g., plate, total joint prosthesis).

After gaining entry into the blood, the microorganisms multiply, resulting in increased pressure because of the nonexpanding nature of most bone. This leads to ischemia and vascular compromise of the periosteum.

- The infection spreads through the bone cortex and marrow cavity, ultimately resulting in cortical devascularization and necrosis.
- The area of devitalized bone eventually separates from surrounding living bone, forming *sequestra.* The part of the periosteum that continues to have a blood supply forms new bone called *involucrum.* It is difficult for blood-borne antibiotics or WBCs to reach the sequestrum. A sequestrum may become a reservoir for microorganisms that spread to other sites, including the lungs and brain. If the sequestrum does not resolve on its own or is debrided surgically, a sinus tract may develop, resulting in chronic, purulent cutaneous drainage.

Acute osteomyelitis refers to the initial infection or an infection of less than 1 month in duration.

Chronic osteomyelitis refers to a bone infection that persists for longer than 1 month or an infection that failed to respond to an initial course of antibiotic therapy. Chronic osteomyelitis is either a continuous, persistent problem (a result of inadequate acute treatment) or a process of exacerbations and remissions. Over time, granulation tissue turns to scar tissue. This avascular scar tissue provides an ideal site for continued microorganism growth that cannot be penetrated by antibiotics.

Clinical Manifestations

Acute Osteomyelitis

Systemic manifestations include fever, night sweats, restlessness, nausea, and malaise.

- Local manifestations include constant bone pain that is unrelieved by rest and worsens with activity; swelling, tenderness, and warmth at the infection site; and restricted movement of the affected part.

- Later signs include drainage from the sinus tracts to the skin and/or fracture site.

Chronic Osteomyelitis

Systemic signs may be diminished, with local signs of infection more common, including constant bone pain and swelling, tenderness, and warmth at the infection site.

Diagnostic Studies

- Bone or soft tissue biopsy is definitive for determining the causative microorganism.
- Blood and/or wound cultures are frequently positive for microorganisms.
- Elevated WBC and erythrocyte sedimentation rate (ESR) may be found.
- X-ray signs suggestive of osteomyelitis usually do not appear until 10 days to weeks after the appearance of clinical symptoms, by which time the disease will have progressed.
- Radionuclide bone scans (gallium and indium) are helpful in diagnosis and usually positive in the area of infection.
- MRI and CT scan may be used to help identify the extent of the infection.

Collaborative Care

Vigorous and prolonged IV antibiotic therapy is the treatment of choice for acute osteomyelitis if bone ischemia has not occurred. If antibiotic therapy is delayed, surgical debridement and decompression are often necessary.

Patients are often discharged to home care with IV antibiotics delivered through a central venous catheter or peripherally inserted central catheter (PICC). IV antibiotic therapy may initially be started in the hospital and continued in the home for 4 to 6 weeks or as long as 3 to 6 months. A variety of antibiotics may be prescribed, depending on the microorganism. These drugs include penicillin, nafcillin (Nafcil), neomycin, vancomycin, and cephalexin (Keflex).

- In adults with chronic osteomyelitis, oral therapy with a fluoroquinolone (ciprofloxacin [Cipro]) for 6 to 8 weeks may be prescribed instead of IV antibiotics.
- Oral antibiotic therapy may also be given after IV therapy is complete to ensure resolution of the infection.
- Patient response to drug therapy is monitored through bone scans and ESR tests.

Surgical treatment for chronic osteomyelitis includes surgical removal of the poorly vascularized tissue and dead bone and extended use of antibiotics. Antibiotic-impregnated polymethylmethacrylate bead chains may also be implanted during surgery.

- Intermittent or constant irrigation of the affected bone with antibiotics may also be initiated.
- Hyperbaric oxygen therapy using 100% oxygen may be administered as an adjunct therapy in refractory cases of chronic osteomyelitis.

Orthopedic prosthetic devices may need to be removed. Muscle flaps or skin grafting provide wound coverage over the dead space (cavity) in the bone. Bone grafts may help to restore blood flow. Amputation of the extremity may be indicated to preserve life or improve quality of life (see Amputation, p. 677).

- Rare complications of osteomyelitis include septicemia, septic arthritis, pathologic fractures, and amyloidosis.

Nursing Management

Goals
The patient with osteomyelitis will have satisfactory pain and fever control, not experience any complications associated with osteomyelitis, cooperate with the treatment plan, and maintain a positive outlook on the disease outcome.

Nursing Diagnoses
- Acute pain
- Impaired physical mobility
- Ineffective self-health management

Nursing Interventions
Control of infections already in the body (e.g., urinary and respiratory tract, deep pressure ulcers) is important in preventing osteomyelitis. Individuals who are immunocompromised, have orthopedic devices, and/or have vascular insufficiencies such as diabetes mellitus are especially at risk.

- Instruct these patients and their families regarding manifestations of osteomyelitis and to immediately report symptoms of bone pain, fever, swelling, and restricted limb movement to the health care provider.

Some immobilization of the affected limb (e.g., splint, traction) is usually indicated to decrease pain. Carefully handle the involved limb to avoid excessive manipulation, which increases pain and may cause a pathologic fracture.

- Assess the patient's pain. Minor to severe pain may be experienced with muscle spasms. Nonsteroidal antiinflammatory drugs (NSAIDs), opioid analgesics, and muscle relaxants may be prescribed to provide patient comfort. Encourage nondrug (e.g., guided imagery, relaxation breathing) approaches to pain.
- Dressings are used to absorb the exudate from draining wounds and to debride devitalized tissue from the wound site when removed. Sterile technique is essential when changing the dressing.

The patient is frequently on bed rest in the early stages of acute infection. Good body alignment and frequent position changes prevent complications associated with immobility and promote comfort.

- Peak and trough blood levels of most antibiotics should be monitored to avoid adverse drug effects.

▼ **Patient and Caregiver Teaching**

- Teach the patient potential adverse and toxic reactions associated with prolonged and high-dose antibiotic therapy, including hearing deficit, fluid retention, and neurotoxicity, which can occur with the aminoglycosides. With cephalosporins (e.g., cefazolin [Ancef]), these reactions include hives, severe or watery diarrhea, blood in stools, and throat or mouth sores.
- Long-term antibiotic therapy can result in an overgrowth of *Candida albicans* and *Clostridium difficile* in the genitourinary and oral cavities. Instruct the patient to report any whitish yellow, curdlike lesions to the health care provider.
- If at home, instruct the patient and family on the management of the venous access device. Also teach how to administer the antibiotic when scheduled and the need for follow-up laboratory testing. Stress the importance of continuing to take antibiotics after the symptoms have subsided.
- If there is an open wound, dressing changes are often necessary. The patient and caregiver may require supplies and instruction in the technique.
- The patient and caregiver are often frightened and discouraged because of the serious nature of the disease, uncertainty of the outcome, and the high cost and lengthy course of treatment. Continued psychologic and emotional support is an integral part of nursing management.

OSTEOPOROSIS

Description

Osteoporosis, or porous bone (fragile bone disease), is a chronic, progressive metabolic bone disease characterized by low bone mass and structural deterioration of bone tissue, leading to increased bone fragility. Over 44 million people in the United States have decreased bone density or osteoporosis. One in two women and one in eight men over the age of 50 will sustain an osteoporosis-related fracture during their lifetime.

Risk factors for osteoporosis are female gender, advancing age (>65), white or Asian ethnicity, family history, low body weight, postmenopausal (estrogen deficiency), sedentary lifestyle, and a diet low in calcium or vitamin D deficiency. Low testosterone levels are a major risk factor in men.

- An initial bone scan is recommended in women before the age of 65 years old. If results are normal and the person is at low risk for osteoporosis, another scan is not needed for 15 years. Testing should start earlier and be done more frequently if a person is at high risk for fractures (e.g., low body weight, smoker, prior fractures).
- Men should be screened before the age of 70 years old and by age 50 if at high risk for fractures (e.g., low body weight, hypogonadism).

Pathophysiology

Peak bone mass (maximum bone tissue) is primarily achieved before age 20 years. It is determined by a combination of four major factors: heredity, nutrition, exercise, and hormone function. Heredity may be responsible for up to 70% of peak bone mass.

- Bone loss from midlife (age 35 to 40 years) onward is inevitable, but the rate of loss varies. At menopause, women experience rapid bone loss when the decline in estrogen production is the sharpest. This rate of loss then slows and eventually matches the rate of bone lost by men 65 to 70 years old.

Bone is continually being deposited by osteoblasts and resorbed by osteoclasts, a process called *remodeling*. Normally the rates of bone deposition and resorption are equal to each other so that the total bone mass remains constant. In osteoporosis, bone resorption exceeds bone deposition.

- Specific diseases associated with osteoporosis include inflammatory bowel disease, intestinal malabsorption, kidney disease, rheumatoid arthritis, hyperthyroidism, chronic alcoholism, cirrhosis of the liver, and diabetes mellitus.
- Many drugs can interfere with bone metabolism, including corticosteroids, antiseizure drugs (phenytoin [Dilantin]), heparin, aluminum-containing antacids, certain cancer treatments, and excessive thyroid hormones. Long-term corticosteroid use is a major contributor to osteoporosis.

Clinical Manifestations

Osteoporosis is often called the "silent disease" because bone loss occurs without symptoms. People may not know they have osteoporosis until their bones become so weak that a sudden strain, bump, or fall causes a hip, wrist, or vertebral fracture.

- The usual first signs of osteoporosis are back pain or spontaneous fractures. The loss of bone substance causes the bone to become mechanically weakened and prone to either spontaneous fractures or fractures from minimal trauma. A person who has one spinal vertebral fracture due to osteoporosis has an increased risk of having a second vertebral fracture within 1 year.

- Over time, wedging and fractures of the vertebrae produce gradual loss of height and a humped back known as *"dowager's hump,"* or *kyphosis.*

Diagnostic Studies

Osteoporosis often goes unnoticed because it cannot be detected by conventional x-ray until more than 25% to 40% of the calcium in the bone is lost.

- Serum calcium, phosphorus, and alkaline phosphatase levels remain normal, although alkaline phosphatase may be elevated after a fracture.
- Bone mineral density (BMD) measurements are used to measure bone density.
  - Quantitative ultrasound (QUS) measures bone density with sound waves in the heel, kneecap, or shin.
  - One of the most common BMD studies is dual-energy x-ray absorptiometry (DXA), which measures bone density in the spine, hips, and forearm (the most common sites of fractures resulting from osteoporosis). DXA studies are also useful to evaluate changes in bone density over time and to assess the effectiveness of treatment.
  - DXA results are reported as T-scores: The T-score is the number of standard deviations below the average for normal bone density. A T-score of >-1 indicates normal bone density. Osteoporosis is defined as a BMD of <-2.5 (at least 2.5 standard deviations) below the mean BMD of young adults.

Osteopenia is defined as bone loss that is more than normal (a T-score between -1 and -2.5), but not yet at the level for a diagnosis of osteoporosis.

Nursing and Collaborative Management

Care of the patient with osteoporosis focuses on proper nutrition, calcium and calcium supplementation, exercise, prevention of falls and fractures, and drugs. Treatment is recommended for postmenopausal women treatment who have (1) a T-score of <-2.5, (2) a T-score between -1 and -2.5 with additional risk factors, or (3) prior history of a hip or vertebral fracture.

- Determining a patient's risk of fracture due to osteoporosis can also be calculated by the Fracture Risk Assessment (FRAX) tool *(www.shef.ac.uk/FRAX).*

Prevention and treatment of osteoporosis focus on adequate calcium intake (1000 mg/day in premenopausal women and postmenopausal women taking estrogen and 1500 mg/day in postmenopausal women who are not receiving supplemental estrogen).

- If dietary intake of calcium is inadequate, supplemental calcium may be recommended. The amount of elemental calcium varies in different calcium preparations (see Table 64-15, Lewis et al.: *Medical-Surgical Nursing,* ed. 9, p. 1556).

- Most people get enough vitamin D from their diet or naturally through synthesis in the skin from exposure to sunlight. Being in the sun for 20 minutes a day is generally enough. However, supplemental vitamin D (800 to 1000 IU) is recommended for postmenopausal women, older adults, those who are home-bound, and those who get minimal sun exposure.

- Regular physical activity is important to build up and maintain bone mass. The best exercises are those that are weight bearing and force an individual to work against gravity, such as walking, weight training, stair climbing, and dancing. Walking (30 minutes, three times per week) is preferred to high-impact aerobics or running, both of which may put too much stress on the bones resulting in fractures.

Vertebroplasty and kyphoplasty are minimally invasive procedures that are used to treat osteoporotic vertebral fractures. In vertebroplasty, bone cement is injected into the collapsed vertebra to stabilize it, but it does not correct the deformity. In kyphoplasty, an air bladder is inserted into the collapsed vertebra and inflated to regain vertebral body height and then bone cement is injected.

Drug Therapy

Estrogen replacement therapy after menopause is no longer given as a primary treatment to prevent osteoporosis because of the associated increased risk of heart disease and breast and uterine cancer. If estrogen therapy is being used to treat menopausal symptoms, it will also protect the woman against bone loss and fractures of the hip and vertebrae. It is believed that estrogen inhibits osteoclast activity, leading to decreased bone resorption.

- Bisphosphonates inhibit osteoclast-mediated bone resorption, thereby increasing BMD and total bone mass. This group of drugs includes etidronate (Didronel), alendronate (Fosamax), pamidronate (Aredia), risedronate (Actonel), clodronate (Bonefos), tiludronate (Skelid), and ibandronate (Boniva). Alendronate is available as a weekly oral tablet, and ibandronate and risedronate are available as once-per-month oral tablet. Zoledronic acid (Reclast) has been approved for a once-yearly IV infusion and been shown to prevent osteoporosis for two years after a single infusion.

- Calcitonin is secreted by the thyroid gland and inhibits osteoclastic bone resorption by directly interacting with active osteoclasts. Salmon calcitonin (Calcimar) is available in intramuscular (IM), subcutaneous, and intranasal forms. When calcitonin is used, calcium supplementation is necessary to prevent secondary hyperparathyroidism.

- Another type of medication used to treat osteoporosis is selective estrogen receptor modulators, such as raloxifene (Evista). These drugs mimic the effect of estrogen on bone by reducing bone resorption without stimulating the tissues of the breast or uterus. Raloxifene may decrease breast cancer risk. Similar to tamoxifen, it blocks the estrogen receptor sites of cancer cells.

- Teriparatide (Forteo) is a portion of human parathyroid hormone that is used for the treatment of osteoporosis by increasing the action of osteoblasts. It is the first drug for osteoporosis that stimulates new bone formation rather than just preventing further bone loss.

- Denosumab (Prolia) may be used for postmenopausal women with osteoporosis who are at high risk for fractures. It is a monoclonal antibody that binds to a protein (RANKL) involved in the formation and function of osteoclasts. Denosumab is given as a subcutaneous injection every 6 months.

Medical management of patients receiving corticosteroids includes prescribing the lowest possible dose of the drug and ensuring an adequate intake of calcium and vitamin D including supplementation when osteoporosis drugs are prescribed. If osteopenia is evident on bone densitometry, treatment with bisphosphonates may be considered.

OVARIAN CANCER

Description

Ovarian cancer is a malignant tumor of the ovaries. It is the fifth leading cause of cancer deaths in women in the United States. Most women with ovarian cancer have advanced disease at diagnosis. It occurs most frequently in women between 55 and 65 years of age. Currently only 20% of ovarian cancers are diagnosed at an early stage.

Women who have mutations of the *BRCA* genes have an increased susceptibility for ovarian (and breast) cancer. The *BRCA* genes are tumor suppressor genes that inhibit tumor growth when functioning normally. Additional risk factors are presented in Table 65. Protective factors decrease the risk of ovarian cancer by

| Table 65 | Risk Factors for Ovarian Cancer |

Increased Risk	Decreased Risk
■ Family or personal history of ovarian, breast, or colon cancer ■ Personal history of hereditary nonpolyposis colorectal cancer ■ Hormone therapy ■ Mutant *BRCA* gene ■ Early menarche and late menopause ■ Increasing age ■ Nulliparity ■ High-fat diet	■ Oral contraceptive use (>5 yr) ■ Breastfeeding ■ Multiple pregnancies ■ Early age at birth of first baby

reducing the number of ovulatory cycles, and thus reduce exposure to estrogen.

Pathophysiology

The cause of ovarian cancer is unknown. About 90% of ovarian cancers are epithelial carcinomas that arise from malignant transformation of the surface epithelial cells. Germ cell tumors account for another 10%. Histologic grading is an important prognostic determinant. Tumor cells are graded according to the level of differentiation, ranging from well differentiated (grade I) to poorly differentiated (grade III) to undifferentiated (grade IV). Grade IV cells carry a poorer prognosis than the other grades.

Intraperitoneal dissemination is a common characteristic of ovarian cancer. It metastasizes to the uterus, bladder, bowel, and omentum. In advanced disease, ovarian cancer may spread to the stomach, colon, and liver.

Clinical Manifestations

Symptoms are vague in the early stages. An accumulation of fluid initially causes abdominal enlargement. Nonspecific symptoms warranting further evaluation include pelvic or abdominal pain, bloating, urinary urgency or frequency, and difficulty in eating or feeling full quickly. Women who have one or more of these symptoms, especially if they are new, persistent, or worsening, need to see their health care provider.

■ Vaginal bleeding rarely occurs, and pain is not an early symptom. Later signs are increased abdominal girth, unexplained weight loss or gain, and menstrual changes.

Diagnostic Studies

- Yearly bimanual pelvic examinations should be performed to identify the presence of an ovarian mass. Abdominal or vaginal ultrasound can be used to detect ovarian masses.
- An exploratory laparotomy may be used to establish the diagnosis and disease stage.
- For women with a high risk of ovarian cancer, a combination of serum CA-125 (a tumor marker) and ultrasound is recommended in addition to a yearly pelvic examination. CA-125 is positive in 80% of women with epithelial ovarian cancer and is used to monitor the disease.

Collaborative Care

Women identified as being at high risk based on family and health history may require counseling regarding options such as prophylactic oophorectomy and oral contraceptives.

Most patients with ovarian cancer have widespread disease at presentation. The initial treatment for all stages of ovarian cancer is surgery, which is usually a total abdominal hysterectomy and bilateral salpingo-oophorectomy with omentectomy and removal of as much of the tumor as possible (i.e., tumor debulking).

Depending on cell differentiation and cancer stage, other treatments may include intraperitoneal and systemic chemotherapy, intraperitoneal instillation of radioisotopes, and external abdominal and pelvic radiation therapy.

Chemotherapy usually consists of a combination of a platinum compound, such as cisplatin (Platinol) or carboplatin (Paraplatin), and a taxane, such as paclitaxel (Taxol) or docetaxel (Taxotere).

Nursing Management: Cancers of the Female Reproductive Tract

See Cervical Cancer, p. 119.

PAGET'S DISEASE

Description

Paget's disease (osteitis deformans) is a chronic skeletal bone disorder in which there is excessive bone resorption followed by replacement of normal marrow by vascular, fibrous connective tissue and new bone that is larger, more disorganized, and weaker. Regions of the skeleton commonly affected are the pelvis, long bones, spine, ribs, sternum, and cranium. The etiology of Paget's disease is unknown, although a viral etiology has been proposed.

Up to 40% of all patients with Paget's disease have a relative with the disorder. Compared with women, men are affected twice as often.

Clinical Manifestations

In milder forms of Paget's disease, patients may remain free of symptoms, and the disease may be discovered incidentally on x-ray or serum chemistry findings of a high alkaline phosphatase level.

- Initial manifestations are usually insidious development of skeletal pain (which may progress to severe intractable pain), fatigue, and progressive development of a waddling gait.
- Headaches, dementia, visual deficits, and loss of hearing can result with an enlarged, thickened skull. Increased bone volume in the spine can cause spinal cord or nerve root compression.

Pathologic fracture is the most common complication and may be the first indication of the disease. Other complications include osteosarcoma, osteoclastoma (giant cell tumor), or fibrosarcoma.

Diagnostic Studies

- Serum alkaline phosphatase (ALP) levels are markedly elevated (indicating high bone turnover) in advanced disease.
- X-rays may demonstrate that the normal contour of the affected bone is curved and the bone cortex is thickened, especially in weight-bearing bones and the cranium.
- Bone scans using a radiolabeled bisphosphate demonstrate increased uptake in the affected skeletal areas.

Nursing and Collaborative Management

Management is usually limited to symptomatic and supportive care and correction of secondary deformities by either surgical intervention or braces.

- Bisphosphonate drugs such as etidronate (Didronel), alendronate (Fosamax), risedronate (Actonel), and ibandronate (Boniva) are also used to retard bone resorption. Zoledronic acid (Reclast) may also be given as a bone-building drug.
- Calcium and vitamin D are often given to decrease hypocalcemia, a common side effect of bisphosphonates.
- Calcitonin therapy is recommended for patients who cannot tolerate bisphosphonate drugs. These drugs include human calcitonin (Cibacalcin) and salmon calcitonin (Calcimar).
- Pain is usually managed by nonsteroidal antiinflammatory drugs (NSAIDs).
- Orthopedic surgery for fractures, hip and knee replacements, and knee realignment may be necessary.

A firm mattress should be used to provide back support and relieve pain. The patient may be required to wear a corset or light brace to relieve back pain and provide support when in the upright position. The patient should be proficient in the correct application of such devices and know how to regularly examine areas of the skin for friction damage.

- Discourage activities such as lifting and twisting. Good body mechanics are essential. Physical therapy may increase muscle strength.
- A properly balanced nutritional program, especially as it pertains to vitamin D, calcium, and protein, is important for bone formation.
- Teach the patient preventive measures such as the use of an assistive device and environmental changes (e.g., removing scatter rugs) to prevent falls and subsequent fractures.

PANCREATIC CANCER

Description

Pancreatic cancer is the fourth leading cause of death from cancer in the United States, with the peak incidence occurring between 65 and 80 years. Most pancreatic tumors are adenocarcinomas. As the tumor grows, the common bile duct becomes obstructed and obstructive jaundice develops. Tumors starting in the body or the tail often remain silent until their growth is advanced.

The majority of cancers have metastasized at the time of diagnosis. Signs and symptoms of pancreatic cancer are often similar to those of chronic pancreatitis. The prognosis of a patient with cancer of the pancreas is poor. The majority of patients die within 5 to 12 months of the initial diagnosis, and the 5-year survival rate is less than 5%.

Pathophysiology

The cause of pancreatic cancer is unknown. Risk factors are diabetes mellitus, chronic pancreatitis, family history of pancreatic cancer, cigarette smoking, high-fat diet, and exposure to chemicals such as benzidine. Smokers are two to three times more likely to develop pancreatic cancer than nonsmokers. The risk is related to both the duration and number of cigarettes smoked.

Clinical Manifestations

Manifestations include abdominal pain (dull or aching), anorexia, rapid and progressive weight loss, nausea, and jaundice.

- The most common manifestations when the cancer occurs in the head of the pancreas are pain, jaundice, and weight loss.
- Pruritus may accompany obstructive jaundice. In general, pain is common and is related to the location of the malignancy.

Extreme, unrelenting pain is related to extension of the cancer into the retroperitoneal tissues and nerve plexuses. The pain is frequently located in the upper abdomen or left hypochondrium and often radiates to the back. It is commonly related to eating, and it also occurs at night.

- Weight loss is due to poor digestion and absorption caused by lack of digestive enzymes from the pancreas.

Diagnostic Studies

- Abdominal ultrasound, spiral CT scan, MRI, and MR cholangio-pancreatography (MRCP) are the most commonly used diagnostic imaging techniques for diagnosing and staging pancreatic cancer.
- Endoscopic retrograde cholangiography (ERCP) allows for visualization and collection of secretions and tissues from the pancreatic duct and biliary system.
- CA19-9 is elevated in pancreatic cancer and is the most commonly used tumor marker.

Collaborative Care

Surgery provides the most effective treatment, but only 15% to 20% of patients have resectable tumors. The classic surgery is a *radical pancreaticoduodenectomy* or *Whipple procedure.* This procedure is a resection of the proximal pancreas (proximal pancreatectomy), the adjoining duodenum (duodenectomy), the distal portion of the stomach (partial gastrectomy), and the distal segment of the common bile duct. An anastomosis of the pancreatic duct, common bile duct, and stomach to the jejunum is done.

- Radiation therapy alters survival rates little, but is effective for pain relief. External radiation is usually used, but implantation of internal radiation seeds into the tumor has also been used.
- The role of chemotherapy in pancreatic cancer is limited. Chemotherapy usually consists of fluorouracil (5-FU) and gemcitabine (Gemzar), either alone or in combination with agents such as capecitabine (Xeloda) or erlotinib (Tarceva). Erlotinib is a targeted therapy.

Nursing Management

Because the patient with pancreatic cancer has many of the same problems as the patient with pancreatitis, nursing care includes the same measures (see Pancreatitis, Acute, on the facing page).

- Provide symptomatic and supportive nursing care, including medications and comfort measures to relieve pain.
- Psychologic support is essential, especially during times of anxiety or depression.

- Adequate nutrition is an important part of the nursing care plan. Frequent and supplemental feedings may be necessary. Measures to stimulate the appetite as much as possible and overcome anorexia, nausea, and vomiting should be included.
- Because bleeding can result from impaired vitamin K production, assess for bleeding from body orifices and mucous membranes.
- A significant component of nursing care is helping the patient and caregiver through the grieving process.

PANCREATITIS, ACUTE

Description

Acute pancreatitis is an acute inflammation of the pancreas, with the degree of inflammation varying from mild edema to severe hemorrhagic necrosis. It is most common in middle-aged men and women, with the rate of pancreatitis three times higher in African Americans than whites.

The severity of the disease varies according to the extent of pancreatic destruction. Some patients recover completely, others have recurring attacks, and still others develop chronic pancreatitis. Acute pancreatitis can be life threatening.

Pathophysiology

Many factors can cause injury to the pancreas. In the United States the most common cause is gallbladder disease (gallstones), which is more common in women. The second most common cause is chronic alcohol intake, which is more common in men. Smoking is an independent risk factor for acute pancreatitis. Biliary sludge, which is a mixture of cholesterol crystals and calcium salts, is found in 20% to 40% of patients with acute pancreatitis. Acute pancreatitis attacks are also associated with hypertriglyceridemia (serum levels over 1000 mg/dL).

Less common causes of acute pancreatitis include trauma (postsurgical, abdominal), viral infections (mumps, HIV), penetrating duodenal ulcers, cysts, abscesses, cystic fibrosis, certain drugs (corticosteroids, sulfonamides, nonsteroidal antiinflammatory drugs [NSAIDs]), and metabolic disorders (hyperparathyroidism, renal failure). In some cases the cause is unknown (idiopathic).

- The most common pathogenic mechanism is believed to be autodigestion of the pancreas. The etiologic factors cause injury to pancreatic cells or activate pancreatic enzymes in the pancreas rather than in the intestine.

The pathophysiologic involvement of acute pancreatitis is classified as either *mild pancreatitis* (also known as edematous or interstitial) or *severe pancreatitis* (also called *necrotizing pancreatitis*).
Patients with severe pancreatitis are at high risk for developing
pancreatic necrosis, organ failure, and septic complications.

Clinical Manifestations

Abdominal pain is the predominant symptom of acute pancreatitis.
The pain is usually located in the left upper quadrant but may be in
the mid-epigastric area. The pain commonly radiates to the back
because of the retroperitoneal location of the pancreas.

- The pain has a sudden onset and is described as severe, deep,
  piercing, and continuous or steady. It is aggravated by eating
  and frequently has its onset when the patient is recumbent; it is
  not relieved by vomiting. The pain may be accompanied by
  flushing, cyanosis, and dyspnea.

Other manifestations of acute pancreatitis include nausea and
vomiting, low-grade fever, leukocytosis, hypotension, tachycardia,
and jaundice. Abdominal tenderness with muscle guarding is common. Bowel sounds may be decreased or absent. Paralytic ileus
may occur and causes marked abdominal distention. The lungs are
frequently involved, with crackles present.

- Intravascular damage from circulating trypsin may cause areas of cyanosis or greenish to yellow-brown discoloration of
  the abdominal wall. Other areas of ecchymoses are the flanks
  (*Grey Turner's spots* or *sign,* a bluish flank discoloration) and
  the periumbilical area (*Cullen's sign,* a bluish periumbilical
  discoloration).
- Shock may occur because of hemorrhage into the pancreas,
  toxemia from the activated pancreatic enzymes, or hypovolemia
  as a result of massive fluid shifts into the retroperitoneal space.

Complications

Local complications of acute pancreatitis are pseudocyst and
abscess.

- A *pancreatic pseudocyst* is an accumulation of fluid, pancreatic
  enzymes, tissue debris, and inflammatory exudates surrounded
  by a wall. Manifestations of pseudocyst are abdominal pain,
  palpable epigastric mass, nausea, vomiting, and anorexia. The
  serum amylase level frequently remains elevated. CT, MRI, and
  endoscopic ultrasound (EUS) may be used in the diagnosis. The
  cysts usually resolve spontaneously within a few weeks but may
  perforate, causing peritonitis, or rupture into the stomach or the
  duodenum. Treatment options include surgical drainage, percutaneous catheter placement and drainage, and endoscopic drainage.

- A *pancreatic abscess* is a collection of pus resulting from extensive necrosis in the pancreas. It may become infected or perforate into adjacent organs. Manifestations include upper abdominal pain, abdominal mass, high fever, and leukocytosis. Pancreatic abscesses require prompt surgical drainage to prevent sepsis.

Systemic complications of acute pancreatitis include pleural effusion, atelectasis, pneumonia, hypotension, and hypocalcemia leading to tetany.

Diagnostic Studies

- Elevations of serum amylase and lipase are primary diagnostic findings.
- Liver enzymes, triglycerides, glucose, and bilirubin are elevated with a decrease in calcium.
- Abdominal ultrasound, x-ray, or contrast-enhanced CT scan can identify pancreatic problems.
- Endoscopic retrograde cholangiopancreatography (ERCP) is used along with EUS, magnetic resonance cholangiopancreatography (MRCP), and angiography to diagnose pancreatic problems.

Collaborative Care

Goals of management for acute pancreatitis include relief of pain, prevention or alleviation of shock, reduction of pancreatic secretions, correction of fluid and electrolyte imbalances, prevention or treatment of infections, and removal of the precipitating cause, if possible.

Conservative therapy is primarily focused on supportive care, including aggressive hydration, pain management, management of metabolic complications, and minimization of pancreatic stimulation. Treatment and control of pain are very important. Morphine may be used and may be combined with an antispasmodic.

- If shock is present, blood volume replacements and expanders such as dextran or albumin may be given.

It is important to reduce or suppress pancreatic enzymes to decrease stimulation of the pancreas and allow it to rest. Usually the patient is NPO, and nasogastric (NG) suction is used to reduce vomiting and prevent gastric digestive juices from entering the duodenum. Drugs that neutralize or suppress formation of HCl in the stomach, such as antacids, histamine H_2-receptor antagonists, and proton pump inhibitors, also help suppress gastric acid secretion.

- Inflamed and necrotic pancreatic tissue is a good medium source for bacterial growth. Antibiotic therapy should be instituted early if an infection occurs.

- With resolution of the pancreatitis, the patient resumes oral intake. For the patient with severe acute pancreatitis who does not resume oral intake, enteral nutrition support may be initiated.

When the acute pancreatitis is related to gallstones, an urgent ERCP plus endoscopic sphincterotomy may be performed. This may be followed by laparoscopic cholecystectomy to reduce the potential for recurrence. Surgical intervention may be indicated when the diagnosis is uncertain and in patients who do not respond to conservative therapy. Patients with severe acute pancreatitis may require drainage of necrotic fluid collections. This can be done surgically, under CT guidance, or endoscopically. Percutaneous drainage of a pseudocyst can be performed, and a drainage tube is left in place.

Several different drugs are used to prevent and treat problems associated with pancreatitis (see Table 44-18, Lewis et al.: *Medical-Surgical Nursing,* ed. 9, p. 1032). Currently there are no drugs that cure pancreatitis.

Nursing Management

Goals

The patient with acute pancreatitis will have relief of pain, normal fluid and electrolyte balance, minimal to no complications, and no recurrent attacks.

Nursing Diagnoses

- Acute pain
- Deficient fluid volume
- Imbalanced nutrition: less than body requirements
- Ineffective self-health management

Nursing Interventions

Encourage early diagnosis and treatment of biliary tract disease, such as cholelithiasis. Encourage the patient to eliminate alcohol intake, especially if there have been any previous episodes of pancreatitis.

During the acute phase, a major focus of your care is the relief of pain. Pain and restlessness can increase the metabolic rate and subsequent stimulation of pancreatic enzymes. Assess and document the duration of pain relief. Measures such as comfortable positioning, frequent changes in position, and relief of nausea and vomiting assist in reducing the restlessness that usually accompanies the pain.

- Assuming positions that flex the trunk and draw the knees up to the abdomen may decrease pain. A side-lying position with the head elevated 45 degrees decreases tension on the abdomen and may help ease the pain.

- For the patient who is on NPO status or has an NG tube, provide frequent oral and nasal care to relieve dryness of the mouth and nose.
- Observe for fever and other manifestations of infection. Respiratory tract infections are common because the retroperitoneal fluid raises the diaphragm, which causes the patient to take shallow, guarded abdominal breaths. Measures to prevent respiratory tract infections include turning, coughing, deep breathing, and assuming a semi-Fowler's position.

Patients may require follow-up home care. Physical therapy may be needed due to loss of muscle strength. Continued care to prevent infection and detect any complications is important.

▽ **Patient and Caregiver Teaching**

- Counseling regarding abstinence from alcohol is important to prevent the patient from experiencing future attacks of acute pancreatitis and development of chronic pancreatitis. Because cigarettes can stimulate the pancreas, smoking should be avoided.
- Dietary teaching should include the restriction of fats because they stimulate the secretion of cholecystokinin, which then stimulates the pancreas. Carbohydrates are less stimulating to the pancreas, so they should be encouraged. Instruct the patient to avoid crash dieting and binge eating because these can precipitate attacks.
- Instruct the patient and caregiver to recognize symptoms of infection, diabetes mellitus, or *steatorrhea* (foul-smelling, frothy stools). These changes indicate possible ongoing destruction of pancreatic tissue.
- Teach the patient and caregiver about the prescribed regimen, including the importance of taking the required medications and following the recommended diet.

PANCREATITIS, CHRONIC

Description

Chronic pancreatitis is a continuous, prolonged, inflammatory, and fibrosing process of the pancreas. The pancreas is progressively destroyed as it is replaced by fibrotic tissue. Strictures and calcifications may also occur in the pancreas. Chronic pancreatitis may follow acute pancreatitis, but it may also occur in the absence of any history of an acute condition.

Chronic pancreatitis can be due to alcohol abuse; obstruction cause by cholelithiasis (gallstones), tumor, pseudocysts, or trauma; and systemic diseases (e.g., systemic lupus erythematosus), autoimmune pancreatitis, and cystic fibrosis.

Pathophysiology

The most common cause of obstructive pancreatitis is inflammation of the sphincter of Oddi associated with cholelithiasis (gallstones). Cancer of the ampulla of Vater, duodenum, or pancreas can also cause this type of chronic pancreatitis.

In nonobstructive pancreatitis there is inflammation and sclerosis, mainly in the head of the pancreas and around the pancreatic duct. This type of chronic pancreatitis is the most common form. In the United States, chronic pancreatitis is found almost exclusively in individuals who abuse alcohol.

Clinical Manifestations

As with acute pancreatitis, a major manifestation of chronic pancreatitis is abdominal pain. The patient may have episodes of acute pain, but it usually is chronic (recurrent attacks at intervals of months or years). The attacks may become more and more frequent until they are almost constant, or they may diminish as the pancreatic fibrosis develops. The pain is located in the same areas as in acute pancreatitis but is usually described as a heavy, gnawing feeling or sometimes as burning and cramplike. The pain is not relieved with food or antacids.

- Other manifestations include symptoms of pancreatic insufficiency, including malabsorption with weight loss, constipation, mild jaundice with dark urine, steatorrhea, and diabetes mellitus. The steatorrhea may become severe with voluminous, foul, fatty stools. Urine and stool may be frothy. Some abdominal tenderness may be found.
- Complications of chronic pancreatitis may include pseudocyst formation, bile duct or duodenal obstruction, pancreatic ascites or pleural effusion, and pancreatic cancer.

Diagnostic Studies

Confirming the diagnosis of chronic pancreatitis can be challenging and is based on the patient's signs and symptoms, lab studies, and imaging.

- Serum amylase and lipase levels may be elevated slightly or not at all.
- Serum bilirubin and alkaline phosphatase levels may be elevated.
- Mild leukocytosis and elevated sedimentation rate may be found.
- Endoscopic retrograde cholangiopancreatography (ERCP) is used to visualize the pancreatic and biliary ductal system.
- CT, MRI, MR cholangiopancreatography (MRCP), abdominal ultrasound, and endoscopic ultrasound may be used in the diagnostic work-up.

Nursing and Collaborative Management

When the patient with chronic pancreatitis experiences an acute attack, the therapy is similar to that for acute pancreatitis. At other times the focus is on the prevention of further attacks, relief of pain, and control of pancreatic exocrine and endocrine insufficiency. Sometimes large, frequent doses of analgesics are needed to relieve the pain.

- Diet, pancreatic enzyme replacement such as pancrelipase (Creon, Zenpep), and control of the diabetes are measures used to control the pancreatic insufficiency. The diet is bland, low in fat, and high in carbohydrates.
- Treatment of chronic pancreatitis sometimes requires endoscopic therapy or surgery. When biliary disease is present or obstruction or pseudocyst develops, surgery may be indicated to divert bile flow or relieve ductal obstruction.

▼ **Patient and Caregiver Teaching**

- Instruct the patient to take measures to prevent further attacks. Dietary control, along with consistency of other treatment measures such as taking pancreatic enzymes, is essential.
- Observe the patient's stools for steatorrhea to help determine the effectiveness of the enzyme replacement. Instruct the patient and caregiver to observe the stools.
- The patient must avoid alcohol and may need assistance with this problem. If the patient is dependent on alcohol, a referral to other agencies or resources may be necessary.
- If diabetes has developed, the patient needs instruction regarding testing of blood glucose levels and drug therapy (see Diabetes Mellitus, p. 175).

PARKINSON'S DISEASE

Description

Parkinson's disease (PD) is a chronic, progressive neurodegenerative disorder characterized by slowness in the initiation and execution of movement *(bradykinesia),* increased muscle tone *(rigidity),* tremor at rest, and gait disturbance. It is the most common form of *parkinsonism* (a syndrome characterized by similar symptoms).

The prevalence of PD is about 160 per 100,000 people. The diagnosis of PD increases with age, with the condition affecting about 2% of people over the age of 60 years. About 15% of those diagnosed with PD are younger than 50 years old. PD is more common in men.

Approximately 20% of PD patients have a family history of PD. Many autosomal dominant and recessive genes have been linked to the development of familial PD.

Pathophysiology

Although the exact cause of PD is unknown, a complex interplay of environmental and genetic factors is involved. Between 10% and 15% of PD patients have a family history of the disease, indicating a strong genetic basis for PD. In other people, exposure to toxins or certain viruses may trigger PD.

There are many forms of parkinsonism other than PD. Parkinsonism-like symptoms have occurred after intoxication with a variety of chemicals, including carbon monoxide and manganese (among copper miners) and the product of meperidine analog synthesis, MPTP.

Drug-induced parkinsonism can follow reserpine (Serpasil), methyldopa (Aldomet), lithium, haloperidol (Haldol), and phenothiazine (Thorazine) therapy. It is also seen following the use of amphetamine and methamphetamine.

- The pathology of PD involves the degeneration of the dopamine-producing neurons in the substantia nigra of the midbrain, which in turn disrupts the normal balance between dopamine (DA) and acetylcholine (ACh) in the basal ganglia.
- Dopamine is a neurotransmitter essential for normal functioning of the extrapyramidal motor system, including control of posture, support, and voluntary motion. Symptoms do not occur until 80% of neurons in the substantia nigra are lost.
- *Lewy bodies,* unusual clumps of protein, are found in the brains of patients with PD. It is not known what causes these bodies to form, but their presence indicates abnormal functioning of the brain.

Clinical Manifestations

Onset of PD is gradual and insidious, with an ongoing progression. Classic manifestations are a triad of tremor, rigidity, and bradykinesia. In the beginning stages, only a mild tremor, slight limp, or decreased arm swing may be evident. Later the patient may have a shuffling, propulsive gait with arms flexed and loss of postural reflexes. Some patients have a slight change in speech patterns.

- *Tremor,* often the first sign, may initially be minimal, so that the patient is the only one who notices it. This tremor is more prominent at rest and is aggravated by emotional stress or increased concentration. The hand tremor is described as "pill rolling" because the thumb and forefinger appear to move in a rotary fashion as if rolling a pill, coin, or other small object. Tremor can involve the diaphragm, tongue, lips, and jaw.

- *Rigidity* is increased resistance to passive motion when the limbs are moved through their range of motion. Parkinsonian rigidity is typified by cogwheel rigidity, or a jerky quality, as if there were intermittent catches in the movement of a cogwheel, when the joint is passively moved.
- *Bradykinesia* (slow and retarded movement) is particularly evident in the loss of automatic movements, which is secondary to the physical and chemical alteration of the basal ganglia. In the unaffected person, automatic movements are involuntary and occur subconsciously; these include the blinking of the eyelids, swinging of the arms while walking, swallowing of saliva, self-expression with facial and hand movements, and minor movement of postural adjustment. The patient with PD does not execute these movements. This lack of spontaneous activity accounts for the "old man" image with stooped posture, masked face ("deadpan" expression), drooling of saliva, and shuffling gait.
- Postural instability is common, and patients may complain of being unable to stop themselves from going forward (propulsion) or backward (retropulsion).
- Nonmotor symptoms include depression, anxiety, apathy, fatigue, pain, impotence, and short-term memory impairment. Sleep problems are common and include difficulty staying asleep at night, restless sleep, nightmares, and drowsiness or sudden sleep onset during the day.

Complications

As the disease progresses, complications may occur including motor symptoms. These include dyskinesias (spontaneous, involuntary movements), weakness, and *akinesia* (total immobility). Neurologic problems (e.g., dementia) and neuropsychiatric problems (e.g., depression, hallucinations, psychosis) may also occur. Dementia is present in up to 70% of patients with PD and is associated with an increase in mortality.

- Swallowing becomes more difficult *(dysphagia);* malnutrition or aspiration may result.
- General debilitation may lead to pneumonia, urinary tract infections, and skin breakdown.
- Orthostatic hypotension may occur in some patients and, along with the loss of postural reflexes, may result in falls or other injury.

Diagnostic Studies

Because there is no specific diagnostic test for PD, the diagnosis is based on the history and clinical features.

- A definitive diagnosis can be made only when at least two of the three characteristic signs of the classic triad are present: tremor, rigidity, and bradykinesia.
- The ultimate confirmation is a positive response to antiparkinsonian drugs.

Collaborative Care

Because there is no cure, management is aimed at relieving symptoms.

Drug Therapy

Drug therapy for PD is aimed at correcting the imbalance of central nervous system (CNS) neurotransmitters. Antiparkinsonian drugs either enhance the release or supply of DA (dopaminergic) or antagonize or block the effects of ACh in the striatum. Levodopa with carbidopa (Sinemet) is often the first drug used. Levodopa is a precursor of dopamine and can cross the blood-brain barrier. It is converted to dopamine in the basal ganglia. Prolonged use of levodopa can often result in dyskinesias and "off/on" periods when the medication will unpredictably start or stop working.

Some health care providers believe that, after a few years of therapy, the effectiveness of Sinemet wears off. Therefore they prefer to initiate therapy with a DA receptor agonist instead. These drugs include bromocriptine (Parlodel), pergolide (Permax), ropinirole (Requip), and pramipexole (Mirapex). These drugs directly stimulate DA receptors. When more moderate to severe symptoms are present, levodopa with carbidopa (Sinemet) is added to the drug regimen.

- Anticholinergic drugs such as trihexyphenidyl (Artane) and benztropine (Cogentin) may also be used. These drugs act by decreasing the activity of acetylcholine, thus providing balance between cholinergic and dopaminergic actions.
- Selegiline (Eldepryl) and rasagiline (Azilect), monoamine oxidase type B (MAO-B) inhibitors, are sometimes used with Sinemet. By inhibiting MAO-B, the degradative enzyme for DA, these agents increase the levels of DA and prolong the half-life of levodopa. Rasagiline can also be used alone as therapy in early PD.
- Entacapone (Comtan) and tolcapone (Tasmar) block the enzyme catechol O-methyl transferase (COMT), which breaks down levodopa in the peripheral circulation, thus prolonging the effect of Sinemet. These drugs are used only as adjuncts to levodopa.
- The antiviral agent amantadine (Symmetrel) is also an effective antiparkinsonian drug.

- Rivastigmine (Exelon) or donepezil (Aricept) is used to treat mild to moderate Parkinson's dementia. Amitriptyline (Elavil) may be used to treat depression.

See Table 59-18 in Lewis et al.: *Medical-Surgical Nursing,* ed. 9, p. 1435, which summarizes drugs commonly used in Parkinson's disease.

Surgical Therapy

Surgical procedures are aimed at relieving symptoms of PD and are usually used in patients who are unresponsive to drug therapy or who have developed severe motor complications. Procedures fall into three categories: ablation (destruction), deep brain stimulation (DBS), and transplantation.

- Ablative procedures have been replaced by DBS, which involves placing an electrode in the thalamus, globus pallidus, or subthalamic nucleus that delivers a specific current that the targeted brain location. Ablative and DBS procedures work by reducing the increased neuronal activity produced by DA depletion. DBS has been shown to improve motor function and reduce dyskinesia and medication usage.

Transplantation of fetal neural tissue into the basal ganglia is designed to provide DA-producing cells in the brain. This form of therapy is still in experimental stages.

Nutritional Therapy

Diet is of major importance because malnutrition and constipation can be serious consequences of inadequate nutrition. Patients who have dysphagia and bradykinesia need appetizing foods that are easily chewed and swallowed. The diet should contain adequate roughage and fruit to avoid constipation. Provide ample time for eating to avoid frustration.

Nursing Management

Goals

The patient with PD will maximize neurologic function, maintain independence in activities of daily living for as long as possible, and optimize psychosocial well-being.

Nursing Diagnoses

- Impaired physical mobility
- Impaired swallowing
- Imbalanced nutrition: less than body requirements

Nursing Interventions

Promotion of physical exercise and a well-balanced diet are major concerns for nursing care. Exercise can limit the consequences of decreased mobility such as muscle atrophy, contractures, and constipation. Overall muscle tone as well as specific exercises to strengthen the muscles involved with speaking and swallowing should be included.

Because PD is a chronic degenerative disorder with no acute exacerbations, focus on teaching and nursing care directed toward the maintenance of good health, encouragement of independence, and avoidance of complications such as contractures.

▼ **Patient and Caregiver Teaching**

- For patients who are at risk for falling and tend to "freeze" while walking, have them think consciously about stepping over imaginary lines on the floor, drop rice kernels and step over them, rock from side to side, lift the toes when stepping, or take one step backward and two steps forward.
- Teach the patient to facilitate getting out of a chair by using an upright chair with arms and placing the back legs on small (2-inch) blocks.
- Encourage environmental alterations, such as removing rugs and excess furniture to avoid stumbling.
- Clothing can be simplified by the use of slip-on shoes and Velcro hook-and-loop fasteners or zippers on clothing instead of buttons and hooks.
- An elevated toilet seat can facilitate getting on and off the toilet.
- As the disease progresses, the impact on the psychologic well-being of the patient also increases. Assist the patient through listening, providing education, encouraging social interactions, and referral to the American Parkinson Disease Association *(www.apdaparkinson.org)*.

Family caregivers (e.g., spouse, children) care for the majority of patients with PD, and as the disease progresses, the caregiver burden increases. This increase has been associated with decreases in caregiver physical and mental health. Strategies to reduce caregiver burden are described in Lewis et al.: *Medical-Surgical Nursing,* ed. 9, pp. 51-52.

PELVIC INFLAMMATORY DISEASE

Description
Pelvic inflammatory disease (PID) is an infectious condition of the pelvic cavity that may involve the fallopian tubes (salpingitis), ovaries (oophoritis), and pelvic peritoneum (peritonitis). PID may be "silent" with no symptoms, whereas other women may be in acute distress. Silent PID is a major cause of infertility. PID may also be a cause of chronic pelvic pain (see Pelvic Pain, Chronic, p. 483). In the United States it is estimated that each year, 1 million women experience an acute episode of PID.

Pathophysiology

PID is often the result of untreated cervicitis. The organism infecting the cervix ascends higher into the uterus, fallopian tubes, ovaries, and peritoneal cavity. The most frequent causative organisms are *Chlamydia trachomatis* and *Neisseria gonorrhoeae.* These organisms, as well as mycoplasma, streptococci, and anaerobes, gain entrance during sexual intercourse or after pregnancy termination, pelvic surgery, or childbirth.

Clinical Manifestations

Women with PID usually go to a health care provider because of lower abdominal pain.

- The pain typically starts gradually and then becomes constant. The intensity may vary from mild to severe. Movement such as walking and intercourse increases the pain.
- Spotting after intercourse and purulent cervical or vaginal discharge are common.
- Fever and chills may also be present.
- Women with less acute symptoms often notice increased cramping pain with menses, irregular bleeding, and some pain with intercourse. Women who have mild symptoms may go untreated either because they did not seek care or the health care provider misdiagnosed their complaints.

Complications

Immediate complications of PID include septic shock and *Fitz-Hugh-Curtis syndrome,* which occurs when PID spreads to the liver and causes acute perihepatitis. The patient has symptoms of right upper quadrant pain, but liver function tests are normal. Tubo-ovarian abscesses may "leak" or rupture, resulting in pelvic or generalized peritonitis.

- As the general circulation is flooded with bacterial endotoxins from the infected areas, septic shock may result. Embolisms may occur as the result of thrombophlebitis of the pelvic veins.

PID can cause adhesions and strictures to develop in the fallopian tubes. After one episode of PID, the risk of having an ectopic pregnancy increases 10-fold. Further damage can obstruct the fallopian tubes and cause infertility.

Diagnostic Studies

A pelvic examination is used to assist in the diagnosis of PID. Women with PID have lower abdominal tenderness, bilateral adnexal tenderness, and positive cervical motion tenderness.

- Diagnostic criteria may also include fever and abnormal vaginal or cervical discharge.

- Cultures for gonorrhea and chlamydia are also obtained.
- A pregnancy test is done to rule out ectopic pregnancy.
- When pain or obesity compromises the pelvic examination and a tubo-ovarian abscess may be present, a vaginal ultrasound is indicated.

Collaborative Care

Treatment of PID is usually on an outpatient basis. The patient is given a combination of antibiotics such as cefoxitin (Mefoxin) and doxycycline (Vibramycin) to provide broad coverage against the causative organisms. The patient must not have intercourse for 3 weeks. Her partner(s) must be examined and treated. Physical rest and oral fluids are also important. Reevaluation in 48 to 72 hours, even if symptoms are improving, is essential.

If outpatient treatment is not successful or the patient is acutely ill or in severe pain, hospital admission is indicated. Maximum doses of parenteral antibiotics are then given with analgesics to relieve pain and IV fluids to prevent dehydration. Corticosteroids may be added to the antibiotic regimen to reduce inflammation. Application of heat to the lower abdomen or sitz baths may be used to improve circulation and decrease pain. Bed rest in semi-Fowler's position promotes pelvic cavity drainage and may prevent the development of abscesses.

An indication for surgery is the presence of abscesses that fail to resolve with IV antibiotics. The abscesses may be drained by laparotomy or laparoscopy. Childbearing function in young women is preserved whenever possible.

Nursing Management

Prevention, early recognition, and prompt treatment of vaginal and cervical infections can help prevent PID and its serious complications. Provide information regarding factors that place a woman at increased risk for PID. Urge women to seek medical attention for any unusual vaginal discharge or possible infection of their reproductive organs.

During hospitalization for PID, you have an important role in implementing drug therapy, monitoring the patient's health status, and providing symptom relief and patient teaching. Explain the need for limited activity, being in a semi-Fowler's position, and increased fluid intake. Assess the degree of abdominal pain to provide information about the effectiveness of drug therapy.

- The patient may feel guilty about having PID, especially if it was associated with a sexually transmitted infection. She may also be concerned about the complications associated with PID, such as adhesions and strictures of the fallopian tubes, infertility, and the increased incidence of ectopic pregnancy. Discuss with the patient her feelings and concerns to assist her to cope more effectively with them.

PELVIC PAIN, CHRONIC

Description

Chronic pelvic pain refers to pain in the pelvic region (below the umbilicus and between the hips) that lasts 6 months or longer. It accounts for 10% of all visits to gynecologists and is the reason for 20% to 30% of all laparoscopies. Up to one third of women who have pelvic inflammatory disease (PID) have chronic pelvic pain. The cause of chronic pelvic pain is often hard to find.

- Gynecologic etiologies include dysmenorrhea, endometriosis, PID, ovarian cysts, uterine fibroids, pelvic adhesions, and ectopic pregnancies.
- Abdominal etiologies include irritable bowel syndrome, interstitial cystitis, appendicitis, and colitis.
- Psychologic factors (e.g., depression, chronic stress, history of sexual or physical abuse) may increase the risk of developing chronic pelvic pain. Emotional distress makes pain worse, and living with chronic pain contributes to emotional distress.

Manifestations and Diagnostic Studies

Manifestations of chronic pelvic pain include severe and steady pain, intermittent pain, dull and achy pain, pelvic pressure or heaviness, and sharp pains or cramping. Pain during intercourse or while having a bowel movement may also occur.

- In addition to a detailed history and physical examination (including a pelvic examination), the patient may be asked to keep a journal of the onset of symptoms and any precipitating factors.
- Diagnostic tests may include cultures from cervix or vagina (used to detect sexually transmitted infections [STIs]), ultrasound, CT scan, or MRI to detect abnormal structures or growths. Laparoscopy may be used to visualize the pelvic organs.

Collaborative Care

If the cause of chronic pelvic pain is found, such as PID, treatment focuses on that cause (see Pelvic Inflammatory Disease, p. 480). If an infection is the source of the problem, antibiotics will be used. If no cause can be found, treatment focuses on managing the pain. Over-the-counter pain medications (e.g., aspirin, ibuprofen, acetaminophen) may provide some relief. Sometimes stronger pain drugs may be needed. Birth control pills or other hormonal medications may help relieve cyclic pelvic pain related to menstrual cycles.

Tricyclic antidepressants (e.g., amitriptyline [Elavil], nortriptyline [Pamelor]) have pain-relieving as well as antidepressant effects. These drugs may help improve pain even in women who do not have depression. The patient may be encouraged to get counseling for any emotional issues.

Laparoscopic surgery may be used to remove pelvic adhesions or endometrial tissue. As a last attempt at treatment, a hysterectomy may be done.

PEPTIC ULCER DISEASE

Description

Peptic ulcer disease is an erosion of the mucosa resulting from the digestive action of hydrochloric acid (HCl) and pepsin. Any portion of the GI tract that comes into contact with gastric secretions is susceptible to ulcer development, including the lower esophagus, stomach, and duodenum, and at the margin of a gastrojejunal anastomosis site after surgical procedures. Approximately 350,000 new cases of ulcers are diagnosed each year.

Peptic ulcers can be classified as acute or chronic, depending on the degree and duration of mucosal involvement, and gastric or duodenal, according to the location.

- An *acute ulcer* is associated with superficial erosion and minimal inflammation. It is of short duration and resolves quickly when the cause is identified and removed.
- A *chronic ulcer* is of long duration, eroding through the muscular wall with the formation of fibrous tissue. It is continuously present for many months or intermittently throughout the person's lifetime. Chronic ulcers are more common than acute erosions.
- *Gastric* and *duodenal* ulcers, although defined as peptic ulcers, are distinctly different in etiology and incidence (Table 66). Generally, the treatment of all ulcer types is similar.

Pathophysiology

Peptic ulcers develop only in the presence of an acid environment. The back-diffusion of HCl into the gastric mucosa results in cellular destruction and inflammation. Histamine is released from the damaged mucosa, resulting in vasodilation and increased capillary permeability and further secretion of acid and pepsin. A variety of agents are known to destroy the mucosal barrier (see Gastritis, p. 241).

Table 66   Comparison of Gastric and Duodenal Ulcers

	Gastric Ulcers	Duodenal Ulcers
Lesion	Superficial, smooth margins. Round, oval, or cone shaped.	Penetrating (associated with deformity of duodenal bulb from healing of recurrent ulcers).
Location of lesion	Predominantly antrum; also in body and fundus of stomach.	First 1-2 cm of duodenum.
Gastric secretion	Normal to decreased.	Increased.
Incidence	Greater in women.	Greater in men, but increasing in women (especially postmenopausal).
	Peak age 50-60 yr.	Peak age 35-45 yr.
	More common in people of lower socioeconomic status.	Associated with psychologic stress.
	↑ With smoking, drug use (aspirin, NSAID), and alcohol use.	↑ With smoking, drug use, and alcohol use.
	↑ With incompetent pyloric sphincter and bile reflux.	Associated with other diseases (e.g., chronic obstructive pulmonary disease, pancreatic disease, hyperparathyroidism, Zollinger-Ellison syndrome, chronic renal failure).

Continued

P

Table 66   Comparison of Gastric and Duodenal Ulcers—cont'd

	Gastric Ulcers	Duodenal Ulcers
Clinical manifestations	Burning or gaseous pressure in high left epigastrium and back and upper abdomen. Pain 1-2 hr after meals. If penetrating ulcer, aggravation of discomfort with food. Occasional nausea and vomiting, weight loss.	Burning, cramping, pressure-like pain across midepigastrium and upper abdomen. Back pain with posterior ulcers. Pain 2-4 hr after meals and midmorning, midafternoon, middle of night. Periodic and episodic. Pain relief with antacids and food. Occasional nausea and vomiting.
Recurrence rate	High.	High.
Complications	Hemorrhage, perforation, gastric outlet obstruction, intractability.	Hemorrhage, perforation, obstruction.

In addition to chronic gastritis, *Helicobacter pylori* is associated with peptic ulcer development. Approximately two thirds of the world's population is infected with *H. pylori*. In the stomach the bacteria can live a long time by colonizing the gastric epithelial cells within the mucosal layer. The bacteria also produce urease, which metabolizes urea-producing ammonium chloride and other damaging chemicals. Urease also activates the immune response with both antibody production and the release of inflammatory cytokines.

- In one patient, *H. pylori* may lead to intestinal metaplasia in the stomach resulting in chronic atrophic gastritis, whereas in other patients *H. pylori* may alter gastric secretion and produce tissue damage leading to peptic ulcer disease. Response to *H. pylori* is likely influenced by many factors, including genetics, environment, and diet.

Clinical Manifestations

Discomfort generally associated with gastric ulcer is located high in the epigastrium and occurs about 1 to 2 hours after meals. The pain is described as burning or gaseous. If the ulcer has eroded through the gastric mucosa, food tends to aggravate rather than alleviate the pain.

Duodenal ulcer symptoms occur when gastric acid comes in contact with the ulcer, generally 2 to 5 hours after a meal. The pain is described as "burning" or "cramplike." It is most often located in the midepigastric region beneath the xiphoid process. Duodenal ulcers can also produce back pain. A characteristic of duodenal ulcer is its tendency to occur continuously for a few weeks or months and then disappear for a time, only to recur some months later.

- Not all patients with gastric or duodenal ulcers experience pain or discomfort. Silent peptic ulcers are more likely to occur in older adults and those taking nonsteroidal antiinflammatory drugs (NSAIDs). The presence or absence of symptoms is not directly related to the size of the ulcer or the degree of healing.

Complications

Major complications of peptic ulcers are hemorrhage, perforation, and gastric outlet obstruction. All are considered emergency situations and may require surgical intervention.

Hemorrhage is the most common complication. Duodenal ulcers account for a greater percentage of upper GI bleeding than gastric ulcers.

Perforation, the most lethal complication, occurs when the ulcer penetrates the serosal surface with spillage of either gastric or duodenal contents into the peritoneal cavity. The contents entering the peritoneal cavity from the stomach or the duodenum may contain saliva, food particles, HCl acid, pepsin, bacteria, bile, and pancreatic enzymes. Bacterial peritonitis may occur within 6 to 12 hours.

- Manifestations of perforation are sudden and dramatic in onset and include severe upper abdominal pain that quickly spreads throughout the abdomen. Respirations become shallow and rapid, and bowel sounds are usually absent.

Gastric outlet obstruction may occur with acute or chronic peptic ulcer disease. Obstruction in the distal stomach and the duodenum is the result of edema, inflammation, or pylorospasm and fibrous scar tissue formation. Symptoms include upper abdomen discomfort and swelling that worsens toward the end of the day, vomiting (often projectile), and constipation.

Diagnostic Studies

- Endoscopy is used to obtain tissue for biopsy, to confirm the absence of a malignancy, to obtain specimens to test for *H. pylori,* and to determine the degree of ulcer healing after treatment.
- Biopsy of the antral mucosa and testing for urease (rapid urease testing) confirms a diagnosis of *H. pylori* infection. Noninvasive tests include a urea breath test, which can identify active infection.
- CBC, urinalysis, liver enzyme studies, serum amylase determination, and stool examination may be performed for further diagnostic information.

Collaborative Care

Conservative Therapy

The aim of treatment is to decrease gastric acidity and enhance mucosal defense mechanisms. The regimen consists of adequate rest, dietary modifications as needed, drug therapy, elimination of smoking, and long-term follow-up care. Strict adherence to the prescribed regimen of drugs is important because ulcers frequently recur.

Drug therapy includes the use of histamine (H_2)-receptor antagonists (e.g., cimetidine [Tagamet], famotidine [Pepcid]), protein pump inhibitors (PPIs) (e.g., omeprazole [Prilosec]), antisecretory agents (e.g., misoprostol [Cytotec]), cytoprotective agents (e.g., sucralfate [Carafate]), antacids, and anticholinergics. Aspirin and NSAIDs are discontinued for 4 to 6 weeks. When aspirin must be continued, co-administration with a PPI, H_2-receptor blocker, or misoprostol (Cytotec) may be prescribed. See Table 42-10, Lewis et al.: *Medical-Surgical Nursing,* ed. 9, p. 934.

The patient is given antibiotics and a PPI for 10 to 14 days to eradicate *H. pylori* infection. Because of the development of antibiotic-resistant organisms, a growing percentage of patients do not have *H. pylori* eradicated with a single round of therapy.

Healing of a peptic ulcer requires many weeks of therapy. Pain disappears after 3 to 6 days, but ulcer healing is much slower. Complete healing may take 3 to 9 weeks, depending on the ulcer size, treatment regimen, and patient adherence.

An acute exacerbation is frequently accompanied by bleeding, increased pain and discomfort, and nausea and vomiting.

- In hemorrhage, management is similar to that described for upper GI bleeding (p. 247). Emergency assessment and management of the patient with a massive hemorrhage is described in Lewis et al.: *Medical-Surgical Nursing,* ed. 9, p. 948.
- In perforation, the focus of therapy is to stop the spillage of gastric contents by nasogastric (NG) tube or surgery. Blood volume is replaced with lactated Ringer's and albumin solutions, and packed RBCs may be necessary. Broad-spectrum antibiotic therapy is started immediately to treat bacterial peritonitis. Pain medication is also given.
- In gastric outlet obstruction, the aim of therapy is to decompress the stomach using an NG tube. IV fluids and electrolytes may be given for dehydration, vomiting, and electrolyte imbalances. Pain relief results from the decompression.

Nutritional Therapy

There are no recommended dietary modifications for peptic ulcer disease. Patients are taught to eat and drink foods and fluids that do not cause any distressing symptoms. Caffeine-containing beverages and foods can increase symptom distress in some patients. Teach the patient to eliminate alcohol because it can delay healing. Foods that commonly cause gastric irritation include hot, spicy foods; pepper; carbonated beverages; and broth (meat extract).

Surgical Therapy

With the use of antisecretory and antibiotic agents, surgery for PUD is uncommon. Surgery is done when the patient has complications unresponsive to medical management or when gastric cancer may be present.

Surgical procedures include partial gastrectomy, vagotomy, or pyloroplasty. Partial gastrectomy with removal of the distal two thirds of the stomach and anastomosis of the gastric stump to the duodenum is called a *gastroduodenostomy* or *Billroth I* operation; removal of the distal two thirds of the stomach with anastomosis of the gastric stump to the jejunum is called a *gastrojejunostomy* or *Billroth II* operation. *Vagotomy* (severing of the vagal nerve) is done to decrease gastric acid secretion. *Pyloroplasty* is the surgical enlargement of the pyloric sphincter to facilitate the passage of contents from the stomach.

Postoperative complications from surgery are dumping syndrome, postprandial hypoglycemia, and bile reflux gastritis.

- *Dumping syndrome* occurs when surgery drastically reduces the reservoir capacity of the stomach and causes loss of control over the amount of gastric chyme entering the small intestine. The large bolus of hypertonic fluid entering the intestine causes a fluid shift into the bowel, creating a decrease in plasma volume along with distention of the bowel lumen and rapid intestinal transit. The patient usually describes feelings of generalized weakness, sweating, palpitations, and dizziness caused by the decrease in plasma volume. The patient also complains of abdominal cramps, borborygmi, and the urge to defecate. The onset of symptoms occurs within 15 to 30 minutes of eating, and symptoms usually last about 1 hour after eating.

- *Postprandial hypoglycemia* is considered a variant of dumping syndrome, because it is the result of uncontrolled gastric emptying of a bolus of fluid high in carbohydrates, resulting in hyperglycemia and the release of excessive amounts of insulin into the circulation. Symptoms are similar to a hypoglycemic reaction, including sweating, weakness, mental confusion, palpitations, and tachycardia. Symptoms generally occur 2 hours after eating.

- Gastric surgery that involves the pylorus can result in reflux of bile into the stomach. The major symptom of reflux alkaline gastritis is continual epigastric distress that increases after meals. Vomiting relieves distress but only temporarily. The administration of cholestyramine (Questran) to bind with the bile salts, either before or with meals, successfully treats this problem.

Because of surgical changes, the stomach's reservoir is diminished and meal size must be reduced accordingly. Advise the patient to reduce fluids drunk with meals. Dry foods with a low carbohydrate content and moderate protein and fat content are better tolerated initially. Dietary changes, along with a short rest period after each meal, reduce the likelihood of dumping syndrome.

Nursing Management

Goals

The patient with peptic ulcer disease will adhere to the prescribed therapeutic regimen, experience a reduction in or absence of discomfort, exhibit no signs of GI complications, have complete healing of the peptic ulcer, and make appropriate lifestyle changes to prevent recurrence.

Nursing Diagnoses
- Acute pain
- Ineffective self-health management
- Nausea

Nursing Interventions

During an acute phase the patient may be NPO for a few days, have an NG tube inserted and connected to intermittent suction, and have IV fluid replacement. Explain the rationale for this therapy to the patient and caregiver. The volume of fluid lost, the patient's signs and symptoms, and laboratory test results determine the type and amount of IV fluids administered. When the stomach is kept empty of gastric secretions, the ulcer pain diminishes and ulcer healing begins. The patient's immediate environment should be quiet and restful.

If the patient has surgery, postoperative care is similar to postoperative care after abdominal laparotomy (see Abdominal Pain, Acute, pp. 4 to 5). Additional considerations for a patient with a partial gastrectomy include:

- Observe the gastric aspirate for color, amount, and odor during the immediate postoperative period.
- It is essential that the NG suction be working and that the tube remain patent so that accumulated gastric secretions do not put a strain on the anastomosis.
- Observe the patient for signs of decreased peristalsis and lower abdominal discomfort that may indicate impending intestinal obstruction.
- Keep the patient comfortable and free of pain by administering prescribed medications and by frequent changes in position.
- Observe the dressing for signs of bleeding or odor and drainage indicative of an infection.
- Encourage early ambulation.
- While the NG tube is connected to suction, maintain IV therapy. Add potassium and vitamin supplements (as ordered) to the infusion until oral feedings are resumed.
- The patient may require cobalamin therapy.

▼ **Patient and Caregiver Teaching**

General instructions should cover aspects of the disease process, drugs, possible changes in lifestyle, and regular follow-up care (Table 67).

- Emphasize the need for long-term follow-up care, and encourage the patient to seek immediate intervention if symptoms return.

Table 67	Patient and Caregiver Teaching Guide *Peptic Ulcer Disease (PUD)*

Include the following when teaching the patient and caregiver about management of PUD.

1. Follow dietary modifications, including avoidance of foods that may cause epigastric distress. This may include black pepper, spicy foods, and acidic foods.
2. Avoid cigarettes. In addition to promoting ulcer development, smoking delays ulcer healing.
3. Reduce or eliminate alcohol intake.
4. Avoid OTC drugs unless approved by the health care provider. Many preparations contain ingredients, such as aspirin, that should not be taken unless approved by the health care provider. Check with the health care provider regarding the use of nonsteroidal antiinflammatory drugs.
5. Do not interchange brands of antacids, H_2-receptor blockers, and proton pump inhibitors that can be purchased OTC without checking with the health care provider. This can lead to harmful side effects.
6. Take all medications as prescribed. This includes both antisecretory and antibiotic drugs. Failure to take medications as prescribed can result in relapse.
7. It is important to report any of the following:
   ▪ Increased nausea or vomiting
   ▪ Increased epigastric pain
   ▪ Bloody emesis or tarry stools
8. Stress can be related to signs and symptoms of PUD. Learn and use stress management strategies (see Chapter 7, Lewis et al.: *Medical-Surgical Nursing*, ed. 9, pp. 93 to 95).
9. Share concerns about lifestyle changes and living with a chronic illness.

PERICARDITIS, ACUTE

Description

Pericarditis is a condition caused by inflammation of the pericardium. The pericardium provides lubrication to decrease friction during systolic and diastolic heart movements and assists in preventing excessive dilation of the heart during diastole.

Pathophysiology

Acute pericarditis is most often idiopathic with a variety of suspected viral causes. The coxsackievirus B group is the most commonly identified virus. Other causes include uremia, bacterial infection, acute myocardial infarction (MI), neoplasm, and trauma.

Pericarditis in the patient with an acute MI may be described as two distinct syndromes. *Acute pericarditis* may occur within the initial 48- to 72-hour period after an MI. The second is *Dressler's syndrome* (late pericarditis), which appears 4 to 6 weeks after an MI.

An inflammatory response is the characteristic pathologic finding in acute pericarditis. There is an influx of neutrophils, increased pericardial vascularity, and eventual fibrin deposition on the pericardium.

Clinical Manifestations

Clinical manifestations include progressive, frequently severe chest pain that is sharp and pleuritic in nature. The pain is generally worse with deep inspiration and when lying supine. It is relieved by sitting up and leaning forward.

- The pain may radiate to the neck, arms, or left shoulder, making it difficult to distinguish from angina. One distinction is that pericarditis pain can be referred to the trapezius muscle (shoulder, upper back).
- Dyspnea that accompanies acute pericarditis is related to the patient's need to breathe in rapid, shallow breaths to avoid chest pain and may be aggravated by fever and anxiety.
- The hallmark finding is a *pericardial friction rub,* which is a scratching, grating, high-pitched sound believed to arise from friction between the roughened pericardial and epicardial surfaces. It is best heard with the stethoscope diaphragm firmly placed at the lower left sternal border of the chest with the patient leaning forward. Because it is difficult to distinguish a pericardial friction rub from a pleural friction rub, ask the patient to hold his or her breath. If you still hear the rub, then it is cardiac. It may require frequent attempts to identify because pericardial friction rubs are often intermittent and short lived.

Complications

Pericardial effusion is buildup of fluid in the pericardium. Large effusions may compress nearby structures. Pulmonary tissue compression can cause cough, dyspnea, and tachypnea. Phrenic nerve compression can induce hiccups, and compression of the recurrent laryngeal nerve may result in hoarseness. Heart sounds are generally distant and muffled. BP is usually maintained.

Cardiac tamponade develops as the pericardial effusion increases in volume, compressing the heart. The patient may report chest pain and is often confused, anxious, and restless.

Heart sounds become muffled, pulse pressure is narrowed, and the patient develops tachypnea, tachycardia, and decreased cardiac output. Neck veins are usually markedly distended because of jugular venous pressure elevation, and a pulsus paradoxus is present. *Pulsus paradoxus* is a decrease in systolic BP with inspiration that is exaggerated in cardiac tamponade. (See Table 37-5, Lewis et al.: *Medical-Surgical Nursing,* ed. 9, p. 816, for measurement technique.)

Diagnostic Studies

- ECG is useful in diagnosis, with changes (e.g., diffuse ST segment elevations) noted in approximately 90% of the cases.
- Echocardiography is used to determine the presence of pericardial effusion or cardiac tamponade.
- Doppler imaging and color M-mode assess diastolic function and help to diagnose constrictive pericarditis.
- Laboratory findings include leukocytosis and elevation of erythrocyte sedimentation rate (ESR) and C-reactive protein (CRP). Troponin levels may be elevated in patients with ST segment elevation and acute pericarditis, which may indicate concurrent myocardial damage.
- CT scan and MRI provide for visualization of the pericardium and pericardial space.

Collaborative Care

Management is directed toward identification and treatment of the underlying problem. Antibiotics treat bacterial pericarditis, and nonsteroidal antiinflammatory drugs (NSAIDs) (e.g., salicylates [aspirin], ibuprofen) control the pain and inflammation of acute pericarditis. Corticosteroids are generally reserved for patients with pericarditis secondary to systemic lupus erythematosus, patients already taking corticosteroids for a rheumatologic or other immune system condition, or those who do not respond to NSAIDs. Colchicine (Colsalide), an antiinflammatory drug used for gout, can be used for patients who have recurrent pericarditis.

- Pericardiocentesis is usually performed for pericardial effusion with acute cardiac tamponade, purulent pericarditis, and suspected neoplasm. Hemodynamic support for the patient undergoing pericardiocentesis may include the administration of volume expanders and inotropic agents (e.g., dopamine [Intropin]) and the discontinuation of any anticoagulants.
- A *pericardial window* can be used for diagnosis or for drainage of excess fluid. It involves cutting a "window" or portion of the pericardium. This allows the fluid to drain continuously into the peritoneum or the chest.

Nursing Management

Management of the patient's pain and anxiety is your primary nursing consideration. Assess the pain to distinguish the pain of myocardial ischemia (angina) from the pain of pericarditis. Pericarditic pain is usually located in the precordium or left trapezius ridge and has a sharp, pleuritic quality that increases with inspiration. Relief from this pain is often obtained by sitting or leaning forward and is worse when lying supine.

- Pain relief measures include maintaining the patient on bed rest with the head of the bed elevated to 45 degrees and providing an overhead table for support.
- Antiinflammatory medications help to alleviate the patient's pain. Because of the risk for GI bleeding, administer these drugs with food and instruct the patient to avoid alcohol.
- Monitor for the signs and symptoms of tamponade and prepare for possible pericardiocentesis.
- Anxiety-reducing measures for the patient include providing simple, complete explanations of all procedures performed. These explanations are particularly important for the patient whose diagnosis is being established and for the patient who has previously experienced angina or an acute MI.

PERIPHERAL ARTERY DISEASE

Description

Peripheral artery disease (PAD) involves thickening of artery walls, which results in a progressive narrowing of the arteries of the upper and lower extremities. PAD is strongly related to other types of cardiovascular disease (CVD) and their risk factors. About 6% of adults ages 40 years and older and 13% of adults ages 60 years and older have PAD.

Pathophysiology

The leading cause of PAD is atherosclerosis, which is a gradual thickening of the *intima* (the innermost layer of the arterial wall) and *media* (middle layer of the arterial wall). This results from the deposit of cholesterol and lipids within the vessel walls and leads to progressive narrowing of the artery. Although the exact cause(s) of atherosclerosis are unknown, inflammation and endothelial injury play a major role.

- Significant risk factors for PAD are hyperlipidemia, uncontrolled hypertension, and diabetes mellitus, with the highest risk being tobacco use.

- Atherosclerosis more commonly affects certain segments of the arterial tree. These include the coronary, carotid, and lower extremity arteries. Clinical symptoms occur when vessels are 60% to 75% blocked.

Peripheral Artery Disease: Lower Extremities

Lower extremity PAD may affect the iliac, femoral, popliteal, tibial, or peroneal arteries, or any combination of these arteries. The femoral popliteal area is the most common site in nondiabetic patients. Patients with diabetes tend to develop PAD in the arteries below the knee. In advanced PAD, multiple levels of occlusions are found.

Clinical Manifestations

Severity of the manifestations generally depends on the site, and extent of the obstruction and the amount of collateral circulation.

- The classic symptom of PAD is *intermittent claudication,* which is ischemic muscle pain that is caused by exercise, resolves within 10 minutes or less with resting, and is reproducible.
- Paresthesia, manifested as numbness or tingling in the toes or feet, may result from nerve tissue ischemia. Reduced blood flow to neurons produces loss of both pressure and deep pain sensation.
- Pallor of the foot is noted in response to leg elevation. *Reactive hyperemia* (redness) develops when the limb is allowed to hang in a dependent position *(dependent rubor).* The skin becomes shiny and taut, and there is hair loss on the lower legs. Pedal, popliteal, or femoral pulses are diminished or absent.
- As PAD progresses and involves multiple arterial segments, continuous pain develops at rest. Rest pain most often occurs in the forefoot or toes and is aggravated by limb elevation.

The most serious complications are nonhealing arterial ulcers and gangrene, which may result in lower extremity amputation. If PAD has been present for an extended period, collateral circulation may prevent gangrene of the extremity.

Diagnostic Studies

- Doppler ultrasound and duplex imaging assess blood flow.
- Segmental BPs are obtained (using Doppler ultrasound and a sphygmomanometer) at the thigh, below the knee, and at ankle level while the patient is supine. A drop in segmental BP of greater than 30 mm Hg suggests PAD.
- Angiography or magnetic resonance angiography (MRA) delineates location and extent of PAD.

Collaborative Care

The first treatment goal is to reduce cardiovascular risk factors in all patients with PAD regardless of the severity of symptoms. Tobacco cessation is essential. Both dietary interventions and drug therapy are needed.

- Statins (e.g., simvastatin [Zocor]) lower low-density lipoprotein (LDL) and triglyceride levels and reduce CVD morbidity and mortality risks. Hypertension and diabetes mellitus also need to be properly controlled.

- Antiplatelet agents are critical for reducing the risks of CVD events and death in PAD patients. Oral antiplatelet therapy should include 75 to 100 mg/day of aspirin for patients with asymptomatic PAD and 75 to 325 mg/day of aspirin for patients with symptomatic PAD. Aspirin-intolerant patients may take clopidogrel (Plavix) daily.

- Two drugs available to treat intermittent claudication are pentoxifylline (Trental) and cilostazol (Pletal). Cilostazol, a phosphodiesterase inhibitor, inhibits platelet aggregation and increases vasodilation. It is recommended as a first-line drug therapy for patients with intermittent claudication who do not respond to exercise therapy or stop using tobacco. Cilostazol does not reduce CVD morbidity and mortality risks, so antiplatelet therapy is also needed.

The primary nondrug treatment for claudication is tobacco cessation in combination with a formal exercise-training program. Walking is the most effective exercise. Instruct the patient to walk to the point of discomfort, stop and rest, and then resume walking until the discomfort recurs. Walking should be done for 30 to 40 minutes per day, three to five times per week.

- Teach PAD patients to adjust their overall caloric intake so that an ideal body weight can be achieved and maintained. Recommend a diet high in fruits, vegetables, and whole grains and low in cholesterol, saturated fat, and salt.

- Patients taking antiplatelet agents, nonsteroidal antiinflammatory drugs, or anticoagulants should consult with their health care provider before using any dietary or herbal supplements because of potential interactions and bleeding risks.

Critical limb ischemia is a condition characterized by chronic ischemic rest pain lasting more than 2 weeks, arterial leg ulcers, or gangrene of the leg as a result of PAD. Conservative management goals for critical limb ischemia include protecting the patient's extremity from trauma, decreasing ischemic pain, preventing and controlling infection, and maximizing perfusion. Carefully inspect, cleanse, and lubricate both feet to prevent cracking of the skin and infection. Optimal therapy is revascularization via bypass surgery.

Interventional radiology catheter-based procedures are alternatives to open surgical approaches for treatment of lower extremity PAD. Determining which intervention to use depends on blockage location and lesion type and severity.

- *Percutaneous transluminal balloon angioplasty* uses a catheter that contains a cylindric balloon at the tip. The end of the catheter is advanced to the stenotic area of the artery. The balloon is inflated, compressing the confining atherosclerotic intimal lining.
- *Stents,* expandable metallic devices, are positioned within the artery immediately after the balloon angioplasty is performed. The stent acts as a scaffold to keep the artery open. The stents may be covered with Dacron or a drug-eluting agent (e.g., paclitaxel) to reduce restenosis by limiting the amount of new tissue growth in the stent.
- *Atherectomy* removes the obstructing plaque. A directional atherectomy device uses a high-speed cutting disk that cuts long strips of the atheroma. Laser atherectomy uses ultraviolet energy to break the atheroma.

Various surgical approaches can be used to improve arterial blood flow beyond a blocked artery. The most common is a peripheral arterial bypass operation with autogenous (native) vein or synthetic graft material to bypass or carry blood around the lesion.

- Other surgical options include *endarterectomy* (opening the artery and removing the obstructing plaque) and *patch graft angioplasty* (opening the artery, removing the plaque, and sewing a patch to the opening to widen the lumen).
- Amputation may be required if tissue necrosis is extensive, gangrene or osteomyelitis develops, or all major arteries in the limb are occluded, precluding the possibility of successful surgery.

Nursing Management

Goals
The patient with lower extremity PAD will have adequate tissue perfusion, relief of pain, increased exercise tolerance, and intact, healthy skin on extremities.

Nursing Diagnoses
- Ineffective peripheral tissue perfusion
- Activity intolerance
- Ineffective self-health management

Nursing Interventions
After surgical or radiologic intervention, check the operative extremity every 15 minutes initially and then hourly for color, temperature,

capillary refill, presence of peripheral pulses, and movement and sensation. Loss of palpable pulses or a change in the Doppler sound over a pulse requires immediate notification of the physician or radiologist and prompt intervention.

After the patient leaves the recovery area, continue to monitor perfusion of the extremities and assess for potential complications such as bleeding, hematoma, thrombosis, embolization, and compartment syndrome. A dramatic increase in pain, loss of previously palpable pulses, extremity pallor or cyanosis, decreasing ankle-brachial indexes (ABIs), numbness or tingling, or a cold extremity suggest blockage of the graft or stent. Report these findings to the physician immediately.

- Knee-flexed positions should be avoided except for exercise. Turn the patient and position frequently with pillows to support the incision. Starting on postoperative day 1, assist patient out of bed several times daily. Discourage prolonged sitting with leg dependency because it may cause pain and edema, increase the risk of venous thrombosis, and place stress on the suture lines.
- If edema develops, position the patient supine and elevate the leg above the heart level. Walking even short distances is desirable.

▼ **Patient and Caregiver Teaching**
- Encourage supervised exercise training after a successful revascularization. Explain that exercise improves a number of CVD risk factors, including hypertension, hyperlipidemia, obesity, and glucose levels.
- Teach foot care to all patients with PAD. Meticulous foot care is especially important in the diabetic patient with PAD.
- Instruct patients to inspect their legs and feet daily for mottling, changes in skin color or texture, and reduction in hair growth. Show patients how to check skin temperature and capillary refill and to palpate pulses.
- Encourage patients to wear clean, all-cotton or all-wool socks and comfortable shoes with rounded (not pointed) toes and soft insoles. Tell patients to lace shoes loosely and to break in new shoes gradually.

PERITONITIS

Description

Peritonitis results from a localized or generalized inflammatory process of the peritoneum. Causes are listed in Table 68. Primary peritonitis occurs when blood-borne organisms enter the peritoneal

Table 68	Causes of Peritonitis

Primary
- Blood-borne organisms
- Genital tract organisms
- Cirrhosis with ascites

Secondary
- Appendicitis with rupture
- Blunt or penetrating trauma to abdominal organs
- Diverticulitis with rupture
- Ischemic bowel disorders
- Pancreatitis
- Perforated intestine
- Perforated peptic ulcer
- Peritoneal dialysis
- Postoperative (breakage of anastomosis)

cavity. For example, the ascites that occurs with cirrhosis of the liver provides an excellent liquid environment for bacteria to flourish. Organisms can also enter the peritoneum during peritoneal dialysis. Secondary peritonitis is more common and occurs when abdominal organs perforate or rupture and release their contents (bile, enzymes, bacteria) into the peritoneal cavity.

Pathophysiology

Intestinal contents and bacteria irritate the normally sterile peritoneum and produce an initial chemical peritonitis which is followed a few hours later by bacterial peritonitis. The resulting inflammatory response leads to massive fluid shifts (peritoneal edema) and adhesions as the body attempts to wall off the infection.

Clinical Manifestations and Complications

- Abdominal pain is the most common symptom.
- A universal sign of peritonitis is tenderness over the involved area. Rebound tenderness, muscular rigidity, and spasm are other major signs of peritoneum irritation.
- Abdominal distention or ascites, fever, tachycardia, tachypnea, nausea, vomiting, and altered bowel habits may also be present.

Complications include hypovolemic shock, sepsis, intraabdominal abscess formation, paralytic ileus, and acute respiratory distress syndrome. If treatment is delayed, peritonitis may be fatal.

Diagnostic Studies

- CBC will determine elevations in WBC count and hemoconcentration from fluid shifts.
- Peritoneal aspiration and analysis for blood, bile, pus, bacteria, fungi, and amylase content.
- Abdominal x-ray may show dilated loops of bowel consistent with paralytic ileus, free air if perforation has occurred, or air and fluid levels if an obstruction is present.
- CT scan and ultrasound may be useful in identifying ascites or abscesses.
- Peritoneoscopy may be helpful in patients without ascites.

Collaborative Care

Patients with milder cases of peritonitis or those who are poor surgical risks may be managed nonsurgically. Treatment consists of antibiotics, nasogastric (NG) suction, analgesics, and IV fluid administration. Surgery is indicated to locate the cause, drain purulent fluid, and repair any damage (e.g., perforated organs).

Nursing Management

Goals

The patient with peritonitis will have resolution of inflammation, relief of abdominal pain, freedom from complications (especially hypovolemic shock and sepsis), and normal nutritional status.

Nursing Interventions

The patient with peritonitis is extremely ill and needs skilled supportive care. An IV line is inserted to replace fluids lost to the peritoneal cavity and as an access for antibiotic therapy. Monitor the patient for pain and response to analgesics. The patient may be positioned with knees flexed to increase comfort. Sedatives may be given to allay anxiety.

- Accurate monitoring of fluid intake and output and electrolyte status is necessary to determine replacement therapy. Monitor vital signs frequently. Low-flow oxygen may be needed.
- Antiemetics may be administered to decrease nausea and vomiting and prevent further fluid and electrolyte losses. The patient is NPO and may have an NG tube in place to decrease gastric distention and further leakage of bowel contents into the peritoneum.
- If the patient has an open surgical procedure, drains are inserted to remove purulent drainage and excess fluid. Postoperative care is similar to that for the patient with an exploratory laparotomy (see Abdominal Pain, Acute, pp. 4 to 5).

PNEUMONIA

Description

Pneumonia is an acute inflammation of the lung parenchyma caused by a microorganism. Despite new antimicrobial agents to treat pneumonia, it is still associated with significant morbidity and mortality rates. Pneumonia can be caused by bacteria, viruses, *Mycoplasma,* fungi, parasites, and chemicals.

A clinically effective way to classify pneumonia is to classify it as *community-acquired pneumonia* (CAP) or *medical care–associated pneumonia* (MCAP). Classifying pneumonia is important because of the differences in the likely causative organisms (Table 69) and the selection of appropriate treatment.

CAP is an acute infection of the lung occurring in patients who have not been hospitalized or resided in a long-term care facility within 14 days of the onset of symptoms.

Table 69	Organisms Causing Pneumonia

Community-Acquired Pneumonia	Medical Care–Associated Pneumonia
■ *Streptococcus pneumoniae**	■ *Pseudomonas aeruginosa*†
■ *Mycoplasma pneumoniae*	■ *Escherichia coli*†
■ *Haemophilus influenzae*	■ *Klebsiella pneumoniae*†
■ Respiratory viruses	■ *Acinetobacter* species†
■ *Chlamydophila pneumoniae*	■ *Haemophilus influenzae*
■ *Chlamydophila psittaci*	■ *Staphylococcus aureus*
■ *Coxiella burnetii*	■ *Streptococcus pneumoniae*
■ *Legionella pneumophila*	■ *Proteus* species
■ Oral anaerobes	■ *Enterobacter* species
■ *Moraxella catarrhalis*	■ Oral anaerobes
■ *Staphylococcus aureus*	
■ *Pseudomonas aeruginosa*	
■ Enteric aerobic gram-negative bacteria (e.g., *Klebsiella* species)	
■ Fungi	
■ *Mycobacterium tuberculosis*	

*Most common cause of community-acquired pneumonia (CAP).
†Most common causes of medical care–associated pneumonia (MCAP).

MCAP encompasses three forms of pneumonia:

- *Hospital-associated pneumonia (HAP)* is pneumonia that occurs 48 hours or longer after hospital admission and was not incubating at the time of hospitalization
- *Ventilator-associated pneumonia (VAP)* refers to pneumonia that occurs more than 48 hours after endotracheal intubation.
- *Health care–associated pneumonia (HCAP)* is a new-onset pneumonia in a patient who (1) was hospitalized in an acute care hospital for 2 days or longer within 90 days of the infection; (2) resided in a long-term care facility; (3) received IV antibiotic therapy, chemotherapy, or wound care within the past 30 days of the current infection; or (4) attended a hospital or hemodialysis clinic.

Pathophysiology

Normally the airway distal to the larynx is sterile because of protective defense mechanisms. Pneumonia is more likely to result when defense mechanisms become incompetent or are overwhelmed by infectious agents including:

- Decreased consciousness that depresses the cough and epiglottal reflexes.
- Tracheal intubation interfering with the normal cough reflex and the mucociliary escalator mechanism.
- Impaired mucociliary mechanism caused by air pollution, cigarette smoking, viral upper respiratory tract infections, and normal aging changes
- Chronic diseases such as cancer, diabetes mellitus, and heart disease that can suppress the immune system's ability to inhibit bacterial growth.

Organisms that cause pneumonia reach the lungs by aspiration from the nasopharynx or oropharynx, inhalation of microbes present in the air, or hematogenous spread from a primary infection elsewhere in the body.

Specific pathophysiologic changes vary according to the offending organism. Most organisms trigger an inflammatory response in the lung. A vascular reaction occurs with increased blood flow and vascular permeability. Neutrophils, the offending organism, and fluid from surrounding blood vessels fill the alveoli, interrupting oxygen transportation, which leads to hypoxia. Mucus production is increased, which can obstruct airflow and further decrease gas exchange.

Consolidation, a feature of bacterial pneumonia, occurs when normally air-filled alveoli are filled with fluid and debris.

Complete resolution and healing occur if there are no complications. Macrophages lyse and process the debris, normal lung tissue is restored, and gas exchange returns to normal.

Clinical Manifestations and Complications

Most common presenting manifestations of pneumonia are cough, fever, shaking chills, dyspnea, tachypnea, and pleuritic chest pain.

- Cough may be or may not be productive. Sputum may appear green, yellow, or rust colored (bloody).
- Viral pneumonia may initially be seen as influenza, with respiratory symptoms appearing and/or worsening 12 to 36 hours after onset.
- In older or debilitated patients, confusion or stupor (possibly related to hypoxia) may be the only finding.

On physical examination, rhonchi and crackles may be auscultated over the affected area. If consolidation is present, bronchial breath sounds, egophony, and increased fremitus may be noted.

Complications include *pleurisy* (inflammation of the pleura), pleural effusion, *atelectasis* (collapsed, airless alveoli), bacteremia, lung abscess, pericarditis, meningitis, sepsis, and acute respiratory failure.

Diagnostic Studies

- History, physical examination, and chest x-ray often provide enough information for making management decisions without further testing.
- Chest x-ray often shows a pattern characteristic of the infecting organism.
- Sputum culture is often done.
- Gram stain of sputum and blood cultures is used to identify the causative organism.
- Arterial blood gases (ABGs) are used to assess for hypoxemia, hypercapnia, and acidosis.
- WBC count often reveals leukocytosis.

Collaborative Care

Pneumococcal vaccine (Pneumovax) is used to prevent *Streptococcus pneumoniae* (pneumococcus) *pneumonia*. Vaccination is recommended for individuals 65 years of age or older and younger patients who are at high risk. A one-time repeat vaccination in 5 years is recommended for those who received their initial vaccination when less than 65 years of age.

Currently, no definitive treatment exits for the majority of viral pneumonias. Care is generally supportive. Prompt treatment with appropriate antibiotics almost always cures bacterial and *Mycoplasma* pneumonia. In uncomplicated cases, the patient responds to drug therapy within 48 to 72 hours. Table 28-6 in Lewis et al.: *Medical-Surgical Nursing,* ed. 9, p. 526, outlines drugs for bacterial CAP.

- Supportive measures may be used, including oxygen therapy, analgesics to relieve chest pain, and antipyretics such as aspirin or acetaminophen. Individualize rest and activity to the patient's tolerance.

- Hydration is important. If the patient has heart failure, fluid intake is carefully monitored. If the patient cannot maintain adequate oral intake, IV administration of fluids and electrolytes may be necessary.
- Small, frequent meals are easier for some patients to tolerate. Offer foods high in calories and nutrients.

Nursing Management

Goals

The patient with pneumonia will have clear breath sounds, normal breathing patterns, no signs of hypoxia, normal chest x-ray, and no complications related to pneumonia.

Nursing Diagnoses

- Impaired gas exchange
- Ineffective breathing pattern
- Acute pain

Nursing Interventions

Interventions focus on preventing the occurrence of pneumonia. If possible, exposure to upper respiratory infections (URIs) should be avoided. If a URI occurs, it should be treated promptly with supportive measures (e.g., rest, fluids). If symptoms persist for more than 7 days, the person should seek medical care. The individual at increased risk for pneumonia should be encouraged to obtain both influenza and pneumococcal vaccines.

In the hospital, priority interventions involve identifying the patient at risk and taking measures to prevent pneumonia.

- Place the patient with altered consciousness in positions (e.g., side-lying, upright) that will prevent or minimize aspiration. Turn and reposition the patient at least every 2 hours to facilitate adequate lung expansion and discourage the pooling of secretions.
- The patient who has a feeding tube requires attention to prevent aspiration.
- In the intensive care unit, strict adherence to "ventilator bundle" interventions has been shown to significantly reduce VAP. These interventions are elevation of the head of the bed 30 to 45 degrees, daily "sedation holidays," assessment of readiness to extubate, peptic ulcer disease and venous thromboembolism prophylaxis, and daily oral care with chlorhexidine.
- The patient who has difficulty swallowing (e.g., a stroke patient) needs assistance in eating, drinking, and taking medication to prevent aspiration. In the patient who has had local anesthesia to the throat, assess for a gag reflex before giving food or fluids.

- Patients with impaired mobility from any cause need assistance with turning and moving as well as encouragement to breathe deeply at frequent intervals.
- Practice strict medical asepsis and adherence to infection control guidelines to reduce the incidence of medical care–associated pneumonia.

▼ **Patient and Caregiver Teaching**
- Teach the patient about the importance of taking every dose of the prescribed antibiotic, any drug–drug and food–drug interactions for the prescribed antibiotic, and the need for adequate rest to continue recovery.
- Instruct the patient to drink plenty of liquids (at least 6 to 10 glasses/day, unless contraindicated) and to avoid alcohol and smoking.
- A cool mist humidifier or warm bath may help the patient breathe easier.
- Teaching should also include information about available influenza and pneumococcal vaccines.

PNEUMOTHORAX

Description
A *pneumothorax* is a complete or partial collapse of a lung as a result of an accumulation of air in the pleural space. Pneumothorax can be classified as *open* (air entering through an opening in the chest wall) or *closed* (no external wound).

Pathophysiology
Normally, negative pressure exists between the visceral pleura (surrounding the lung) and the parietal pleura (lining the thoracic cavity), allowing the lungs to be filled by chest wall expansion. The pleural space contains only a few milliliters of lubricating fluid to reduce friction when the tissues move. When air enters the pleural space, the change in pressure (from negative to positive) causes a partial or complete lung collapse. As the volume of air in the pleural space increases, the lung volume decreases. This condition should be suspected after any blunt trauma to the chest wall.

Types
Spontaneous pneumothorax typically occurs as a result of the rupture of small blebs (air-filled blisters) located on the apex of the lung. These blebs can occur in healthy, young individuals (primary spontaneous pneumothorax) or as a result of lung disease such

as chronic obstructive pulmonary disease (COPD), asthma, cystic fibrosis, and pneumonia (secondary spontaneous pneumothorax). Smoking increases the risk for bleb formation. Other risk factors include being tall and thin, male gender, family history, and previous spontaneous pneumothorax.

Traumatic pneumothorax can occur from either penetrating (open) or nonpenetrating (closed) chest trauma. Penetrating trauma allows air to enter the pleural space through an opening in the chest wall. Examples include stab or gunshot wounds and surgical thoracotomy. A penetrating chest wound may be referred to as a *sucking chest wound,* because air enters the pleural space through the chest wall during inspiration.

Tension pneumothorax occurs when air enters the pleural space but cannot escape. The continued accumulation of air in the pleural space causes increasingly elevated intrapleural pressures. This results in compression of the lung on the affected side and pressure on the heart and great vessels, pushing them away from the affected side (Fig. 12). The mediastinum shifts toward the unaffected side, compressing the "good" lung, which further compromises oxygenation. As pressure increases, venous return is decreased and cardiac output falls. Tension pneumothorax may result from either an open or a closed pneumothorax.

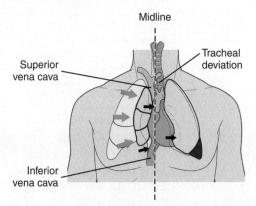

Fig. 12. Tension pneumothorax. As pleural pressure on the affected side increases, mediastinal displacement ensues, with resultant respiratory and cardiovascular compromise. Tracheal deviation is an external manifestation of the mediastinal shift.

Hemothorax is an accumulation of blood in the pleural space resulting from injury to the chest wall, diaphragm, lung, blood vessels, or mediastinum. The patient with a traumatic hemothorax requires immediate insertion of a chest tube for evacuation of the blood, which can be recovered and reinfused for a short time after the injury.

Clinical Manifestations

If the pneumothorax is small, only mild tachycardia and dyspnea may be present. If it is a large pneumothorax, shallow, rapid respirations, dyspnea, air hunger, and oxygen desaturation may occur.

- Chest pain and a cough with or without hemoptysis may be present.
- On auscultation, no breath sounds are detected over the affected area.
- Chest x-ray shows air or fluid in the pleural space and reduction in lung volume.

Collaborative Care

Tension pneumothorax is a medical emergency, requiring urgent needle compression followed by chest tube insertion to water-seal drainage.

If the patient is stable and minimal air and fluid is accumulated in the intrapleural space, no treatment may be needed because the condition may resolve spontaneously, or the pleural space can be aspirated with a large-bore needle (thoracentesis).

The most common treatment for a pneumothorax and hemothorax is to insert a chest tube and connect it to water-seal drainage (see Chest Tubes and Pleural Drainage, p. 700). Repeated spontaneous pneumothoraces may need to be treated surgically by a partial pleurectomy, stapling, or pleurodesis to promote the adherence of pleurae to one another.

POLYCYSTIC KIDNEY DISEASE

Polycystic kidney disease (PKD) is the most common life-threatening genetic disease in the world, affecting 600,000 people in the United States. There are two forms of PKD. The *childhood form* is a rare autosomal recessive disorder that is often rapidly progressive. The *adult form* of PKD is an autosomal dominant disorder.

Adult PKD is latent for many years and is usually manifested between 30 and 40 years of age. It involves both kidneys. The cortex and the medulla are filled with large, thin-walled cysts that are several millimeters to several centimeters in diameter. The cysts enlarge and destroy surrounding tissue by compression.

Early in PKD, patients are usually asymptomatic. Symptoms appear when the cysts begin to enlarge. Often the first manifestations are hypertension, hematuria (from rupture of cysts), or a feeling of heaviness in the back, side, or abdomen. On physical examination, palpable bilateral enlarged kidneys are often found.

- Sometimes the first manifestations are a urinary tract infection (UTI) or urinary calculi.
- Chronic pain is one of the most common problems, and in some people it can be constant and quite severe.
- Usually the disease progresses to end-stage kidney disease (ESKD) occurring by age 60 in 50% of patients.
- PKD can also affect the liver (liver cysts), heart (abnormal heart valves), blood vessels (aneurysms), and intestines (diverticulosis). The most serious complication is a cerebral aneurysm, which can rupture.

Diagnosis is based on clinical manifestations, family history, ultrasound (best screening measure), intravenous pyelogram (IVP), or CT scan.

There is no specific treatment for PKD. A major treatment aim is to prevent infections of the urinary tract or to treat them with appropriate antibiotics if they occur. Nephrectomy may be necessary if pain, bleeding, or infection becomes a chronic, serious problem. When the patient begins to experience progressive renal failure, interventions are determined by the remaining renal function. Dialysis and kidney transplant may be needed to treat ESKD.

Nursing measures are those used for management of end-stage kidney disease (see Kidney Disease, Chronic, p. 377). They include diet modification, fluid restriction, medications (e.g., antihypertensives), and assisting the patient and family in coping with the chronic disease process and financial concerns.

- The patient who has adult PKD often has children by the time the disease is diagnosed. The patient needs appropriate counseling regarding plans for having more children. In addition, genetic counseling should be provided for the children.

POLYCYTHEMIA

Description

Polycythemia is the production and presence of increased number of RBCs. The increase in RBCs can be so great that blood circulation is impaired as a result of the increased blood viscosity (hyperviscosity) and volume (hypervolemia).

Pathophysiology

The two types of polycythemia are primary polycythemia (polycythemia vera) and secondary polycythemia (Fig. 13). Their etiologies and pathogeneses differ, although their complications and clinical manifestations are similar.

Polycythemia vera is a chronic myeloproliferative disorder. Therefore not only are RBCs involved, but also WBCs and platelets, leading to increased production of each of these blood cells. The disease develops insidiously and follows a chronic, vacillating course. The median age at diagnosis is 60 years. Patients have enhanced blood viscosity and blood volume and congestion of organs and tissues with blood. Splenomegaly and hepatomegaly are common.

- Polycythemia vera is associated with mutations in a gene that provides instructions for making a protein that promotes proliferation of cells, especially blood cells from hematopoietic stem cells.

Secondary polycythemia can be either hypoxia driven or hypoxia independent. In *hypoxia-driven polycythemia*, hypoxia stimulates erythropoietin (EPO) production in the kidney, which in turn stimulates RBC production. The need for O_2 may result from high altitude, pulmonary and cardiovascular disease, defective O_2 transport, or tissue hypoxia. In *hypoxia-independent polycythemia*, EPO is produced by a malignant or benign tumor tissue.

Clinical Manifestations

- Initial manifestations from hypertension caused by hypervolemia and hyperviscosity include complaints of headache, vertigo, dizziness, tinnitus, and visual disturbances.
- Manifestations caused by blood vessel distention, circulatory stasis, thrombosis, and tissue hypoxia include angina, heart failure (HF), intermittent claudication, and thrombophlebitis.
- The most common serious acute complication is stroke secondary to thrombosis.
- Hemorrhage caused by either vessel rupture from overdistention or inadequate platelet function may result in petechiae, ecchymoses, epistaxis, or GI bleeding.

Other clinical manifestations include:

- Generalized pruritus that may be a striking symptom and is related to histamine release from an increased number of basophils.
- Hepatomegaly and splenomegaly may contribute to patient complaints of satiety and fullness.
- Pain from peptic ulcer caused by increased gastric secretions.

P

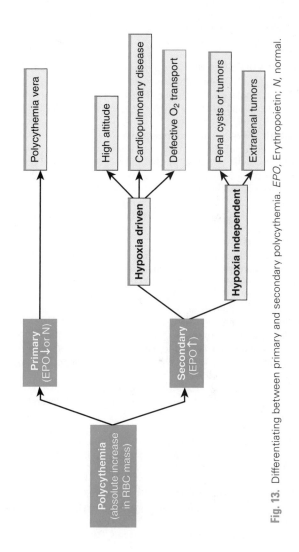

Fig. 13. Differentiating between primary and secondary polycythemia. *EPO*, Erythropoietin; *N*, normal.

- Paresthesia and erythromelalgia (painful burning and redness of the hands and feet).
- Plethora (ruddy complexion) may be present.
- Hyperuricemia resulting from the increase in RBC destruction that accompanies excessive RBC production; may cause gout.

Diagnostic Studies

Diagnostic study abnormalities include:

- Elevated hemoglobin (Hgb) and RBC count with microcytosis
- Low to normal EPO level (polycythemia vera). High EPO level (secondary polycythemia)
- Elevated WBC count with basophilia
- Elevated platelets (thrombocytosis) and platelet dysfunction
- Elevated leukocyte alkaline phosphatase, uric acid, and cobalamin levels
- Elevated histamine levels

Bone marrow examination in polycythemia vera shows hypercellularity of RBCs, WBCs, and platelets.

Collaborative Care

Treatment is directed toward reducing blood volume and viscosity and bone marrow activity. Phlebotomy is the mainstay of treatment. At the time of diagnosis, 300 to 500 mL of blood may be removed every other day until the hematocrit (Hct) level is reduced to normal. An individual managed with repeated phlebotomies eventually becomes iron deficient, although this effect is rarely symptomatic. Avoid iron supplementation.

- Hydration therapy is used to reduce the blood's viscosity.
- Myelosuppressive agents such as busulfan (Myleran), hydroxyurea (Hydrea), and imatinib (Gleevec) are used.
- Low-dose aspirin is used to prevent clotting.
- Interferon-alpha (IFN-α) is used in women of childbearing age or those with intractable pruritus.
- Anagrelide (Agrylin) may be used to reduce the platelet count and inhibit platelet aggregation.
- Allopurinol (Zyloprim) may reduce the number of acute gouty attacks.

Nursing Management

Primary polycythemia vera is not preventable. However, because secondary polycythemia is caused by hypoxia, maintaining adequate oxygenation may prevent problems. Therefore controlling chronic pulmonary disease, stopping smoking, and avoiding high altitudes may be important.

When acute exacerbations of polycythemia vera develop, assist with or perform phlebotomies, depending on the institution's policies.

- Evaluate fluid intake and output during hydration therapy to avoid fluid overload (which further complicates circulatory congestion) and underhydration (which can make the blood even more viscous).
- If myelosuppressive agents are used, administer the drugs as ordered, observe the patient, and teach the patient about medication side effects.
- Assess the patient's nutritional status because inadequate food intake can result from GI symptoms of fullness, pain, and dyspepsia.
- Begin activities and/or medications to decrease thrombus formation. Initiate active or passive leg exercises and ambulation when possible.
- Because of its chronic nature, polycythemia vera requires ongoing evaluation. Phlebotomy may need to be done every 2 to 3 months. Evaluate the patient for complications.

PRESSURE ULCER

Description

A *pressure ulcer* is localized injury to the skin and/or underlying tissue (usually over a bony prominence) as a result of pressure or pressure in combination with shear and/or friction. The most common site for pressure ulcers is the sacrum, with heels being second.

Factors influencing pressure ulcer development include amount of pressure (intensity), length of time pressure is exerted on skin (duration), and ability of patient's tissue to tolerate externally applied pressure. *Shearing force* (pressure exerted on skin when it adheres to the bed and skin layers slide in direction of body movement), friction (two surfaces rubbing against each other), and excessive moisture also contribute to pressure ulcer formation.

- Risk factors for the development of pressure ulcers include patients who are bed- or wheelchair-bound, older, incontinent, or recovering from spinal cord injuries.

Clinical Manifestations

Pressure ulcers are graded or staged according to their deepest level of tissue damage. Table 70 illustrates the pressure ulcer

Table 70	Staging of Pressure Ulcers

Definition and Description	**Clinical Presentation***
Suspected Deep Tissue Injury Purple or maroon localized area of discolored intact skin or blood-filled blister caused by damage of underlying soft tissue from pressure and/or shear. The area may be painful, firm, mushy, boggy, warmer, or cooler compared with adjacent tissue.	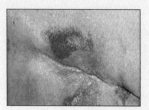
Stage I Intact skin with nonblanchable redness of a localized area, usually over a bony prominence. Darkly pigmented skin may not have visible blanching. Its color may differ from the surrounding area.	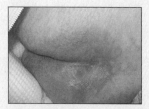
Stage II Partial-thickness loss of dermis manifesting as a shallow open ulcer with a red-pink wound bed, without slough. May also manifest as an intact or open/ruptured serum-filled blister.	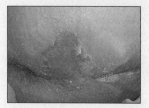
Stage III Full-thickness tissue loss. Subcutaneous fat may be visible, but bone, tendon, and muscle are not exposed. Slough may be present but does not obscure the depth of tissue loss. May include undermining and tunneling.	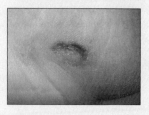

Photos used with permission of the National Pressure Ulcer Advisory Panel.

Table 70	Staging of Pressure Ulcers—cont'd

Definition and Description	Clinical Presentation*
Stage IV Full-thickness tissue loss with exposed bone, tendon, or muscle. Slough or eschar may be present on some parts of the wound bed. Often includes undermining and tunneling.	
Unstageable Ulcer Full-thickness tissue loss in which the base of the ulcer is covered by slough (yellow, tan, gray, green, or brown) and/or eschar (tan, brown, or black) in the wound bed. The true depth and stage of the ulcer cannot be determined until enough slough and eschar are removed. Stable (dry, adherent, intact without erythema or fluctuance) eschar on the heels provides a natural biologic cover and should not be removed.	

*Color images are available in Table 12-13, Lewis et al.: *Medical-Surgical Nursing*, ed. 9, p. 185.

stages. A pressure ulcer may be unstageable. If the pressure ulcer becomes infected, signs of systemic infection, such as leukocytosis and fever, may occur.

Nursing and Collaborative Management

Pressure ulcer management requires local wound care as well as support measures such as adequate nutrition, pain management, and pressure relief. Both conservative and surgical strategies are used in the treatment of pressure ulcers, depending on the ulcer's stage and condition.

Nursing Management

Goals

The patient with a pressure ulcer will have no deterioration of the ulcer, reduce or eliminate the factors that lead to pressure ulcers, not develop an infection in the pressure ulcer, have healing of pressure ulcers, and have no recurrence.

Nursing Diagnosis

- Impaired skin integrity

Nursing Interventions

Assess patients for pressure ulcer risk on admission and at periodic intervals. Reposition patients frequently to prevent pressure ulcers (usually every 2 hours). Devices such as alternating pressure mattresses, foam mattresses with adequate stiffness and thickness, wheelchair cushions, padded commode seats, foam boots, and lift sheets are useful in reducing pressure and shearing force.

- Once a person has been identified as being at risk for a pressure ulcer, prevention strategies should be implemented. Table 71 and eNCP 12-2 (available on the website for Lewis et al.: *Medical-Surgical Nursing,* ed. 9) list guidelines for preventing pressure ulcers.

Once a pressure ulcer has developed, initiate interventions based on the ulcer's characteristics (e.g., size, stage, location, presence of infection or pain) and the patient's general status. Also document the size of the ulcer.

Local ulcer care may involve debridement, wound cleaning, relief of pressure, and the application of a dressing.

- A pressure ulcer with necrotic tissue or eschar (except for dry, stable necrotic heels) must have the tissue removed by surgical, mechanical, enzymatic, or autolytic debridement methods. Once the pressure ulcer has been successfully debrided and has a clean granulating base, the goal is to provide an appropriate wound environment that supports moist wound healing and prevents disruption of newly formed granulation tissue.
- Reconstruction of the pressure ulcer site by operative repair, including skin grafting, skin flaps, musculocutaneous flaps, or free flaps, may be necessary.
- Pressure ulcers should be cleaned with noncytotoxic solutions that do not kill or damage cells, especially fibroblasts.
- After the pressure ulcer has been cleansed, it needs to be covered with an appropriate dressing. (Dressings are discussed in Table 12-10, Lewis et al.: *Medical-Surgical Nursing,* ed. 9, p. 182.)
- Maintenance of adequate nutrition is an important nursing responsibility for the patient with a pressure ulcer. Often the patient is debilitated and has a poor appetite secondary to inactivity.
- Oral feedings must be adequate in calories, protein, fluids, vitamins, and minerals to meet the patient's nutritional requirements.

Table 71	Patient and Caregiver Teaching Guide *Pressure Ulcer*

When teaching the patient or caregiver to prevent and care for pressure ulcers, do the following.

1. Identify and explain risk factors and etiology of pressure ulcers to patient and caregiver.
2. Assess all at-risk patients at the time of first hospital and/or home visit or whenever the patient's condition changes. Thereafter assess at regular intervals based on care setting (every 24 hours for acute care or every visit in home care).
3. Teach the caregiver techniques for incontinence. If incontinence occurs, cleanse skin at time of soiling and use absorbent pads or briefs.
4. Demonstrate correct positioning to decrease risk of skin breakdown. Instruct caregiver to reposition a bed-bound patient at least every 2 hours, a chair-bound patient every hour. NEVER position the patient directly on the pressure ulcer.
5. Assess resources (i.e., caregiver's availability and skill, finances, equipment) of patients requiring pressure ulcer care at home. When selecting ulcer care dressing, consider cost and amount of caregiver time required.
6. Teach patient and/or caregiver to place clean dressings over sterile dressings using "no touch" technique when changing dressings. Instruct caregiver on disposal of contaminated dressings.
7. Teach patient and caregiver to inspect skin daily. Tell them to report any significant changes to the health care provider.
8. Teach patient and caregiver the importance of good nutrition to enhance ulcer healing.
9. Evaluate program effectiveness.

- Enteral feedings can be used to supplement oral feedings. If necessary, parenteral nutrition may be used.

▼ **Patient and Caregiver Teaching**

Because recurrence of pressure ulcers is common, it is extremely important to teach both the patient and caregiver about prevention techniques (see Table 71).

- Teach caregiver about the etiology of pressure ulcers, prevention techniques, early signs, nutritional support, and care techniques for pressure ulcers.
- Because the patient with a pressure ulcer often requires extensive care for other health problems, it is important that you support the caregiver.

PROSTATE CANCER

Description

Prostate cancer is a malignant tumor of the prostate gland. It is the most common form of cancer in men excluding skin cancer, with one in six men developing prostate cancer at some point in their lives. It is the second leading cause of cancer death in men after lung cancer. Most cases occur in men older than age 65 years, but many cases occur in younger men, who sometimes have a more aggressive type of cancer.

- African American men have a higher incidence of prostate cancer than any other male group worldwide (except Jamaican men of African descent).

Pathophysiology

Prostate cancer is an androgen-dependent adenocarcinoma that is usually slow growing. Tumor spread is by three routes: direct extension, through the lymph system, or through the bloodstream. Spread by direct extension involves the seminal vesicles, urethral mucosa, bladder wall, and external sphincter. Later spread occurs through the lymphatic system to the regional lymph nodes. The bloodstream appears to the mode of spread to the pelvic bones, head of the femur, lower lumbar spine, liver, and lungs.

- The incidence of prostate cancer increases markedly after age 50, with a median age at diagnosis of 67 years old.
- Dietary factors and obesity may be associated with prostate cancer. A diet high in red and processed meat and high-fat dairy products along with a low intake of vegetables and fruits may increase the risk of prostate cancer.
- Some genes or gene mutations are more common in men diagnosed with prostate cancer.

Clinical Manifestations

Prostate cancer is usually asymptomatic in the early stages. Eventually the patient may have symptoms similar to those of benign prostatic hyperplasia (BPH), including dysuria, hesitancy, dribbling, frequency, urgency, hematuria, nocturia, retention, interruption of urinary stream, and inability to urinate.

- Pain in the lumbosacral area that radiates down to the hips or legs, when coupled with urinary symptoms, may indicate metastasis. As the cancer spreads to the bones, pain can become severe, especially in the back and legs, because of spinal cord compression and bone destruction.

Diagnostic Studies

Most men in the United States with prostate cancer are diagnosed by prostate-specific antigen (PSA) screening. Although specific recommendations regarding PSA screening vary, there is general agreement that men should be informed about the potential risks (e.g., subsequent evaluation and treatment that may be unnecessary) and benefits (early detection of prostate cancer) of PSA screening before being tested.

- Mild elevations in PSA may occur with aging, BPH, recent ejaculation, acute or chronic prostatitis, or after long bike rides. Decreases in the PSA level can occur with drugs such as finasteride (Proscar) and dutasteride (Avodart).
- When treatment has been successful in removing prostate cancer, PSA levels should fall to undetectable levels.
- In a digital rectal examination (DRE) of the prostate gland, it may feel hard, nodular, and asymmetric.
- Elevated prostatic acid phosphatase (PAP) levels are specific for prostate cancer.
- Biopsy using transrectal ultrasound can confirm the diagnosis.
- CT scan, bone scan, or MRI can assess cancer spread.
- Elevated serum alkaline phosphatase may indicate bone metastasis.

Collaborative Care

The management of prostate cancer depends on the stage and overall health of the patient. The most common classification system for determining the extent of the prostate cancer is the tumor, node, and metastasis (TNM) system (Table 72).

The tumor is graded on the basis of tumor histology using the Gleason scale: Grade 1 represents the most well-differentiated or lowest grade (most like original cells), and grade 5 represents the most poorly differentiated (unlike original cells) or highest grade. The two most commonly occurring patterns of cells are graded with the two scores, then added together to create a Gleason score.

- The patient's Gleason score and PSA level at diagnosis are used with the TNM system to determine the stage of the tumor.
- Most patients (90%) with prostate cancer are initially diagnosed when the cancer is in either a local or regional stage. The 5-year survival rate with an initial diagnosis at these stages is 100%.

At all stages, there is more than one possible treatment option. The decision of which treatment course to pursue should be made jointly by patients, their partners, and the health care team. Various

Table 72   Staging of Prostate Cancer

Stage	Tumor Size	Lymph Node Involvement	Metastasis	PSA Level	Gleason Score
I	Not felt on DRE. Not seen by visual imaging.	No	No	<10	≦6
II	Felt on DRE. Seen by imaging. Tumor confined to prostate.	No	No	10-20	6-7
III	Cancer outside prostate. Possible spread to seminal vesicles.	No	No	Any level	Any score
IV	Any size.	Any nodal involvement	Yes	Any level	Any score

Adapted from American Cancer Society: How is prostate cancer staged? Retrieved from *www.cancer.org/Cancer/ProstateCancer/DetailedGuide/prostate-cancer-staging*; and National Cancer Institute: Stages of prostate cancer. Retrieved from *www.cancer.gov/cancertopics/pdq/treatment/prostate*. *DRE*, Digital rectal examination; *PSA*, prostate-specific antigen.

treatment options are summarized in Table 55-6, Lewis et al.: *Medical-Surgical Nursing,* ed. 9, p. 1317.

- A conservative approach to slow-growing tumors is active surveillance or "watchful waiting." This strategy is appropriate when there is (1) a life expectancy of less than 10 years (low risk of dying of the disease), (2) the presence of a low-grade, low-stage tumor, and (3) serious coexisting medical conditions. Patients are monitored and typically followed with frequent PSA testing and DREs to monitor the progress of the disease. Significant changes in PSA, DRE, or symptoms warrant a reevaluation of treatment options.

Surgical Therapy

With radical prostatectomy, the entire prostate gland, seminal vesicles, and part of the bladder neck (ampulla) are removed. In addition, a retroperitoneal lymph node dissection is usually done as a separate procedure. Surgery is usually not considered an option for advanced-stage disease (except to relieve symptoms associated with obstruction) because metastasis has already occurred.

- Traditional approaches for radical prostatectomy are retropubic (low abdominal incision) and perineal (incision between the scrotum and anus).
- After surgery, the patient has a large indwelling catheter with a 30-mL balloon placed in the bladder via the urethra. A drain is left in the surgical site to aid in the removal of drainage from the area.

Two major adverse outcomes following a radical prostatectomy are erectile dysfunction and urinary incontinence. The incidence of erectile dysfunction is dependent on the patient's age, preoperative sexual functioning, whether nerve-sparing surgery was performed, and the expertise of the surgeon. A nerve-sparing technique is sometimes used to reduce the risk of erectile dysfunction. Problems with urinary control may occur for the first few months because the bladder must be reattached to the urethra after the prostate is removed. Over time, the bladder adjusts and most men regain control.

Cryotherapy is a surgical technique that destroys cancer cells by freezing. The treatment takes about 2 hours, with the patient under general or spinal anesthesia.

A bilateral orchiectomy is the surgical removal of the testes that may be done alone or in combination with prostatectomy. For advanced stages of prostate cancer, an orchiectomy is one treatment option for cancer control.

Radiation Therapy

Radiation therapy is a common option for prostate cancer. Radiation therapy may be offered as the only treatment, or it may be offered in combination with surgery or hormonal therapy. Salvage radiation therapy given for cancer recurrence after a radical prostatectomy may improve survival for some men.

- External beam radiation is the most widely used method. Brachytherapy using radioactive seed implants placed in the prostate gland is best suited for patients with early-stage disease.

Drug Therapy

The types of drug therapy available for the treatment of prostate cancer are androgen deprivation (hormone) therapy, chemotherapy, or a combination of both.

Prostate cancer growth is largely dependent on the presence of androgens. Androgen deprivation therapy (ADT) is focused on reducing the levels of circulating androgens in order to reduce the tumor growth. One of the biggest challenges with ADT is that almost all tumors treated will become resistant to this therapy *(hormone refractory)* within a few years. Androgen deprivation can be produced by inhibiting androgen production or blocking androgen receptors. See Table 55-7, Lewis et al.: *Medical-Surgical Nursing,* ed 9, p. 1319, for mechanisms of action and side effects from androgen deprivation therapy.

- Luteinizing hormone–releasing hormone (LHRH) agonists (e.g., leuprolide [Lupron, Eligard, Viadur], goserelin [Zoladex], triptorelin [Trelstar], buserelin [Suprefact]) produce a chemical castration similar to the effects of an orchiectomy.
- Androgen receptor blockers (e.g., flutamide [Eulexin], nilutamide [Nilandron], enzalutamide (Xtandi), bicalutamide [Casodex]) compete with circulating androgens at the receptor sites.
- Combining an androgen receptor blocker with an LHRH agonist is an often-used treatment that results in combined androgen blockade.

Chemotherapy is generally reserved for those with hormone-refractory prostate cancer (HRPC) in late-stage disease. In HRPC the cancer is progressing despite treatment. This occurs in patients who have taken an antiandrogen for a certain period of time. The goal of chemotherapy is mainly palliative.

- Men with advanced prostate cancer who have HRPC may receive a vaccine (sipuleucel-T [Provenge]). The vaccine stimulates the patient's system against the cancer and may prolong survival.

Nursing Management

Goals

The patient with prostate cancer will be an active participant in the treatment plan, have satisfactory pain control, follow the therapeutic plan, understand the effect of the therapeutic plan on sexual function, and find a satisfactory way to manage the impact on bladder or bowel function.

Nursing Diagnoses

- Decisional conflict
- Acute pain
- Urinary retention and impaired urinary elimination
- Sexual dysfunction
- Anxiety

Nursing Interventions

One of your most important roles is to encourage patients (in consultation with their health care provider) to have an annual prostate screening (PSA and DRE) starting at the age of 50 years or younger if risk factors are present.

- Provide sensitive, caring support for the patient and the family to help them cope with the cancer diagnosis.
- Care during the preoperative and postoperative phases of radical prostatectomy is similar to surgical procedures for Benign Prostatic Hyperplasia (see pp. 77 to 78).
- Refer to nursing interventions for the patient undergoing radiation therapy (p. 730) and chemotherapy (p. 694).
- Pain control is the primary nursing intervention for the terminally ill patient. It is managed through ongoing pain assessment, administration of prescribed medications (both opioid and nonopioid agents), and the use of nonpharmacologic methods of pain relief (e.g., relaxation breathing).
- In advanced prostate cancer, hospice care is often appropriate and beneficial to the patient and family. (Hospice care is discussed in Chapter 10, Lewis et al.: *Medical-Surgical Nursing,* ed. 9.)

▼ **Patient and Caregiver Teaching**

Teach appropriate catheter care if the patient is discharged with an indwelling catheter in place.

- Instruct the patient to clean the urethral meatus with soap and water once each day; maintain a high fluid intake; keep the collecting bag lower than the bladder at all times; keep the catheter securely anchored to the inner thigh or abdomen; and report any signs of bladder infection, such as bladder spasms, fever, or hematuria.
- If urinary incontinence is a problem, the patient should be encouraged to practice pelvic floor muscle exercises (Kegel) at every urination and throughout the day. Continuous practice during the 4- to 6-week healing process has been shown to improve the success rate.

PSORIATIC ARTHRITIS

Psoriatric arthritis (PsA) is a progressive, inflammatory disease affecting about 10% of the 3 million people with psoriasis. *Psoriasis* is a common, benign, inflammatory skin disorder characterized by the presence of red, irritated, and scaly patches.

- Both PsA and psoriasis appear to have a genetic link with the human leukocyte antigen (HLA) in many patients. Although the exact cause of PsA is unknown, a combination of immune, genetic, and environmental factors is suspected.

PsA can occur in different forms including (1) arthritis involving primarily the small joints of the hands and feet (distal phalangeal [DIP]), (2) asymmetric arthritis involving joints of the extremities, (3) symmetric polyarthritis resembling rheumatoid arthritis, and (4) arthritis of the sacroiliac joints and spine (psoriatic spondylitis).

- On x-ray, cartilage loss and erosion resemble that of rheumatoid arthritis. Advanced cases of PsA often reveal widened joint spaces.
- A "pencil in cup" deformity is common in the DIP joints as a result of osteolysis. In this deformity, the narrowed end(s) of the metacarpals or phalanges insert into the expanded end of the other (adjacent) bone sharing the joint.
- Elevated erythrocyte sedimentation rate (ESR), mild anemia, and elevated blood uric acid levels can be seen in some patients. Therefore the diagnosis of gout must be excluded.

Treatment includes splinting, joint protection, and physical therapy. Nonsteroidal antiinflammatory drugs (NSAIDs) given early in the course of the disease may help with inflammation. Drug therapy also includes the disease-modifying antirheumatic drugs (DMARDs) such as methotrexate, which is effective for both articular and cutaneous manifestations. Sulfasalazine (Azulfidine) and cyclosporine may be used for treating PsA. In addition, biologic and targeted therapy, such as etanercept (Enbrel), golimumab (Simponi), adalimumab (Humira), and infliximab (Remicade), may also be used.

PULMONARY EMBOLISM

Description

Pulmonary embolism (PE) is the blockage of pulmonary arteries by a thrombus, fat, or air embolus or tumor tissue. Risk factors for PE include immobility, surgery within the last 3 months (especially pelvic and lower extremity surgery), history of deep vein thrombosis (DVT), malignancy, obesity, heavy cigarette smoking, and pregnancy.

Approximately 10% of patients with PE die within the first hour. An additional 30% die from recurrent embolism. Treatment with anticoagulants reduces the mortality rate to less than 5%.

Pathophysiology

Most PEs arise from DVT in the deep leg veins. *Venous thromboembolism* (VTE) is the preferred terminology to describe the spectrum of pathologic conditions from DVT to pulmonary embolism (PE).

Lethal pulmonary emboli most commonly originate in the femoral or iliac veins. *Emboli* are mobile clots that generally do not stop moving until they lodge at a narrowed part of the circulatory system. Because of a higher blood flow, the lower lobes of the lung are commonly affected.

Clinical Manifestations

Manifestations of PE are varied and nonspecific, making diagnosis difficult.

- Dyspnea is the most common presenting symptom. Hypoxemia with a low $PaCO_2$ is a common finding.
- Other signs are tachypnea, cough, chest pain, hemoptysis, crackles, wheezing, fever, accentuation of the pulmonic heart sound, tachycardia, syncope, and sudden change in mental status as a result of hypoxemia.
- Massive emboli may produce abrupt hypotension and shock. The mortality rate for massive PE and shock is 30% to 60%.

Small emboli may go undetected or produce vague, transient symptoms. The exception to this is the patient with underlying cardiopulmonary disease, in whom even small or medium-sized emboli may result in severe cardiopulmonary compromise.

Complications

Pulmonary infarction (death of lung tissue) is most likely when (1) the occlusion is of a large or medium-sized pulmonary vessel (more than 2 mm in diameter), (2) there is insufficient collateral blood flow from the bronchial circulation, or (3) preexisting lung disease is present. Infarction results in alveolar necrosis and hemorrhage. Concomitant pleural effusion is frequent.

Pulmonary hypertension results from hypoxemia or involvement of more than 50% of the area of the normal pulmonary bed. As a single event, an embolus does not cause pulmonary hypertension unless it is massive. Recurrent emboli may result in chronic pulmonary hypertension. Pulmonary hypertension eventually results in dilation and hypertrophy of the right ventricle. Depending on the degree of pulmonary hypertension and its rate of development, outcomes can vary, with some patients dying within months of the diagnosis and others living for decades (see Pulmonary Hypertension on the facing page).

Diagnostic Studies
- Spiral (or helical) CT scan is the most frequently used test for PE. If the patient cannot have the contrast media used in a spiral CT, then a ventilation-perfusion (V/Q) scan is done.
- D-dimer testing assists in screening for an embolism.
- Pulmonary angiography is the most sensitive and specific test for emboli.
- Arterial blood gases (ABGs) are abnormal with pulmonary occlusion but are not diagnostic of PE.

Collaborative Care
Objectives of treatment are to (1) prevent further growth or multiplication of thrombi in the lower extremities, (2) prevent embolization from the upper or lower extremities to the pulmonary vascular system, and (3) provide cardiopulmonary support if indicated. Supportive therapy for the patient's cardiopulmonary status varies according to the severity of the PE.
- Administration of O_2 is by mask or cannula with the concentration determined by ABG analysis. In some situations, endotracheal intubation and mechanical ventilation may be needed to maintain adequate oxygenation.
- Respiratory measures such as turning, coughing, and deep breathing are important to help prevent or treat atelectasis.
- If shock is present, vasopressor agents may be necessary to support perfusion. If heart failure is present, diuretics are used.

Immediate coagulation is required for patients with PE. Subcutaneous administration of low–molecular-weight heparin (LMWH) (e.g., enoxaparin [Lovenox]) has been found to be safer and more effective than using unfractionated heparin. Warfarin (Coumadin) should be initiated within the first 3 days of heparinization and is typically administered for 3 to 6 months. Some health care providers use factor Xa inhibitors and direct thrombin inhibitors in treating PE.
- Fibrinolytic agents, such as tissue plasminogen activator (tPA [Activase]) or alteplase (Activase) dissolve the PE as well as the thrombus source.

Hemodynamically unstable patients with massive PE with contraindications for fibrinolytic therapy are candidates for immediate pulmonary embolectomy. This can be done via a vascular (catheter) or surgical approach. Pulmonary embolectomy has a high mortality rate and is thus not recommended for patients who can be successfully treated otherwise.

- To prevent further emboli, an inferior vena cava (IVC) filter may be surgically placed in the vena cava to prevent migration of large clots from the lower extremities into the pulmonary system.

Nursing Management

Nursing measures aimed at prevention of pulmonary embolism are similar to those for prevention of DVT (see Venous Thrombosis, p. 670).

The prognosis of a patient with pulmonary emboli is good if therapy is promptly instituted. Keep the patient in bed in a semi-Fowler's position to facilitate breathing. Maintain an IV line for medications and fluid therapy. Administer O_2 therapy as ordered. Carefully monitor vital signs, ABGs, cardiac rhythm, pulse oximetry, and lung sounds to assess the patient's status.

- The patient is usually anxious because of pain, inability to breathe, and fear of death. Carefully explain the situation and provide emotional support and reassurance to help relieve the patient's anxiety.

▼ **Patient and Caregiver Teaching**

- Long-term management is similar to that for the patient with DVT (see pp. 670 to 671).
- Patient teaching regarding long-term anticoagulant therapy is critical. Anticoagulant therapy continues for at least 3 to 6 months. Patients with recurrent emboli are treated indefinitely. INR (international normalized ratio) levels are obtained at intervals, and warfarin dosage is adjusted accordingly.
- Discharge planning is aimed at limiting the progression of the condition and preventing complications and recurrence. Reinforce the need for the patient to return to the health care provider for regular follow-up examinations.

PULMONARY HYPERTENSION

Description

Pulmonary hypertension is elevated pulmonary pressures resulting from an increase resistance to blood flow through the pulmonary circulation. Pulmonary hypertension can occur as a primary disease (idiopathic pulmonary arterial hypertension) or as a secondary complication of a respiratory, cardiac, autoimmune, hepatic, or connective tissue disorder (secondary pulmonary arterial hypertension).

Idiopathic pulmonary arterial hypertension (IPAH) is pulmonary hypertension that occurs without an apparent cause. (It was previously known as *primary pulmonary hypertension* [PPH].) If untreated, this disorder can be rapidly progressive, causing right-sided heart failure and death within a few years. Although new drug therapy has greatly improved survival, the disease remains incurable.

Pathophysiology
The etiology of IPAH is unknown. It affects females more than males. The pathophysiology of IPAH is poorly understood. Some type of insult (e.g., hormonal, mechanical) to the pulmonary endothelium may occur, causing a cascade of events leading to vascular scarring, endothelial dysfunction, and smooth muscle proliferation.

Clinical Manifestations
Classic manifestations are dyspnea on exertion and fatigue. Exertional chest pain, dizziness, and exertional syncope are other symptoms. Eventually, as the disease progresses, dyspnea occurs at rest. Pulmonary hypertension increases the workload of the right ventricle and causes right ventricular hypertrophy (a condition called *cor pulmonale*) (see Cor Pulmonale, p. 159) and eventually heart failure (see Heart Failure, p. 280).
- Right-sided cardiac catheterization is the definitive test to diagnose any type of pulmonary hypertension.
- Confirmation of IPAH requires a thorough workup to exclude conditions that may cause secondary pulmonary arterial hypertension. Diagnostic evaluation includes ECG, chest x-ray, pulmonary function tests, echocardiogram, and CT scans.

Nursing and Collaborative Management
Although IPAH has no cure, treatment can relieve symptoms, improve quality of life, and prolong life. Drug therapy consists of several drug classifications that promote vasodilation of the pulmonary blood vessels, reduce right ventricular overload, and reverse remodeling. See Table 28-27, Lewis et al.: *Medical-Surgical Nursing,* ed. 9, p. 555.
- Diuretics are used to manage peripheral edema.
- Anticoagulants are beneficial in pulmonary complications related to thrombus formation.
- Hypoxia is a potent pulmonary vasoconstrictor, and use of low-flow oxygen provides symptomatic relief.

Surgical interventions for pulmonary hypertension include atrial septostomy (AS) and lung transplantation. AS is a palliative procedure that involves the creation of an intraatrial right-to-left shunt to decompress the right ventricle. It is used for a select group of patients awaiting lung transplantation. Lung transplantation is indicated for patients who do not respond to drug therapy and progress to severe right-sided heart failure. Recurrence of the disease has not been reported in individuals who have undergone transplantation.

- A patient teaching and support site for pulmonary hypertension is located at www.phassociation.org.

Secondary Pulmonary Arterial Hypertension

Secondary pulmonary arterial hypertension (SPAH) occurs when a primary disease causes a chronic increase in pulmonary artery pressures. SPAH can develop as a result of parenchymal lung disease, left ventricular dysfunction, intracardiac shunts, chronic pulmonary thromboembolism, or systemic connective tissue disease. The specific primary disease pathology can result in anatomic or vascular changes causing pulmonary hypertension.

Symptoms can reflect the underlying disease, but some are directly attributable to SPAH, including dyspnea, fatigue, lethargy, and chest pain. Diagnosis of SPAH is similar to that of IPAH.

- Treatment of SPAH consists mainly of treating the underlying primary disorder. When irreversible pulmonary vascular damage has occurred, therapies used for IPAH are initiated.

PYELONEPHRITIS

Description

Pyelonephritis is an inflammation of the renal parenchyma and collecting system (including the renal pelvis). *Urosepsis* is a systemic infection arising from a urologic source. Its prompt diagnosis and effective treatment are critical because it can lead to septic shock, the outcome of unresolved bacteremia involving a gram-negative organism (see Shock, p. 566).

Pathophysiology

Pyelonephritis usually begins with colonization and infection of the lower urinary tract via the ascending urethral route. Bacteria normally found in the intestinal tract, such as *Escherichia coli*, frequently cause pyelonephritis.

A preexisting factor is often present, such as *vesicoureteral reflux* (retrograde or backward movement of urine from lower to upper urinary tract) or dysfunction of lower urinary tract function, such as obstruction from benign prostatic hyperplasia or a urinary stone. For residents of long-term care facilities, urinary tract catheterization and the use of indwelling catheters are common causes of pyelonephritis and urosepsis.

Acute pyelonephritis commonly starts in the renal medulla and spreads to the adjacent cortex. Recurring episodes of pyelonephritis, especially in the presence of obstructive abnormalities, can lead to chronic pyelonephritis.

Chronic pyelonephritis is usually the result of recurring infections involving the upper urinary tract. However, it may also occur in the absence of an existing infection, recent infection, or history of urinary tract infections (UTIs). In chronic pyelonephritis, the kidneys become small, atrophic, and shrunken and lose function because of fibrosis (scarring). It often progresses to end-stage kidney disease when both kidneys are involved, even if the underlying infection or problem is successfully eradicated (see Kidney Disease, Chronic, p. 373).

Clinical Manifestations

Acute pyelonephritis manifestations vary from mild fatigue to the sudden onset of chills, fever, vomiting, malaise, flank pain, and costovertebral tenderness on the affected side. Dysuria, urinary urgency, and frequency may also be present. *Costovertebral tenderness* to percussion (costovertebral angle [CVA] pain) is typically present on the affected side. Acute manifestations generally subside within a few days even without specific therapy, although bacteriuria or pyuria usually persists.

Diagnostic Studies

- Urinalysis shows pyuria, bacteriuria, hematuria, and WBC casts.
- CBC count with WBC differential is done to identify leukocytosis.
- Urine and blood cultures may also be obtained.
- Ultrasound is used to identify anatomic abnormalities, hydronephrosis, renal abscesses, or stones.

Chronic pyelonephritis is diagnosed by radiologic and biopsy rather than clinical features. Biopsy results indicate the loss of functioning nephrons, infiltration of the parenchyma with inflammatory cells, and fibrosis.

Collaborative Care

Patients with severe infections or complicating factors such as nausea and vomiting with dehydration require hospital admission. Parenteral antibiotics are often given initially in the hospital to rapidly establish high serum and urinary drug levels.

The patient with mild symptoms may be treated as an outpatient with antibiotics for 14 to 21 days. Symptoms and signs typically improve or resolve within 48 to 72 hours after starting therapy. Relapses may be treated with a 6-week course of antibiotics. Antibiotic prophylaxis may also be used for recurrent infections.

Nursing Management

Goals

The patient with pyelonephritis will have normal renal function, normal body temperature, no complications, relief of pain, and no recurrence of symptoms.

See eNCP 46-1 for the patient with a UTI on the website for Lewis et al.: *Medical-Surgical Nursing,* ed. 9.

Nursing Diagnoses/Collaborative Problem

- Impaired urinary elimination
- Readiness for enhanced self-health management
- Potential complication: urosepsis

Nursing Interventions

It is important that the patient receive early treatment for cystitis to prevent ascending infections. Because the patient with structural abnormalities of the urinary tract is at increased risk for infection, emphasize the need for regular medical care.

Nursing interventions vary depending on symptom severity. These interventions include teaching the patient about the disease process with emphasis on continuing medications as prescribed, having a follow-up urine culture, and recognizing manifestations of recurrence or relapse.

- In addition to antibiotic therapy, encourage the patient to drink at least eight glasses of fluid every day, even after the infection has been treated.
- Rest will increase patient comfort.
- The patient with frequent relapses or reinfections may be treated with long-term, low-dose antibiotics. Understanding the rationale for therapy is important to enhance patient adherence.

RAYNAUD'S PHENOMENON

Description

Raynaud's phenomenon is an episodic vasospastic disorder of the small cutaneous arteries, most frequently involving the fingers and toes. It occurs primarily in young women (typically between 15 and 40 years old). The pathogenesis is due to abnormalities in the vascular, intravascular, and neuronal mechanisms that cause an imbalance between vasodilation and vasoconstriction.

Raynaud's phenomenon may occur in isolation or in association with an underlying disease (e.g., rheumatoid arthritis, scleroderma, or systemic lupus erythematosus). Other contributing factors include occupation-related conditions, such as use of vibrating machinery or work in cold environments, and exposure to heavy metals (e.g., lead).

Clinical Manifestations

Exposure to cold, emotional upsets, tobacco use, and caffeine often bring on symptoms.

- The disorder is characterized by vasospasm-induced color changes (white, red, and blue) of fingers, toes, ears, and nose. Decreased perfusion results in pallor (white). The digits then appear cyanotic (bluish purple). These changes are subsequently followed by rubor (red) caused by the hyperemic response that occurs when blood flow is restored.
- The patient usually describes cold and numbness in the vaso-constrictive phase, with throbbing and aching pain, tingling, and swelling in the hyperemic phase. An episode usually lasts only minutes, but in severe cases it may persist for several hours.
- After frequent, prolonged attacks, the skin may become thickened and the nails brittle. Complications include punctate (small hole) lesions of the fingertips and superficial gangrenous ulcers in advanced stages.
- Diagnosis is based on persistent symptoms for at least 2 years.

Nursing and Collaborative Management

When conservative management is ineffective, drug therapy is considered. Sustained-release calcium channel blockers (e.g., nife-dipine [Procardia]) are the first-line drug therapy. Calcium channel blockers relax smooth muscles of the arterioles by blocking the influx of calcium into the cells. This reduces the frequency and severity of vasospastic attacks.

Prompt intervention is needed for patients with digital ulceration and/or critical ischemia. Treatment options include IV prostanoid therapy (e.g., iloprost), antibiotics, analgesics, and possibly an en-dothelin receptor antagonist (e.g., bosentan [Tracleer]) and surgical debridement of necrotic tissue. Sympathectomy is considered only in advanced cases.

▼ **Patient and Caregiver Teaching**

Teaching should be directed toward preventing recurrent episodes.

- Loose, warm clothing should be worn for protection from cold, including gloves when a refrigerator or freezer is used or cold objects are being handled.

- Temperature extremes should be avoided. Immersing hands in warm water often decreases the spasm.
- Patients should stop using all tobacco products and avoid caffeine and other drugs with vasoconstrictive effects (e.g., pseudoephedrine).
- Provide patients with information about stress management techniques as appropriate.

REACTIVE ARTHRITIS

Reactive arthritis (Reiter's syndrome) is associated with a symptom complex that includes urethritis or cervicitis, conjunctivitis, and mucocutaneous lesions. It occurs more commonly in young men as compared with young women.

- Although the exact etiology is unknown, reactive arthritis appears to be a reaction triggered in the body after exposure to specific genitourinary or GI tract infections. *Chlamydia trachomatis* is most often implicated in sexually transmitted reactive arthritis.
- Reactive arthritis is also associated with GI infections with *Shigella*, Salmonella, Campylobacter, or *Yersinia* species and other microorganisms.

Individuals with inherited HLA-B27 are at increased risk of developing reactive arthritis after sexual contact or exposure to certain enteric pathogens, supporting the likelihood of a genetic predisposition.

- Urethritis develops within 1 to 2 weeks after sexual contact or GI infection. Low-grade fever, conjunctivitis, and arthritis may occur over the next several weeks.
- This arthritis tends to be asymmetric, frequently involving large joints of the lower extremities and toes. Lower back pain may occur with severe disease.
- Mucocutaneous lesions commonly occur as small, painless, superficial ulcerations on the tongue, oral mucosa, and glans penis. Soft tissue manifestations commonly include enthesopathies such as Achilles tendinitis or plantar fasciitis.
- Few laboratory abnormalities occur, although the erythrocyte sedimentation rate (ESR) may be elevated.

Prognosis is favorable, with most patients recovering after 2 to 16 weeks. Because reactive arthritis is often associated with *Chlamydia trachomatis* infection, treatment of patients and their sexual partners with doxycycline (Vibramycin) is widely recommended. Drug therapy may also include nonsteroidal antiinflammatory drugs (NSAIDs), methotrexate, and sulfasalazine. Physical therapy may be helpful during disease recovery.

REFRACTIVE ERRORS

Refractive errors are the most common visual problem. This defect prevents light rays from converging into a single focus on the retina. Defects are a result of corneal curvature irregularities, lens-focusing power, or eye length. Types of refractive errors include the following:

- *Myopia* (nearsightedness), the most common refractive error, is caused by light rays focusing in front of the retina, resulting in an inability to accommodate for objects at a distance.
- *Hyperopia* (farsightedness) is caused by light rays focusing behind the retina and requires the person to use accommodation to focus the light rays on the retina for near and far objects.
- *Presbyopia* is a loss of accommodation resulting from age, with the crystalline lens becoming larger, firmer, and less elastic. This condition generally appears about the age of 40 years and results in an inability to focus on near objects.
- *Astigmatism* is caused by an irregular corneal curvature so that incoming light rays are bent unequally and light rays do not come to a single point of focus on the retina. Astigmatism can occur in conjunction with any of the other refractive errors.

The major symptom of refractive errors is blurred vision. Additional complaints may include ocular discomfort, eye strain, or headaches. Management of refractive errors is correction, which may include eyeglasses, contact lenses, refractive surgery, or surgical implantation of an artificial lens.

RESPIRATORY FAILURE, ACUTE

Description

The major function of the respiratory system is gas exchange, which involves the transfer of oxygen (O_2) and carbon dioxide (CO_2) between inhaled tidal volumes and circulating blood volume within the pulmonary capillary bed. Respiratory failure results when one or both of these gas-exchanging functions are inadequate.

Respiratory failure is not a disease but a symptom of an underlying pathology affecting lung tissue function, O_2 delivery, cardiac output (CO), or the baseline metabolic state. It is a condition that occurs because of one or more diseases involving the lungs or other body systems (Table 73). Respiratory failure is classified as hypoxemic or hypercapnic. Many patients experience both hypoxemic and hypercapnic respiratory failure.

- *Hypoxemic respiratory failure* is also referred to as oxygenation failure because the primary problem is inadequate O_2 transfer

Table 73	Causes of Hypoxemic and Hypercapnic Respiratory Failure*

Hypoxemic Respiratory Failure	Hypercapnic Respiratory Failure
Respiratory System ■ Acute respiratory distress syndrome (ARDS) ■ Toxic inhalation (e.g., smoke inhalation) ■ Pneumonia ■ Hepatopulmonary syndrome (e.g., low-resistance flow state, V/Q mismatch) ■ Massive pulmonary embolism (e.g., thrombus emboli, fat emboli) ■ Pulmonary artery laceration and hemorrhage ■ Inflammatory state and related alveolar injury	**Respiratory System** ■ Asthma ■ COPD ■ Cystic fibrosis **Central Nervous System** ■ Brainstem injury or infarction ■ Sedative and opioid overdose ■ Spinal cord injury ■ Severe head injury **Chest Wall** ■ Thoracic trauma (e.g., flail chest) ■ Kyphoscoliosis ■ Pain ■ Severe obesity
Cardiac System ■ Anatomic shunt (e.g., ventricular septal defect) ■ Cardiogenic pulmonary edema ■ Shock (decreasing blood flow through pulmonary vasculature) ■ High cardiac output states: diffusion limitation	**Neuromuscular System** ■ Myasthenia gravis ■ Critical illness polyneuropathy ■ Acute myopathy ■ Toxin exposure or ingestion (e.g., tree tobacco, acetylcholinesterase inhibitors, carbamate or organophosphate poisoning) ■ Amyotrophic lateral sclerosis ■ Phrenic nerve injury ■ Guillain-Barré syndrome ■ Poliomyelitis ■ Muscular dystrophy ■ Multiple sclerosis

V/Q, Ventilation-perfusion.
*This list is not all inclusive.

between the alveoli and the pulmonary capillaries. Although no universal definition exists, hypoxemic respiratory failure is commonly defined as a partial pressure of oxygen in arterial blood (PaO_2) of 60 mm Hg or less when the patient is receiving an inspired O_2 concentration of at least 60%.

- *Hypercapnic respiratory failure* is also referred to as ventilatory failure because the primary problem is insufficient CO_2 removal. Hypercapnic respiratory failure is commonly defined as a partial pressure of carbon dioxide in arterial blood (Pa CO_2) greater than 45 mm Hg in combination with acidemia (pH less than 7.35).

Pathophysiology

Hypoxemic Respiratory Failure

Four physiologic mechanisms may cause hypoxemia and subsequent hypoxemic respiratory failure: (1) mismatch between ventilation (V) and perfusion (Q) commonly referred to as V/Q mismatch, (2) shunt, (3) diffusion limitation, and (4) hypoventilation. The most common causes are V/Q mismatch and shunt.

- Many diseases and conditions cause *V/Q mismatch.* The most common are those in which increased secretions are present in the airways (e.g., chronic obstructive pulmonary disease [COPD]) or alveoli (e.g., pneumonia) or when bronchospasm is present (e.g., asthma). V/Q mismatch may also result when alveoli collapse (atelectasis) or as a result of pain.
- *Shunt* occurs when blood exits the heart without having participated in gas exchange. A shunt can be viewed as an extreme V/Q mismatch. There are two types of shunt: anatomic and intrapulmonary. O_2 therapy alone may be ineffective in increasing the PaO_2 if hypoxemia is caused by shunt.
- *Diffusion limitation* occurs when gas exchange across the alveolar-capillary interface is compromised by a process that thickens, damages, or destroys the alveolar membrane or affects blood flow through the pulmonary capillaries. Diffusion limitation is worsened by disease states affecting the pulmonary vascular bed, such as severe emphysema or recurrent pulmonary emboli. Some diseases cause the alveolar-capillary membrane to become thicker (fibrotic), which slows gas transport. These diseases include pulmonary fibrosis, interstitial lung disease, and acute respiratory distress syndrome (ARDS). The classic sign of diffusion limitation is hypoxemia that is present during exercise but not at rest.
- *Alveolar hypoventilation* is a generalized decrease in ventilation that results in an increase in the $PaCO_2$ and a consequent decrease in PaO_2. Alveolar hypoventilation may be the result of restrictive lung disease, central nervous system (CNS) disease, chest wall dysfunction, or neuromuscular disease.

Frequently, hypoxemic respiratory failure is caused by a combination of V/Q mismatch, shunt, diffusion limitation, and alveolar hypoventilation.

Hypercapnic Respiratory Failure

Hypercapnic respiratory failure results from an imbalance between ventilatory supply and ventilatory demand. Normally, ventilatory supply far exceeds ventilatory demand. However, patients with preexisting lung disease such as severe COPD cannot effectively increase lung ventilation in response to exercise or metabolic demands. Hypercapnic respiratory failure is sometimes called ventilatory failure because the primary problem is the inability of the respiratory system to remove sufficient CO_2 to maintain a normal $PaCO_2$.

- Many diseases can cause a limitation in ventilatory supply (see Table 73). They can be grouped into four categories: (1) abnormalities of the airways and alveoli, (2) abnormalities of the CNS, (3) abnormalities of the chest wall, and (4) neuromuscular conditions.

Clinical Manifestations

Respiratory failure may develop suddenly (minutes or hours) or gradually (several days or longer). A sudden decrease in PaO_2 or a rapid rise in $PaCO_2$ implies a serious condition that can rapidly become a life-threatening emergency.

Manifestations are related to the extent of the change in PaO_2 and $PaCO_2$, the rapidity of change (acute versus chronic), and the ability to compensate to overcome this change. When the patient's compensatory mechanisms fail, respiratory failure occurs. Because manifestations are variable, it is important to monitor trends in arterial blood gas (ABG) values and/or pulse oximetry to evaluate the extent of change.

- Mental status changes such as restlessness, confusion, and combative behavior will occur early, frequently before ABG results indicate changes.
- Tachycardia, tachypnea, and mild hypertension are also early signs. A severe morning headache may suggest that hypercapnia occurred during the night. Rapid shallow breaths suggest that the tidal volume may be inadequate to remove CO_2 from the lungs.
- As the PaO_2 decreases and acidosis increases, the myocardium becomes dysfunctional, resulting in angina and dysrhythmias. Permanent brain damage may occur if the hypoxia is severe and prolonged. Renal function may be impaired, and sodium retention, edema formation, acute tubular necrosis, and uremia may occur.

The patient may have a rapid, shallow breathing pattern or a respiratory rate that is slower than normal. A change from a rapid to a slower rate in a patient in acute respiratory distress suggests extreme progression of respiratory fatigue and increased possibility of respiratory arrest.

- Respiratory behaviors such as assumption of tripod position, pursed-lip breathing, and two- or three-word dyspnea also indicate respiratory distress.

- There may be a change in the inspiratory (I) to expiratory (E) (I/E) ratio. Normally the I/E ratio is 1:2. In patients in respiratory distress, the ratio may increase to 1:3 or 1:4. This change signifies airflow obstruction.
- You may observe *retraction* (inward movement) of the intercostal spaces or the supraclavicular area and the use of accessory muscles during inspiration or expiration. Use of the accessory muscles signifies moderate distress. Paradoxic breathing indicates severe distress.

Immediately report any change in mental status, such as agitation, confusion, or a decreased level of consciousness (LOC), because this change may indicate the onset of rapid deterioration and the need for mechanical ventilation.

Diagnostic Studies

- ABGs determine the levels of $PaCO_2$, PaO_2, bicarbonate, and pH.
- Chest x-ray helps to identify possible causes of respiratory failure.
- A catheter may be inserted into a peripheral artery for monitoring BP and obtaining ABGs.
- Pulse oximetry monitors oxygenation status but reveals little about lung ventilation.
- Other studies may include CBC, serum electrolytes, urinalysis, and ECG.
- Sputum and blood cultures are obtained as necessary to determine sources of possible infection.
- If pulmonary embolus is suspected, a V/Q lung scan or CT scan may be done.

In severe respiratory failure requiring endotracheal intubation, end-tidal CO_2 ($ETCO_2$) may be used to assess tube placement within the trachea immediately following intubation. $ETCO_2$ may also be used during ventilator management to assess trends in lung ventilation. A central venous or pulmonary artery (PA) catheter is often used to measure hemodynamic parameters (e.g., central venous pressure, PA pressures, CO, pulmonary artery wedge pressure, central/mixed venous O_2 saturation [$ScvO_2$/SvO_2]).

Nursing and Collaborative Management

Because many different problems can cause respiratory failure, specific care of these patients varies. Goals and related interventions to maximize O_2 delivery are essential to improving the patient's oxygenation and ventilation status. The primary goal is to treat the underlying cause of the respiratory failure. Other supportive goals include maintaining an adequate CO and hemoglobin concentration.

- Interventions are directed toward reversing the disease process that resulted in the development of acute respiratory failure.

- Decreased cardiac output is treated by administration of IV fluids, medications, or both.
- If hemoglobin concentration is less than 9 g/dL (less than 90 g/L), packed RBCs may be transfused.

Nursing Diagnoses
- Impaired gas exchange
- Ineffective airway clearance
- Ineffective breathing pattern

Respiratory Therapy

The major goals of care for acute respiratory failure include maintaining adequate oxygenation and ventilation. Interventions include O_2 therapy, mobilization of secretions, and positive pressure ventilation (PPV).

O_2 Therapy. The primary goal of O_2 therapy is to correct hypoxemia (see Oxygen Therapy, p. 717). If hypoxemia is secondary to V/Q mismatch, supplemental O_2 administered at 1 to 3 L/min by nasal cannula or 24% to 32% by simple face mask or Venturi mask should improve the PaO_2 and SaO_2. Hypoxemia secondary to an intrapulmonary shunt is usually not responsive to high O_2 concentrations, and the patient usually requires PPV (see Mechanical Ventilation, p. 711).

- Patients with chronic hypercapnia should receive O_2 through a low-flow device, such as a nasal cannula at 1 to 2 L/min or a Venturi mask at 24% to 28%. Closely monitor these patients for changes in mental status, respiratory rate, and ABG results until their PaO_2 level has reached their baseline normal value.

Mobilization of Secretions. Retained pulmonary secretions may cause or exacerbate acute respiratory failure by blocking O_2 movement into the alveoli and the removal of CO_2. Secretions can be mobilized through effective coughing, adequate hydration and humidification, chest physical therapy, ambulation when possible, and tracheal suctioning.

Effective Coughing and Positioning. If secretions are obstructing the airway, encourage the patient to cough. The patient with a neuromuscular weakness from disease or exhaustion may not be able to generate sufficient airway pressures to produce an effective cough. *Augmented coughing (quad coughing)* may be helpful. Perform augmented coughing by placing the palm of your hand (or the palms of both hands) on the patient's abdomen below the xiphoid process. As the patient ends a deep inspiration and begins the expiration, move your hands forcefully downward, increasing abdominal pressure and facilitating the cough.

- Positioning the patient by elevating the head of the bed to at least 45 degrees or using a reclining chair bed may help maximize thoracic expansion.

- Lateral or side-lying positioning may be used in patients with disease involving only one lung. This position, termed *good lung down,* allows for improved V/Q matching in the affected lung. All patients should be side-lying if there is a possibility that the tongue will obstruct the airway or aspiration may occur. Keep an oral or nasal artificial airway at the bedside for use if necessary.

Hydration and Humidification. Thick and viscous secretions are difficult to expel. Adequate fluid intake (2 to 3 L/day) keeps secretions thin and easier to remove. If the patient is unable to take sufficient fluids orally, IV hydration is used. Assess for signs of fluid overload by clinical evaluation (e.g., crackles, dyspnea) and invasive monitoring (e.g., increased central venous pressure) at regular intervals.

Airway Suctioning. If the patient is unable to expectorate secretions, nasopharyngeal, oropharyngeal, or nasotracheal suctioning is done. Suctioning through an artificial airway, such as an endotracheal tube, is also performed as needed. At all times, suction cautiously and closely monitor the patient for complications (e.g., hypoxia, increased intracranial pressure, dysrhythmias).

Positive Pressure Ventilation. If intensive measures fail to improve ventilation and oxygenation, and the patient continues to show signs of acute respiratory failure, ventilatory assistance may be initiated (see Mechanical Ventilation, p. 711). PPV may be provided invasively through orotracheal or nasotracheal intubation or noninvasively through a nasal or face mask.

Drug Therapy

Goals of drug therapy for patients in acute respiratory failure include relief of bronchospasm, reduction of airway inflammation and pulmonary congestion, treatment of pulmonary infection, and reduction of severe anxiety and restlessness.

Relief of Bronchospasm. Relief of bronchospasm increases alveolar ventilation. Short-acting bronchodilators, such as metaproterenol (Alupent) and albuterol (Ventolin), reverse bronchospasm, using either a hand-held nebulizer or a metered-dose inhaler with a spacer. These drugs may be given at 15- to 30-minute intervals until you determine that a response is occurring.

Reduction of Airway Inflammation. Corticosteroids (e.g., methylprednisolone [Solu-Medrol]) may be used in conjunction with bronchodilating agents when bronchospasms and inflammation are present. Inhaled corticosteroids require 4 to 5 days for optimum therapeutic effects and are not used for acute respiratory failure.

Reduction of Pulmonary Congestion. IV diuretics (e.g., furosemide [Lasix]) and nitroglycerin (e.g., Tridil) are used to decrease the pulmonary congestion caused by heart failure. If atrial fibrillation is also present, calcium channel blockers and β-adrenergic blockers are used to decrease heart rate and improve cardiac output.

Treatment of Pulmonary Infections. Pulmonary infections can either cause or exacerbate acute respiratory failure. IV antibiotics, such as azithromycin (Zithromax) or ceftriaxone (Rocephin), are often given to treat infections.

Reduction of Severe Anxiety and Restlessness. Anxiety, restlessness, and agitation result from hypoxia. In addition, fear caused by the inability to breathe and a sense of loss of control may increase anxiety. Anxiety, pain, and agitation increase O_2 consumption, which may worsen the degree of hypoxemia. Anxiety, pain, and agitation also increase CO_2 production, affect ventilator management, and increase morbidity.

- Sedation and analgesia with drug therapy are used to decrease anxiety, agitation, and pain.

Nutritional Therapy

Maintenance of protein and energy stores is especially important because nutritional depletion causes a loss of muscle mass, including the respiratory muscles, and may prolong recovery. During the acute manifestations of respiratory failure, the risk of aspiration typically prevents oral intake. Enteral or parenteral nutrition may be administered until acute manifestations subside.

RESTLESS LEGS SYNDROME

Description

Restless legs syndrome (RLS), also known as *Willis-Ekbom disease (WED),* is characterized by unpleasant sensory (paresthesias) and motor abnormalities of one or both legs. Prevalence rates vary from 5% to 15%, although the numbers may be higher, because the condition is underdiagnosed.

There are two distinct types of RLS, primary (idiopathic) and secondary. The majority of cases are primary, and many patients with this type of RLS report a positive family history. Secondary RLS can be seen in metabolic abnormalities associated with iron deficiency, renal failure, polyneuropathy associated with diabetes mellitus, rheumatoid arthritis, or pregnancy. Anemia, pregnancy, and certain medications can cause or worsen symptoms.

Pathophysiology

Although the exact pathophysiology of primary RLS is unknown, it is believed that RLS is related to a dysfunction in the brain's basal ganglia circuits that use the neurotransmitter dopamine, which controls movements. In RLS, this dysfunction causes the urge to move the legs. Abnormal iron metabolism or brain iron deficiencies may result in abnormalities of the dopamine system, thus leading to RLS.

Clinical Manifestations

The severity of RLS sensory symptoms ranges from infrequent minor discomfort (paresthesias including numbness, tingling, "pins and needles") to severe pain. Sensory symptoms often appear first and are manifested as an annoying and uncomfortable (but usually not painful) sensation in the legs.

- Some describe the sensations as bugs creeping or crawling on the skin.
- The leg pain is localized within the calf muscles.
- Patients can also experience pain in the upper extremities and trunk that occurs when the patient is sedentary and usually in the evening or at night.
- Pain at night can produce sleep disruptions and is often relieved by physical activity such as walking, stretching, rocking, or kicking.

Over time, RLS advances to more frequent and severe episodes.

Diagnostic Studies

RLS is a clinical diagnosis based in large part on the patient's history or the report of the bed partner related to nighttime activities. Diagnostic criteria include (1) desire to move the extremities, often associated with paresthesias; (2) motor restlessness; (3) worsening of symptoms at rest with at least temporary relief from activity; and (4) worsening of symptoms in the evening or night.

- Polysomnography studies during sleep distinguish RLS from other clinical conditions (e.g., sleep apnea) that disturb sleep.
- CBC, serum ferritin levels, and renal function tests (e.g., serum creatinine) may help to exclude secondary causes of RLS.

Nursing and Collaborative Management

The goal of collaborative management is to reduce patient discomfort and distress and improve sleep quality. When RLS is secondary to uremia or iron deficiency, treatment of these conditions will decrease symptoms.

- Nondrug approaches include establishing regular sleep habits, encouraging exercise, avoiding activities that cause symptoms, and eliminating aggravating factors such as alcohol, caffeine, and certain drugs (antipsychotics, lithium, antihistamines, antidepressants).

If nondrug measures fail to provide symptom relief, drug therapy is an option. The main drugs used in RLS are dopaminergic agents such as carbidopa-levodopa (Sinemet) and dopamine agonists (e.g., ropinirole [Requip]), pramipexole [Mirapex]) to increase the amount of dopamine in the brain. The antiseizure drug gabapentin enacarbil (Horizant) is used to decrease the sensory sensations. If the patient has iron deficiency or low serum ferritin levels, iron supplementation is considered.

Other drugs that may be used include antiseizure drugs and benzodiazepines. Low doses of opioids (e.g., oxycodone) are usually reserved for those patients with severe symptoms who fail to respond to other drug therapies.

RETINAL DETACHMENT

Description

Retinal detachment is a separation of the sensory retina and underlying pigment epithelium with fluid accumulation between the two layers. Almost all patients with an untreated, symptomatic retinal detachment become blind in the involved eye. Risk factors include increasing age, severe myopia, cataract surgery, eye trauma, and family or personal history of retinal detachment.

Pathophysiology

The most common cause is a retinal break, which is an interruption in the full thickness of the retinal tissue. Retinal holes are spontaneous atrophic breaks, and retinal tears occur when the vitreous shrinks with aging and pulls on the retina.

Once there is a retinal break, liquid vitreous enters between the sensory and retinal pigment epithelium layers, causing detachment. Untreated retinal detachment leads to blindness in the involved eye.

Clinical Manifestations

Symptoms of a detaching retina include photopsia ("light flashes"), floaters, and a "cobweb" or ring in the vision field. Once the retina is detached, a painless loss of peripheral or central vision occurs.

Diagnostic Studies

- Direct and indirect ophthalmoscopy or slit lamp microscopy
- Ultrasound to help identify a detachment

Collaborative Care

Some retinal breaks are not likely to progress to detachment. In these situations the ophthalmologist monitors the patient, giving precise information about warning signs and symptoms of impending detachment and instructing the patient to seek immediate evaluation if any of those signs or symptoms are recognized. The ophthalmologist usually refers the patient with a detachment to a retinal specialist.

Treatment objectives are to seal any retinal breaks and relieve inward traction on the retina. Surgical treatment to seal breaks may include laser photocoagulation and cryopexy. Management of inward retinal traction can involve scleral buckling, pneumatic retinopexy, and vitrectomy.

- Reattachment of the retina is successful in 90% of all cases, with visual prognosis dependent on the extent, length, and area of detachment.

Nursing Management

In most cases, retinal detachment is an urgent situation, and the patient is confronted suddenly with the need for surgery. The patient needs emotional support, especially during the immediate preoperative period.

- With postoperative pain, administer prescribed pain medications and teach the patient to take medication as necessary when discharged.
- Discharge planning is important. Begin this process as early as possible because the patient may not be hospitalized long.

▼ **Patient and Caregiver Teaching**

- Instruct the patient with an increased risk of retinal detachment about the signs and symptoms of detachment and to seek immediate evaluation if any of these occur.
- Promote the use of proper protective eyewear to help avoid retinal detachments related to trauma.
- After eye surgery for retinal detachment, review the signs and symptoms of retinal detachment with the patient because the risk of detachment in the other eye is increased.

Patient and caregiver teaching after eye surgery is discussed in Table 22, p. 117.

RHEUMATIC FEVER AND HEART DISEASE

Description

Rheumatic fever (RF) is an acute inflammatory disease of the heart. *Rheumatic heart disease* is a chronic condition resulting from RF that is characterized by scarring and deformity of the heart valves.

Pathophysiology

RF is a complication that occurs as a delayed result (usually after 2 to 3 weeks) after a group A streptococcal pharyngitis. Symptoms of RF appear to be related to an abnormal immunologic response to group A streptococcal cell membrane antigens. RF affects the heart, skin, joints, and central nervous system (CNS).

About 40% of RF episodes are marked by carditis, and all layers of the heart (endocardium, myocardium, pericardium) are involved.

- Rheumatic endocarditis is found mainly in the valves, with swelling and erosion of the valve leaflets. Vegetations form and initially create a fibrous thickening of the valve leaflets, fusion of commissures and chordae tendineae, and fibrosis of the papillary muscle. Stenosis and regurgitation may occur in valve leaflets. The mitral and aortic valves are most commonly affected.
- Nodules, called *Aschoff's bodies,* are formed by a reaction to inflammation with accompanying swelling and fragmentation of collagen fibers. As the Aschoff's bodies age, they become more fibrous, and scar tissue forms in the myocardium.
- Rheumatic pericarditis develops and affects both layers of the pericardium, which becomes thickened and covered with a fibrinous exudate.

The lesions of RF are systemic and involve the skin, joints, and CNS. Painless subcutaneous nodules, arthralgias or arthritis, and chorea may develop.

Clinical Manifestations

The presence of two major criteria, or one major and two minor criteria, plus evidence of a preceding group A streptococcal infection indicates a high probability of RF.

Major Criteria

- *Carditis* is the most important manifestation of RF and results in three signs: (1) an organic heart murmur or murmurs of mitral or aortic regurgitation, or mitral stenosis; (2) cardiac enlargement and heart failure (HF) occurring secondary to myocarditis; and (3) pericarditis resulting in distant heart sounds, chest pain, a pericardial friction rub, or signs of effusion.
- *Monoarthritis or polyarthritis,* the most common finding in RF, involves swelling, warmth, redness, tenderness, and limitation of motion. The larger joints (particularly the knees, ankles, elbows, and wrists) are most affected.
- *Sydenham's chorea* is the major CNS manifestation. It is characterized by involuntary movements (especially of the face and limbs), muscle weakness, and disturbances of speech and gait.
- *Erythema marginatum* lesions are a less common feature. The bright pink, nonpruritic, maplike macular lesions occur mainly on the trunk and proximal extremities and may be exacerbated by heat (e.g., warm bath).
- *Subcutaneous nodules* are firm, small, hard, painless swellings found most commonly over extensor surfaces of the joints, especially the knees, wrists, and elbows.

Minor Criteria

Minor clinical manifestations are frequently present and helpful in diagnosing the disease. These include fever, polyarthralgia, and certain laboratory tests (e.g., elevated C-reactive protein, elevated WBC count).

Evidence of Infection

Evidence of a preceding group A streptococcal infection include a positive rapid antigen test for group A streptococci, an elevated antistreptolysin-O titer, or a positive throat culture.

Diagnostic Studies

- Chest x-ray may show an enlarged heart if HF is present.
- Echocardiogram may show valvular insufficiency and pericardial fluid or thickening.
- ECG reveals a prolonged PR interval with delayed atrioventricular (AV) conduction.

Collaborative Care

Treatment consists of drug therapy and supportive measures. Antibiotic therapy does not change the course of the acute disease or the development of carditis, but it does eliminate residual group A streptococci remaining in the tonsils and pharynx and prevents the spread of organisms to close contacts. Salicylates, nonsteroidal antiinflammatory drugs (NSAIDs), and corticosteroids are effective in controlling the fever and joint manifestations. Corticosteroids are also used if severe carditis is present.

Nursing Management

Goals

The patient with RF and rheumatic heart disease will have normal or baseline heart function, resumption of daily activities without joint pain, and verbalization of the ability to manage the disease sequelae.

Nursing Diagnoses

- Activity intolerance
- Decreased cardiac output
- Ineffective self-health management

Nursing Interventions

RF is a preventable disease that involves the early detection and immediate treatment of group A streptococcal pharyngitis. Adequate treatment of streptococcal pharyngitis prevents initial attacks of RF. Your role is to teach people in the community to seek medical attention for symptoms of streptococcal pharyngitis and emphasize the need for prompt and adequate treatment.

The primary goals of managing a patient with RF are to control and eradicate the infecting organism; prevent cardiac complications; and relieve joint pain, fever, and other symptoms.

- Administer antibiotics as ordered and teach the patient that oral antibiotics require adherence to the full course of therapy.
- Administer antipyretics, NSAIDs, and corticosteroids and monitor fluid intake.
- Promoting optimal rest is essential to reduce cardiac workload and the body's metabolic needs. After acute symptoms have subsided, the patient without carditis should ambulate.
- If the patient has carditis with HF, strict bed rest restrictions apply. Encourage nonstrenuous activities once recovery has begun.

▼ **Patient and Caregiver Teaching**

- Teach the patient with a previous history of RF about the disease process, possible sequelae, and the need for continuous prophylactic antibiotics.
- Patient teaching should include good nutrition, hygiene practices, and adequate rest.
- Caution the patient about the possibility of developing valvular heart disease. Teach the patient to seek medical attention if symptoms such as excessive fatigue, dizziness, palpitations, or exertional dyspnea develop.

RHEUMATOID ARTHRITIS

Description

Rheumatoid arthritis (RA) is a chronic, systemic autoimmune disease characterized by inflammation of connective tissue in the diarthrodial (synovial) joints, typically with periods of remission and exacerbation. RA is frequently accompanied by extraarticular manifestations.

RA occurs globally, affecting all ethnic groups. It can occur at any time of life, but the incidence increases with age, peaking between 30 and 50 years old. An estimated 1.3 million adult Americans are affected by RA. Women are more likely than men to have the disease.

Pathophysiology

Although the exact cause of rheumatoid arthritis is unknown, it probably results from a combination of genetics and environmental triggers. An autoimmune etiology, which is currently the most widely accepted, suggests that changes associated with RA begin when a genetically susceptible person has an initial immune response to an antigen. Although a bacteria or virus has been proposed as a possible antigen, to date no infection or organism has been identified as the cause.

The antigen, which is probably not the same in all patients, triggers the formation of an abnormal immunoglobulin G (IgG). RA is characterized by the presence of autoantibodies against this abnormal IgG. The autoantibodies are known as *rheumatoid factor* (RF), and they combine with IgG to form immune complexes that initially deposit on synovial membranes or superficial articular cartilage in the joints.

- Immune complex formation leads to the activation of complement, and an inflammatory response results. Neutrophils are attracted to the site of inflammation, where they release proteolytic enzymes that damage articular cartilage and cause the synovial lining to thicken.
- Other inflammatory cells include T helper (CD4) cells and proinflammatory cytokines, such as interleukin-1 (IL-1), interleukin-6 (IL-6), and tumor necrosis factor (TNF).
- Genetic predisposition is important in the development of RA.

If unarrested, the disease progresses through four stages, which are identified in Table 74.

| Table 74 | Anatomic Stages of Rheumatoid Arthritis |

Stage	Characteristics
I: Early	No destructive changes on x-ray. Possible x-ray evidence of osteoporosis.
II: Moderate	X-ray evidence of osteoporosis, with or without slight bone or cartilage destruction. No joint deformities (although possibly limited joint mobility). Adjacent muscle atrophy. Possible presence of extraarticular soft tissue lesions (e.g., nodules, tenosynovitis).
III: Severe	X-ray evidence of cartilage and bone destruction in addition to osteoporosis. Joint deformity, such as subluxation, ulnar deviation, or hyperextension, without fibrous or bony ankylosis. Extensive muscle atrophy. Possible presence of extraarticular soft tissue lesions (e.g., nodules, tenosynovitis).
IV: Terminal	Fibrous or bony ankylosis with stage III criteria.

Note: These findings describe spontaneous remission or drug-induced disease suppression. Data from American College of Rheumatology: Classification criteria for determining progression of rheumatoid arthritis. Retrieved from *www.hopkins-arthritis.org/physician-corner/education/acr/acr.html#class_rheum*.

Clinical Manifestations

RA typically develops insidiously. Nonspecific manifestations such as fatigue, anorexia, weight loss, and generalized stiffness may precede the onset of arthritic complaints. The stiffness becomes more localized after weeks to months. Some patients report a history of a precipitating stressful event, such as infection, work stress, physical exertion, childbirth, surgery, or emotional upset.

Articular Manifestations

Articular involvement is manifested by pain, stiffness, limitation of motion, and signs of inflammation (heat, swelling, tenderness). Joint symptoms occur symmetrically and frequently affect the small joints of the hands and feet, as well as the larger peripheral joints, including wrists, elbows, shoulders, knees, hips, ankles, and jaw.

- The patient characteristically has joint stiffness after periods of inactivity. (See Table 74 for a comparison of the manifestations of RA and osteoarthritis [OA].)
- As RA progresses, inflammation and fibrosis of the joint capsule and supporting structures may lead to deformity and disability. Atrophy of muscles and destruction of tendons around the joint cause one articular surface to slip past the other *(subluxation)*. Typical hand deformities include "ulnar drift," "swan neck," and boutonniere deformities.

Extraarticular Manifestations

RA can affect nearly every system in the body. Extraarticular manifestations of RA are depicted in Fig. 65-5, Lewis et al.: *Medical-Surgical Nursing,* ed. 9, p. 1572.

Rheumatoid nodules develop in up to 20% to 30% of all patients with RA. They appear subcutaneously as firm, nontender, granuloma-type masses and are usually found over the extensor surfaces of joints such as the fingers and elbows. Nodules at the base of the spine and back of the head are common in older adults.

Sjögren's syndrome is seen in 10% to 15% of patients with RA. Sjögren's syndrome can occur as a disease by itself or in conjunction with other arthritic disorders, such as RA and systemic lupus erythematosus (SLE). Affected patients have diminished lacrimal and salivary gland secretion, leading to complaints of burning, gritty, and itchy eyes with decreased tearing and photosensitivity (see Sjögren's Syndrome, p. 582).

Felty syndrome occurs most commonly in patients with severe, nodule-forming RA. It is characterized by splenomegaly and leukopenia.

Flexion contractures and hand deformities cause diminished grasp strength and affect the patient's ability to perform self-care tasks. Nodular myositis and muscle fiber degeneration can lead to pain similar to that of vascular insufficiency. Cataract development and loss of vision can result from scleral nodules. Depression may occur, which is often related to the chronic pain associated with RA.

Diagnostic Studies

A diagnosis is often made based on history and physical findings, but some laboratory tests are useful for confirmation and to monitor disease progression.

- Erythrocyte sedimentation rate (ESR) and C-reactive protein are general indicators of active inflammation.
- Positive RF occurs in 80% of patients and titers rise during active disease.
- Antinuclear antibody (ANA) titers may increase in some patients.
- Anti–citrullinated protein antibody (ACPA) testing is another important test. Levels of ACPA are more specific than RF for rheumatoid arthritis and, in some cases, may allow for an earlier and more accurate diagnosis.
- Synovial fluid analysis in early disease often shows a straw-colored fluid with many fibrin flecks. The WBC count of synovial fluid is elevated (up to $25,000/\mu L$).
- Inflammatory changes in the synovium can be confirmed by tissue biopsy.
- X-ray findings (not specifically diagnostic) may reveal bone demineralization and soft tissue swelling during the early months of RA. Later, narrowing of the joint space, destruction of articular cartilage, erosion, subluxation, and deformity are seen. Malalignment and ankylosis are seen in advanced disease.

Collaborative Care

Care of the patient with RA begins with a comprehensive program of education and drug therapy. Teaching regarding drug therapy includes correct administration, reporting of side effects, and frequent medical and laboratory follow-up visits. Physical therapy maintains joint motion and muscle strength. Occupational therapy develops upper-extremity function and encourages joint protection through the use of splints, pacing techniques, and assistive devices.

Drug Therapy

Drugs remain the cornerstone of RA treatment. Because irreversible joint changes can occur as early as the first year of RA, health care providers aggressively prescribe disease-modifying antirheumatic drugs (DMARDs). These drugs have the potential to lessen the permanent effects of RA, such as joint erosion and deformity. Choice of drug is based on disease activity, patient's level of function, and lifestyle considerations, such as the desire to bear children.

- Treatment of early RA often involves methotrexate (Rheumatrex) because it reduces clinical symptoms in days to weeks, is inexpensive, and has a lower toxicity compared with other drugs.

- Sulfasalazine (Azulfidine) and the antimalarial drug hydroxychloroquine (Plaquenil) may be effective DMARDs for mild to moderate disease.
- Leflunomide (Arava) is a synthetic DMARD that blocks immune cell overproduction and has efficacy similar to that of methotrexate and sulfasalazine.
- Tofacitinib (Xeljanz) is used to treat moderate to severe active rheumatoid arthritis. This drug is from a new class of medications called JAK (Janus kinase) inhibitors. The drug interferes with the JAK enzymes that contribute to the joint inflammation.

Biologic and targeted therapy drugs (e.g., etanercept [Enbrel], infliximab [Remicade], adalimumab [Humira]) are also used to slow disease progression in patients with moderate to severe disease who have not responded to DMARDs or in combination therapy with an established DMARD.

- Tumor necrosis factor inhibitors include etanercept (Enbrel), infliximab (Remicade), adalimumab (Humira), certolizumab (Cimzia), and golimumab (Simponi). Other biologic and targeted inhibitors that may be used include anakinra (Kineret), tocilizumab (Actemra), abatacept (Orencia), and rituximab (Rituxan).

Additional drugs used infrequently for treating RA include antibiotics (minocycline [Minocin]), immunosuppressants (azathioprine [Imuran]), penicillamine (Cuprimine), and gold compounds (auranofin [Ridaura], gold sodium thiomalate [Myochrysine]).

Corticosteroid therapy can be used to aid in symptom control. Intraarticular injections may temporarily relieve the pain and inflammation associated with disease flare-ups.

Various NSAIDs and salicylates are included in the drug regimen to treat arthritis pain and inflammation. Enteric-coated aspirin is often used in high dosages of four to six per day (10 to 18 tablets). The newer generation of NSAIDs, COX-2 inhibitors, is effective in RA as well as in OA. Celecoxib (Celebrex) is currently the only available COX-2 inhibitor.

Nursing Management

Goals

The patient with RA will have satisfactory pain relief and minimal loss of functional ability of the affected joints, participate in planning and carrying out the therapeutic regimen, maintain a positive self-image, and perform self-care to the maximum amount possible.

Nursing Diagnoses
- Chronic pain
- Impaired physical mobility
- Disturbed body image

Nursing Interventions

Prevention of RA is not possible at this time. However, community education programs should include information on symptom recognition to promote early diagnosis and treatment. The primary goals in the management of RA are reduction of inflammation, management of pain, maintenance of joint function, and prevention or correction of joint deformity.

Interventions begin with a careful physical assessment (joint pain, swelling, range of motion, general health status), psychosocial assessment (family support, sexual satisfaction, emotional stress, financial constraints, vocation and career limitations), and environmental concerns (transportation, home, and work modifications).

- Suppression of inflammation may be effectively achieved through the administration of NSAIDs, DMARDs, and biologic/targeted therapies. Discuss the action and side effects of each drug and the importance of necessary laboratory monitoring. Make the drug regimen as understandable as possible.
- Nondrug management may include the use of therapeutic heat and cold, rest, relaxation techniques, joint protection, biofeedback, transcutaneous electrical nerve stimulation (TENS), and hypnosis.
- Lightweight splints may be prescribed to rest an inflamed joint and prevent deformity from muscle spasms and contractures. Remove the splints at regular intervals to give the skin care and perform range-of-motion (ROM) exercises. Reapply the splints as prescribed.
- Plan your care and procedures around the patient's morning stiffness. Sitting or standing in a warm shower, sitting in a tub with warm towels around the shoulders, or soaking the hands in a basin of warm water may help to relieve joint stiffness and allow the patient to perform activities of daily living comfortably.
- Alternating scheduled rest periods with activity throughout the day helps relieve fatigue and pain. Help the patient identify ways to modify activities to avoid overexertion.
- Good body alignment while resting can be maintained through the use of a firm mattress or bed board. Encourage positions of extension and teach the patient to avoid positions of flexion. Pillows should never be placed under the knees. A small, flat pillow may be used under the head and shoulders.

Protecting joints from stress is important. Nursing interventions include helping the patient identify ways to modify tasks. Sample activities that protect small joints are listed in Table 65-10, Lewis et al.: *Medical-Surgical Nursing,* ed. 9, p. 1575.

- Patient independence may be increased by occupational therapy training with assistive devices that help simplify tasks, such as built-up utensils, button hooks, and raised toilet seats. A cane or a walker offers support and relief of pain when walking.
- Heat and cold therapy helps to relieve stiffness, pain, and muscle spasm. Application of ice may be beneficial during periods of disease exacerbation, whereas moist heat appears to offer better relief of chronic stiffness.
- Reinforce participation in an exercise program and ensure correct performance of the exercises. Gentle range-of-motion (ROM) exercises are usually done daily to keep the joints functional.

▼ **Patient and Caregiver Teaching**

Self-management and adherence to an individualized home program can only be accomplished if the patient has a thorough understanding of RA, the nature and course of the disease, and the goals of therapy. In addition, consider the patient's value system and perception of the disease.

- Help the patient recognize fears and concerns faced by all people living with a chronic illness. Evaluation of the family support system is important.
- Financial planning may be necessary. Community resources such as a home care nurse, homemaker services, and vocational rehabilitation may be considered. Self-help groups are beneficial for some patients.

SCLERODERMA

Description

Scleroderma (systemic sclerosis) is a disorder of the connective tissue characterized by fibrotic, degenerative, and occasionally inflammatory changes in the skin, blood vessels, synovium, skeletal muscle, and internal organs. Two types of scleroderma exist: *limited cutaneous disease,* which is more common, and *diffuse cutaneous disease*. Both forms are systemic with the degree and type of organ involvement and disease progression distinctly different.

Although symptoms may begin at any time, the usual age of onset is between 30 and 50 years, and most cases occur in women.

Pathophysiology

The exact cause of scleroderma is unknown. Immunologic dysfunction and vascular abnormalities are believed to play a role in the development of widespread systemic disease. Excessive production of collagen leads to progressive tissue fibrosis and occlusion of blood vessels. Proliferation of collagen disrupts the normal functioning of internal organs, such as the lungs, kidney, heart, and GI tract.

- Vascular alterations, which primarily involve the small arteries and arterioles, are almost always present in scleroderma. These changes are some of the earliest alterations in scleroderma.
- Other risk factors associated with skin thickening include environmental or occupational exposure to coal, plastics, and silica dust.

Clinical Manifestations

Manifestations range from a diffuse cutaneous thickening with rapidly progressive and widespread organ involvement to the more benign limited cutaneous form. Signs of limited disease appear on the face and hands, whereas diffuse disease initially involves the trunk and extremities.

Clinical manifestations can be described by the acronym *CREST:* **C**alcinosis (painful calcium deposits in skin), **R**aynaud's phenomenon, **E**sophageal dysfunction (difficulty swallowing), **S**clerodactyly (tightening of the skin on the fingers), and **T**elangiectasia (red spots on the hands, face, and lips).

Raynaud's phenomenon (paroxysmal vasospasm of the digits) is the most common initial complaint in limited systemic sclerosis. Raynaud's phenomenon may precede the onset of systemic disease by months, years, or even decades (see Raynaud's Phenomenon, p. 531).

Symmetric painless swelling or thickening of the skin of the fingers and hands may progress to diffuse scleroderma of the trunk. In limited disease, skin thickening generally does not extend above the elbow or above the knee, although the face can be affected in some individuals. In more diffuse disease, the skin loses elasticity and becomes taut and shiny, producing a typical expressionless face with tightly pursed lips.

About 20% of people with scleroderma develop secondary *Sjögren's syndrome,* a condition associated with dry eyes and dry mouth (see Sjögren's Syndrome, p. 582). Dysphagia, gum disease, and dental caries can result. Frequent reflux of gastric acid also can occur as a result of esophageal fibrosis.

Lung involvement includes pleural thickening, pulmonary fibrosis, pulmonary artery hypertension, and pulmonary function abnormalities.

Primary heart disease consists of pericarditis, pericardial effusion, and cardiac dysrhythmias. Myocardial fibrosis resulting in heart failure occurs most frequently in people with diffuse scleroderma.

Renal disease was previously a major cause of death in diffuse scleroderma. Recent improvements in dialysis, bilateral nephrectomy in patients with uncontrollable hypertension, and kidney transplantation have offered hope to patients with renal failure. In particular, the use of angiotensin-converting enzyme (ACE) inhibitors (e.g., lisinopril [Prinivil]) has had a marked impact on the ability to treat renal disease.

Diagnostic Studies

- Blood studies may reveal mild hemolytic anemia.
- Antinuclear antibodies (ANA) are found in most patients.
- Scleroderma antibody SCL-70 and serum rheumatoid factor (RF) may be found in patients with diffuse disease. Anticentromere antibody is seen in many patients with CREST.
- If renal involvement is present, urinalysis may show proteinuria, microscopic hematuria, and casts.
- X-ray evidence of subcutaneous calcification, distal esophageal hypomotility, and/or bilateral pulmonary fibrosis are diagnostic of scleroderma.
- Pulmonary function studies reveal decreased vital capacity and lung compliance.

Collaborative Care

Management of scleroderma offers no specific treatment. Supportive care is directed toward attempts to prevent or treat the secondary complications of involved organs. Physical therapy helps maintain joint mobility and preserve muscle strength. Occupational therapy assists the patient in maintaining functional abilities.

Drug Therapy

No specific drugs or combinations of drugs have shown to be effective. Vasoactive agents are prescribed in early disease, and calcium channel blockers (nifedipine [Adalat, Procardia] and diltiazem [Cardizem]) are now a common treatment choice for Raynaud's phenomenon. Other vasoactive drugs include reserpine (Serpasil) and losartan (Cozaar). Bosentan (Tracleer), an endothelin receptor antagonist, and epoprostenol (Flolan), a vasodilator, may assist in preventing and treating digital ulcers while improving exercise capacity and heart and lung dynamics.

Topical agents may provide some relief from joint pain. Capsaicin cream may be useful, not only as a local analgesic, but also as a vasodilator. Other therapies are prescribed to treat specific systemic problems, such as tetracycline for diarrhea resulting from bacterial overgrowth, and histamine H_2-receptor blockers (e.g., cimetidine [Tagamet]) and proton pump inhibitors (e.g., omeprazole [Prilosec]) for esophageal symptoms. An antihypertensive agent (e.g., captopril [Capoten], propranolol [Inderal], methyldopa [Aldomet]) may be used to treat hypertension with renal involvement. Immunosuppressive drugs (e.g., cyclophosphamide [Cytoxan], mycophenolate mofetil [CellCept]) may also be used to treat the disease.

Nursing Management

Because prevention is not possible, nursing interventions often begin during hospitalization for diagnostic purposes. Emotional stress and cold ambient temperatures may aggravate Raynaud's phenomenon.

Instruct patients not to have finger-stick blood testing because of compromised circulation and poor healing of the fingers. Teach the patient to protect the hands and feet from cold exposure and possible burns or cuts that might heal slowly. Smoking should be avoided because of its vasoconstricting effect. Lotions may help to alleviate skin dryness and cracking but must be rubbed in for an unusually long time because of skin thickness.

- Dysphagia may be reduced by eating small, frequent meals, chewing carefully and slowly, and drinking fluids. Heartburn may be minimized by using antacids 45 to 60 minutes after each meal and by sitting upright for at least 2 hours after eating.
- Job modifications are often necessary because stair climbing, typing, writing, and cold exposure may pose particular problems.
- Emphasize daily oral hygiene because neglect may lead to increased tooth and gingival problems.
- Biofeedback training and relaxation techniques may be used to reduce tension and improve sleeping habits.

The patient must actively carry out therapeutic exercises at home. Reinforce the use of moist heat applications, assistive devices, and organization of activities to preserve strength and reduce disability. Sexual dysfunction resulting from body changes, pain, muscular weakness, limited mobility, decreased self-esteem, and decreased vaginal secretions may require sensitive counseling by the nurse.

SEIZURE DISORDERS

Description

A *seizure* is a paroxysmal, uncontrolled electrical discharge of neurons in the brain that interrupts normal function. Seizures may accompany a variety of disorders, or they may occur spontaneously without any apparent cause.

- Metabolic disturbances that cause seizures include acidosis, electrolyte imbalances, hypoglycemia, hypoxia, alcohol and barbiturate withdrawal, dehydration, and water intoxication.
- Extracranial disorders that can cause seizures include heart, lung, liver, and kidney disease; systemic lupus erythematosus; diabetes mellitus (DM); hypertension; and septicemia.

Epilepsy is a condition in which a person has spontaneously recurring seizures caused by a chronic underlying condition. National trends show that incidence of epilepsy is increasing in older adults. Some populations are at higher risk to develop epilepsy, including those with Alzheimer's disease, stroke, and people with a parent who has epilepsy.

Pathophysiology

The most common causes of seizure during the first 6 months of life are severe birth injury, congenital defects involving the central nervous system (CNS), infections, and inborn errors of metabolism.

In people between 20 and 30 years old, a seizure disorder usually occurs as a result of structural lesions such as trauma, brain tumors, or vascular disease. After the age of 50 years, primary causes of seizure are stroke and metastatic brain tumors. Nearly 30% of all epilepsy cases are idiopathic. Some types of epilepsy tend to run in families, suggesting a genetic influence.

The etiology of recurring seizures (epilepsy) has long been attributed to a group of abnormal neurons (seizure focus) that undergo spontaneous firing. This firing spreads by physiologic pathways to involve adjacent or distant areas of the brain. The factor that causes this abnormal firing is not clear. Any stimulus that causes the cell membrane of the neuron to depolarize induces a tendency to spontaneous firing. Often the brain area from which epileptic activity arises is found to have scar tissue *(gliosis)*. Scarring is believed to interfere with the normal chemical and structural environment of brain neurons, making them more likely to fire abnormally.

In addition to neuronal alterations, changes in the function of astrocytes may play several key roles in recurring seizures. Activation of astrocytes by hyperactive neurons is one of the crucial factors that predisposes neurons nearby to the generation of an epileptic discharge.

Clinical Manifestations

Clinical manifestations are determined by the site of the electrical disturbance. The preferred method of classifying epileptic seizures is presented in Table 59-6, in Lewis et al.: *Medical-Surgical Nursing,* ed. 9, p. 1420. This system is based on the clinical and electroencephalographic (EEG) manifestations of seizures and divides seizures into two major classes, *generalized* and *focal.*

Depending on the type, a seizure may progress through several phases: (1) *prodromal phase* with signs or activity that precedes a seizure, (2) *aural phase* with a sensory warning, (3) *ictal phase* with full seizure, and (4) *postictal phase,* which is the period of recovery after the seizure.

Generalized Seizures

Generalized seizures involve both sides of the brain and are characterized by bilateral synchronous epileptic discharge in the brain. In most cases the patient loses consciousness for a few seconds to several minutes.

- *Tonic-clonic* (formerly known as grand mal) seizures are the most common generalized seizures. This type of seizure is characterized by a loss of consciousness and falling to the ground if the patient is upright, followed by stiffening of the body (tonic phase) for 10 to 20 seconds and subsequent jerking of the extremities (clonic phase) for another 30 to 40 seconds. Cyanosis, excessive salivation, tongue or cheek biting, and incontinence may accompany the seizure. In the postictal phase the patient usually has muscle soreness, is very tired, and may sleep for several hours. The patient has no memory of the seizure activity.
- *Typical absence* (petit mal) seizures usually occur only in children and rarely continue beyond adolescence. This type of seizure may cease altogether as the child ages, or it may evolve into another type of seizure. The typical clinical manifestation is a brief staring spell resembling "daydreaming" that lasts only a few seconds. When untreated, the seizures may occur up to 100 times each day. The EEG demonstrates a 3-Hz (cycles per second) spike-and-wave pattern that is unique to this type of seizure. Hyperventilation and flashing lights can precipitate absence seizures.
- *Atypical absence* seizures are another type of generalized seizure characterized by a staring spell. A brief warning, peculiar behavior during the seizure and confusion after the seizure are also common.
- Other types of generalized seizures include myoclonic, atonic, tonic, and clonic seizures.

Focal Seizures

Focal seizures (formerly called partial seizures) begin in one hemisphere of the brain in a specific region of the cortex, as indicated by the EEG. They produce signs and symptoms related to the function of the area of the brain involved. For example, if the discharging focus is located in the medial aspect of the postcentral gyrus, the patient may experience paresthesias and tingling or numbness in the leg on the side opposite the focus.

Focal seizures are divided according to their clinical expressions into simple focal seizures (the person remains conscious) and complex focal seizures (the person has a change or loss of consciousness).

Focal seizures may be confined to one side of the brain and remain focal in nature, or they may spread to involve the entire brain, culminating in a generalized tonic-clonic seizure.

Complications

Status epilepticus is a state of continuous seizure activity or a condition in which seizures recur in rapid succession without return to consciousness between seizures. It can occur with any type of seizure. Status epilepticus is the most serious complication of epilepsy and is a neurologic emergency.

- During repeated seizures, the brain uses more energy than can be supplied. Neurons become exhausted and cease to function. Permanent brain damage may result.
- Tonic-clonic status epilepticus is the most dangerous because it can cause ventilatory insufficiency, hypoxemia, cardiac dysrhythmias, and systemic acidosis, all of which can be fatal.
- Severe injury and even death can result from trauma experienced during a seizure. Patients who lose consciousness during a seizure are at greatest risk.

Perhaps the most common complication of seizure disorder is the effect it has on a patient's lifestyle. Although attitudes have improved in recent years, epilepsy still carries a social stigma that can lead to discrimination in employment and educational opportunities. Transportation may also be difficult because of legal sanctions against driving.

Diagnostic Studies

- Most important in diagnosis are accurate and comprehensive descriptions of the seizures and the patient's health history.
- EEG is useful only if it shows abnormalities. It is not a definitive test because some patients who do not have seizure disorders have abnormal EEG patterns, whereas many patients with seizure disorders have normal EEGs between seizures.
- CBC, serum chemistries, studies of liver and kidney function, and urinalysis can rule out metabolic disorders.
- CT scan and MRI can rule out a structural lesion.

- Cerebral angiography, single-photon emission computed tomography (SPECT), magnetic resonance spectroscopy (MRS), magnetic resonance angiography (MRA), and positron emission tomography (PET) may be used in selected situations.

Collaborative Care

Most seizures do not require professional emergency medical care because they are self-limiting and rarely cause body injury. However, if status epilepticus occurs, significant body harm occurs, or the event is a first-time seizure, medical care should be sought immediately. Table 59-8, Lewis et al.: *Medical-Surgical Nursing,* ed. 9, p. 1423, summarizes the emergency care of the patient with a generalized tonic-clonic seizure.

Drug Therapy

Seizure disorders are treated primarily with antiseizure drugs (see Table 59-9, Lewis et al.: *Medical-Surgical Nursing,* ed. 9, p. 1423). Medications generally act by stabilizing the nerve cell membranes and preventing the spread of the epileptic discharge.

The principle of drug therapy is to begin with a single drug based on patient age and weight with consideration of the type, frequency, and cause of seizure and increase the dosage until the seizures are controlled or toxic side effects occur. If seizure control is not achieved with a single drug, the drug dosage and timing or administration may be changed or a second drug may be added.

- Primary drugs to treat generalized tonic-clonic and focal seizures are phenytoin (Dilantin), carbamazepine (Tegretol), phenobarbital, divalproex (Depakote), and primidone (Mysoline). The drugs used to treat absence and myoclonic seizures include ethosuximide (Zarontin), divalproex (Depakote), and clonazepam (Klonopin).
- Other antiseizure drugs include gabapentin (Neurontin), lamotrigine (Lamictal), topiramate (Topamax), tiagabine (Gabitril), levetiracetam (Keppra), and zonisamide (Zonegran). Some of these drugs are broad spectrum and appear to be effective for multiple seizure types.
- Treatment of status epilepticus requires initiation of a rapid-acting antiseizure medication given IV. Drugs most commonly used are lorazepam (Ativan) and diazepam (Valium).
- Antiseizure drugs should not be discontinued abruptly after long-term use, because this can precipitate seizures.

Surgical interventions for patients whose epilepsy cannot be controlled with drug therapy include anterior temporal lobe resection; extratemporal resection and lesionectomies; hemispherectomies; multilobar resections; and corpus callosum sections. These surgeries remove the epileptic focus or prevent spread of epileptic activity in the brain.

- Alternative therapies, such as vagal nerve stimulation and biofeedback, may also be used.

Nursing Management

Goals
The patient with seizures will be free from injury during a seizure, have optimal mental and physical functioning while taking antiseizure drugs, and have satisfactory psychosocial functioning.

Nursing Diagnoses
- Ineffective breathing pattern
- Risk for injury
- Ineffective self-health management

Nursing Interventions
The patient with a seizure disorder should practice good general health habits (e.g., maintaining a proper diet, getting adequate rest, exercising). Help the patient to identify events or situations that precipitate the seizures and give suggestions for avoiding them or handling them better.

Nursing care for a hospitalized patient or for a person who has had seizures as a result of metabolic factors should focus on observation and treatment of the seizure, education, and psychosocial intervention.

- When a seizure occurs, you should carefully observe and record all aspects of the event because the diagnosis and subsequent treatment depend on the seizure description. The description should include the exact onset of the seizure (which body part was affected first and how); the course and nature of the seizure activity (loss of consciousness, tongue biting, automatisms, stiffening, jerking, total lack of muscle tone); the body parts involved and their sequence of involvement; and the presence of autonomic signs (dilated pupils, excessive salivation, altered breathing, cyanosis, flushing, diaphoresis, or incontinence).
- Assessment of the postictal period should include a detailed description of the level of consciousness (LOC), vital signs, memory loss, muscle soreness, speech disorders (aphasia, dysarthria), weakness or paralysis, sleep period, and the duration of each sign or symptom.
- During the seizure you should do the following: maintain a patent airway for the patient, protecting the patient's head, turn the patient to the side, loosen constrictive clothing, and ease the patient to the floor if seated. After the seizure, the patient may require suctioning and oxygen.

- A seizure can be a frightening experience for the patient and for others who may witness it. Assess the level of their understanding and provide information about how and why the event occurred.

▼ **Patient and Caregiver Teaching**

Prevention of recurring seizures is the major goal in the treatment of epilepsy. Drugs must be taken regularly and continually, often for a lifetime. You have an important role in teaching the patient and caregiver. Guidelines for teaching are shown in Table 75.

- Caution the patient not to adjust drug dosages without professional guidance, because this can increase seizure frequency and even cause status epilepticus.
- Ensure that the patient knows the specifics of the drug regimen and what to do if a dose is missed.
- Encourage the patient to report any drug side effects and keep regular appointments with the health care provider.
- Teach the caregiver, family members, and significant others the emergency management of tonic-clonic seizures.
- Provide support for the patient through teaching and by helping to identify effective coping mechanisms.

Table 75	Patient and Caregiver Teaching Guide *Seizure Disorders and Epilepsy*

Include the following information in the teaching plan for the patient with a seizure disorder.

- Take drugs as prescribed. Report any and all side effects of drugs to the health care provider. When necessary, blood is drawn to ensure that therapeutic levels are maintained.
- Use nondrug techniques, such as relaxation therapy and biofeedback training, to potentially reduce the number of seizures.
- Be aware of availability of resources in the community.
- Wear a Medic Alert bracelet or necklace, and carry an identification card.
- Avoid excessive alcohol intake, fatigue, and loss of sleep.
- Eat regular meals and snacks in between if feeling shaky, faint, or hungry.

Caregivers should receive the following information.

- For first aid treatment of tonic-clonic seizure, it is not necessary to call an ambulance or send the patient to the hospital after a single seizure unless the seizure is prolonged, another seizure immediately follows, or extensive injury has occurred.
- During an acute seizure, it is important to protect the patient from injury. his may involve supporting and protecting the head, turning the patient to the side, loosening constrictive clothing, and easing the patient to the floor, if seated.

SEXUALLY TRANSMITTED INFECTIONS

Sexually transmitted infections (STIs) are infectious diseases commonly acquired through sexual contact. Common infections that are transmitted sexually are listed in Table 76.

Infections that are associated with sexual transmission can also be contracted by other routes, such as through blood, blood products, and autoinoculation. See Gonorrhea, p. 255; Syphilis, p. 611; Herpes, Genital, p. 309; Warts, Genital, p. 672; and Chlamydial Infections, p. 124.

An estimated 65 million people in the United States are currently infected with one or more STIs. In the United States, all gonorrhea and syphilis and, in most states, chlamydial infection must be reported to the state or local public health authorities. In spite of this requirement, there are many unreported cases of these infections.

S

| Table 76 | Causes of Sexually Transmitted Infections |

Sexually Transmitted Infection	Cause
Bacterial	
Gonorrhea	*Neisseria gonorrhoeae*
Syphilis	*Treponema pallidum*
Nongonococcal urethritis (NGU), cervicitis, lymphogranuloma venereum	*Chlamydia trachomatis*
Viral	
Genital herpes	Herpes simplex virus (HSV)
Genital warts; cervical, vulvar, vaginal, penile, anal, and oropharyngeal cancers	Human papillomavirus (HPV)
Human immunodeficiency virus (HIV) infection, acquired immunodeficiency syndrome (AIDS)	HIV virus (see Chapter 15)
Hepatitis B and C	Hepatitis B and C viruses (see Chapter 44)
Encephalitis, esophagitis, retinitis, pneumonitis in immunocompromised patients	Cytomegalovirus (CMV)

Many factors are related to the current STI rates. Earlier reproductive maturity and increased longevity has resulted in a longer sexual life span. An increase in the total population has resulted in an increase in the number of susceptible hosts.

- Other factors include greater sexual freedom, lack of barrier methods (e.g., condoms) during sexual activity, and an increased emphasis on sexuality in the media.
- Changes in the methods of contraception are also reflected in the incidence of STIs. The condom is considered to be the best form of protection (other than abstinence) against STIs. Although condom use has increased, condoms are still not used frequently in the general population.
- The preference for oral contraceptives and intrauterine devices (IUDs) that offer no protection against STIs over barrier contraceptives such as condoms increases the risk of transmission of infection.

Nursing Management: Sexually Transmitted Infections

Goals

The patient with an STI will demonstrate understanding of the mode of transmission and the risk posed by STIs, complete treatment and return for appropriate follow-up care, notify or assist in notification of sexual contacts about their need for testing and treatment, abstain from intercourse until infection is resolved, and demonstrate knowledge of safer sex practices.

Nursing Diagnoses

- Risk for infection
- Ineffective health maintenance
- Anxiety

Nursing Interventions

The diagnosis of an STI may be met with a variety of emotions, such as shame, guilt, anger, and a desire for vengeance. Provide counseling and encourage the patient to verbalize feelings. A referral for professional counseling to explore ramifications of an STI may be indicated.

All patients should return to the treatment center for a repeat culture from infected sites or serologic testing at designated times to determine effectiveness of treatment.

- Explain to the patient that cures are not always obtained on the first treatment to reinforce the need for a follow-up visit.
- Advise the patient to inform sexual partners of the need for treatment, regardless of whether they are free of symptoms or experiencing symptoms.

Emphasize to the patient with an STI the importance of certain hygiene measures. An important measure is frequent hand washing and bathing.

- Bathing and cleaning of involved areas can provide local comfort and prevent secondary infection.
- Douching may spread infection and is therefore contraindicated.
- Sexual abstinence is indicated during the communicable phase of the infection. If sexual activity occurs before the patient has completed treatment, the use of condoms may prevent spread of infection and reinfection.

▼ **Patient Teaching**

Be prepared to discuss "safe" sex practices with all patients, not only those who are perceived to be at risk. These practices include abstinence, monogamy with an uninfected partner, avoidance of certain high-risk sexual practices, and use of condoms and other barriers to limit contact with potentially infectious body fluids or lesions. A patient teaching guide related to the patient with a STI is presented in Table 53-9, Lewis et al.: *Medical-Surgical Nursing,* ed. 9, p. 1272.

Initiate a discussion to assess the risk for contracting an STI. Questions to ask include number of partners, type of birth control used, use of condoms, history of an STI, use of IV drugs, and sexual preference. Do not assume that older people are not at risk, as an increasing number of older people are becoming infected.

- All sexually active women should be screened for cervical cancer using a Pap test. Women with a history of STIs are at greater risk for cervical cancer.
- An inspection of the sexual partner's genitals before coitus is recommended. The presence of discharge, sores, blisters, or rash should be viewed with concern.
- Tell men that some protection is provided if they void immediately after intercourse and wash their genitals and adjacent areas with soap and water.
- Women may also benefit from postcoital voiding and washing. Spermicidal jellies and creams have not been shown to reduce STI risk.
- Proper use of a condom provides a highly effective barrier to infection. The condom should be undamaged and correctly in place throughout all phases of sexual activity.
- Actively encourage communities to provide better education related to STIs for their citizens. Teenagers, who are known to have a high incidence of infection, should be a prime target for such educational programs.
- The human papillomavirus (HPV) vaccine that protects against cervical cancer and genital warts should be encouraged before the start of sexual activity.

S

SHOCK

Description

Shock is a syndrome characterized by decreased tissue perfusion and impaired cellular metabolism. The four main categories of shock are cardiogenic, hypovolemic, distributive, and obstructive.

- Although the cause, initial presentation, and management strategies vary for each type of shock, the physiologic responses of the cells to hypoperfusion are similar.

Cardiogenic Shock

Cardiogenic shock occurs when either systolic or diastolic dysfunction of the pumping action of the heart results in reduced cardiac output (CO). The heart's inability to pump the blood forward is classified as systolic dysfunction. The most common cause of systolic dysfunction is acute myocardial infarction (MI). Cardiogenic shock is the leading cause of death from acute MI. The patient experiences impaired tissue perfusion and cellular metabolism because of cardiogenic shock.

- The patient presents with tachycardia, hypotension, and a narrowed pulse pressure. A low CO (less than 4 L/min) and cardiac index (less than 2.5 L/min/m^2) result when systolic dysfunction is present.
- The patient has tachypnea and pulmonary congestion that is evident by the presence of crackles. An increase in the pulmonary artery wedge pressure (PAWP) and pulmonary vascular resistance is also noted.
- Signs of peripheral hypoperfusion (e.g., cyanosis, pallor, diaphoresis, diminished pulses, decreased capillary refill time) are apparent.
- Decreased renal blood flow results in sodium and water retention and decreased urine output. Anxiety, confusion, and agitation may develop as cerebral perfusion is impaired.

Studies helpful in diagnosing cardiogenic shock include laboratory studies (e.g., cardiac enzymes, b-type natriuretic peptide [BNP]), troponin levels), electrocardiogram (ECG), chest x-ray, and echocardiogram.

Hypovolemic Shock

Hypovolemic shock occurs when there is a loss of intravascular fluid volume. The volume loss may be either an absolute or a relative volume loss.

- *Absolute hypovolemia* results when fluid is lost through hemorrhage, GI loss (e.g., vomiting, diarrhea), fistula drainage, diabetes insipidus, or diuresis.

- In *relative hypovolemia*, fluid volume moves out of the vascular space into the extravascular space (e.g., intracavity space). This fluid shift is called *third spacing*. One example of relative volume loss is leakage of fluid from the vascular space to the interstitial space from increased capillary permeability, as seen in burns.

In hypovolemic shock, the size of the vascular compartment remains unchanged while the volume of blood or plasma decreases. A reduction in intravascular volume results in decreased venous return to the heart, decreased preload, decreased stroke volume, and decreased CO. A cascade of events results in decreased tissue perfusion and impaired cellular metabolism, the hallmarks of shock (Fig. 14).

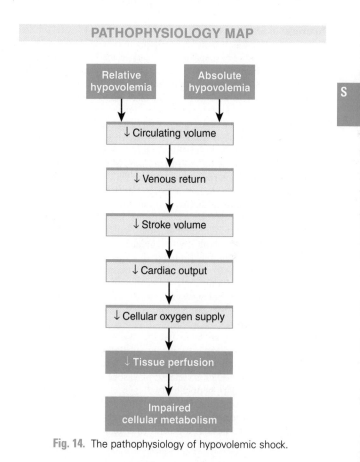

PATHOPHYSIOLOGY MAP

Fig. 14. The pathophysiology of hypovolemic shock.

A total blood loss of 15% to 30% results in a sympathetic nervous system (SNS)–mediated response that causes an increase in heart rate, CO, and respiratory rate and depth. If hypovolemia is corrected at this time, tissue dysfunction is generally reversible.

■ If volume loss is greater than 30%, blood volume must be immediately replaced with blood products. A loss of more than 40% of the total blood volume results in irreversible tissue destruction.

Laboratory studies include serial measurements of hemoglobin and hematocrit levels, electrolytes, lactate, blood gases, and central venous oxygenation ($ScvO_2$), as well as hourly urine outputs.

Distributive Shock (Neurogenic, Anaphylactic, Septic)

Neurogenic Shock

Neurogenic shock is a hemodynamic phenomenon that can occur within 30 minutes after a spinal cord injury at the fifth thoracic (T5) vertebra or above and last up to 6 weeks. The injury results in a massive vasodilation without compensation because of the loss of SNS vasoconstrictor tone. This leads to a pooling of blood in the blood vessels, tissue hypoperfusion, and ultimately impaired cellular metabolism.

In addition to spinal cord injury, spinal anesthesia can also block transmission of impulses from the SNS. Depression of the vasomotor center of the medulla from drugs (e.g., opioids, benzodiazepines) may result in decreased vasoconstrictor tone of the peripheral blood vessels, resulting in neurogenic shock.

■ Clinical manifestations are hypotension (from massive vasodilation) and bradycardia (from unopposed parasympathetic stimulation).

The patient in neurogenic shock may not be able to regulate body temperature. The inability to regulate temperature, combined with massive vasodilation, promotes heat loss. Initially, the patient's skin will be warm because of the massive dilation. As the heat disperses, the patient is at risk for hypothermia.

The pathophysiology of neurogenic shock is described in Fig. 67-4, Lewis et al.: *Medical-Surgical Nursing,* ed. 9, p. 1636.

Anaphylactic Shock

Anaphylactic shock is an acute and life-threatening hypersensitivity (allergic) reaction to a sensitizing substance, such as a drug, chemical, vaccine, food, or insect venom. The reaction quickly causes massive vasodilation, release of vasoactive mediators, and an increase in capillary permeability.

■ As capillary permeability increases, fluid leaks from the vascular space into the interstitial space. Anaphylactic shock can lead to respiratory distress as a result of laryngeal edema or severe bronchospasm, and circulatory failure as a result of massive vasodilation.

- Patients present with a sudden onset of symptoms, including dizziness, chest pain, incontinence, swelling of the lips and tongue, wheezing, and stridor. Skin changes include flushing, pruritus, urticaria, and angioedema.
- A patient can develop a severe allergic reaction, possibly leading to anaphylactic shock, after contact, inhalation, ingestion, or injection with an antigen (allergen) to which the person has previously been sensitized.

Septic Shock

Septic shock is the presence of *sepsis* (systemic inflammatory response to infection) with hypotension despite fluid resuscitation along with the presence of inadequate tissue perfusion resulting in tissue hypoxia. The main organisms that cause sepsis are gram-negative and gram-positive bacteria. Parasites, fungi, and viruses can also lead to the development of sepsis and septic shock. The pathophysiology of septic shock is described in Fig. 67-5, Lewis et al.: *Medical-Surgical Nursing,* ed. 9, p. 1638.

- When a microorganism enters the body, the normal immune/inflammatory cascade responses start. However, in severe sepsis and septic shock, the body's response to the microorganism is exaggerated. There is an increase in inflammation and coagulation and a decrease in fibrinolysis. Endotoxins from the microorganism cell wall stimulate the release of cytokines and other proinflammatory mediators. The combined effects of the mediators result in damage to the endothelium, vasodilation, increased capillary permeability, and neutrophil and platelet aggregation and adhesion to the endothelium.
- Clinical manifestations include an initial decreased ejection fraction with the ventricles dilating so as to maintain stroke volume. The ejection fraction typically improves and the ventricular dilation resolves over 7 to 10 days. Persistence of a high CO and a low systemic vascular resistance (SVR) beyond 24 hours is an ominous finding and is often associated with an increased development of hypotension and multiple organ dysfunction syndrome (MODS) (see Multiple Organ Dysfunction Syndrome, p. 614).
- Respiratory failure is common. The patient initially hyperventilates, resulting in respiratory alkalosis. Once the patient can no longer compensate, respiratory acidosis develops.
- Other clinical signs include decreased urine output, alteration in neurologic status, and GI dysfunction, such as GI bleeding and paralytic ileus.

Obstructive Shock

Obstructive shock develops when a physical obstruction to blood flow occurs with a decreased CO. This can be caused from a restriction to diastolic filling of the right ventricle because of compression (e.g., cardiac tamponade, tension pneumothorax, pulmonary embolism, superior vena cava syndrome). The pathophysiology of obstructive shock is described in Fig. 67-6, Lewis et al.: *Medical-Surgical Nursing,* ed. 9, p. 1638.

■ Patients experience a decreased CO, increased afterload, and variable left ventricular filling pressures depending on the obstruction. Other clinical signs include jugular venous distention and pulsus paradoxus. Rapid assessment and immediate treatment are important to prevent further hemodynamic compromise and possibly cardiac arrest.

Stages of Shock

The shock continuum begins with the initial stage that occurs at a cellular level and is usually not clinically apparent. Metabolism changes at the cellular level from aerobic to anaerobic cause lactic acid buildup. The removal of lactic acid by the liver requires oxygen, which is unavailable because of decreased tissue perfusion.

Shock is categorized into three clinically apparent but overlapping stages: compensatory stage, progressive stage, and irreversible stage.

Compensatory Stage

In the *compensatory stage,* the body activates neural, hormonal, and biochemical mechanisms to overcome the increasing consequences of anaerobic metabolism and maintain homeostasis.

■ One of the classic signs of shock is a drop in BP. The SNS stimulates vasoconstriction and the release of the potent vasoconstrictors epinephrine and norepinephrine. Blood flow to the most essential organs, the heart and brain, is maintained; blood flow to the kidneys, GI tract, and lungs is shunted or diverted.

■ The myocardium responds to SNS stimulation and the increase in oxygen demand by increasing heart rate and contractility.

■ Shunting blood from the lungs has an important effect on the patient in shock. Areas of the lungs participating in ventilation are not perfused because of decreased blood flow to the lungs. The patient has a compensatory increase in the rate and depth of respirations.

■ Decreased blood flow to the kidneys activates the renin-angiotensin-aldosterone system, resulting in vasoconstriction and sodium and water reabsorption.

If the cause of shock is corrected at this stage, the patient recovers with few or no residual effects. If the cause of shock is not corrected and the body is unable to compensate, the patient goes on to the progressive stage of shock.

Progressive Stage

The *progressive stage* of shock begins as compensatory mechanisms fail. Continued decreased cellular perfusion and resulting altered capillary permeability are the distinguishing features of this stage. The patient may have diffuse and profound edema (*anasarca*). In this stage, aggressive interventions are necessary to prevent the development of MODS.

- CO begins to fall, with a resultant decrease in BP and peripheral perfusion, including a decrease in coronary artery, cerebral, and peripheral perfusion. Myocardial dysfunction from decreased perfusion results in dysrhythmias, myocardial ischemia, and possibly myocardial infarction.
- The combined effects of pulmonary vasoconstriction and bronchoconstriction are impaired gas exchange, decreased compliance, and worsening ventilation-perfusion mismatch. The patient presents with tachypnea, crackles, and an overall increased work of breathing.
- As the blood supply to the GI tract is decreased, the normally protective mucosal barrier becomes ischemic, which predisposes the patient to ulcers and GI bleeding.
- The patient has a decreased urine output and an elevated blood urea nitrogen (BUN) and serum creatinine. Metabolic acidosis occurs from an inability to excrete acids and reabsorb bicarbonate.
- Loss of the functional ability of the liver leads to a failure to metabolize drugs and waste products such as ammonia and lactate. Jaundice results from an accumulation of bilirubin.
- Dysfunction of the hematologic system places the patient at risk for the development of disseminated intravascular coagulation (DIC) (see Disseminated Intravascular Coagulation, p. 195).

Irreversible Stage

In the final stage of shock, the *irreversible stage,* decreased perfusion from peripheral vasoconstriction and decreased cardiac output exacerbate anaerobic metabolism. The loss of intravascular volume worsens hypotension and tachycardia and decreases coronary blood flow. Cerebral blood flow cannot be maintained, and cerebral ischemia results.

- The patient demonstrates profound hypotension and hypoxemia. In this final stage, recovery is unlikely. The organs are in failure, and the body's compensatory mechanisms are overwhelmed.

Diagnostic Studies

- Obtaining a thorough medical and surgical history and a history of recent events (e.g., surgery, chest pain, trauma) provides valuable data.

- Blood studies may include CBC, DIC screen, cardiac enzymes, BUN, glucose, electrolytes, arterial blood gases (ABGs), lactate, blood cultures, and liver enzymes.
- Twelve-lead ECG, continuous cardiac monitoring, chest x-ray, continuous pulse oximetry, and hemodynamic monitoring (e.g., arterial pressure, central venous or pulmonary artery [PA] pressure, $ScvO_2/SvO_2$).

See Table 67-3, Lewis et al.: *Medical-Surgical Nursing,* ed. 9, p. 1635, for further information.

Collaborative Care: General Measures

Critical factors in management are early recognition and treatment. Prompt intervention in the early stages may prevent the decline to the progressive or irreversible stage. Successful management includes (1) identification of patients at risk for shock; (2) integration of the patient's history, physical examination, and clinical findings to establish a diagnosis; (3) interventions to control or eliminate the cause of the decreased perfusion; (4) protection of target and distal organs from dysfunction; and (5) provision of multisystem supportive care.

Emergency care of the patient in shock is presented in Table 77. General management strategies begin with ensuring that the patient has a patent airway. Once the airway is established, with either a natural airway or an endotracheal tube, oxygen delivery must be optimized.

- Supplemental oxygen and mechanical ventilation may be necessary to support the delivery of oxygen to maintain an arterial oxygen saturation of at least 90% (PaO_2 greater than 60 mm Hg) to avoid hypoxemia (see Artificial Airways: Endotracheal Tubes, p. 679, Oxygen Therapy, p. 717, and Mechanical Ventilation, p. 711). The mean arterial pressure and circulating blood volume are optimized with fluid replacement and drug therapy (see Table 67-8 in Lewis et al.: *Medical-Surgical Nursing,* ed. 9, p. 1643).

Collaborative Care: Specific Measures

In addition to general management of shock, there are specific interventions for different types of shock (Table 78).

Nursing Management

Goals

The patient with shock will have evidence of adequate tissue perfusion, restoration of normal or baseline BP, return/recovery of organ function, avoidance of complications from prolonged states of hypoperfusion, and prevention of health care–acquired complications of disease management and care.

Table 77 Emergency Management
Shock

Etiology*	Assessment Findings	Interventions
Surgical ■ Postoperative bleeding ■ Ruptured organ or vessel ■ Gastrointestinal bleeding ■ Aortic dissection ■ Vaginal bleeding ■ Ruptured ectopic pregnancy or ovarian cyst **Medical** ■ Myocardial infarction ■ Dehydration ■ Addisonian crisis ■ Diabetes insipidus ■ Sepsis ■ Diabetes mellitus ■ Pulmonary embolus	■ Restlessness ■ Confusion ■ Anxiety ■ Feeling of impending doom ■ Decreased level of consciousness ■ Weakness ■ Rapid, weak, thready pulses ■ Dysrhythmias ■ Hypotension ■ Narrowed pulse pressure ■ Cool, clammy skin (warm skin in early onset of septic and neurogenic shock) ■ Tachypnea, dyspnea, or shallow, irregular respirations ■ Decreased O₂ saturation ■ Extreme thirst ■ Nausea and vomiting	**Initial** ■ Assess ABCs. ■ Stabilize cervical spine as appropriate. ■ Administer high-flow O₂ (100%) by non-rebreather mask or bag-valve-mask. ■ Anticipate need for intubation and mechanical ventilation. ■ Establish IV access with two large-bore catheters (14- to 16-gauge) or assist with insertion of central line and begin fluid resuscitation with crystalloids (e.g., 1 L normal saline solution over 30 min). ■ Draw blood for laboratory studies (e.g., blood cultures, lactate, WBC). ■ Control any external bleeding with direct pressure or pressure dressing. ■ Assess for life-threatening injuries (e.g., cardiac tamponade, liver laceration, tension pneumothorax).

*See Table 67-1 in Lewis, et al.: *Medical-Surgical Nursing,* ed. 9, p. 1632, for additional etiologies of shock.

Continued

S

Table 77 Emergency Management

Shock—cont'd

Etiology*	Assessment Findings	Interventions
Trauma ■ Ruptured or lacerated vessel or organ (e.g., spleen) ■ Fractures, spinal injury ■ Multiorgan injury	■ Chills ■ Pallor ■ Cyanosis ■ Obvious hemorrhage or injury ■ Temperature dysregulation	■ Consider vasopressor therapy if hypotension persists after fluid resuscitation. ■ Insert an indwelling urinary catheter and nasogastric tube. ■ Administer antibiotic therapy after blood cultures if sepsis is suspected. ■ Treat dysrhythmias. **Ongoing Monitoring** ■ Level of consciousness ■ Vital signs, including pulse oximetry; peripheral pulses, capillary refill, skin color and temperature ■ Respiratory status ■ Cardiac rhythm ■ Urine output

Table 78 Collaborative Care
Shock

Oxygenation	Circulation	Drug Therapies	Supportive Therapies
Cardiogenic Shock			
■ Provide supplemental O$_2$ (e.g., nasal cannula, non-rebreather mask) ■ Intubation and mechanical ventilation, if necessary ■ Monitor SvO$_2$ or ScvO$_2$	■ Restore blood flow with thrombolytics, angioplasty with stenting, emergent coronary revascularization ■ Reduce workload of the heart with circulatory assist devices: IABP, VAD	■ Nitrates (e.g., nitroglycerin) ■ Inotropes (e.g., dobutamine) ■ Diuretics (e.g., furosemide) ■ β-Adrenergic blockers (contraindicated with ↓ ejection fraction)	■ Correct dysrhythmias
Hypovolemic Shock			
■ Provide supplemental O$_2$ ■ Monitor SvO$_2$ or ScvO$_2$	■ Restore fluid volume (e.g., blood or blood products, crystalloids) ■ Rapid fluid replacement using two large-bore (14- to 16-gauge) peripheral IV lines or central venous catheter ■ End points of fluid resuscitation: ■ CVP 15 mm Hg ■ PAWP 10-12 mm Hg	■ No specific drug therapy	■ Correct the cause (e.g., stop bleeding, GI losses) ■ Use warmed IV fluids, including blood products (if appropriate)

CO, Cardiac output; *CVP*, central venous pressure; *IABP*, intraaortic balloon pump; *PAWP*, pulmonary artery wedge pressure; *VAD*, ventricular assist device.

Continued

S

Table 78	Collaborative Care *Shock*—cont'd		
Oxygenation	**Circulation**	**Drug Therapies**	**Supportive Therapies**
Septic Shock			

■ Provide supplemental O_2
■ Intubation and mechanical ventilation, if necessary
■ Monitor SvO_2 or $ScvO_2$
	■ Aggressive fluid resuscitation (e.g., 1 L crystalloids every 30-60 min as long as hemodynamic improvement is noted)
	■ End points of fluid resuscitation:
	    ■ CVP 15 mm Hg
	    ■ PAWP 10-12 mm Hg
		■ Antibiotics as ordered
		■ Vasopressors (e.g., norepinephrine)
		■ Inotropes (e.g., dobutamine)
		■ Anticoagulants (e.g., low–molecular-weight heparin)
			■ Obtain cultures (e.g., blood, wound) before beginning antibiotics
			■ Monitor temperature
			■ Control blood glucose
			■ Stress ulcer prophylaxis

Neurogenic Shock			
Maintain patent airway Provide supplemental O_2 Intubation and mechanical ventilation (if necessary)	Cautious administration of fluids	Vasopressors (e.g., phenylephrine) Atropine (for bradycardia)	Minimize spinal cord trauma with stabilization Monitor temperature

Anaphylactic Shock

Maintain patent airway Optimize oxygenation with supplemental O_2 Intubation and mechanical ventilation, if necessary	Aggressive fluid resuscitation with colloids	Epinephrine (IM or IV) Antihistamines (e.g., diphenhydramine) Histamine (H_2)-receptor blockers (e.g., famotidine [Pepcid]) Bronchodilators: nebulized (e.g., albuterol) Corticosteroids (if hypotension persists)	Identify and remove offending cause Prevention via avoidance of known allergens Premedication with history of prior sensitivity (e.g., contrast media)

Obstructive Shock

Maintain patent airway Provide supplemental O_2 Intubation and mechanical ventilation, if necessary	Restore circulation by treating cause of obstruction Fluid resuscitation may provide temporary improvement in CO and BP	No specific drug therapy	Treat cause of obstruction (e.g., pericardiocentesis for cardiac tamponade, needle decompression or chest tube insertion for tension pneumothorax, embolectomy for pulmonary embolism)

CO, Cardiac output; *CVP,* central venous pressure; *IABP,* intraaortic balloon pump; *PAWP,* pulmonary artery wedge pressure; *VAD,* ventricular assist device.

Nursing Diagnoses
- Ineffective peripheral tissue perfusion
- Anxiety

Nursing Interventions

To prevent shock, you need to identify people at risk. In general, patients who are older, those with debilitating diseases, and those who are immunocompromised are at increased risk. Any person who has surgery or trauma is at risk of shock resulting from conditions such as hemorrhage, spinal cord injury, and sepsis.

Your role in shock involves (1) monitoring the patient's ongoing physical and emotional status, (2) identifying trends to detect changes in the patient's condition, (3) planning and implementing nursing interventions and therapy, (4) evaluating the patient's response to therapy, (5) providing emotional support to the patient and caregiver, and (6) collaborating with other members of the health team to coordinate care.

Do not overlook or underestimate the effects of fear and anxiety on the patient and caregiver when faced with a critical, life-threatening situation. Fear, anxiety, and pain may aggravate respiratory distress and increase the release of catecholamines.

- Provide medications to decrease anxiety and pain as appropriate. Continuous infusions of a benzodiazepine (e.g., lorazepam [Ativan]) and an opioid or anesthetic (e.g., morphine, propofol [Diprivan]) are extremely helpful in decreasing anxiety and pain.
- Talk to the patient and encourage the caregiver to talk to the patient, even if the patient is intubated, sedated, or appears comatose. Hearing is often the last sense to be reduced, and even if the patient cannot respond, he or she may still be able to hear. If the intubated patient is capable of writing, provide a "magic slate" or a pencil and paper.
- Do not overlook the patient's spiritual needs. One way to provide support is to offer to call a member of the clergy rather than wait for the patient or caregiver to express a wish for spiritual counseling.

Caregivers can have a therapeutic effect on the patient. To perform this role, they need to be supportive and comforting. Encourage caregivers to perform simple comfort measures if desired. Provide privacy and assure the patient and caregivers that assistance is readily available if needed.

Rehabilitation of the patient who has experienced critical illness necessitates correction of the precipitating cause, prevention or early treatment of complications, and education focused on disease management and/or prevention of recurrence based on initial cause of shock.

- Continue to monitor the patient for indications of complications throughout recovery, including decreased range of motion, decreased physical endurance, renal failure following acute tubular necrosis, and the development of fibrotic lung disease because of acute respiratory distress syndrome (ARDS).

- Patients recovering from shock may require diverse services after discharge. These can include admission to transitional care units (e.g., for mechanical ventilation weaning), rehabilitation centers (inpatient or outpatient), or home health care agencies. Anticipate and facilitate a safe transition from the hospital to home, starting when the patient is admitted to the hospital.

SICKLE CELL DISEASE

Description

Sickle cell disease (SCD) is a group of inherited, autosomal recessive disorders characterized by an abnormal form of hemoglobin (Hgb) in the erythrocyte. This abnormal hemoglobin, *hemoglobin S* (Hgb S), causes the erythrocyte to stiffen and elongate, taking on a sickle shape in response to low oxygen (O_2) levels.

SCD is usually identified during infancy or early childhood. It is an incurable disease that is often fatal by middle age from renal or pulmonary failure and/or stroke. The disease affects about 100,000 Americans and is most common in African Americans, occurring in an estimated prevalence of 1 in about 500 live births.

Pathophysiology

Types of SCD include sickle cell anemia, sickle cell-thalassemia, sickle cell Hgb C disease, and sickle cell trait. *Sickle cell anemia*, the most severe of the SCD syndromes, occurs when a person is homozygous for hemoglobin S (Hgb SS). The person has inherited Hgb S from both parents.

Sickle cell-thalassemia and *sickle cell Hgb C* occur when a person inherits Hgb S from one parent and another type of abnormal hemoglobin (e.g., thalassemia or hemoglobin C) from the other parent. Both of these forms of SCD are less common and less severe than sickle cell anemia.

Sickle cell trait occurs when a person is heterozygous for hemoglobin S (Hgb AS). The person has inherited hemoglobin S from one parent and normal hemoglobin (hemoglobin A) from the other parent. Sickle cell trait is typically a mild to asymptomatic condition.

The major pathophysiologic event of SCD is sickling of erythrocytes. Sickling episodes are most commonly triggered by low O_2 tension in the blood. Hypoxia or deoxygenation of the erythrocytes can be caused by viral or bacterial infection (most common factor), high altitude, emotional stress, surgery, and blood loss. Other triggering events include dehydration, increased hydrogen ion concentration (acidosis), decreased plasma volume, or low body temperature. A sickling episode can also occur without an obvious cause.

- Sickled RBCs become rigid and take on an elongated, crescent shape. Sickled cells cannot easily pass through capillaries or other small vessels and can cause vascular occlusion, leading to acute or chronic tissue injury. The resulting hemostasis promotes a self-perpetuating cycle of local hypoxia, deoxygenation of more erythrocytes, and more sickling.
- Circulating sickled cells are hemolyzed by the spleen, leading to anemia. Initially the sickling of cells is reversible with reoxygenation, but eventually the condition becomes irreversible because of cell membrane damage from recurrent sickling.

Sickle cell crisis is a severe, painful, acute exacerbation of erythrocyte sickling causing a vaso-occlusive crisis. As blood flow is impaired by sickled cells, vasospasm occurs, further restricting blood flow. Tissue ischemia, infarction, and necrosis eventually occur from lack of oxygen. Shock is a possible life-threatening consequence because of severe oxygen depletion of the tissues and a reduction of the circulating fluid volume. Sickle cell crisis can begin suddenly and persist for days to weeks.

- The frequency, extent, and severity of sickling episodes are highly variable and unpredictable, but largely depend on the percentage of Hgb S present. Individuals with sickle cell anemia have the most severe form because erythrocytes contain a high percentage of Hgb S.

Clinical Manifestations

The manifestations of SCD vary greatly from person to person. Many people with sickle cell anemia are in reasonably good health most of the time. However, they may have chronic health problems and pain because of organ tissue hypoxia and damage (e.g., involving the kidneys or liver). The typical patient is anemic but asymptomatic except during sickling episodes.

- Because most individuals with sickle cell anemia have dark skin, pallor is more readily detected by examining the mucous membranes. The skin may have a grayish cast. Because of the hemolysis, jaundice is common and patients are prone to gallstones (cholelithiasis).
- The primary symptom associated with sickling is pain. During sickle cell crisis the pain is quite severe as a result of tissue ischemia. The back, chest, extremities, and abdomen are most commonly affected. Pain episodes are accompanied by fever, swelling, tenderness, tachypnea, hypertension, and nausea and vomiting.

Complications

With repeated episodes of sickling there is gradual involvement of all body systems, especially the spleen, lungs, kidneys, and brain.

- Infection is a major cause of morbidity and mortality in patients with sickle cell disease. Pneumonia is the most common infection.
- The spleen becomes infarcted, dysfunctional, and small because of repeated scarring.
- *Acute chest syndrome* is a pulmonary complication that includes pneumonia, tissue infarction, and fat embolism, resulting in pulmonary hypertension, myocardial infarction (MI), and ultimately cor pulmonale.
- The kidneys may be injured from the lack of oxygen, resulting in renal failure.
- Stroke can result from thrombosis and infarction of cerebral blood vessels.
- The heart may become ischemic and enlarged, leading to heart failure.
- Retinal vessel obstruction may result in hemorrhage, scarring, retinal detachment, and blindness.
- Bone changes may include osteoporosis and osteosclerosis after infarction. Chronic leg ulcers can result from hypoxia.

Diagnostic Studies

- Peripheral blood smear may reveal sickled cells and abnormal reticulocytes.
- Hgb S can be diagnosed by the sickling test, which uses erythrocytes (in vitro) and exposes them to a deoxygenation agent.
- Findings of hemolysis (jaundice, elevated serum bilirubin levels) and abnormal laboratory test results (see Table 9, p. 33) may be present.
- Skeletal x-rays, MRI, and Doppler studies may be indicated to assess for bone and joint deformities, stroke, and deep vein thromboses, respectively.

Nursing and Collaborative Management

Care is directed toward alleviating the symptoms from complications of the disease, minimizing end-organ damage, and promptly treating serious sequelae, such as acute chest syndrome. Teach patients with SCD to avoid high altitudes, maintain adequate fluid intake, and treat infections promptly.

- Pneumovax, *Haemophilus influenzae,* influenza, and hepatitis immunizations should be administered.
- Chronic leg ulcers may be treated with bed rest, antibiotics, warm saline soaks, mechanical or enzyme debridement, and grafting if necessary.

- Sickle cell crises may require hospitalization. O_2 may be administered to treat hypoxia and control sickling. Rest may be instituted to reduce metabolic requirements, and fluids and electrolytes are administered to reduce blood viscosity and maintain renal function.

- Transfusion therapy is indicated when an aplastic crisis occurs. These patients, like those with thalassemia major, may require chelation therapy to reduce transfusion-produced iron overload.

- During an acute crisis, optimal pain control usually includes large doses of continuous (rather than as-needed [prn]) opioid analgesics along with breakthrough analgesia, often in the form of patient-controlled analgesia (PCA).

- Infection must be treated. Patients with acute chest syndrome are treated with broad-spectrum antibiotics, O_2 therapy, and fluid therapy.

- Although many antisickling agents have been tried, hydroxyurea (Hydrea) is the only one shown to be clinically beneficial. This drug increases the production of hemoglobin F (fetal hemoglobin), which is accompanied by a reduction in hemolysis, an increase in hemoglobin concentration, and a decrease in sickled cells and painful crises.

- Hematopoietic stem cell transplantation (HSCT) is the only available treatment that can cure some patients with SCD.

▼ **Patient and Caregiver Teaching**

Patient teaching and support is important in the long-term care of the patient. The patient and caregiver need to understand the basis of the disease and the reasons for supportive care.

- Teach the patient ways to avoid crises, including taking steps to avoid dehydration and hypoxia, such as avoiding high altitudes and seeking medical attention quickly to counteract problems including upper respiratory tract infections.

- Also teach about pain control, because the pain during a crisis may be severe and often requires considerable analgesia.

SJÖGREN'S SYNDROME

Sjögren's syndrome is a relatively common autoimmune disease that targets moisture-producing glands, leading to the common symptoms of xerostomia (dry mouth) and keratoconjunctivitis sicca (dry eyes). The nose, throat, airways, and skin can also become dry. The disease can also affect the stomach, pancreas, and intestines. The disease is usually diagnosed in women after age 40 years.

In *primary Sjögren's syndrome,* symptoms are related to problems with the lacrimal and salivary glands. The patient with primary disease is likely to have antibodies against the cytoplasmic antigens SS-A and SS-B, as well as antinuclear antibody (ANA). The patient with *secondary Sjögren's syndrome* typically has had another autoimmune disease (e.g., rheumatoid arthritis, systemic lupus erythematosus) before Sjögren's develops.

- Sjögren's syndrome appears to be caused by genetic and environmental factors. The trigger may be a viral or bacterial infection that adversely stimulates the immune system, causing lymphocytes to attack and damage the lacrimal and salivary glands.

Decreased tearing leads to a "gritty" sensation in the eyes, burning, blurred vision, and photosensitivity. Dry mouth produces buccal membrane fissures, altered sense of taste, dysphagia, and increased frequency of mouth infections or dental caries.

- Dry skin and rashes, joint and muscle pain, and thyroid problems may also be present. Other exocrine glands can be affected. For example, vaginal dryness may lead to dyspareunia (painful intercourse).
- Autoimmune thyroid disorders are common, including Graves' disease or Hashimoto's thyroiditis.
- The disease may become more generalized and involve the lymph nodes, bone marrow, and visceral organs (pseudolymphoma). People with severe Sjögren's syndrome have a 5% risk of developing non-Hodgkin's lymphoma.

Ophthalmologic examination (Schirmer's test), salivary flow rates, and lower lip biopsy of minor salivary glands confirm the diagnosis.

Treatment is symptomatic, including instillation of artificial tears (e.g., cyclosporine [Restasis]) as necessary to maintain adequate hydration and lubrication, surgical occlusion of the puncta lacrimalia, and increased fluids with meals.

- Pilocarpine (Salagen) and cevimeline (Evoxac) can be used to treat symptoms of dry mouth.
- Increased humidity at home may reduce respiratory infections. Vaginal lubrication with a water-soluble product such as K-Y jelly may increase comfort during intercourse.

SPINAL CORD INJURY

Description

Spinal cord injury (SCI) is caused by trauma or damage to the spinal cord. It can result in either a temporary or permanent alteration in the function of the spinal cord. About 12,000 Americans suffer SCIs each year. About 260,000 people in the United States are living with SCI.

■ The population at highest risk for SCI is young adult men between the ages of 16 and 30 years. SCIs are usually due to trauma, including motor vehicle collisions, falls, violence, and sports injuries.

Pathophysiology

The extent of the neurologic damage caused by an SCI results from primary injury (actual physical disruption of axons) and secondary injury (ischemia, hypoxia, hemorrhage, and edema).

Primary Injury

The initial mechanical disruption of axons as a result of stretch or laceration is referred to as the *primary injury.* SCI can be due to cord compression by bone displacement, interruption of blood supply to the cord, or traction resulting from pulling on the cord. Penetrating trauma, such as gunshot and stab wounds, can result in tearing and transection.

Secondary Injury

Secondary injury refers to the ongoing, progressive damage that occurs after the primary injury. Several theories exist on what causes this ongoing damage, including free radical formation, uncontrolled calcium influx, ischemia, and lipid peroxidation.

■ *Apoptosis* (cell death) occurs and sometimes may continue for weeks or months after the initial injury. Thus the complete cord damage (previously thought to be transection) in severe trauma is related to autodestruction of the cord. This ongoing destructive process makes it critical that the initial care and management of the patient with an SCI be initiated as soon as possible to limit further destruction of the spinal cord.

Figure 15 illustrates the cascade of events causing secondary injury following traumatic spinal cord injury. The resulting hypoxia reduces oxygen tension below the level that meets the metabolic needs of the spinal cord. Lactate metabolites and an increase in vasoactive substances, including norepinephrine, serotonin, and dopamine, are noted. At high levels, these vasoactive substances cause vasospasms and hypoxia, leading to subsequent necrosis. Unfortunately, the spinal cord has minimal ability to adapt to vasospasm.

■ Because secondary injury processes occur over time, the extent of injury and prognosis for recovery are most accurately determined at 72 hours or more after injury.

Spinal and Neurogenic Shock

About 50% of people with acute SCI experience a temporary neurologic syndrome known as *spinal shock* that is characterized by

PATHOPHYSIOLOGY MAP

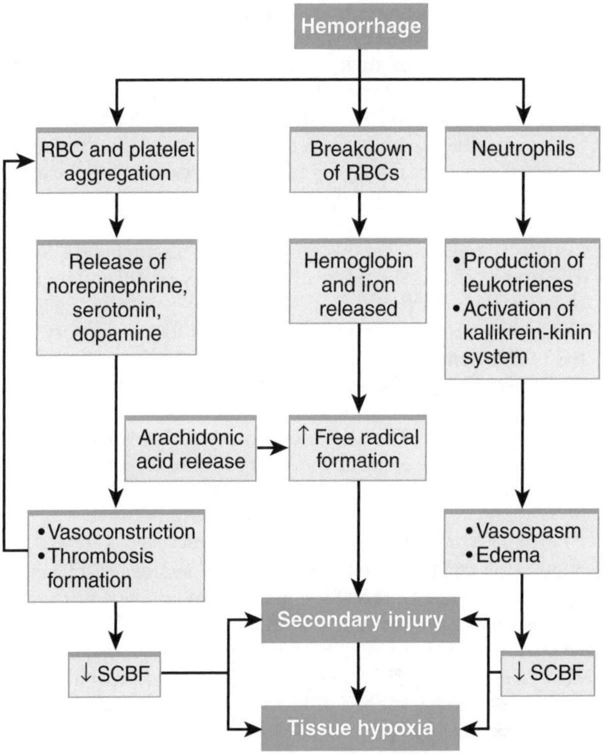

Fig. 15. Cascade of metabolic and cellular events that leads to spinal cord ischemia and hypoxia of secondary injury. *SCBF,* spinal cord blood flow.

decreased reflexes, loss of sensation, and flaccid paralysis below the level of the injury. This syndrome lasts days to months and may mask postinjury neurologic function.

Neurogenic shock results from the loss of vasomotor tone caused by injury and is characterized by hypotension and bradycardia. Loss of sympathetic innervation causes peripheral vasodilation, venous pooling, and decreased cardiac output. These effects are generally associated with a cervical or high thoracic injury (T6 or higher).

Classification

SCIs are classified by the mechanism of injury, level of injury, and degree of injury. The major mechanisms of injury are flexion, hyperextension, flexion-rotation, extension-rotation, and compression. The level of injury may be cervical, thoracic, lumbar, or sacral. Cervical and lumbar injuries are the most common because these levels are associated with the greatest flexibility and movement.

- If the cervical cord is involved, paralysis of all four extremities occurs, resulting in *tetraplegia* (formerly termed *quadriplegia*). However, when the damage is low in the cervical cord, the arms are rarely completely paralyzed.
- If the thoracic, lumbar, or sacral spinal cord is damaged, the result is *paraplegia* (paralysis and loss of sensation in the legs). The degree of spinal cord involvement may be either complete or incomplete (partial).
- *Complete cord involvement* results in total loss of sensory and motor function below the level of the injury.
- *Incomplete cord involvement* (partial transection) results in a mixed loss of voluntary motor activity and sensation and leaves some tracts intact. The degree of sensory and motor loss varies depending on the level of the injury and reflects the specific nerve tracts damaged.

Clinical Manifestations

Manifestations of SCI are related to the level and degree of injury. The patient with an incomplete lesion may demonstrate a mixture of symptoms—the higher the injury, the more serious the effects because of the proximity of the cervical cord to the medulla and brainstem.

Movement and rehabilitation potential related to specific locations of the SCI are described in Table 61-4, Lewis et al.: *Medical-Surgical Nursing,* ed. 9, p. 1473. In general, sensory function closely parallels motor function at all levels.

Complications

Respiratory System

Cervical injuries above the level of C4 present with a total loss of respiratory muscle function. Mechanical ventilation is required to keep the patient alive. Injury or fracture below the level of C4 can result in diaphragmatic breathing with respiratory insufficiency and hypoventilation.

Cardiovascular System

Any cord injury above the level of T6 greatly decreases the influence of the sympathetic nervous system. Bradycardia and peripheral vasodilation result. Cardiac monitoring is necessary.

Urinary System

Urinary retention is common in acute SCI and spinal shock. While the patient is in spinal shock, the bladder is atonic and becomes overdistended. An indwelling catheter is inserted to drain the bladder. In the postacute phase, the bladder may become hyperirritable, with a loss of inhibition from the brain resulting in reflex emptying.

Gastrointestinal System

If SCI has occurred above the level of T5, the primary GI problems are related to hypomotility. Decreased GI activity contributes to the development of a paralytic ileus and gastric distention. A nasogastric (NG) tube for intermittent suctioning may relieve the gastric distention. Histamine H_2-receptor blockers and proton pump inhibitors are frequently used to prevent the development of stress ulcers.

- Loss of voluntary neurologic control over the bowel results in a *neurogenic bowel*. With an injury level of T12 or below, the bowel is areflexic and sphincter tone is decreased, resulting in constipation. As reflexes return, the bowel becomes reflexic, sphincter tone is enhanced, and reflex emptying occurs. Bowel programs can be used to manage both types of neurogenic bowel.

Integumentary System

A major consequence of lack of movement is the potential for skin breakdown over bony prominences in areas of decreased sensation. Pressure ulcers can occur quickly and lead to major infection or sepsis.

Thermoregulation

Poikilothermism (adjustment of body temperature to the room temperature) occurs because the interruption of the sympathetic nervous system prevents peripheral temperature sensations from reaching the hypothalamus. With spinal cord disruption, there is also decreased ability to sweat or shiver below the level of injury, which also affects the ability to regulate body temperature.

Peripheral Vascular Problems

Venous thromboembolism (VTE) is a common problem accompanying SCI in the first 3 months. Pulmonary embolism is one of the leading causes of death in patients with SCI.

Autonomic Dysreflexia

Autonomic dysreflexia is a massive uncompensated cardiovascular reaction mediated by the sympathetic nervous system. It involves stimulation of sensory receptors below the level of the SCI. The intact sympathetic nervous system below the SCI responds to the stimulation by increasing BP, but the parasympathetic nervous system is unable to directly counteract these responses via the injured spinal cord. Baroreceptors in the carotid sinus and the aorta sense the hypertension and stimulate the parasympathetic system. This results in a decreased heart rate, but the visceral and peripheral vessels do not dilate because efferent impulses cannot pass through the injured spinal cord.

- The condition is a life-threatening situation that requires immediate resolution. If resolution does not occur, this condition can lead to status epilepticus, myocardial infarction, stroke, and even death.
- A common precipitating cause is a distended bladder or rectum, although any sensory stimulation may cause autonomic dysreflexia.
- Manifestations include hypertension (up to 300 mm Hg systolic), blurred vision, throbbing headache, marked diaphoresis above the level of the lesion, bradycardia (30 to 40 beats per minute), piloerection (erection of body hair), nasal congestion, and nausea. It is important to measure BP when a patient with an SCI complains of a headache.
- You should elevate the head of the bed 45 degrees or sit the patient upright, notify the physician, and determine the cause. If symptoms persist after the source has been relieved, an α-adrenergic blocker (e.g., phentolamine [Regitine]) or an arterial vasodilator (e.g., nifedipine [Procardia]) is administered.
- Teach the patient and caregiver the causes and symptoms of autonomic dysreflexia (see Table 61-8, Lewis et al.: *Medical-Surgical Nursing,* ed. 9, p. 1480). They must understand the life-threatening nature of this dysfunction and know how to relieve the cause.

Diagnostic Studies
- CT scan is the preferred imaging study to diagnose the location and degree of injury and degree of spinal canal compromise. Cervical x-rays are obtained when CT scan is not readily available.
- MRI is used to assess soft tissue and neurologic changes and for neurologic deficits or worsening of neurologic status.
- Comprehensive neurologic examination is done along with assessment of head, chest, and abdomen for additional injuries or trauma.
- Patients with cervical injuries who demonstrate altered mental status may need vertebral angiography to rule out vertebral artery damage.

Collaborative Care
After stabilization at the injury scene, the person is transferred to a medical facility. A thorough assessment is done to specifically evaluate the degree of deficit and establish the level and degree of injury. The patient may go directly to surgery after initial immobilization and assessment or to the ICU for monitoring and management.

Nonoperative Stabilization
Nonoperative treatments are focused on stabilization of the injured spinal segment and decompression, either through traction

or realignment, to prevent secondary spinal cord damage caused by repeated contusion or compression.

Surgical Therapy

When cord compression is certain or the neurologic disorder progresses, immediate surgery may be beneficial. Surgery stabilizes the spinal column. Early cord decompression may result in reduced secondary injury to the spinal cord and therefore improved outcomes. Other criteria for early surgery include (1) evidence of cord compression, (2) progressive neurologic deficit, (3) compound fracture of the vertebrae, (4) bony fragments (may dislodge and penetrate the cord), and (5) penetrating wounds of the spinal cord or surrounding structures.

- A fusion procedure involves attaching metal screws, plates, or other devices to the bones of the spine to help keep them properly aligned. This is usually done when two or more vertebrae have been injured. Small pieces of bone may also be attached to the injured bones to help them fuse into one solid piece.

Drug Therapy

Methylprednisolone (MP), which was used for many years for the treatment of acute SCI, is no longer recommended. This drug has been associated with harmful side effects including immunosuppression, increased frequency of upper GI bleeding, increased risk of infection, sepsis, longer stays in the ICU, and sometimes death.

- Low–molecular-weight heparin (e.g., enoxaparin [Lovenox]) is used to prevent VTE unless contraindicated.
- Vasopressor agents such as dopamine (Intropin) are used in the acute phase as adjuvants to treatment. These agents maintain mean arterial pressure at a level greater than 90 mm Hg so that perfusion to the spinal cord is improved.

Nursing Management

Goals

The patient with an SCI will maintain an optimal level of neurologic functioning; have minimal or no complications of immobility; learn new skills, gain new knowledge, and acquire new behaviors to be able to care for self or successfully direct others to do so; and return to home and the community at an optimal level of functioning.

Nursing Diagnoses

- Ineffective breathing pattern
- Impaired skin integrity
- Constipation
- Impaired urinary elimination
- Risk for autonomic dysreflexia

Nursing Interventions

High cervical injury resulting from flexion-rotation is the most complex SCI and is discussed in this section. Interventions for this type of injury can be modified for patients with less severe problems.

Immobilization. Proper immobilization of the neck involves maintenance of a neutral position. For cervical injuries, skeletal traction is used less frequently with the development of better surgical stabilization. When skeletal traction is used, realignment or reduction of the injury is usually provided by Crutchfield, Vinke, Gardner-Wells, or other types of skull tongs.

- Infection at the sites of tong insertion is a potential problem. Preventive care includes cleansing the sites twice each day with normal saline solution and applying an antibiotic ointment that acts as a mechanical barrier to the bacteria.
- Special beds are often used to provide frequent turning to prevent pressure sores.

After cervical fusion or other stabilization surgery, a hard cervical collar or sternal-occipital-mandibular immobilizer brace can be worn. In a stable injury for which surgery is not done, a halo fixation apparatus may be applied.

Respiratory Dysfunction. If the patient is exhausted from labored breathing or arterial blood gases (ABGs) deteriorate (indicating inadequate oxygenation), initiate endotracheal intubation or tracheostomy and mechanical ventilation. (See Artificial Airways: Endotracheal Tubes, p. 679, Tracheostomy, p. 732, and Mechanical Ventilation, p. 711.) The possibility of respiratory arrest requires careful monitoring and prompt action should it occur. Pneumonia and atelectasis are potential problems because of reduced vital capacity and the loss of intercostal and abdominal muscle function.

- Regularly assess breath sounds, ABGs, tidal volume, vital capacity, skin color, breathing patterns (especially the use of accessory muscles), subjective comments about the ability to breathe, and the amount and color of sputum.
- In addition to monitoring, you can intervene in maintaining ventilation by the administration of O_2 until ABGs stabilize, chest physiotherapy and assisted coughing, incentive spirometry, and tracheal suctioning.

Cardiovascular Instability. If bradycardia is symptomatic, an anticholinergic medication such as atropine is administered. A pacemaker may be inserted in some patients (see Pacemakers, p. 725). Hypotension is managed with a vasopressor agent, such as dopamine, and fluid replacement.

- Sequential compression devices or compression gradient stockings can be used to prevent thromboemboli and promote venous return.

- Perform range-of-motion (ROM) exercises and stretching regularly. Assess the thighs and calves of the legs every shift for the signs of deep vein thrombosis (DVT).
- Monitor the patient for indications of hypovolemic shock secondary to hemorrhage.

Fluid and Nutritional Maintenance. During the first 48 to 72 hours after the injury, the GI tract may stop functioning (paralytic ileus) and an NG tube must be inserted.

- Once bowel sounds are present or flatus is passed, gradually introduce oral food and fluids. Because of severe catabolism, a high-protein, high-calorie diet is necessary for energy and tissue repair.
- In patients with high cervical cord injuries, evaluate swallowing before starting oral feedings. If the patient is unable to resume eating, enteral nutrition may be started to provide nutritional support.

Bowel and Bladder Management. An indwelling catheter is usually inserted as soon as possible after injury. Ensure its patency by irrigation and frequent inspection. Strict aseptic technique for catheter care is essential to avoid introducing infection.

- Urinary tract infections (UTIs) are a common problem. The best method for preventing UTIs is regular and complete bladder drainage.
- Constipation is generally a problem during spinal shock because no voluntary or involuntary (reflex) evacuation of the bowels occurs. A bowel program should be started during acute care. This consists of a rectal stimulant (suppository or mini-enema) inserted daily at a regular time of day followed by gentle digital stimulation or manual evacuation.

Temperature Control. Because there is no vasoconstriction, piloerection, or heat loss through perspiration below the level of injury, temperature control is largely external to the patient. Monitor the environment closely to maintain an appropriate temperature. Also monitor body temperature regularly.

Stress Ulcers. Stress ulcers are a problem because of the physiologic response to severe trauma, psychologic stress, and high-dose corticosteroids. Peak incidence is 6 to 14 days after injury. Test stool and gastric contents daily for blood, and monitor hematocrit for a slow drop. When corticosteroids are given, administer with antacids or food. Histamine (H_2)-receptor blockers (e.g., ranitidine [Zantac]) or proton pump inhibitors (e.g., omeprazole [Prilosec]) may be given prophylactically to decrease HCl acid secretion.

Sensory Deprivation. You need to compensate for the patient's absent sensations to prevent sensory deprivation. Do this by stimulating the patient above the level of injury. Conversation, music, strong aromas, and interesting foods should be a part of nursing care. Provide prism glasses so the patient can read and watch television. Make every effort to prevent the patient from withdrawing from the environment.

Reflexes. Once spinal shock is resolved, reflexes often return with hyperactive and exaggerated responses. Penile erections can occur from a variety of stimuli, causing embarrassment and discomfort. Spasms ranging from mild twitches to convulsive movements below the level of the lesion may also occur. Reflex activity may be interpreted by the patient or caregiver as a return of function. Tactfully explain the reason for the activity. Spasms may be controlled with antispasmodic medications, such as baclofen (Lioresal), dantrolene (Dantrium), or tizanidine (Zanaflex).

Rehabilitation. Physiologic and psychologic rehabilitation is complex. Many of the problems identified in the acute period become chronic and continue throughout life. Rehabilitation focuses on refined retraining of physiologic processes and extensive patient, caregiver, and family teaching about how to manage the physiologic and life changes resulting from injury.

Rehabilitation and long-term management of the SCI patient are further described in Chapter 61 of Lewis et al.: *Medical-Surgical Nursing,* ed. 9.

SPINAL CORD TUMORS

Description

Spinal cord tumors account for 0.5% to 1% of all neoplasms. These tumors are classified as *primary* (arising from some component of cord, dura, nerves, or vessels) or *secondary* (from primary growths that have metastasized to the spinal cord).

Spinal cord tumors are further classified as *extradural tumors* (outside the spinal cord), *intradural-extramedullary tumors* (within the dura but outside the actual spinal cord), and *intradural-intramedullary tumors* (within the spinal cord itself) (see Fig. 61-13 and Table 61-15, Lewis et al.: *Medical-Surgical Nursing,* ed. 9, pp. 1484 and 1485).

Because many of these tumors are slow growing, their symptoms are due to the mechanical effects of slow compression and irritation of nerve roots, displacement of the cord, or gradual obstruction of the vascular supply. Slowness of growth does not cause autodestruction as in traumatic lesions. Therefore complete functional restoration may be possible when the tumor is removed.

Clinical Manifestations

A common early symptom of a spinal cord tumor is back pain, with the location of the pain depending on the level of compression. The pain worsens with activity, coughing, straining, and lying down.

- Sensory disruption is later manifested by coldness, numbness, and tingling in an extremity or several extremities.
- Motor weakness accompanies sensory disturbances and consists of slowly increasing clumsiness, weakness, and spasticity. Paralysis can develop. The sensory and motor disturbances are ipsilateral to (on the same side as) the lesion.
- Bladder disturbances are marked by urgency with difficulty in starting the flow and progressing to retention with overflow incontinence.

Diagnostic Studies

Extradural tumors are seen on routine spinal x-rays, whereas intradural and intramedullary tumors require MRI or CT scans for detection. Cerebrospinal fluid (CSF) analysis may reveal tumor cells.

Nursing and Collaborative Management

Compression of the spinal cord is an emergency. Relief of the ischemia related to the compression is the goal of therapy. Corticosteroids, usually dexamethasone (Decadron) in large doses, are generally prescribed immediately to relieve tumor-related edema.

Indications for surgery vary depending on the type of tumor. Primary spinal tumors may be removed with the goal of cure. In patients with metastatic tumors, treatment is primarily palliative, with the goal of restoring or preserving neurologic function, stabilizing the spine, and alleviating pain.

Radiation therapy after surgery is fairly effective. Chemotherapy may be used in conjunction with radiation therapy.

- Relief of pain and return of function are the ultimate goals of treatment. Be aware of the patient's neurologic status before and after treatment. Ensuring that the patient receives pain medication as needed is an important nursing responsibility.
- Depending on the amount of neurologic dysfunction exhibited, the patient may need to be cared for as though recovering from a spinal cord injury. Rehabilitation of patients with spinal cord tumors is also similar to spinal cord injury rehabilitation.

SPLEEN DISORDERS

The spleen can be affected by many illnesses, most of which can cause some degree of *splenomegaly* (enlarged spleen).

- The degree of splenic enlargement varies with the disease. For example, massive splenic enlargement occurs with chronic myelogenous leukemia and thalassemia major, whereas mild splenic enlargement occurs with heart failure and systemic lupus erythematosus. When the spleen enlarges, its normal filtering and sequestering capacity increases. Consequently, there is often a reduction in the number of circulating blood cells.

A slight to moderate enlargement of the spleen is usually asymptomatic and found during routine examination of the abdomen. Massive splenomegaly can be well tolerated, but patients may complain of abdominal discomfort and early satiety. In addition to physical examination, other techniques to assess spleen size include radionuclide colloid liver-spleen scan, CT or PET scan, MRI, and ultrasound scan.

Occasionally laparoscopy or open laparotomy and splenectomy are indicated in the evaluation or treatment of splenomegaly. Another indication for splenectomy is splenic rupture. The spleen may rupture from trauma, inadvertent tearing during other surgical procedures, and diseases such as mononucleosis, malaria, and lymphoid neoplasms. After a splenectomy there can be a dramatic increase in increasing peripheral RBC, WBC, and platelet counts.

Nursing responsibilities for patients with spleen disorders vary depending on the problem.

- Splenomegaly may be painful and require analgesic administration; care in moving, turning, and positioning; and evaluation of lung expansion, because spleen enlargement may impair diaphragmatic excursion.
- If anemia, thrombocytopenia, or leukopenia develops from splenic enlargement, institute nursing measures to support the patient and prevent life-threatening complications.
- If splenectomy is performed, observe the patient for hemorrhage and shock.
- Postsplenectomy patients may develop immunologic deficiencies and have a lifelong risk for infection from encapsulated organisms, such as pneumococcus. This risk is reduced by immunization with polyvalent pneumococcal vaccine (Pneumovax).

STOMACH CANCER

Description

Stomach (gastric) cancer is an adenocarcinoma of the stomach wall. The rate of stomach cancer has been steadily declining in the United States since the 1930s. Most individuals are between ages 65 and 80 when diagnosed. More than 50% have advanced metastatic disease at the time of diagnosis. The 5-year survival rate is less than 30% in those with advanced disease and 80% in patients with early-stage cancer confined to the stomach.

Pathophysiology

Many factors have been implicated in stomach cancer. Stomach cancer probably begins with a nonspecific mucosal injury as a result of autoimmune-related inflammation, repeated exposure to irritants such as bile, antiinflammatory agents, or tobacco use. Stomach cancer has also been associated with diets containing smoked foods, salted fish and meat, and pickled vegetables. *Helicobacter pylori* infection, especially at an early age, is considered a risk factor for stomach cancer. Other predisposing factors are obesity, family history, atrophic gastritis, pernicious anemia, adenomatous and hyperplastic polyps, and achlorhydria. Whole grains and fresh fruits and vegetables are associated with reduced rates of stomach cancer.

Stomach cancer spreads by direct extension and typically infiltrates rapidly to the surrounding tissue and liver. Seeding of tumor cells into the peritoneal cavity occurs later in the disease.

Clinical Manifestations

Stomach cancers often spread to adjacent organs before any distressing symptoms occur. Clinical manifestations may include unexplained weight loss, early satiety, indigestion, abdominal discomfort or pain, and signs and symptoms of anemia.

- Anemia commonly occurs with chronic blood loss as the lesion erodes the stomach mucosa. The patient appears pale and weak with fatigue, dizziness, weakness, and positive occult stools.
- Supraclavicular lymph nodes that are hard and enlarged suggest metastasis via the thoracic duct. The presence of ascites is a poor prognostic sign.

Diagnostic Studies

- Upper GI endoscopy is the best diagnostic tool.
- Endoscopic ultrasound and CT and positron emission tomography (PET) scans can be used to stage the disease.

- Laparoscopy can be done to determine peritoneal spread.
- Blood studies detect anemia and its severity and also elevations in liver enzymes and serum amylase, which may indicate liver and pancreatic involvement.
- Stool examination provides evidence of occult or gross bleeding.

Collaborative Care

Treatment of choice is surgical removal of the tumor. Surgical procedures used are similar to those used for peptic ulcer disease (see Peptic Ulcer Disease, pp. 489 to 490).

- Preoperative management focuses on the correction of nutritional deficits and transfusions of packed RBCs to treat anemia. Gastric decompression may be necessary if gastric outlet obstruction is present, and special preparation of the bowel is needed if the tumor has involved the colon.
- Therapy for localized stomach cancer is surgical resection followed by chemotherapy agents used in combination including continuous-infusion fluorouracil, epirubicin, cisplatin, etoposide, irinotecan, capecitabine (Xeloda), docetaxel, and oxaliplatin (Eloxatin) (see Chemotherapy, p. 694).
- The surgical aim is to remove as much of the stomach as necessary to remove the tumor and a margin of normal tissue. When the lesion is located in the fundus, a total gastrectomy with esophagojejunostomy is performed. Lesions located in the antrum or the pyloric region are generally treated by either a Billroth I or II procedure. When metastasis has occurred to adjacent organs, such as the spleen, ovaries, or bowel, the surgical procedure is modified and extended as necessary.

Radiation therapy may be used as a palliative measure to decrease tumor mass and provide temporary relief of obstruction (see Radiation Therapy, p. 730).

Nursing Management

Goals

The patient with stomach cancer will experience minimal discomfort, achieve optimal nutritional status, and maintain a degree of spiritual and psychologic well-being appropriate to the disease stage.

Nursing Diagnoses

- Imbalanced nutrition: less than body requirements
- Anxiety
- Acute pain
- Grieving

Nursing Interventions

Your role in the early detection of stomach cancer is focused on the identification of patients at risk such as those with *H. pylori* infection, pernicious anemia, or achlorhydria. Encourage patients who have a positive family history of stomach cancer to undergo diagnostic evaluation if manifestations of anemia, peptic ulcer disease, or vague epigastric distress are present.

When diagnostic tests confirm a malignancy, offer emotional and physical support, provide information, and clarify test results. The preoperative teaching plan is similar to that for peptic ulcer disease surgery (see Peptic Ulcer Disease, p. 492).

Postoperative care is also similar to that following a Billroth I or II procedure for peptic ulcer disease. When a total gastrectomy is done, closely observe the patient for signs of fluids leaking at the site of anastomosis, as evidenced by an elevation in temperature and increasing dyspnea. Dumping syndrome may also occur with this procedure (see p. 490 under Peptic Ulcer Disease).

- Postoperative wound healing may be impaired because of inadequate dietary intake. This necessitates IV or oral replacement of C, D, K, and B-complex vitamins and IM or intranasal administration of cobalamin.

Your role when radiation therapy or chemotherapy is used is to provide detailed instructions, reassure the patient, and ensure completion of the designated number of treatments. Teach the patient about skin care, the need for good nutrition and fluid intake during therapy, and appropriate use of antiemetic drugs.

▼ **Patient and Caregiver Teaching**

Before discharge, instruct the patient and caregiver about comfort measures and the use of analgesics. Additional considerations include:

- Teach wound care, if needed, to the primary caregiver in the home setting.
- Dressings, special equipment, or special services that may be required for the patient's continued care at home.
- Provide a list of community agencies that are available for assistance.

STROKE

Description

Stroke occurs when there is ischemia to a part of the brain or hemorrhage into the brain that results in brain cell death. Functions, such as movement, sensation, or emotions, that were controlled by the affected brain area are lost or impaired. The severity of the loss of function varies according to the location and extent of the brain damage.

- Stroke is the fourth most common cause of death behind cancer, heart disease, and lung disease. Strokes are considered a major public health problem in the United States in terms of mortality and morbidity, because an estimated 800,000 people experience strokes annually.
- More than 275,000 deaths occur annually from stroke. Of those who survive, 50% to 70% will be functionally independent and 15% to 30% will live with permanent disability.

Risk factors associated with stroke can be divided into non-modifiable and modifiable. Stroke risk increases with multiple risk factors.

Nonmodifiable risk factors include age, ethnicity or race, and family history or heredity. Two thirds of all strokes occur in individuals older than 65 years, but stroke can occur at any age. Strokes are more common in men, but more women die from stroke than men.

- African Americans have a higher incidence of stroke and a higher death rate than whites, which may be related in part to an increased incidence of hypertension, obesity, and diabetes mellitus (DM).
- People with a family history of stroke are also at higher risk for stroke.

Modifiable risk factors are hypertension, cardiovascular disease, DM, obesity, sickle cell disease, and certain lifestyle habits, such as cigarette smoking, a diet high in fat, and excessive alcohol consumption. Hypertension is the single most important modifiable risk factor, and its treatment can reduce the risk of stroke by up to 50%.

Transient Ischemic Attack

A *transient ischemic attack* (TIA) is a transient episode of neurologic dysfunction caused by focal brain, spinal cord, or retinal ischemia, but without acute infarction of the brain. Clinical symptoms typically last less than 1 hour. TIAs may be caused by microemboli that temporarily block the blood flow and are a warning sign of progressive cerebrovascular disease.

Most TIAs resolve. However, it is important to teach the patient to seek treatment for any stroke symptoms, as there is no way to predict if a TIA will resolve or if it is in fact the development of a stroke. In general, one third of individuals who experience a TIA will not experience another event, one third will have additional TIAs, and one third will progress to stroke.

TIA signs and symptoms depend on the blood vessel involved and the brain area that is ischemic.

- If the carotid system is involved, patients may have a temporary loss of vision in one eye, transient hemiparesis, numbness or loss of sensation, or a sudden inability to speak.
- Signs and symptoms of a TIA involving the vertebrobasilar system may include tinnitus, vertigo, darkened or blurred vision, ptosis, dysphagia, ataxia, and unilateral or bilateral numbness or weakness.

TIAs should be treated as medical emergencies. Teach people at risk for TIA to seek medical attention immediately with any stroke-like symptom and to identify the time of symptom onset.

Pathophysiology

Strokes are classified as ischemic or hemorrhagic based on the cause and underlying pathophysiology (Fig. 16 and Table 79).

Ischemic Stroke

An *ischemic stroke* results from inadequate blood flow to the brain from partial or complete occlusion of an artery. Nearly 80% of all strokes are ischemic. A TIA is usually a precursor to ischemic stroke. Ischemic strokes are further divided into thrombotic and embolic.

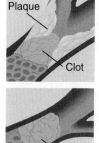

Thrombotic stroke. The process of clot formation (thrombosis) results in a narrowing of the lumen, which blocks the passage of the blood through the artery.

Embolic stroke. An embolus is a blood clot or other debris circulating in the blood. When it reaches an artery in the brain that is too narrow to pass through, it lodges there and blocks the flow of blood.

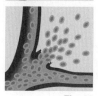

Hemorrhagic stroke. A burst blood vessel may allow blood to seep into and damage brain tissues until clotting shuts off the leak.

Fig. 16. Major causes of stroke.

Table 79 Types of Stroke

Gender and Age	Warning and Onset	Prognosis
Ischemic		
Thrombotic		
Men more than women Oldest median age	*Warning:* TIA (30%–50% of cases) *Onset:* Often during or after sleep	Stepwise progression, signs and symptoms develop slowly, usually some improvement, recurrence in 20%-25% of survivors.
Embolic		
Men more than women	*Warning:* TIA (uncommon) *Onset:* Lack of relationship to activity, sudden onset	Single event, signs and symptoms develop quickly, usually some improvement, recurrence common without aggressive treatment of underlying disease.
Hemorrhagic		
Intracerebral		
Slightly higher in women	*Warning:* Headache (25% of cases) *Onset:* Activity (often)	Progression over 24 hr. Poor prognosis, fatality more likely with presence of coma.
Subarachnoid		
Slightly higher in women Youngest median age	*Warning:* Headache (common) *Onset:* Activity (often), sudden onset, most commonly related to head trauma	Usually single sudden event, fatality more likely with presence of coma.

TIA, Transient ischemic attack.

Thrombotic Stroke

A *thrombotic stroke* occurs from injury to a blood vessel wall and formation of a blood clot. The lumen of the blood vessel becomes narrowed and, if it becomes occluded, infarction occurs. It is the most common cause of stroke.

■ Two thirds of thrombotic strokes are associated with hypertension or DM. Both of these conditions accelerate the atherosclerotic process.

The extent of the stroke depends on rapidity of onset, size of lesion, and presence of collateral circulation.

■ Most patients do not have a decreased level of consciousness in the first 24 hours unless it is caused by a brainstem stroke or other conditions, such as seizures, increased intracranial pressure, or hemorrhage.

■ Ischemic stroke symptoms may progress in the first 72 hours as infarction and cerebral edema increase.

Embolic Stroke

Embolic stroke occurs when an embolus lodges in and occludes a cerebral artery, resulting in infarction and edema of the area supplied by the involved vessel. Embolism is the second most common cause of stroke.

Most emboli originate in the heart. The embolus travels to the cerebral circulation and lodges where a vessel narrows. Heart conditions associated with emboli are atrial fibrillation, myocardial infarction (MI), and inflammatory and valvular heart conditions.

■ The embolic stroke often occurs rapidly, giving little time to accommodate by developing collateral circulation. The patient usually remains conscious, although a headache may develop.

■ Recurrence is common unless the underlying cause is aggressively treated.

Hemorrhagic Stroke

A *hemorrhagic stroke* results from bleeding into the brain tissue itself (intracerebral or intraparenchymal hemorrhage) or into the subarachnoid space or ventricles (subarachnoid hemorrhage). These account for 15% of all strokes.

Intracerebral Hemorrhage

Intracerebral hemorrhage is bleeding within the brain caused by a rupture of a blood vessel. Hypertension is the most important cause of intracerebral hemorrhage. Other causes include vascular malformations, coagulation disorders, anticoagulant drugs, trauma, and ruptured aneurysms.

■ Hemorrhage commonly occurs during periods of activity. Most often there is a sudden onset of symptoms, and progression occurs over minutes to hours as a result of ongoing bleeding.

- Manifestations include neurologic deficits, headache, nausea, vomiting, decreased level of consciousness, and hypertension. Extent of the symptoms varies depending on the amount, location, and duration of bleeding.
- Prognosis of patients with intracerebral hemorrhage is poor, with 40% to 80% of patients dying within 30 days, and 50% of the deaths occurring within the first 48 hours.

Subarachnoid Hemorrhage

Subarachnoid hemorrhage occurs when there is intracranial bleeding into the cerebrospinal fluid-filled space between the arachnoid and pia mater membranes on the surface of the brain. Subarachnoid hemorrhage is commonly caused by rupture of a cerebral aneurysm (congenital or acquired weakness and ballooning of vessels). Other causes of subarachnoid hemorrhage include arteriovenous malformations (AVMs), trauma, and illicit drug (cocaine) abuse.

- The patient may have warning symptoms if the ballooning artery applies pressure to brain tissue, or minor warning symptoms may result from leaking of an aneurysm before major rupture. Sudden onset of a severe headache that is different from a previous headache and typically the "worst headache of one's life" is a characteristic symptom of a ruptured aneurysm.
- Loss of consciousness may or may not occur, and the patient's level of consciousness may range from alert to comatose, depending on the severity of the bleeding.
- Other manifestations include focal neurologic deficits (including cranial nerve deficits), nausea, vomiting, seizures, and stiff neck.
- Despite improvements in surgical techniques and management, many patients with subarachnoid hemorrhage die or are left with significant disability.

Clinical Manifestations

Manifestations seen with specific cerebral artery involvement are listed in Table 58-3, Lewis et al.: *Medical-Surgical Nursing,* ed. 9, p. 1393. Figure 17 illustrates manifestations of right- and left-sided stroke.

Motor Function. Motor deficits are the most obvious effect of stroke. Motor deficits include impairment of (1) mobility, (2) respiratory function, (3) swallowing and speech, (4) gag reflex, and (5) self-care abilities. Symptoms are caused by the destruction of motor neurons in the pyramidal pathway (nerve fibers from the brain that pass through the spinal cord to the motor cells). Because the pyramidal pathway crosses at the level of the medulla, a lesion on one side of the brain affects motor function on the opposite side of the brain (contralateral).

- The initial *hyporeflexia* (depressed reflexes) progresses to *hyperreflexia* (hyperactive reflexes) for most patients.

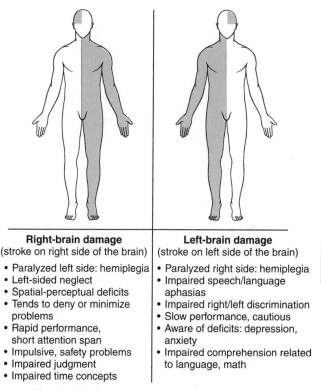

Right-brain damage (stroke on right side of the brain)	**Left-brain damage** (stroke on left side of the brain)
• Paralyzed left side: hemiplegia • Left-sided neglect • Spatial-perceptual deficits • Tends to deny or minimize problems • Rapid performance, short attention span • Impulsive, safety problems • Impaired judgment • Impaired time concepts	• Paralyzed right side: hemiplegia • Impaired speech/language aphasias • Impaired right/left discrimination • Slow performance, cautious • Aware of deficits: depression, anxiety • Impaired comprehension related to language, math

Fig. 17. Manifestations of right- and left-brain stroke.

Communication. The left hemisphere is dominant for language skills in all right-handed people and most left-handed people.

■ Language disorders involve the expression and comprehension of written or spoken words. A*phasia* (total loss of comprehension and use of language) occurs when a stroke damages the dominant hemisphere of the brain.

■ Many stroke patients also experience *dysarthria,* a disturbance in the muscular control of speech.

Affect. Patients who have had a stroke may have difficulty expressing their emotions. Emotional responses may be exaggerated or unpredictable. Depression and feelings associated with changes in body image and loss of function can make this worse. Patients may also be frustrated by mobility and communication problems.

Diagnostic Studies

When manifestations of a stroke occur, diagnostic studies are done to confirm that it is a stroke and not another brain lesion and to identify the likely cause of the stroke. Tests also guide decisions about therapy.

- CT or MRI rapidly distinguish between ischemic and hemorrhagic stroke and help determine the size and location of the stroke.
- CT angiography (CTA) provides visualization of cerebral blood vessels and an estimate of perfusion. CTA also detects filling defects in the cerebral arteries.
- Magnetic resonance angiography (MRA) can detect vascular lesions and blockages similar to CTA.
- Angiography can identify cervical and cerebrovascular occlusion, atherosclerotic plaques, and malformation of vessels.
- Intraarterial digital subtraction angiography (DSA) involves injection of a contrast agent to visualize vessels in the neck and the circle of Willis.
- Transcranial Doppler (TCD) ultrasonography has been effective in detecting microemboli and vasospasm in the major cerebral arteries.
- If the suspected cause of the stroke includes emboli from the heart, diagnostic cardiac tests should be done.

The LICOX system, which measures brain oxygenation and temperature, may be used as a diagnostic tool to evaluate the progression of stroke.

Collaborative Care

Prevention

The goals of stroke prevention include management of modifiable risk factors to prevent a stroke. Health promotion focuses on (1) healthy diet, (2) weight control, (3) regular exercise, (4) no smoking, (5) limiting alcohol consumption, and (6) routine health assessments. Patients with known risk factors such as diabetes mellitus, hypertension, obesity, high serum lipids, or cardiac dysfunction require close management.

- Measures to prevent the development of a thrombus or embolus are used in patients with TIAs as they are at high risk for stroke. Antiplatelet drugs are usually the chosen treatment to prevent stroke in patients who have had a TIA. Aspirin at a dose of 81 to 325 mg/day is the most frequently used antiplatelet agent. Other drugs include ticlopidine (Ticlid), clopidogrel (Plavix), dipyridamole (Persantine), and combined dipyridamole and aspirin (Aggrenox). For patients who have atrial fibrillation, oral anticoagulation can include warfarin (Coumadin), rivaroxaban (Xarelto), and dabigatran etexilate (Pradaxa). Statins (simvastatin [Zocor], lovastatin [Mevacor]) have also been shown to be effective in the prevention of stroke for individuals who have experienced a TIA in the past.

- Surgical therapy for the patient with TIAs from carotid disease includes carotid endarterectomy, transluminal angioplasty, stenting, and extracranial-intracranial (EC-IC) bypass.

Acute Care: Ischemic Stroke

The goals of acute care are preserving life, preventing further brain damage, and reducing disability. Acute care begins with managing the airway, breathing, and circulation. Oxygen administration, artificial airway insertion, intubation, and mechanical ventilation may be required. Table 58-7, Lewis et al.: *Medical-Surgical Nursing,* ed. 9, p. 1398, outlines emergency management of the patient with a stroke.

- Baseline neurologic assessment is carried out, and patients are monitored closely for signs of increasing neurologic deficit.
- Elevated BP is common immediately after a stroke and may be a protective response to maintain cerebral perfusion. Immediately following ischemic stroke in those patients who do not receive fibrinolytic therapy, the use of drugs to lower BP is recommended only if BP is markedly increased (systolic BP greater than 220 mm Hg or diastolic greater than 120 mm Hg).
- Fluid and electrolyte balance must be controlled carefully. Although the goal is to maintain perfusion to the brain, overhydration may compromise perfusion by increasing cerebral edema. Adequate fluid intake during acute care via oral, IV, or tube feedings is a priority. Also monitor urine output.

Management of increased intracranial pressure (ICP) includes practices that improve venous drainage such as elevating the head of the bed, maintaining head and neck in alignment, and avoiding hip flexion.

- Additional measures for reducing ICP include management of hyperthermia (goal temperature of 96.8° to 98.6° F [36° to 37° C]), drug therapy to prevent seizures, pain management, avoidance of hypervolemia, and management of constipation. Cerebrospinal fluid drainage may be used in some patients to reduce ICP.

Drug Therapy. Recombinant tissue plasminogen activator (tPA) is administered IV to reestablish blood flow and prevent cell death for patients with acute onset of ischemic stroke. This drug must be administered within 3 to 4.5 hours of the onset of clinical signs. Patients are screened carefully before tPA can be given, including a CT or MRI scan to rule out hemorrhagic stroke, blood tests for coagulation disorders, and screening for recent history of GI bleeding, head trauma, or major surgery.

- During infusion, closely monitor the patient's vital signs to assess for improvement or deterioration related to intracerebral hemorrhage.

- Control of BP is critical during treatment and for 24 hours following.
- Aspirin may be initiated within 24 to 48 hours of an ischemic stroke. Other platelet inhibitors and anticoagulants may also be used to prevent further clot formation. Platelet inhibitors include aspirin, ticlopidine (Ticlid), clopidogrel (Plavix), and dipyridamole (Persantine).

Surgical Therapy. Stent retrievers (e.g., Solitaire FR, Trevo) are a way of opening blocked arteries in the brain by using a removable stent system. Another surgical approach is to use a corkscrew-like device that is twisted into the clot, after which the clot is gently pulled out. The mechanical embolus removal in cerebral ischemia (MERCI) retriever (a corkscrew-like device) allows physicians to go inside the blocked artery of patients who are experiencing ischemic strokes.

Acute Care: Hemorrhagic Stroke

Drug Therapy. Anticoagulants and platelet inhibitors are contraindicated in patients with hemorrhagic strokes. The main drug therapy for patients with hemorrhagic stroke is the management of hypertension. Oral and IV agents may be used to maintain BP within a normal to high-normal range (systolic BP less than 160 mm Hg).

- Seizure prophylaxis in the acute period after intracerebral and subarachnoid hemorrhages is situation specific.

Surgical Therapy. Surgical interventions for hemorrhagic stroke include immediate evacuation of aneurysm-induced hematomas or cerebellar hematomas larger than 3 cm. Individuals who have an arteriovenous malformation (AVM) may experience a hemorrhagic stroke if the AVM ruptures.

- Treatment of AVM is surgical resection and/or radiosurgery (i.e., gamma knife). Both may be preceded by interventional neuroradiology to embolize the blood vessels that supply the AVM.

Subarachnoid hemorrhage is usually caused by a ruptured aneurysm. Approximately 20% of patients will have multiple aneurysms. Treatment of an aneurysm involves clipping or coiling the aneurysm to prevent rebleeding.

- Following aneurysmal occlusion via clipping or coiling, hyperdynamic therapy (hemodilution induced-hypertension using vasoconstricting agents such as phenylephrine or dopamine [Intropin] and hypervolemia) may be instituted in an effort to increase the mean arterial pressure and increase cerebral perfusion. Volume expansion is achieved via crystalloid or colloid solution.
- The calcium channel blocker nimodipine (Nimotop) is given to patients with subarachnoid hemorrhage to decrease the effects of vasospasm and minimize cerebral damage.

- Subarachnoid and intracerebral hemorrhage can involve bleeding into the ventricles of the brain. Insertion of a ventriculostomy for cerebrospinal fluid drainage can dramatically improve these situations.

Rehabilitation Care

After the stroke has stabilized for 12 to 24 hours, care shifts from preserving life to lessening disability and attaining optimal function. Many of the interventions discussed in the acute phase are maintained during this phase.

Nursing Management

Goals

Establish the goals of nursing care together with the patient, caregiver, and family. Typical goals are that the patient will (1) maintain a stable or improved level of consciousness, (2) attain maximum physical functioning, (3) attain maximum self-care abilities and skills, (4) maintain stable body functions (e.g., bladder control), (5) maximize communication abilities, (6) maintain adequate nutrition, (7) avoid complications of stroke, and (8) maintain effective personal and family coping.

See NCP 58-1 for the patient with a stroke, Lewis et al.: *Medical-Surgical Nursing,* ed. 9, pp. 1402 to 1404.

Nursing Diagnoses

- Decreased intracranial adaptive capacity
- Risk for aspiration
- Impaired physical mobility
- Impaired verbal communication
- Unilateral neglect
- Impaired urinary elimination
- Impaired swallowing
- Situational low self-esteem

Nursing Interventions

Respiratory System. During the acute phase after a stroke, management of respiratory function is a nursing priority. An oropharyngeal airway may be used in comatose patients to prevent the tongue from falling back and obstructing the airway and to provide access for suctioning. Alternatively, a nasopharyngeal airway may be used to provide airway protection and access. Interventions include frequently assessing airway patency and function, providing oxygenation, suctioning, promoting patient mobility, positioning the patient to prevent aspiration, and encouraging deep breathing.

Neurologic System. The primary clinical assessment tool to evaluate and document neurologic status in acute stroke patients is the NIH Stroke Scale (NIHSS) that measures stroke severity (see NIHSS in

Table 58-9, Lewis et al.: *Medical-Surgical Nursing,* ed. 9, p. 1401).
A decreasing level of consciousness may indicate increasing ICP.

Cardiovascular System. Nursing goals for the cardiovascular system are aimed at maintaining homeostasis. Interventions include (1) monitoring vital signs frequently; (2) monitoring cardiac rhythms; (3) calculating intake and output, noting imbalances; (4) regulating IV infusions; (5) adjusting fluid intake to the individual needs of the patient; (6) monitoring lung sounds for crackles and rhonchi indicating pulmonary congestion; and (7) monitoring heart sounds for murmurs or for S_3 or S_4 heart sounds.

- After a stroke, the patient is at risk for venous thromboembolism (VTE), especially in the weak or paralyzed lower extremity. The most effective prevention is to keep the patient moving. Teach active range-of-motion (ROM) exercises if the patient has voluntary movement in the affected extremity. For the patient with hemiplegia, perform passive ROM exercises several times each day.
- Other measures to prevent VTE include positioning to minimize the effects of dependent edema and the use of elastic compression gradient stockings or support hose.

Musculoskeletal System. The goal for the musculoskeletal system is to maintain optimal function, which is accomplished by prevention of joint contractures and muscle atrophy.

- In the acute phase, ROM exercises and positioning are important interventions. Passive ROM exercise is begun on the first day of hospitalization. Muscle atrophy secondary to lack of innervation and inactivity can develop after a stroke, so exercise is an important intervention for rehabilitation and recovery.

Interventions to optimize musculoskeletal function include (1) trochanter roll at the hip to prevent external rotation; (2) hand cones (not rolled washcloths) to prevent hand contractures; (3) arm supports with slings and lap boards to prevent shoulder displacement; (4) avoidance of pulling the patient by the arm to avoid shoulder displacement; (5) posterior leg splints, footboards, or high-top tennis shoes to prevent foot drop; and (6) hand splints to reduce spasticity.

Integumentary System. Interventions for prevention of skin breakdown include (1) pressure relief by position changes, special mattresses, or wheelchair cushions; (2) good skin hygiene; (3) emollients applied to dry skin; and (4) early mobility. An example of a position change schedule is side-back-side, with a maximum duration of 2 hours for any position.

- Position the patient on the weak or paralyzed side for only 30 minutes. If an area of redness develops and does not return to normal color within 15 minutes of pressure relief, the epidermis and dermis are damaged.

▪ Do not massage the damaged area, because this may cause additional damage. Control of pressure is the single most important factor in both the prevention and treatment of skin breakdown.

Gastrointestinal System. The most common bowel problem is constipation. Physical activity also promotes bowel function. Laxatives, suppositories, or additional stool softeners may be ordered if the patient does not respond to increased fluid and fiber. Bowel retraining may be needed and continues into the rehabilitation phase.

Urinary System. In the acute stage of stroke, the primary urinary problem is poor bladder control, resulting in incontinence.

▪ Take steps to promote normal bladder function and avoid the use of an indwelling catheter.

▪ Long-term use of an indwelling catheter is associated with urinary tract infections and delayed bladder retraining. An intermittent catheterization program may be used for patients with urinary retention.

Nutrition. The patient may initially receive IV infusions to maintain fluid and electrolyte balance and to administer drugs. Patients with severe impairment may require enteral or parenteral nutrition support. Patients should have their nutritional needs addressed in the first 72 hours of admission to the hospital, because nutrition is important for recovery and healing.

▪ To assess swallowing ability, elevate the head of the bed to an upright position (unless contraindicated) and give the patient a small amount of crushed ice or ice water to swallow. If the gag reflex is present and the patient is able to swallow safely, you may proceed with feeding.

▪ Place food on the unaffected side of the mouth. Feedings must be followed by scrupulous oral hygiene because food may collect on the affected side of the mouth.

Communication. During the acute stage your role in meeting the psychologic needs of the patient is primarily supportive.

▪ An alert patient is usually anxious because of a lack of understanding of what has happened and the inability to communicate. Give the patient extra time to comprehend and respond to communication.

Sensory-Perceptual Alterations. *Homonymous hemianopsia* (blindness in the same half of each visual field) is a common problem after a stroke.

▪ Initially, help the patient to compensate by arranging the environment within the patient's perceptual field, such as arranging the food tray so that all food is on the right side or the left side to accommodate for field of vision.

- Later, the patient learns to compensate for the visual defect by consciously attending or scanning the neglected side. The weak or paralyzed extremities are carefully checked for adequacy of dressing, hygiene, and trauma.

Other visual problems may include diplopia, loss of the corneal reflex, and ptosis, especially if the stroke is in the vertebrobasilar distribution. Diplopia is often treated with an eye patch. If the corneal reflex is absent, the patient is at risk for a corneal abrasion and should be observed closely and protected against eye injuries.

Coping. A stroke is usually a sudden, extremely stressful event for the patient, caregiver, and significant others.

- Reactions vary considerably but may involve fear, apprehension, denial of severity of the stroke, depression, anger, and sorrow.
- During the acute phase of caring for the patient and family, nursing interventions designed to facilitate coping involve providing information and emotional support.
- Explanations to the patient about what has happened and diagnostic and therapeutic procedures should be clear and understandable. Decision making and upholding the patient's wishes during this challenging time are of utmost importance.
- Because family members usually have not had time to prepare for the illness, they may need assistance in arranging care for family members or pets and arranging transportation and finances.

Home Care and Rehabilitation. The patient is usually discharged from the acute care setting to home, an intermediate or long-term care facility, or a rehabilitation facility. You have an excellent opportunity to prepare the patient and family for hospital discharge through teaching, demonstration and return demonstration, practice, and evaluation of self-care skills before discharge. Total care is considered in discharge planning in relation to medications, nutrition, mobility, exercises, hygiene, and toileting.

Follow-up care is carefully planned to permit continuing nursing, physical, occupational, and speech therapy, as well as medical care.

Rehabilitation requires a team approach so patient and caregiver can benefit from the combined, expert care of a stroke team. The team must communicate and coordinate care to achieve the patient's goals. You are in a good position to facilitate this process and are often the key to successful rehabilitation efforts.

The rehabilitation nurse assesses the patient, caregiver, and family with attention to (1) rehabilitation potential of the patient, (2) physical status of all body systems, (3) presence of complications caused by the stroke or other chronic conditions, (4) cognitive status of the patient, (5) family resources and support, and (6) expectations of the patient and caregiver related to the rehabilitation program.

Rehabilitation and long-term management of the stroke patient are further described in Chapter 58 of Lewis et al.: *Medical-Surgical Nursing,* ed. 9.

▼ **Patient and Caregiver Teaching**

- Provide the caregiver with instruction and practice in the necessary areas of home care while the patient is hospitalized. This allows for support and encouragement, as well as opportunities for feedback. Adjustments in the home environment, such as the removal of a door to accommodate a wheelchair, can be made before discharge.
- Your instruction related to home care should include exercise and ambulation techniques; dietary requirements; recognition of signs indicating the possibility of another stroke (e.g., headache, vertigo, numbness, visual disturbances); understanding of emotional lability and the possibility of depression; medication routine; and time, place, and frequency of follow-up activities, such as occupational therapy and physical therapy.
- Assist the caregiver to stay healthy after the patient is discharged. Emphasize the importance of planning for respite or time away from caregiving activities on a regular basis.

SYPHILIS

Description

Syphilis is a sexually transmitted infection (STI) in which many organs and tissues can become infected by *Treponema pallidum,* a spirochete. The incidence of syphilis reported in the United States in 2000 was at its lowest rate since reporting started in 1941. During the past decade, syphilis rates increased until 2010, when the rate slightly decreased. Many new cases of syphilis are being seen in men who have sex with men.

Pathophysiology

The organism *T. pallidum* is thought to enter the body through very small breaks in the skin or mucous membranes. Its entry is facilitated by the minor abrasions that often occur during sexual intercourse. The infection causes the production of antibodies that also react with normal tissues. *T. pallidum* is extremely fragile and is easily destroyed by drying, heating, or washing.

- Not all people who are exposed to syphilis acquire the infection; about one third become infected after intercourse with an infected person.
- In addition to sexual contact, syphilis may be spread through contact with infectious lesions and through the sharing of needles among IV drug users.

- Congenital syphilis is transmitted from an infected mother to the fetus in utero after the 10th week of pregnancy.

There is an association between syphilis and human immunodeficiency virus (HIV) infection. People at increased risk for acquiring syphilis are also at increased risk for acquiring HIV. Often, both infections may be present in the same person. Therefore the evaluation of all patients with syphilis should include serologic testing for HIV with the patient's consent. Conversely, HIV patients should be tested at least annually for syphilis.

Clinical Manifestations

Syphilis has a variety of signs and symptoms that can mimic a number of other infections. Consequently, compared with other STIs, it is more difficult to recognize syphilis. If it is not treated, specific clinical stages are characteristic of the infection progression.

- In the *primary stage, chancres* (painless indurated lesions found on the penis, vulva, and lips and in the mouth, vagina, and rectum) occur 10 to 90 days after inoculation. During this time the draining of the microorganisms into the lymph nodes causes regional lymphadenopathy. Genital ulcers may also be present. Without treatment, the infection progresses to the secondary stage.
- In the *secondary stage,* syphilis is systemic. During this stage blood-borne bacteria spread to all major organ systems. Manifestations include flu-like symptoms and generalized adenopathy. Cutaneous lesions include a bilateral, symmetric rash usually involving the trunk, palms, and soles; mucous patches in the mouth, tongue, or cervix; and condylomata lata (moist papules) in the anal and genital area.
- *Latent* syphilis follows the secondary stage and is a period during which the immune system is able to suppress the infection. There are no signs or symptoms of syphilis during this time.
- The *late or tertiary stage* of syphilis is the most severe, which appears 3 to 20 years after initial infection. Because antibiotics can cure syphilis, manifestations of late syphilis are rare. When late syphilis does occur, however, it is responsible for significant morbidity and mortality. *Gummas* (destructive skin, bone, and soft tissue lesions associated with late syphilis) are probably caused by a severe hypersensitivity reaction to the microorganism. Within the cardiovascular system, late syphilis may cause aneurysms, heart valve insufficiency, and heart failure. Within the central nervous system, the presence of *T. pallidum* in cerebrospinal fluid (CSF) may cause manifestations of neurosyphilis.

Complications

Complications mostly occur in late syphilis. The gummas of late syphilis may produce irreparable damage to bone, liver, or skin.

- In cardiovascular syphilis, the resulting aneurysm may press on structures such as the intercostal nerves, causing pain. Scarring of the aortic valve results in aortic valve insufficiency and eventually heart failure.
- Neurosyphilis causes degeneration of the brain with mental deterioration. Problems related to sensory nerve involvement are a result of *tabes dorsalis* (progressive locomotor ataxia). There may be sudden attacks of pain anywhere in the body. Loss of vision and position sense in the feet and legs can also occur. Walking may become even more difficult as joint stability is lost.

Diagnostic Studies

- Detailed and accurate sexual history is important.
- Dark-field microscopy and direct fluorescent antibody tests of lesion exudate or tissue can confirm the diagnosis.
- To screen for syphilis, Venereal Infection Research Laboratory (VDRL) and rapid plasma reagin (RPR) testing can detect non-specific antitreponemal antibodies, which are usually positive 10 to 14 days after chancre appearance.
- To confirm a diagnosis of syphilis, the fluorescent treponemal antibody absorption (FTA-ABS) test and the *T. pallidum* particle agglutination (TP-PA) test can detect specific antitreponemal antibodies.

Collaborative Care

Management is aimed at eradicating all syphilitic organisms. However, treatment cannot reverse damage that is already present in the late stage of the disease.

- Penicillin G benzathine (Bicillin) or aqueous penicillin G procaine is the treatment of choice for all stages of syphilis. When penicillin is contraindicated, doxycycline (Vibramycin) or tetracycline may be used.
- Patients having persistent or recurring symptoms after drug therapy has ended should be reevaluated.
- It is important that all sexual contacts in the last 90 days be treated.
- Patients with neurosyphilis must be carefully monitored with periodic serologic testing, clinical evaluation at 6-month intervals, and repeat CSF examinations for at least 3 years.

Nursing Management: Syphilis

See Nursing Management: Sexually Transmitted Infections, p. 564.

SYSTEMIC INFLAMMATORY RESPONSE SYNDROME (SIRS) AND MULTIPLE ORGAN DYSFUNCTION SYNDROME (MODS)

Description

Systemic inflammatory response syndrome (SIRS) is a systemic inflammatory response to a variety of insults, including infection (referred to as sepsis), ischemia, infarction, and injury. Generalized inflammation in organs remote from the initial insult characterizes SIRS. Many mechanisms can trigger a systemic inflammatory response, including:

- *Mechanical tissue trauma*: burns, crush injuries, surgical procedures
- *Abscess formation*: intraabdominal, extremities
- *Ischemic or necrotic tissue*: pancreatitis, vascular disease, myocardial infarction
- *Microbial invasion*: bacteria, viruses, fungi, parasites
- *Endotoxin release*: gram-negative and -positive bacteria
- *Global perfusion deficits*: post–cardiac resuscitation, shock states
- *Regional perfusion deficits*: distal perfusion deficits

Multiple organ dysfunction syndrome (MODS) is failure of two or more organ systems in an acutely ill patient such that homeostasis cannot be maintained without intervention. MODS results from SIRS, but the transition from SIRS to MODS does not occur in a clear-cut manner.

- Prognosis for the patient with MODS is poor, with mortality rates at 70% to 80% when three or more organ systems fail.

Pathophysiology and Clinical Manifestations

When the inflammatory response is activated, consequences occur including activation of inflammatory cells and release of mediators, direct damage to the endothelium, and hypermetabolism.

- An increase in vascular permeability allows mediators and protein to leak out of the endothelium and into the interstitial space.
- WBCs begin to digest the foreign debris, and the coagulation cascade is activated.
- Hypotension, decreased perfusion, microemboli, and redistributed or shunted blood flow eventually compromise organ perfusion.

The respiratory system is often the first system to show signs of dysfunction in SIRS and MODS. Inflammatory mediators have a direct effect on the pulmonary vasculature. Endothelial damage from the release of inflammatory mediators results in increased capillary permeability. Fluid then moves to the alveoli, causing alveolar edema. The alveoli collapse, and the end result is acute respiratory distress syndrome (ARDS, see p. 13).

Cardiovascular changes include myocardial depression and massive vasodilation in response to increasing tissue demands. To compensate for hypotension, heart rate and stroke volume increase, but increased capillary permeability diminishes venous return and thus preload. Eventually, either perfusion of vital organs becomes insufficient or the cells are unable to use oxygen and their function is further compromised.

Neurologic dysfunction commonly manifests as mental status changes, which can be an early sign of SIRS or MODS. Confusion, agitation, disorientation, lethargy, or coma may occur. These changes may be caused by hypoxemia, the direct effect of inflammatory mediators, or impaired perfusion.

Acute kidney injury is frequently seen in SIRS and MODS. Hypoperfusion and the effects of the mediators can cause acute kidney injury. Antibiotics commonly used to treat gram-negative bacteria (e.g., aminoglycosides) can be nephrotoxic. Careful monitoring of drug levels is essential to avoid the nephrotoxic effects.

In the early stages of SIRS and MODS, blood is shunted away from the GI mucosa, making it highly vulnerable to ischemic injury. Decreased perfusion leads to a breakdown of the mucosal barrier, thereby increasing the risk for ulceration and GI bleeding.

- Breakdown of the mucosal barrier of the gut also results in the potential for bacterial movement from the GI tract into the circulation.

Metabolic changes are pronounced in SIRS and MODS. Both syndromes trigger a hypermetabolic response. The net result is a catabolic state, and lean body mass (muscle) is lost.

- The hypermetabolism may last for days and results in liver dysfunction.
- The liver is unable to synthesize albumin that is necessary to maintain plasma oncotic pressure, adding to the loss of intravascular fluid to the interstitial space.
- As the state of hypermetabolism persists, the patient is unable to convert lactate to glucose, and lactate accumulates (lactic acidosis). Eventually the liver is unable to maintain a glucose level, and the patient becomes hypoglycemic.

Disseminated intravascular coagulation (DIC) may result from dysfunction of the coagulation system. DIC results in simultaneous microvascular clotting and bleeding because of the depletion of clotting factors and platelets in addition to excessive fibrinolysis (see Disseminated Intravascular Coagulation, p. 195).

Electrolyte imbalances are common and result from hormonal and metabolic changes and fluid shifts. These changes exacerbate mental status changes, neuromuscular dysfunction, and dysrhythmias.

- Release of antidiuretic hormone and aldosterone results in sodium and water retention; aldosterone increases urinary potassium loss, and catecholamines cause potassium to move into the cells, resulting in hypokalemia.
- Metabolic acidosis results from impaired tissue perfusion, hypoxia, a shift to anaerobic metabolism, and progressive renal dysfunction.
- Hypocalcemia, hypomagnesemia, and hypophosphatemia are common.

The clinical manifestations of MODS are presented in Table 67-10, Lewis et al.: *Medical-Surgical Nursing,* ed. 9, p. 1651.

Nursing and Collaborative Management: SIRS and MODS

The most important goal in the management of SIRS and MODS is to prevent the progression of SIRS to MODS. A critical component of the nursing role is vigilant assessment and ongoing monitoring to detect early signs of deterioration or organ dysfunction.

Collaborative care of patients with MODS focuses on prevention and treatment of infection, maintenance of tissue oxygenation, nutritional and metabolic support, and appropriate support for individual failing organs.

- Aggressive infection control is essential to decrease the risk for hospital-acquired infections. Early, aggressive surgery is recommended to remove necrotic tissue (e.g., early debridement of burn tissue) that can provide a culture medium for microorganisms. Aggressive pulmonary management, including early ambulation, can reduce the risk of infection. Strict asepsis can decrease infections related to intraarterial lines, endotracheal tubes, urinary catheters, IV lines, and other invasive devices or procedures.
- Hypoxemia frequently occurs in patients with SIRS or MODS. Interventions to decrease oxygen demand and increase oxygen delivery are essential. Sedation, mechanical ventilation, analgesia, and rest may decrease oxygen demand and should be considered.
- Hypermetabolism in SIRS or MODS can result in profound weight loss, cachexia, and further organ failure. Nutritional support is vital to preserve organ function. Providing early and adequate nutrition decreases morbidity and mortality. The use of the enteral route is preferred to parenteral nutrition.

Support of any failing organ is a primary goal of therapy. For example, the patient with ARDS requires aggressive oxygen therapy and mechanical ventilation. Renal failure may require dialysis or continuous renal replacement therapy.

A final consideration may be that further interventions are futile. It is important to maintain communication between the health care team and, in most cases, the patient's caregiver regarding realistic goals and likely outcomes for the patient with MODS. It may be that withdrawal of life support is the best option for the patient.

SYSTEMIC LUPUS ERYTHEMATOSUS

Description

Systemic lupus erythematosus (SLE) is a multisystem inflammatory autoimmune disease. It typically affects the skin; joints; serous membranes (pleura, pericardium); and renal, hematologic, and neurologic systems. SLE is characterized by a chronic unpredictable course marked by alternating periods of exacerbations and remissions. Women are 10 times more likely to develop SLE than men. It is observed more often in African Americans, Asian Americans, and Native Americans than in whites.

Pathophysiology

The etiology of SLE is unknown, but it is thought to result from interactions among genetic, hormonal, environmental, and immunologic factors. Multiple susceptibility genes from the human leukocyte antigen (HLA) complex show associations with SLE.

- Hormones are also known to play a role in the etiology of SLE. Onset or exacerbation of disease symptoms sometimes occurs after the onset of menarche, with the use of oral contraceptives, and during and after pregnancy. SLE tends to worsen in the immediate postpartum period.
- Environmental factors believed to contribute to the occurrence of SLE include sun exposure and sunburns and exposure to infectious agents and certain drugs such as procainamide (Pronestyl), hydralazine (Apresoline), and some antiseizure drugs.

SLE is characterized by the production of a large variety of autoantibodies against nucleic acids (e.g., single- and double-stranded deoxyribonucleic acid [DNA]), erythrocytes, coagulation proteins, lymphocytes, and platelets. Autoimmune reactions are characteristically directed against constituents of the cell nucleus (antinuclear antibodies [ANA]), particularly DNA.

Circulating immune complexes containing antibody against DNA are deposited in the basement membranes of capillaries in the kidneys, heart, skin, brain, and joints. The overaggressive antibody response is also related to B and T cell hyperactivity. Specific manifestations of SLE depend on which cell types or organs are involved.

Clinical Manifestations and Complications

No characteristic pattern occurs in the progressive organ involvement. General complaints, including fever, weight loss, arthralgia, and excessive fatigue, may precede an exacerbation of disease activity.

Dermatologic Manifestations. Cutaneous vascular lesions can appear in any location but are most likely to develop in sun-exposed areas. Severe skin reactions can occur in people who are photosensitive. The classic butterfly rash over the cheeks and bridge of the nose occurs in 50% of patients with SLE.

- Ulcers of the oral or nasopharyngeal membranes can occur.
- Alopecia is common, and the scalp becomes dry, scaly, and atrophied.

Musculoskeletal Problems. Polyarthralgia with morning stiffness is often the patient's first complaint and may precede the onset of multisystem disease by many years. Arthritis occurs in 90% of all patients with SLE. Diffuse swelling is accompanied by joint and muscle pain.

- Lupus-related arthritis is generally nonerosive, but it may cause deformities such as swan neck, ulnar deviation, and subluxation with hyperlaxity of the joints.

Cardiopulmonary Problems. Tachypnea and cough in patients with SLE are suggestive of restrictive lung disease. Cardiac involvement may include dysrhythmias resulting from fibrosis of the sinoatrial (SA) and atrioventricular (AV) nodes. This occurrence is an ominous sign of advanced disease.

- Hypertension and hypercholesterolemia require aggressive therapy and careful monitoring.

Renal Problems. Lupus nephritis (LN) occurs in about 40% of patients with SLE. Manifestations of renal involvement vary from mild proteinuria to rapid, progressive glomerulonephritis. Treatment typically includes corticosteroids, cytotoxic agents (cyclophosphamide [Cytoxan]), and immunosuppressive agents (azathioprine [Imuran], cyclosporine, and mycophenolate mofetil [CellCept]).

Nervous System Problems. Seizures are the most common neurologic manifestation. They are generally controlled by corticosteroids or antiseizure drug therapy.

- Cognitive dysfunction may result from the deposition of immune complexes within the brain tissue. It is characterized by disordered thought processes, disorientation, memory deficits, and psychiatric symptoms, such as severe depression and psychosis. Occasionally a stroke or aseptic meningitis may be attributable to

SLE. Headaches are common and can become severe during a flare (exacerbation).

Hematologic Problems. The formation of antibodies against blood cells such as erythrocytes, leukocytes, thrombocytes, and coagulation factors is a common feature. Anemia, mild leukopenia, and thrombocytopenia are often present. Some patients develop a tendency toward coagulopathy involving either excessive bleeding or blood clot development.

Infection. Patients appear to have increased susceptibility to infections, possibly related to defects in their ability to phagocytize invading bacteria, deficiencies in the production of antibodies, and the immunosuppressive effect of many antiinflammatory drugs. Infection is a major cause of death, with pneumonia being the most common infection.

Diagnostic Studies

The diagnosis of SLE is based on the presence of distinct criteria revealed through patient history, physical examination, and laboratory findings.

- SLE is marked by the presence of antinuclear antibody (ANA) in 97% of people with the disease. Other antibodies include anti-DNA, antineuronal, anticoagulant, anti-WBC, anti–red blood cell (RBC), antiplatelet, antiphospholipid, and anti–basement membrane.
- Anti–double-stranded DNA antibodies are found in half of people with SLE. The anti-Smith (Sm) antibodies are found in 30% to 40% of people with lupus.
- The lupus erythematosus (LE) cell prep test is a nonspecific test for SLE and is positive in other rheumatic diseases.
- Elevated erythrocyte sedimentation rate (ESR) and C-reactive protein (CRP) levels are not diagnostic of SLE but may be used to monitor disease activity.

Collaborative Care

A major challenge in SLE treatment is to manage the active phase of the disease while preventing complications of treatment. The prognosis of SLE can be improved with early diagnosis, prompt recognition of serious organ involvement, and effective therapeutic regimens.

Drug Therapy

Nonsteroidal antiinflammatory drugs (NSAIDs) are an important intervention, especially for patients with mild polyarthralgia or polyarthritis. Antimalarial agents such as hydroxychloroquine (Plaquenil) are also often used to treat fatigue and moderate skin and joint problems, as well as prevent flares.

Corticosteroid exposure should be limited, but tapering doses of IV methylprednisolone may be useful in controlling severe exacerbations of polyarthritis. Steroid-sparing immunosuppressants (e.g., methotrexate) can serve as an alternate treatment.

Immunosuppressive drugs such as azathioprine (Imuran) and cyclophosphamide (Cytoxan) may be prescribed to reduce the need for long-term corticosteroid therapy or treat severe organ-system disease, such as lupus nephritis.

- Topical immunomodulators are an alternative to corticosteroids for treating serious skin conditions. Tacrolimus (Protopic) and pimecrolimus (Elidel) suppress immune activity in the skin, including the butterfly rash and possibly discoid (round, coin-shaped) lesions.

Nursing Management
Goals
The patient with SLE will have satisfactory pain relief, adhere to the therapeutic regimen to achieve maximum symptom management, demonstrate awareness of and avoid activities that induce disease exacerbation, and maintain optimal role function and a positive self-image.
Nursing Diagnoses
- Fatigue
- Impaired comfort
- Impaired skin integrity
Nursing Interventions
During an exacerbation, patients may become abruptly and dramatically ill. Nursing interventions include accurately recording the severity of symptoms and documenting response to therapy. Specifically assess fever pattern, joint inflammation, limitation of motion, location and degree of discomfort, and fatigue.

- Monitor the patient's weight and fluid intake and output if corticosteroids are prescribed because of the fluid-retention effect of these drugs and the possibility of renal failure. Collection of 24-hour urine for protein and creatinine clearance may be ordered.
- Observe for signs of bleeding that result from drug therapy, such as pallor, skin bruising, petechiae, or tarry stools.
- Careful assess the patient's neurologic status. Observe for visual disturbances, headaches, personality changes, and forgetfulness. Psychosis may indicate central nervous system disease or may be the effect of corticosteroid therapy. Irritation of the nerves of the extremities (peripheral neuropathy) may produce numbness, tingling, and weakness of the hands and feet.

- Explain the nature of the disease, modes of therapy, and all diagnostic procedures. Emotional support for the patient and family is essential.

▼ **Patient and Caregiver Teaching**

It is important to emphasize the importance of patient cooperation for successful home management. Help the patient understand that even strong adherence to the treatment plan is not a guarantee against exacerbation, because the course of the disease is unpredictable. However, a variety of factors may increase disease activity, such as fatigue, sun exposure, emotional stress, infection, drugs, and surgery. Also assist the patient and caregiver to eliminate or minimize exposure to precipitating factors. Patient and caregiver teaching is outlined in Table 80. Counsel the patient and caregiver that SLE has a good prognosis for the majority of people.

- Many couples require pregnancy and sexual counseling. For the best outcome, pregnancy should be planned at a point when the disease activity is minimal.
- Pain and fatigue may interfere with quality of life. Pacing techniques and relaxation therapy can help the patient remain involved in day-to-day activities.

Table 80	Patient and Caregiver Teaching Guide *Systemic Lupus Erythematosus*

Include the following information in the teaching plan for a patient with systemic lupus erythematosus and the caregiver.

- Disease process
- Names of drugs, actions, side effects, dosage, administration
- Pain management strategies
- Energy conservation and pacing techniques
- Therapeutic exercise, use of heat therapy (for arthralgia)
- Avoidance of physical and emotional stress
- Avoidance of exposure to individuals with infection
- Avoidance of drying soaps, powders, household chemicals
- Use of sunscreen protection (at least SPF 15) and protective clothing, with minimal sun exposure from 11:00 AM to 3:00 PM
- Regular medical and laboratory follow-up
- Marital and pregnancy counseling as needed
- Community resources and health care agencies

SPF, Sun protection factor.

TESTICULAR CANCER

Description

Testicular cancer is rare, but it is the most common type of cancer in young men between 15 and 35 years of age. Testicular tumors are more common in men who have had undescended testicles (cryptorchidism) or a family history of testicular cancer or anomalies.

- Other predisposing factors include orchitis, human immunodeficiency virus (HIV) infection, maternal exposure to diethylstilbestrol (DES), and testicular cancer in the contralateral testis.
- Most testicular cancers develop from embryonic germ cells and include seminomas and nonseminomas.

Clinical Manifestations

Testicular cancer may have a slow or rapid onset depending on the tumor.

- The patient may notice a painless lump in his scrotum, as well as scrotal swelling and a feeling of heaviness. The scrotal mass is usually nontender and very firm.
- Some patients complain of a dull ache or heavy sensation in the lower abdomen, perianal area, or scrotum.
- Manifestations associated with metastasis include lower back and/or chest pain, cough, and dyspnea.

Diagnostic Studies

- Palpation of scrotal contents is used to assess for masses and swelling.
- Ultrasound of the testes is indicated whenever testicular cancer is suspected.
- Blood serum levels of α-fetoprotein (AFP), lactate dehydrogenase (LDH), and human chorionic gonadotropin (hCG) are done if testicular cancer is suspected.
- Chest x-ray and CT scan of the abdomen and pelvis are used to detect metastasis.

Nursing and Collaborative Management

The scrotum is easily examined, and tumors are usually palpable. Teach and encourage every man to perform a monthly testicular self-examination for the purpose of detecting testicular tumors or other scrotal abnormalities such as varicoceles. (See Table 55-9 and Fig. 55-11 for scrotum self-examination guidelines, Lewis et al.: *Medical-Surgical Nursing,* ed. 9, p. 1326).

- The man may indicate some reluctance to examine his own genitals, but with encouragement he can learn this simple procedure.

Encourage him to perform self-examinations frequently until he is comfortable with the procedure. The scrotum should be examined once each month.

Collaborative management generally involves a radical orchiectomy (surgical removal of the affected testis, spermatic cord, and regional lymph nodes). Retroperitoneal lymph node dissection and removal may also be done.

- Postorchiectomy treatment may involve surveillance, radiation therapy, or chemotherapy, depending on the cancer stage. Chemotherapy protocols use combination therapy of various agents including bleomycin (Blenoxane), etoposide (VePesid), ifosfamide (Ifex), and cisplatin (Platinol).

The prognosis for patients with testicular cancer has improved, and 95% of all patients obtain complete remission if the disease is detected in the early stages. All patients with testicular cancer, regardless of pathology or stage, require meticulous follow-up monitoring and regular physical examinations, chest x-ray, CT scan, and assessment of hCG and AFP. The goal is to detect relapse when tumor burden is minimal.

- Because of the high risk for infertility due to chemotherapy and/ or pelvic radiation, the cryopreservation of sperm in a sperm bank before treatment begins should be discussed and recommended for the man with testicular cancer.

THALASSEMIA

Description

Thalassemia is a group of diseases involving inadequate production of normal hemoglobin, and therefore decreased erythrocyte production. Hemolysis also occurs in thalassemia.

- Thalassemia is commonly found in members of ethnic groups whose origins are near the Mediterranean Sea and equatorial or near-equatorial regions of Asia, the Middle East, and Africa.

Pathophysiology

Thalassemia has an autosomal recessive genetic basis that results in an absent or reduced globulin protein. α-Globin chains are absent or reduced in α-thalassemia, and β-globin chains are absent or reduced in β-thalassemia. An individual with thalassemia may have a heterozygous or homozygous form of the disease.

- *In thalassemia minor (thalassemic trait),* a person is heterozygous with one thalassemic gene and one normal gene. Thalassemia minor is a mild form of the disease.
- In *thalassemia major,* a person is homozygous with two thalassemic genes. Thalassemia major is a severe form of the disease.

Clinical Manifestations

- The patient with thalassemia minor is frequently asymptomatic, with mild to moderate anemia with microcytosis (small cells) and hypochromia (pale cells).
- The patient who has thalassemia major is pale and displays other general manifestations of anemia (see Anemia, pp. 31, 35). In addition, the person has marked splenomegaly, hepatomegaly, and jaundice from hemolysis of RBCs. Chronic bone marrow hyperplasia leads to expansion of the marrow space. This may cause thickening of the cranium and maxillary cavity.
- Thalassemia major is a life-threatening disease in which growth, both physical and mental, is often retarded.

Collaborative Care

The laboratory findings in thalassemia major are summarized in Table 9, p. 33.

- Thalassemia minor requires no treatment because the body adapts to the reduction of normal Hgb.
- Thalassemia major is managed with blood transfusions or exchange transfusions in conjunction with oral deferasirox (Exjade) or IV or subcutaneous deferoxamine (Desferal) (chelating agents that bind to iron) to reduce the iron overloading (hemochromatosis) that occurs with chronic transfusion therapy. Because RBCs are sequestered in the enlarged spleen, thalassemia may be treated by splenectomy.
- Although hematopoietic stem cell transplantation remains the only cure for patients with thalassemia, the risk of this procedure may outweigh its benefits.

THROMBOANGIITIS OBLITERANS

Thromboangiitis obliterans (Buerger's disease) is a nonatherosclerotic, segmental, recurrent inflammatory vaso-occlusive disorder of the small- and medium-sized arteries and veins of the upper and lower extremities. The disorder occurs predominantly in young men (less than 45 years of age) with a long history of tobacco use, but without other cardiovascular disease (CVD) risk factors (e.g., hypertension, hyperlipidemia, diabetes).

In the acute phase of Buerger's disease, an inflammatory thrombus forms and blocks the vessel. Over time, the thrombus becomes more organized, and the inflammation subsides.

During the chronic phase, thrombosis and fibrosis occur in the vessel, causing tissue ischemia. The symptom complex of Buerger's disease is often confused with peripheral artery disease (PAD) and other autoimmune diseases (e.g., scleroderma).

- Patients may have intermittent claudication of the feet, hands, or arms. As the disease progresses, rest pain and ischemic ulcerations develop.
- Other signs and symptoms may include color and temperature changes of the limbs, paresthesia, superficial vein thrombosis, and cold sensitivity.

There are no laboratory or diagnostic tests specific to Buerger's disease. Diagnosis is based on the age of onset, history of tobacco use, clinical symptoms, involvement of distal vessels, presence of ischemic ulcerations, and exclusion of disorders, including diabetes, autoimmune disease, thrombophilia, and other source of emboli.

Treatment is the complete cessation of tobacco use in any form. Conservative management includes avoiding limb exposure to cold temperatures, a supervised walking program, antibiotics to treat any infected ulcers, and analgesics to manage the ischemic pain. Teach patients to avoid trauma to the extremities.

Painful ulcerations may require finger or toe amputations. Amputation below the knee may occur in severe cases. The amputation rate of patients who continue tobacco use after diagnosis is much higher than in those who stop.

THROMBOCYTOPENIA

Description

Thrombocytopenia is a reduction of platelets below 150,000/μL (150 $\times$ 10^9/L). Acute, severe, or prolonged decreases from this normal range can result in abnormal hemostasis that manifests as prolonged bleeding from minor trauma or spontaneous bleeding without injury.

Platelet disorders can be inherited (e.g., Wiskott-Aldrich syndrome), but the vast majority are acquired. A common cause of acquired disorders is the ingestion of certain herbs or drugs (see Tables 31-11 and 31-12, Lewis et al.: *Medical-Surgical Nursing,* ed. 9, p. 650). Antibodies attack the platelets when the offending agent binds to the platelet surface.

Immune Thrombocytopenic Purpura

Immune thrombocytopenic purpura (ITP), the most common acquired thrombocytopenia, is a syndrome of abnormal destruction of circulating platelets. ITP is an autoimmune disease.

- In ITP, platelets are coated with antibodies. Although these platelets function normally, when they reach the spleen the antibody-coated platelets are recognized as foreign and destroyed by macrophages. Platelets normally survive 8 to 10 days, but in ITP survival is shortened.

- Chronic ITP occurs most commonly in women between 15 and 40 years old. Chronic ITP has a gradual onset, and transient remissions occur.

Thrombotic Thrombocytopenic Purpura

Thrombotic thrombocytopenic purpura (TTP) is an uncommon syndrome characterized by hemolytic anemia, thrombocytopenia, neurologic abnormalities, fever (in the absence of infection), and renal abnormalities. TTP is almost always associated with hemolytic-uremic syndrome (HUS).

- The disease is associated with enhanced agglutination of platelets, which form microthrombi that deposit in arterioles and capillaries.
- In most cases, the syndrome is caused by the deficiency of a plasma enzyme (ADAMTS13) that usually breaks down the von Willebrand (vWF) clotting factor into normal size.
- TTP is seen primarily in adults between the ages of 20 and 50 years old.
- The syndrome may be idiopathic (autoimmune disorder against ADAMTS13), caused by certain drug toxicities (e.g., chemotherapy, cyclosporine, quinine, oral contraceptives, valacyclovir [Valtrex], clopidogrel [Plavix]), pregnancy or preeclampsia, infection, or known autoimmune disorder such as systemic lupus erythematosus or scleroderma.
- TTP is a medical emergency because bleeding and clotting occur simultaneously.

Clinical Manifestations

Many patients with thrombocytopenia are usually asymptomatic.

- The most common symptom is bleeding, usually mucosal or cutaneous. Mucosal bleeding may manifest as epistaxis and gingival bleeding, and large bullous hemorrhages may appear on the buccal mucosa. Bleeding into the skin is manifested as petechiae, purpura, or superficial ecchymoses.
- Prolonged bleeding after routine procedures such as venipuncture or IM injection may indicate thrombocytopenia. Because bleeding may be internal, be aware of manifestations that reflect this type of blood loss, including weakness, fainting, dizziness, tachycardia, abdominal pain, and hypotension.

The major complication of thrombocytopenia is hemorrhage. It may occur in any area of the body, including the joints, retina, and brain. Cerebral hemorrhage may be fatal.

Diagnostic Studies

- Platelet count is decreased below 150,000/μL (150 $\times$ 10^9/L). Spontaneous life-threatening hemorrhages (e.g., intracranial bleeding) may occur with counts below 20,000/μL (20 $\times$ 10^9/L).
- Specific assays for antigens help differentiate ITP from other types of thrombocytopenia.
- Bone marrow analysis may show normal or increased megakaryocytes (precursors of platelets). It is done to rule out leukemia, aplastic anemia, and other myeloproliferative disorders.
- Flow cytometry can be used to detect antiplatelet antibodies.

Collaborative Care

Immune Thrombocytopenic Purpura

Multiple therapies are used to manage the patient with ITP. If the patient is asymptomatic, therapy may not be used unless the platelet count is below 30,000/μL. Corticosteroids (e.g., prednisone) are used initially to suppress the phagocytic response of splenic macrophages.

Splenectomy may be indicated if the patient is not responding to the conservative treatments. Approximately 60% to 70% of patients benefit from splenectomy, resulting in a complete or partial remission. High doses of IV immunoglobulin (IVIG) and a component of IVIG, anti-Rh$_o$(D) (anti-D, WinRho), may be used in the patient who is unresponsive to corticosteroids or splenectomy, or for whom splenectomy is not an option.

- Romiplostim (Nplate) and eltrombopag (Promacta) are used for chronic ITP patients who have had an insufficient response to the other treatments or have a contraindication to splenectomy. These drugs are thrombopoietin receptor agonists and increase platelet production.
- Immunosuppressive therapy may be used in refractory cases including rituximab (Rituxan), cyclophosphamide (Cytoxan), azathioprine (Imuran), and mycophenolate mofetil (CellCept).
- Platelet transfusions are not indicated until the count is less than 10,000/μL (10 $\times$ 10^9/L) or if there is anticipated bleeding before a procedure.

Thrombotic Thrombocytopenic Purpura

TTP may be treated in a variety of ways. The first step is to treat the underlying disorder (e.g., infection) or remove the causative agent, if identified. If untreated, TTP usually results in irreversible renal failure and death. Plasma exchange (plasmapheresis) may be needed to aggressively reverse the process. Treatment should be continued daily until the patient's platelet counts normalize and hemolysis has ceased.

Corticosteroids may be added to this treatment. Rituximab has been used for patients who are refractory to plasma exchange.

Other immunosuppressants such as cyclosporine or cyclophospha-mide may also be used. Splenectomy may be considered in patients who are refractory to plasma exchange or immunosuppression. Administration of platelets is generally contraindicated because it may lead to new vWF-platelet complexes and increased clotting.

Nursing Management

Goals

The patient with thrombocytopenia will have no gross or occult bleeding, maintain vascular integrity, and manage home care to prevent any complications related to an increased risk for bleeding.

See eNCP 31-1 for the patient with thrombocytopenia, available on the website for Lewis et al.: *Medical-Surgical Nursing,* ed. 9.

Nursing Diagnoses

- Impaired oral mucous membrane
- Risk for bleeding
- Deficient knowledge

Nursing Interventions

Discourage excessive use of over-the-counter (OTC) medications known to be possible causes of acquired thrombocytopenia. Many medications contain aspirin as an ingredient. Aspirin reduces plate-let adhesiveness, thus potentially contributing to bleeding.

Encourage people to have a complete medical evaluation if manifestations of bleeding tendencies (e.g., prolonged epistaxis, petechiae) develop. Observe for early signs of thrombocytopenia in patients receiving cancer chemotherapy drugs.

The goal during acute episodes of thrombocytopenia is to pre-vent or control hemorrhage. In the patient with thrombocytopenia, bleeding is usually from superficial sites. Deep bleeding (into the muscles, joints, and abdomen) usually occurs only when clotting factors are diminished. Emphasize that a seemingly minor nose-bleed or new petechiae may indicate potential hemorrhage and the health care provider should be notified.

- In a woman with thrombocytopenia, menstrual blood loss may exceed the usual amount and duration. Counting sanitary nap-kins used during menses is an important intervention to detect excess blood loss.
- Proper administration of platelet transfusions is an important nursing responsibility.
- Monitor patients with ITP for response to therapy.

▼ Patient and Caregiver Teaching

Teach the person with acquired thrombocytopenia to avoid caus-ative agents when possible. If causative agents cannot be avoided (e.g., chemotherapy), the patient should learn to avoid injury or trauma during these periods and detect the clinical signs and symptoms of bleeding caused by thrombocytopenia.

- Patients with either ITP or acquired thrombocytopenia should have planned periodic medical evaluations to assess their status and to treat situations in which exacerbations and bleeding are likely to occur.
- The impact of either an acute or chronic condition on the patient's quality of life should also be addressed.

For a more complete listing of precautions that patients should take when their platelet count is low, see Table 31-16, Lewis et al.: *Medical-Surgical Nursing,* ed. 9, p. 654.

THYROID CANCER

Description

Thyroid cancer is the most common type of cancer of the endocrine system. An estimated 56,500 new cases of thyroid cancer occur annually. The incidence of thyroid cancer has risen significantly in the past 25 years. Thyroid cancer affects more women, and the incidence is higher in Asian Americans.

Radiation exposure significantly increases the risk for thyroid cancer. Adults at higher risk for thyroid cancer include those who were given radiation treatment during childhood for lymphoma, Wilms' tumor, and neuroblastoma. Having a personal or family history of goiter also increases a person's risk.

Four main types of thyroid cancer are papillary, follicular, medullary, and anaplastic.

- *Papillary thyroid cancer* is the most common type, accounting for about 70% to 80% of all thyroid cancers. Papillary cancer tends to grow slowly and spreads initially to lymph nodes in the neck.
- *Follicular thyroid cancer* makes up about 10% to 15% of all thyroid cancers and tends to occur in older patients. Follicular cancer first grows into the cervical lymph nodes, then spreads to the lungs and bones.
- *Medullary thyroid cancer,* which accounts for up to 10% of all thyroid cancers, is more likely to occur in families and be associated with other endocrine problems. It is diagnosed by genetic testing for *a protooncogene* called RET. Medullary thyroid cancer is a type of multiple endocrine neoplasia. This type of cancer is often poorly differentiated and associated with early metastasis.
- *Anaplastic thyroid cancer,* which is found in fewer than 2% of patients with thyroid cancer, is the most advanced and

aggressive thyroid cancer. It is the least likely to respond to treatment and has a poor prognosis.

Clinical Manifestations

The primary sign of thyroid cancer is a painless, palpable nodule or nodules in an enlarged thyroid gland. Patients or health care providers discover most of these nodules during routine palpation of the neck.

Diagnostic Studies

Nodular thyroid gland enlargement or palpation of a mass requires further evaluation.

- Ultrasound is often the first test used. CT, MRI, positron emission tomography (PET), and ultrasound-guided fine-needle aspiration (FNA) are other diagnostic options.
- A thyroid scan may be done to evaluate for a malignancy. The scan shows whether nodules on the thyroid are "hot" or "cold." If the nodule does not take up the radioactive iodine, it appears as "cold" and has a higher risk of being malignant.
- Elevations in serum calcitonin are associated with medullary thyroid cancer. In papillary and follicular cancers, serum thyroglobulin is elevated.

Nursing and Collaborative Management

Surgical removal of the tumor is usually indicated for thyroid cancer. Surgical procedures may range from unilateral total lobectomy with removal of the isthmus to near total thyroidectomy with bilateral lobectomy.

Radioactive iodine (RAI) may be given to some patients to destroy any remaining cancer cells after surgery. External beam radiation may be given as palliative treatment for patients with metastatic thyroid cancer.

Many thyroid cancers are thyroid-stimulating hormone (TSH) dependent, and thyroid hormone therapy in high doses is often prescribed to inhibit pituitary secretion of TSH. Chemotherapy including doxorubicin (Adriamycin) and cyclophosphamide (Cytoxan) may be used for advanced disease. Vandetanib (Caprelsa) and cabozantinib (Cometriq) are targeted therapies used for medullary thyroid cancer that has metastasized. These drugs inhibit tyrosine kinases, which are enzymes that are involved in growth of cancer cells.

Nursing care for the patient with thyroid cancer is similar to that for a patient undergoing thyroidectomy (see Hyperthyroidism, surgical therapy, p. 338). Because of the surgical site location and the potential for hypocalcemia, the patient requires frequent post-operative assessment. Assess the patient for airway obstruction, bleeding, and tetany because the parathyroid gland may have been disturbed or moved during surgery.

TRIGEMINAL NEURALGIA

Description

Trigeminal neuralgia (tic douloureux) is sudden, usually unilateral, severe, brief, stabbing, recurrent, episodes of pain in the distribution of the trigeminal nerve. It is seen twice as often in women as men. The majority of cases are in people older than 40 years.

- Risk factors are multiple sclerosis and hypertension. Other factors that may cause neuralgia include herpes virus infection, infection of the teeth and jaw, and a brainstem infarct.

Pathophysiology

The trigeminal nerve is the fifth cranial nerve (CN V) and has both motor and sensory branches. The sensory branches, primarily the maxillary and mandibular branches, are involved.

- The cause of trigeminal neuralgia is not fully understood. One theory is that blood vessels, especially the superior cerebellar artery, become compressed, resulting in chronic irritation of the trigeminal nerve at the root entry zone. This irritation leads to increased firing of the afferent or sensory fibers.

Clinical Manifestations

The classic feature of trigeminal neuralgia is an abrupt onset of paroxysms of excruciating pain described as burning or knifelike, or a lightning-like shock in the lips, upper or lower gums, cheek, forehead, or side of the nose.

- Intense pain, twitching, grimacing, and frequent blinking and tearing of the eye occur during the acute attack (giving rise to the term *tic*). Some patients may also experience facial sensory loss.
- The attacks are usually brief, lasting seconds to 2 or 3 minutes, and are generally unilateral.
- Recurrences are unpredictable. They may occur several times each day or weeks or months apart.
- After the refractory (pain-free) period, a phenomenon known as *clustering* can occur; it is characterized by a cycle of pain and refractoriness that continues for hours.

The painful episodes are usually initiated by a triggering mechanism of light touch at a specific point (trigger zones) along the distribution of the nerve branches.

- Precipitating stimuli include chewing, tooth brushing, feeling a hot or cold blast of air on the face, washing the face, yawning, or even talking.
- As a result, the patient may not eat properly, neglect hygienic practices, wear a cloth over the face, and withdraw from interaction with other individuals. The patient may sleep excessively as a means of coping with the pain.

Diagnostic Studies

- CT scan or MRI of the brain is used to rule out any lesions, tumors, or vascular abnormalities.
- Neurologic assessment includes audiologic evaluation, although the results are usually normal.

Collaborative Care

The goal of treatment is relief of pain either medically or surgically.

Drug Therapy

Antiseizure drug therapy may reduce pain by stabilizing the neuronal membrane and blocking nerve firing. These first-line drugs include carbamazepine (Tegretol), oxcarbazepine (Trileptal), topiramate (Topamax), clonazepam (Klonopin), phenytoin (Dilantin), lamotrigine (Lamictal), and divalproex (Depakote). Gabapentin (Neurontin) or baclofen (Lioresal) can be used in combination with any of the antiseizure drugs if a single agent is not effective. Tricyclic antidepressants such as amitriptyline (Elavil) or nortriptyline (Pamelor, Aventyl) can be used to treat constant burning or aching pain. Analgesics or opioids are usually not effective in controlling pain.

- Nerve blocking with local anesthetics is a treatment option. Relief of pain is temporary, lasting 6 to 18 months.
- Some patients use complementary and alternative therapies, usually in combination with drug treatment. These techniques include acupuncture, biofeedback, vitamin therapy, nutritional therapy, and electrical stimulation of the nerves.

Surgical Therapy

Surgical therapy is available if a conservative approach (including drug therapy) is not effective.

- *Glycerol rhizotomy* is a percutaneous procedure that consists of an injection of glycerol through the foramen ovale into the trigeminal cistern.
- *Percutaneous radiofrequency rhizotomy* (electrocoagulation) consists of placing a needle into the trigeminal rootlets that are adjacent to the pons and destroying the area by means of a

radiofrequency current. This can result in facial numbness (although some degree of sensation may be retained), corneal anesthesia, and trigeminal motor weakness.

- *Microvascular decompression* of the trigeminal nerve is performed by displacing and repositioning blood vessels that appear to be compressing the nerve at the root-entry zone where it exits the pons. This procedure relieves pain without residual sensory loss but is potentially dangerous.
- Gamma knife radiosurgery is another surgical treatment.

Nursing Management

Monitor the patient's response to drug therapy and note any side effects. Alternative pain-relief measures, such as acupuncture and biofeedback, should be explored for the patient who is not a surgical candidate and whose pain is not controlled by other measures.

Environmental management is essential during an acute period to decrease triggering stimuli. Keep the room at an even, moderate temperature and free of drafts.

Teach the patient about the importance of nutrition, hygiene, and oral care. Convey understanding if previous neglect is apparent.

- A small, very soft-bristled toothbrush or a warm mouthwash assists in promoting oral care.
- Hygiene activities are best carried out when analgesia is at its peak.
- Food should be high in protein and calories and easy to chew. It should be served lukewarm and offered frequently. When oral intake is sharply reduced and the patient's nutritional status is compromised, a nasogastric (NG) tube can be inserted on the unaffected side for enteral feedings.

For the patient who has had surgery, compare the patient's postoperative pain with the preoperative level. Frequently evaluate the corneal reflex, extraocular muscles, hearing, sensation, and facial nerve function. General postoperative nursing care after a craniotomy is appropriate if intracranial surgery is performed.

- After a percutaneous radiofrequency procedure, apply an ice pack to the jaw on the operative side for 3 to 5 hours. To avoid injuring the mouth, the patient should not chew on the operative side until sensation has returned.

▼ Patient and Caregiver Teaching

Plan for regular follow-up care and instruct the patient regarding the dosage and side effects of medications. Encourage the patient to keep environmental stimuli to a moderate level and use stress reduction methods.

Long-term management after surgical intervention depends on the residual effects of the procedure used. If anesthesia is present or the corneal reflex is altered, the patient should be taught to (1) chew on the unaffected side, (2) avoid hot foods or beverages that can burn the mucous membranes, (3) check the oral cavity after meals to remove food particles, (4) practice meticulous oral hygiene and continue with semiannual dental visits, (5) protect the face against extremes of temperature, (6) use an electric razor, (7) wear a protective eye shield, and (8) examine eye regularly for symptoms of infection or irritation.

TUBERCULOSIS

Description

Tuberculosis (TB) is an infectious disease caused by *Mycobacterium tuberculosis*. It usually involves the lungs, but any organ can be infected. TB is a primary cause of death worldwide. It is the leading cause of mortality in patients with HIV/acquired immunodeficiency syndrome (AIDS). Worldwide, more than 2 billion people (one third of the population) are currently infected with TB. Although the prevalence of TB has increased in Europe, in the United States it has steadily declined since reaching a resurgence peak in 1992.

In the United States people at risk include the homeless, residents of inner-city neighborhoods, foreign-born individuals, those living or working in institutions (long-term care facilities, prisons), IV drug users, people at poverty level, and those with poor access to health care.

- Once a strain of *M. tuberculosis* develops resistance to isoniazid and rifampin, it is defined as multidrug-resistant tuberculosis (MDR-TB). Resistance can result from incorrect prescribing, lack of public health case management, and patient nonadherence to the prescribed regimen.

Pathophysiology

M. tuberculosis is a gram-positive, acid-fast bacillus that is usually spread from person to person via airborne droplets produced by speaking, breathing, sneezing, and coughing.

- TB is not highly infectious, and transmission usually requires close, frequent, or prolonged exposure. The disease cannot be spread by touching, sharing food utensils, kissing, or any other type of physical contact.
- Once inhaled, these small particles lodge in the bronchiole and alveolus.
- The organisms find favorable environments for growth primarily in the lungs, kidneys, epiphyses of the bone, cerebral cortex, and adrenal glands.

Classification

Several systems can be used to classify TB. The American Thoracic Society classifies TB based on development of the disease (Table 81). TB can also be classified according to its (1) presentation (primary, latent, or reactivated) and (2) whether it is pulmonary or extrapulmonary.

Primary infection occurs when the bacteria are inhaled but there is an effective immune response and the bacteria become inactive.

Table 81	Classification of Tuberculosis (TB)	
Class	**Exposure or Infection**	**Description**
Class 0	No TB exposure	No TB exposure, not infected (no history of exposure, negative tuberculin skin test)
Class 1	TB exposure, no infection	TB exposure, no evidence of infection (history of exposure, negative tuberculin skin test)
Class 2	Latent TB infection, no disease	TB infection without disease (significant reaction to tuberculin skin test, negative bacteriologic studies, no x-ray findings compatible with TB, no clinical evidence of TB)
Class 3	TB, clinically active	TB infection with clinically active disease (positive bacteriologic studies or both a significant reaction to tuberculin skin test and clinical or x-ray evidence of current disease)
Class 4	TB, but not clinically active	No current disease (history of previous episode of TB or abnormal, stable x-ray findings in a person with a significant reaction to tuberculin skin test; negative bacteriologic studies if done; no clinical or x-ray evidence of current disease)
Class 5	TB suspect	TB suspect (diagnosis pending); person should not be in this classification for >3 mo

Source: American Thoracic Society.

Most people have an effective immune response to encapsulate these organisms for the rest of their lives.

Latent TB infection (LTBI) occurs in a person who does not have active TB. An estimated 10 to 15 million Americans have LTBI. Up to 10% of them will develop active TB disease at some point in their lives. Therefore treatment of LTBI is important.

Active TB disease results if the initial immune response is not adequate, the body cannot contain the organisms, and the bacteria replicate. When active disease develops within the first 2 years of infection, it is termed *primary TB*. Postprimary TB, or *reactivation TB*, is defined as TB disease occurring 2 or more years after the initial infection.

Clinical Manifestations

People with LTBI have a positive skin test but are asymptomatic.

- Active TB disease may initially manifest with fatigue, malaise, anorexia, unexplained weight loss, low-grade fevers, and night sweats.
- Sometimes TB has more acute, sudden presentation. The patient may have a high fever, chills, generalized flu-like symptoms, pleuritic pain, and a productive cough.
- In patients with HIV, classic manifestations of TB such as fever, cough, and weight loss may be wrongly attributed to *Pneumocystis jiroveci* pneumonia (PCP) or other HIV-associated opportunistic diseases.
- The clinical manifestations of extrapulmonary TB depend on the organs infected. For example, renal TB can cause dysuria and hematuria. Bone and joint TB may cause severe pain. Headaches, vomiting, and lymphadenopathy may be present with TB meningitis.

Complications

Miliary TB is the widespread dissemination of the mycobacterium. The infection is characterized by a large amount of TB bacilli and may be fatal if left untreated.

- Clinical manifestations may slowly progress over a period of days, weeks, or months. Symptoms vary depending on which organs are infected.
- Hepatomegaly, splenomegaly, and generalized lymphadenopathy may also be present.

Pleural TB can result from either primary disease or reactivation of a latent infection. *Empyema* is less common than effusion but may occur from large numbers of tubercular organisms in the pleural space.

Acute pneumonia may result when large amounts of tubercle bacilli are discharged from granulomas into the lungs or lymph nodes. Manifestations are similar to those of bacterial pneumonia, including chills, fever, productive cough, pleuritic pain, and leukocytosis.

Diagnostic Studies

- Tuberculin skin test (TST): Induration (not redness) at the injection site means the person has been exposed to TB and has developed antibodies. See Table 26-11 and Chapter 26, Lewis et al.: *Medical-Surgical Nursing,* ed. 9, for guidelines in performing and interpreting TSTs.
- Interferon-γ release assays: Detect IFN-γ released from T cells in response to mycobacterial antigens.
- Chest x-ray: Diagnosis cannot be based solely on x-ray because other diseases may mimic TB.
- Bacteriologic studies: Stained sputum smears for acid-fast bacilli (AFB test) can identify tubercle bacilli; cultures to grow tubercle bacilli confirm diagnosis.

Collaborative Care

Most patients with TB are treated on an outpatient basis and continue to work and maintain their lifestyles with few changes. Hospitalization may be needed for severely ill or debilitated patients.

Drug Therapy

The mainstay of TB treatment is drug therapy.

Active TB Disease. Because of the growing prevalence of MDR-TB, it is important to manage the patient with active TB aggressively. Drug therapy is divided into two phases: initial and continuation (see Tables 28-11 and 28-12, Lewis et al.: *Medical-Surgical Nursing,* ed. 9, p. 531). In most circumstances the treatment regimen for patients with previously untreated TB consists of a 2-month initial phase with four-drug therapy (isoniazid [INH], rifampin, pyrazinamide [PZA], and ethambutol).

- *Directly observed therapy* (DOT) involves providing the antituberculous drugs directly to patients and watching as they swallow the medications.
- Nonadherence is a major factor in the emergence of multidrug resistance and treatment failures. Many individuals do not adhere to the treatment program in spite of understanding that nonadherence can lead to reactivation of TB and multidrug-resistant TB.

Latent TB Infection. In people with LTBI, drug therapy helps prevent a TB infection from developing into active TB disease. The standard treatment regimen for LTBI is 9 months of daily INH.

Bacille Calmette-Guérin (BCG) vaccine is given to infants in parts of the world with a high prevalence of TB. The BCG vaccine should be considered only for select individuals who meet specific criteria (e.g., health care workers who are continually exposed to patients with MDR-TB and when infection control precautions are not successful).

Nursing Management

Goals
The patient with tuberculosis will comply with the therapeutic regimen, have no recurrence of disease, have normal pulmonary function, and take appropriate measures to prevent the spread of the disease.

Nursing Diagnoses
- Ineffective breathing pattern
- Nonadherence
- Ineffective airway clearance

Nursing Interventions
The ultimate goal is to eradicate TB worldwide.
- Screening programs in known high-risk groups are of value in detecting people with TB.
- Chest x-rays to assess for the presence of TB in people with a positive TST should be encouraged.
- Reducing HIV infection, poverty, overcrowded living conditions, malnutrition, smoking, and drug and alcohol abuse can help minimize TB infection rates.

If hospitalization is needed for patients suspected of having TB, special measures should be taken.
- Airborne infection isolation is indicated for the patient with pulmonary or laryngeal TB until the patient is noninfectious (defined as effective drug therapy, clinical improvement, and three negative AFB smears).
- High-efficiency particulate air (HEPA) masks are worn whenever entering the patient's room.

▼ Patient and Caregiver Teaching
- Teach hospitalized patients to cover their nose and mouth with paper tissues every time they cough, sneeze, or produce sputum.
- Teach the patient and caregiver about adherence to the prescribed regimen. Strategies to improve adherence include teaching and counseling, reminder systems, incentives or rewards, contracts, and DOT.
- Because about 5% of individuals experience relapses, teach the patient to recognize symptoms that indicate the recurrence of TB. If these symptoms occur, immediate medical attention should be sought.
- Also teach the patient about factors that could reactivate TB, such as immunosuppression and malignancy.

ULCERATIVE COLITIS

Description

Ulcerative colitis is an autoimmune disorder that, along with Crohn's disease, is referred to as *inflammatory bowel disease* (IBD). See Inflammatory Bowel Disease, p. 352, for a discussion of the disorder.

URETHRITIS

Urethritis is an inflammation of the urethra. Causes of urethritis include a bacterial or viral infection, trichomonal and monilial infection (especially in women), chlamydial infection, and gonorrhea (especially in men).

In men, purulent discharge usually indicates a gonococcal urethritis. A clear discharge typically signifies a nongonococcal urethritis. Urethritis also produces bothersome lower urinary tract symptoms, including dysuria, urgency, and frequent urination, similar to those seen with cystitis.

In women, urethritis is difficult to diagnose. It frequently produces bothersome lower urinary tract symptoms, but urethral discharge may not be present.

Nursing and Collaborative Management

Treatment is based on identifying and treating the cause and providing symptomatic relief.

- Sulfamethoxazole with trimethoprim (Bactrim, Septra) and nitrofurantoin (Furadantin) are examples of medications used for bacterial infections. Metronidazole (Flagyl) and clotrimazole (Mycelex) may be used for trichomonal infection. Medications such as nystatin (Mycostatin) or fluconazole (Diflucan) may be prescribed for monilial infections. In chlamydial infections, doxycycline (Vibramycin) may be used.
- Women with negative urine cultures and no pyuria usually do not respond to antibiotics. Warm sitz baths may temporarily relieve bothersome symptoms.

Teach patients to avoid using vaginal deodorant sprays, properly cleanse the perineal area after bowel movements and urination, and avoid sexual intercourse until symptoms subside. Teach patients with sexually transmitted urethritis to refer their sex partners for evaluation and testing if they had sexual contact in the 60 days preceding onset of the symptoms or diagnosis.

U

URINARY INCONTINENCE

Description

Urinary incontinence (UI), an involuntary leakage of urine, affects an estimated 17 million people in the United States. Although its prevalence is higher among older women and men, it is not a natural consequence of aging. An estimated 80% of incontinence can be cured or significantly improved.

Pathophysiology

UI can result from anything that interferes with bladder or urethral sphincter control.

- Using the acronym *DRIP,* the causes include *D:* delirium, dehydration, depression; *R:* restricted mobility, rectal impaction; *I:* infection, inflammation, impaction; and *P:* polyuria, polypharmacy.
- UI disorders include stress, urge, overflow, and reflex incontinence. (For a complete description of UI, see Table 46-17, Lewis et al.: *Medical-Surgical Nursing,* ed. 9, p. 1088.)
- Patients may have more than one type of incontinence.

Diagnostic Studies

- A focused history, physical assessment, and a voiding record provide information about the onset of UI, factors that provoke urinary leakage, and associated conditions.
- Pelvic examination assesses for organ prolapse and evaluates pelvic floor muscle strength.
- Urinalysis identifies possible factors contributing to transient incontinence or urinary retention (e.g., urinary infection, diabetes mellitus).
- Measure postvoid residual (PVR) urine in the patient undergoing evaluation for UI. The PVR volume is obtained by asking the patient to urinate, followed by catheterization or use of a bladder ultrasound within a relatively brief period (preferably 10 to 20 minutes).
- Urodynamic testing is indicated in selected cases of UI.
- Imaging studies of the upper urinary tract (e.g., ultrasound) are obtained when incontinence is associated with urinary tract infections or there is evidence of upper urinary tract involvement.

Collaborative Care

Transient, reversible factors are corrected initially, followed by management of the type of UI. In general, less invasive treatments are attempted before more invasive methods (e.g., surgery) are used.

Several behavioral therapies may be used including (1) pelvic floor muscle training (Kegel exercises) to help some patients manage stress, urge, or mixed UI, and (2) biofeedback to assist the patient to identify, isolate, contract, and relax the pelvic muscles.

Drug Therapy

Drug therapy varies according to UI type.

- In *stress UI,* drugs have a limited role in management. α-Adrenergic agonists can be used to increase bladder sphincter tone and urethral resistance but have limited benefit.
- In *urge* and *reflex UI,* drugs play a key management role. Anticholinergic drugs and muscarinic receptor antagonists relax the bladder muscle and inhibit overactive detrusor contractions. These preparations include immediate- and extended-release tolterodine (Detrol, Detrol LA); immediate, extended, and transdermal oxybutynin (Ditropan, Ditropan XL, Oxytrol TDS); twice-daily trospium chloride (Sanctura); extended-release solifenacin (VESIcare); and darifenacin (Enablex). Botox (onabotulinumtoxinA) can be used in the treatment of UI as a result of detrusor overactivity. Botox is injected into the bladder, resulting in relaxation of the bladder, an increase in its storage capacity, and a decrease in UI.

Surgical Therapy

Surgical techniques also vary according to the type of UI.

- Surgical correction of stress UI may reposition the urethra and/ or create a backboard of support or otherwise stabilize the urethra and bladder neck and make them more receptive to changes in intraabdominal pressure.
- Another technique for stress UI augments the urethral resistance of the intrinsic sphincter unit with a sling or periurethral injectables.
- Retropubic colposuspension and pubovaginal sling placement appear to be most effective. Typically, both procedures are performed through low transverse incisions.
- Placement of a suburethral sling, using autologous fascia, cadaveric fascia, or a synthetic material, is also used to correct stress UI in women.
- An artificial urethral sphincter can be used in men with intrinsic sphincter deficiency and severe stress UI.
- Alternatively, one of several bulking agents can be injected underneath the mucosa of the urethra to correct stress UI in women or men.

Nursing Management

You need to recognize both the physical and the emotional problems associated with incontinence. Maintain and enhance the patient's dignity, privacy, and feelings of self-worth.

- This is a two-step approach involving containment devices to manage existing urinary leakage and a definitive plan to reduce or resolve the factors leading to incontinence.

- Emphasize consumption of an adequate volume of fluids and reduction or elimination of bladder irritants (particularly caffeine and alcohol) from the diet.
- Advise the patient to maintain a regular, flexible schedule of urination (usually every 2 to 3 hours while awake).
- Also advise patients to quit smoking, because it increases the risk of stress UI.
- Aggressive management of constipation is recommended, beginning with ensuring adequate fluid intake, increasing dietary fiber, lightly exercising, and judiciously using stool softeners.
- Behavioral treatments include bladder retraining and pelvic floor muscle training. (A patient teaching guide for pelvic floor muscle exercise is found in Table 46-19, Lewis et al.: *Medical-Surgical Nursing,* ed. 9, p. 1090.)
- Assess strategies the patient uses to contain UI and share information on products specifically designed to contain urine.
- In inpatient or long-term care facilities, nursing management of UI includes maximizing toilet access. This assistance may take the form of offering the urinal or bedpan or assisting the patient to the bathroom every 2 to 3 hours or at scheduled times. Ensure that toilets are accessible to patients and there is adequate privacy to allow effective urine elimination.

URINARY RETENTION

Description

Urinary retention is the inability to empty the bladder despite micturition or the accumulation of urine in the bladder because of an inability to urinate. In certain cases, it is associated with urinary leakage or postvoid dribbling, called overflow urinary incontinence (UI).

- Acute urinary retention, which is the total inability to pass urine via micturition, is a medical emergency. Chronic urinary retention is defined as incomplete bladder emptying despite urination.

Pathophysiology

Urinary retention is caused by two different dysfunctions of the urinary system: bladder outlet obstruction and deficient detrusor (bladder muscle) contraction strength.

- Bladder outlet obstruction leads to urinary retention when the blockage is so severe that the bladder can no longer evacuate its contents despite a detrusor contraction. A common cause of obstruction in men is an enlarged prostate.
- Common causes of deficient detrusor (bladder wall muscle) contraction strength are neurologic diseases affecting the sacral

segments 2, 3, and 4; long-standing diabetes mellitus; overdistention; long-term alcoholism; and drugs (e.g., anticholinergic drugs).

Diagnostic Studies

The diagnostic studies for urinary retention are the same as the ones for UI (see Urinary Incontinence, p. 640).

Collaborative Care

Behavioral therapies that were described for UI also may be used in the management of urinary retention. Scheduled toileting and double voiding may be effective in chronic urinary retention with moderate postvoid residual volumes.

- Double voiding is an attempt to maximize bladder evacuation by having the patient urinate, sit on the toilet for 3 to 4 minutes, and urinate again before exiting the bathroom.
- If catheterization is required for acute or chronic urinary retention, intermittent catheterization is preferred. It allows the patient to remain free of an indwelling catheter with its associated risk of urinary tract infection (UTI) and urethral irritation.

Drug Therapy

Several drugs may be administered to promote bladder evacuation. For patients with obstruction at the level of the bladder neck, an α-adrenergic antagonist may be prescribed. These drugs relax the smooth muscle of the bladder neck, prostatic urethra, and possibly dual-innervated rhabdosphincter, diminishing urethral resistance.

Surgical Therapy

Surgical interventions are used to manage urinary retention caused by obstruction. Transurethral or open surgical techniques are used to treat benign or malignant prostatic enlargement, bladder neck contracture, urethral strictures, or dyssynergia of the bladder neck.

- Pelvic reconstruction using an abdominal or transvaginal approach can correct bladder outlet obstruction in women with severe pelvic organ prolapse.

Unfortunately, surgery has a minimal role in the management of urinary retention caused by deficient detrusor contraction strength.

Nursing Management

Acute urinary retention is a medical emergency that requires prompt recognition and bladder drainage. You should insert a catheter (as ordered) unless otherwise directed.

- Teach the patient with acute urinary retention to minimize risk, including avoiding intake of large volumes of fluid over a brief period.
- Advise the patient who is unable to urinate to drink a cup of coffee or brewed caffeinated tea to maximize urinary urgency

and sit in a tub of warm water or take a warm shower and attempt to urinate while in the tub or shower.

- If these measures do not lead to successful urination, advise the patient to seek immediate care.

Patients with chronic urinary retention may be managed by behavioral methods, an indwelling or intermittent catheterization, surgery, or drugs. Scheduled toileting and double voiding are the primary behavioral interventions used for chronic retention.

URINARY TRACT CALCULI

Description

Each year an estimated 1 to 2 million people in the United States have *nephrolithiasis* (kidney stone disease). Except for struvite stones, associated with urinary tract infection (UTI), stone disorders are more common in men than women. The majority of patients are between 20 and 55 years old.

- The incidence is also higher in people with a family history of stone formation. Stones can recur in up to 50% of patients.
- Stone formation occurs more often in the summer months, thus supporting the role of dehydration in this process.
- The term *calculus* refers to the stone, and *lithiasis* refers to stone formation.

Pathophysiology

Many factors are involved in the incidence and type of stone formation, including metabolic, dietary, genetic, climatic, lifestyle, and occupational influences. Many theories have been proposed to explain the formation of stones in the urinary tract.

- Crystals, when in a supersaturated concentration, can precipitate and unite to form a stone. Keeping urine dilute and free flowing reduces the risk of recurrent stone formation in many individuals.
- Urinary pH, solute load, and inhibitors in the urine affect the formation of stones. The higher the pH, the less soluble are calcium and phosphate. The lower the pH, the less soluble are uric acid and cystine.

Other important factors in stone development include obstruction with urinary stasis and UTI with urea-splitting bacteria (e.g., *Proteus, Klebsiella, Pseudomonas,* and some species of staphylococci). These bacteria cause the urine to become alkaline and contribute to the formation of struvite (calcium-magnesium-ammonium phosphate) stones.

- Infected stones, entrapped in the kidney, may assume a staghorn configuration as they enlarge. These stones can lead to hydronephrosis, renal infection, and loss of kidney function.

- There are five major categories of stones: calcium phosphate, calcium oxalate, uric acid, cystine, and struvite. Stone composition may be mixed, although calcium stones are the most common.

Clinical Manifestations

The first symptom is usually severe pain that begins suddenly. Typically, a person feels a sharp pain in the flank area, back, or lower abdomen. People describe the pain as the most excruciating that a person can endure.

- *Renal colic* is the term used for the sharp, severe pain, which results from the stretching, dilation, and spasm of the ureter in response to the obstructing stone. Nausea and vomiting may also occur.
- Urinary stones cause manifestations when they obstruct urinary flow. The type of pain is determined by the location of the stone. If the stone is nonobstructing, pain may be absent. If it produces obstruction in a calyx or at the ureteropelvic junction (UPJ), the patient may experience dull costovertebral flank pain or even colic. Pain resulting from the passage of a calculus down the ureter is intense and colicky. The patient may be in mild shock with cool, moist skin. As a stone nears the ureterovesical junction (UVJ), pain will be felt in the lateral flank and sometimes down into the testicles, labia, or groin.
- Manifestations may also include those of a UTI with dysuria, fever, and chills.

Diagnostic Studies

- Noncontrast spiral CT (also called a CT/KUB [kidneys, ureters, bladder]), ultrasound, and intravenous pyelogram (IVP) may be used.
- Urinalysis is used to assess for hematuria, crystalluria, and urine pH. Urine pH checks for struvite stones and renal tubular necrosis (tendency to alkaline pH) and uric acid stones (tendency to acidic pH).
- Retrieval and analysis of the stones are important in the diagnosis of the underlying problem contributing to stone formation.
- Serum calcium, phosphorus, sodium, potassium, bicarbonate, uric acid, and creatinine levels and blood urea nitrogen (BUN) are also measured.

Collaborative Care

Evaluation and management of the patient with renal lithiasis consist of two concurrent approaches. The *first approach* is directed toward management of the acute attack by treating the pain, infection, or obstruction. Administer opioids to relieve renal colic pain. Many stones are 4 mm or less in size and will pass spontaneously. However, such a stone may take weeks to pass. Tamsulosin (Flomax) or terazosin (Hytrin), α-adrenergic blockers that relax the smooth muscle in the ureter, can be used to facilitate stone passage.

The *second approach* is evaluation of the cause of the stone formation and prevention of further stone development. Information obtained from the patient includes family history of stone formation, geographic residence, nutritional assessment (including intake of vitamins A and D), activity pattern (active or sedentary), history of periods of prolonged illness with immobilization or dehydration, and history of disease or surgery involving the GI or genitourinary (GU) tract.

Adequate hydration, dietary sodium restrictions, dietary changes, and drugs minimize urinary stone formation.

- Various drugs are prescribed that prevent stone formation by altering urine pH, preventing excessive urinary excretion of a substance, or correcting a primary disease (e.g., hyperparathyroidism).

Treatment of struvite stones requires control of infection. Acetohydroxamic acid inhibits the chemical action caused by persistent bacteria and thus retards struvite stone formation. If infection cannot be controlled, the stone may have to be surgically removed.

Indications for open surgical, endourologic, or lithotripsy stone removal include:

- Stones too large for spontaneous passage (usually larger than 7 mm), associated with bacteriuria or symptomatic infection, or causing impaired renal function, persistent pain, nausea, or paralytic ileus
- Inability of the patient to be treated medically
- Patient with only one kidney

Endourologic procedures include the use of endoscopes to access stones in the urinary tract. *Cystoscopy* can remove small stones in the bladder. For large stones, a *cystolitholapaxy* is performed using a lithotrite to crush stones. A *cystoscopic lithotripsy* uses an ultrasonic lithotrite to pulverize stones. Complications with these cystoscopic procedures include hemorrhage, retained stone fragments, and infection. Flexible *ureteroscopes* can be used to remove stones from the renal pelvis and upper urinary tract with the use of ultrasonic, laser, or electrohydraulic lithotripsy. The same types of lithotripsy can be used during a percutaneous nephrolithotomy by way of a nephroscope inserted through the skin into the kidney pelvis.

Lithotripsy is a procedure for eliminating calculi from the urinary tract. Specific lithotripsy techniques include percutaneous ultrasonic lithotripsy, electrohydraulic lithotripsy, laser lithotripsy, and extracorporeal shock wave lithotripsy. Extracorporeal shock wave lithotripsy and laser lithotripsy are the most common.

Hematuria is common after lithotripsy procedures. A self-retaining ureteral stent is often placed after this outpatient procedure to promote passage of sand (shattered stone) and prevent obstruction caused by sand buildup in the ureter. The stent is often removed 2 weeks after lithotripsy.

- If a stone is large or positioned in the mid or distal ureter, additional treatment such as surgery may be necessary.

A small group of patients require open surgical procedures including patients with pain, obstruction, and infection. The type of open surgery (e.g., nephrolithotomy, pyelolithotomy, ureterolithotomy) depends on location of the stone. For open surgery on the kidney or ureter, a flank incision directly below the diaphragm and across the side is usually the preferred approach.

Nutritional Therapy

A high fluid intake (at least 3 L/day) is recommended after an episode of urolithiasis to produce a urine output of at least 2 L/day and prevent stone formation.

- Limit consumption of colas, coffee, and tea because high intake of these beverages tends to increase the risk of recurring urinary calculi.
- A low-sodium diet is recommended, because high sodium intake increases calcium excretion in the urine. Foods high in calcium, oxalate, and purines are presented in Table 46-12, Lewis et al.: *Medical-Surgical Nursing,* ed. 9, p. 1080.

Nursing Management

Goals

The patient with urinary tract calculi will have relief of pain, no urinary tract obstruction, and an understanding of measures to prevent recurrence of stones.

Nursing Diagnoses

- Acute pain
- Impaired urinary elimination
- Deficient knowledge

Nursing Interventions

Preventive measures related to the person who is on bed rest or is relatively immobile for a prolonged time include maintaining an adequate fluid intake, turning the patient every 2 hours, and helping the patient sit or stand if possible to maximize urinary flow.

Pain management and patient comfort are primary nursing responsibilities when managing a person with an obstructing stone and renal colic.

- To ensure that any spontaneously passed stones are retrieved, strain all urine voided by the patient using gauze or a urine strainer.

U

- Encourage ambulation to promote movement of the stone from the upper to the lower urinary tract. To ensure safety, tell the patient not to walk unattended while experiencing acute renal colic, particularly if opioid analgesics are being given.

▼ **Patient and Caregiver Teaching**

- Prevention of stone recurrence includes adequate fluid intake to produce a urine output of approximately 2 L/day.
- Dietary restriction of purines may be helpful for the patient at risk for developing uric acid stones.
- Teach the patient the dosage, scheduling, and potential side effects of drugs used to reduce the risk of stone formation.
- Selected patients may be taught to self-monitor urinary pH or urinary output.

URINARY TRACT INFECTIONS

Description

Urinary tract infections (UTIs) are the most common bacterial infection in women. *Escherichia coli (E. coli)* is the most common pathogen causing a UTI.

- Bacterial counts in the urine of 10^5 colony-forming units per milliliter (CFU/mL) or higher typically indicate a UTI. However, bacterial counts as low as 10^2 to 10^3 CFU/mL in a person with symptoms are also indicative of UTI.
- Fungal and parasitic UTIs are uncommon and are seen most frequently in the patient who is immunosuppressed, has diabetes mellitus (DM), or has taken multiple courses of antibiotics.

Classification

A UTI can be broadly classified as upper and lower UTI according to its location within the urinary system. Infection of the upper urinary tract (involving the renal parenchyma, pelvis, and ureters) typically causes fever, chills, and flank pain, whereas a UTI confined to the lower urinary tract does not usually have systemic manifestations.

Specific terms are used to further delineate UTI location. For example, *pyelonephritis* implies inflammation usually caused by infection of the renal parenchyma and collecting system, *cystitis* indicates inflammation of the bladder wall, and *urethritis* is inflammation of the urethra. *Urosepsis* is a UTI that has spread systemically and is a life-threatening condition requiring emergency treatment.

Classifying a UTI as uncomplicated or complicated is also useful.

- *Uncomplicated infections* are those that occur in an otherwise normal urinary tract and usually involve only the bladder.

- *Complicated infections* include those infections with coexisting obstruction, stones, or catheters; the existence of DM or neurologic diseases; or recurrent infection. The individual with a complicated infection is at an increased risk of renal damage.

Pathophysiology

The urinary tract above the urethra is normally sterile, and organisms that cause UTIs are usually introduced by way of the ascending route from the urethra. Most infections are caused by gram-negative aerobic bacilli normally found in the GI tract. Table 82 lists predisposing factors for UTIs.

- A common factor contributing to ascending infection is urologic instrumentation (e.g., catheterization, cystoscopic examinations). Instrumentation allows bacteria that are normally present at the opening of the urethra to enter the urethra or bladder.
- Sexual intercourse promotes "milking" of bacteria from the vagina and perineum and may cause minor urethral trauma that predisposes women to UTIs.
- Rarely do UTIs result from a hematogenous route, where blood-borne bacteria secondarily invade the kidneys, ureters, or bladder from elsewhere in the body.

An important source of UTIs is health care–associated infections (HAIs), previously called nosocomial infections. The cause is often *E. coli* and, less frequently, *Pseudomonas* organisms. Catheter-acquired UTIs are the most common HAI infections and are caused by development of bacterial biofilms that are found on the catheter's inner surface.

Clinical Manifestations

Lower urinary tract symptoms are seen in UTIs of both the upper and lower urinary tracts.

- Symptoms include dysuria, frequent urination (more often than every 2 hours), urgency, and suprapubic discomfort or pressure. Older adults tend to experience nonlocalized abdominal discomfort rather than dysuria and suprapubic pain.
- The urine may contain grossly visible blood (hematuria) or sediment, giving it a cloudy appearance.
- Flank pain, chills, and fever indicate an infection involving the upper urinary tract (pyelonephritis).

Multiple factors may produce lower urinary tract symptoms similar to a UTI. For example, patients with bladder tumors or those receiving intravesical chemotherapy or pelvic radiation usually experience urinary frequency, urgency, and dysuria. Interstitial cystitis also produces urinary symptoms that are similar to and sometimes confused with a UTI (see Interstitial Cystitis/Painful Bladder Syndrome, p. 360).

Table 82 Risk Factors for Urinary Tract Infections

Factors Increasing Urinary Stasis
- Intrinsic obstruction (stone, tumor of urinary tract, urethral stricture, BPH)
- Extrinsic obstruction (tumor, fibrosis compressing urinary tract)
- Urinary retention (including neurogenic bladder and low bladder wall compliance)
- Renal impairment

Foreign Bodies
- Urinary tract calculi
- Catheters (indwelling, external condom catheter, ureteral stent, nephrostomy tube, intermittent catheterization)
- Urinary tract instrumentation (cystoscopy, urodynamics)

Anatomic Factors
- Congenital defects leading to obstruction or urinary stasis
- Fistula (abnormal opening) exposing urinary stream to skin, vagina, or fecal stream
- Shorter female urethra and colonization from normal vaginal flora
- Obesity

Factors Compromising Immune Response
- Aging
- Human immunodeficiency virus infection
- Diabetes mellitus

Functional Disorders
- Constipation
- Voiding dysfunction with detrusor sphincter dyssynergia

Other Factors
- Pregnancy
- Hypoestrogenic state (menopause)
- Multiple sex partners (women)
- Use of spermicidal agents or contraceptive diaphragm (women)
- Poor personal hygiene
- Habitual delay of urination ("nurse's bladder," "teacher's bladder")

BPH, Benign prostatic hyperplasia.

Diagnostic Studies

- Dipstick urinalysis is obtained initially to identify presence of nitrites (indicating bacteriuria), WBCs, and leukocyte esterase (an enzyme present in WBCs indicating pyuria).
- After confirmation of bacteriuria and pyuria, a urine culture with sensitivity may be obtained.
- A CT urogram or ultrasound may be obtained when obstruction of the urinary system is suspected.

Collaborative Care

Drug Therapy

Once a UTI has been diagnosed, appropriate antimicrobial therapy is initiated. Uncomplicated cystitis can be treated by a short-term course of antibiotics, typically for 1 to 3 days. In contrast, complicated UTIs require longer-term treatment, lasting 7 to 14 days or even longer.

- Trimethoprim-sulfamethoxazole (TMP-SMX, Bactrim) or nitrofurantoin (Macrodantin) is often used to empirically treat uncomplicated or initial UTIs.
- Fluoroquinolones (e.g., ciprofloxacin [Cipro], levofloxacin [Levaquin], gatifloxacin [Tequin]) are used to treat complicated UTIs.
- Other antibiotics used to treat uncomplicated UTI include ampicillin, amoxicillin, and cephalosporins.
- A urinary analgesic such as oral phenazopyridine (Pyridium) may be used to relieve discomfort caused by severe dysuria.

Prophylactic or suppressive antibiotics are sometimes administered to patients who experience repeated UTIs. Although suppressive therapy is often effective on a short-term basis, this strategy is limited because of the risk of antibiotic resistance.

Nursing Management

Goals

The patient with a UTI will have relief from bothersome lower urinary tract symptoms, prevention of upper urinary tract involvement, and prevention of recurrence.

Nursing Diagnoses

- Impaired urinary elimination
- Readiness for enhanced self-health management

Nursing Interventions

Health promotion activities, especially for individuals who are at an increased risk for UTI, include teaching preventive measures such as (1) emptying the bladder regularly and completely, (2) evacuating the bowel regularly, (3) wiping the perineal area from front to back after urination and defecation, and (4) drinking an adequate amount of liquid each day.

U

- Daily intake of cranberry or cranberry tablets may reduce the number of UTIs.
- You have a major role in the prevention of HAI infections with avoidance of unnecessary catheterization and early removal of indwelling catheters.

In most cases, acute intervention for a patient with a UTI includes adequate fluid intake. Fluid intake flushes out bacteria before they have a chance to colonize in the bladder. Caffeine, alcohol, citrus juices, chocolate, and highly spiced foods or beverages should be avoided because they may irritate the bladder.

- Application of local heat to the suprapubic area or lower back may relieve the discomfort associated with a UTI. A warm shower or sitting in a tub of warm water filled above the waist can also provide temporary relief.

▼ **Patient and Caregiver Teaching**

Instruct the patient about the prescribed drug therapy including side effects. Emphasize the importance of taking the full course of antibiotics.

- Instruct the patient to monitor for signs of improvement (e.g., cloudy urine becomes clear) and a decrease in or cessation of symptoms.
- Teach patients to promptly report any of the following to their health care provider: (1) persistence of bothersome lower urinary tract symptoms beyond the antibiotic treatment course, (2) onset of flank pain, or (3) fever.
- Teach the patient and caregiver about the need for ongoing care, including taking antimicrobial drugs as ordered, maintaining adequate daily fluid intake, voiding regularly (approximately every 3 to 4 hours), urinating before and after intercourse, and temporarily discontinuing the use of a diaphragm.

If treatment is complete and symptoms are still present, instruct the patient to get follow-up care. Recurrent symptoms because of bacterial persistence or inadequate treatment typically occur within 1 to 2 weeks after completion of therapy.

VAGINAL, CERVICAL, AND VULVAR INFECTIONS

Definition

Infection and inflammation of the vagina, cervix, and vulva commonly occur when the natural defenses of the acid vaginal secretions (maintained by sufficient estrogen level) and the presence of *Lactobacillus* are disrupted. A woman's resistance may also be decreased as a result of aging, poor nutrition, and the use of drugs (e.g., antibiotics, hormones) that alter the bacterial flora or mucosa.

Pathophysiology

Organisms gain entrance to these areas through contaminated hands, clothing, and douche tips and during intercourse, surgery, and childbirth. Table 83 presents the etiology, clinical manifestations, diagnostic methods, and collaborative care of common infections of the lower genital tract.

- Most lower genital tract infections are related to sexual intercourse. Vulvar infections, such as herpes and genital warts, can be sexually transmitted when no lesions are present (see Herpes, Genital, p. 309, and Warts, Genital, p. 672).
- Oral contraceptives, antibiotics, and corticosteroids may produce changes in the vaginal pH and trigger an overgrowth of the organisms present. For example, *Candida albicans* may be present in small numbers in the vagina. An overgrowth of this organism causes vulvovaginitis.

Clinical Manifestations

- Abnormal vaginal discharge and reddened vulvar lesions are common.
- In addition to a thick, white, curdy discharge, women with vulvovaginal candidiasis (VVC) often experience intense itching and dysuria.
- The hallmark of bacterial vaginosis is the fishy odor of the discharge.
- Women with cervicitis may notice spotting after intercourse.

Postmenopausal older women may develop gynecologic problems, such as *lichen sclerosis,* a chronic inflammatory condition associated with intense itching in the genital skin area. The lesions are white with a "tissue paper" appearance initially, although scratching produces changes in the appearance.

V

Diagnostic Studies

- History, physical examination, and sexual history.
- Culture ulcerative lesions for herpes.
- Vulvar dystrophies are examined by colposcope with biopsy specimens taken.
- Microscopy and culture of vaginal discharge are done.
- Bacterial vaginosis, VVC, and trichomoniasis are diagnosed by a wet mount.
- For cervicitis, endocervical cultures are obtained for chlamydia and gonorrhea. If purulent discharge is observed coming from the cervix, endocervical cells may be taken to do a Gram stain.

Collaborative Care

Antibiotics taken as directed will cure bacterial infections. Antifungal preparations (in oral or cream preparations) are indicated for VVC.

Table 83 Infections of the Lower Genital Tract

Infection and Etiology	Manifestations and Diagnostic Methods	Drug Therapy
Vulvovaginal Candidiasis (VVC) (Monilial Vaginitis)		
Candida albicans (fungus)	Commonly found in mouth, GI tract, and vagina. Pruritus, thick white curdlike discharge. KOH microscopic examination: pseudohyphae, pH 4.0-4.7.	Antifungal agents (e.g., miconazole [Monistat], clotrimazole [Gyne-Lotrimin, Mycelex] [available over the counter, in cream or suppository]) Fluconazole (Diflucan).
Trichomonas Vaginitis		
Trichomonas vaginalis (protozoa)	Sexually transmitted. Pruritus, frothy greenish or gray discharge. Hemorrhagic spots on cervix or vaginal walls. Saline microscopic examination: swimming trichomonads, pH >4.5.	Metronidazole (Flagyl) for patient and partner.

Bacterial Vaginosis *Gardnerella vaginalis* *Corynebacterium vaginale*	Mode of transmission unclear. Watery discharge with fishy odor. May or may not have other symptoms. Saline microscopic examination: epithelial cells, pH >4.5.	Oral or vaginal metronidazole (Flagyl) or clindamycin (Clindesse). Examine and treat partner. *Lactobacillus acidophilus* taken orally by diet (e.g., yogurt, fermented soy products) or supplements can decrease unwanted vaginal bacteria.
Cervicitis *Chlamydia trachomatis*	Sexually transmitted; mucopurulent discharge with postcoital spotting from cervical inflammation. Culture for *Chlamydia* and *Neisseria gonorrhoeae*.	Azithromycin (Zithromax). Treat patient and partner.
Severe Recurrent Vaginitis *C. albicans* (most often)	May be indication of HIV infection. All women who are unresponsive to first-line treatment should be offered HIV testing.	Drug appropriate to opportunistic organism.

KOH, Potassium hydroxide.

Women with vaginal conditions or cervical infection should abstain from intercourse for at least 1 week. Douching should be avoided as it has been adversely linked to pelvic inflammatory disease, sexually transmitted infections, and ectopic pregnancy. Sexual partners must be evaluated and treated if the patient is diagnosed with trichomoniasis, chlamydia, gonorrhea, syphilis, or HIV.

Treatment of vulvar dystrophies is symptomatic and involves controlling the itching and hence the scratching. Interrupting the "itch-scratch cycle" prevents further secondary damage to the skin.

Nursing Management

Teach women about common genital conditions and how to reduce their risks. Recognize symptoms that indicate a problem and help women seek care in a timely manner.

When a woman is diagnosed with a genital condition, ensure that she fully understands the directions for treatment. Taking the full course of medication is especially important to decrease the chance of relapse. Because genitals are such a private area, use of graphs and models is especially helpful for patient teaching.

When a woman is using a vaginal medication such as an antifungal cream for the first time, show her the applicator and how to fill it. Also teach where and how the applicator should be inserted by using visual aids or models. Vaginal creams should be inserted before going to bed so that the medication will remain in the vagina for a long period of time. Women using vaginal creams or suppositories may wish to use panty liners during the day when the residual medication may drain out.

VALVULAR HEART DISEASE

Description

Valvular heart disease is defined according to the affected valve or valves (mitral, aortic, tricuspid, pulmonary) and the type of functional alteration: *stenosis* or *regurgitation*.

- The pressure on either side of an open valve is normally equal. However, in *stenosis* the valve opening is smaller, impeding the forward flow of blood and creating a pressure difference on the two sides of the open valve. The degree of stenosis (constriction or narrowing) is reflected in the pressure differences (i.e., the higher the gradient, the greater the stenosis).
- In *regurgitation* (also called incompetence or insufficiency), incomplete closure of valve leaflets results in a backward flow of blood.

Valve disorders occur in children and adolescents mainly from congenital conditions. Aortic stenosis and mitral regurgitation are the common valve disorders in older adults. Other causes of valve disease in adults include disorders related to acquired immunodeficiency syndrome (AIDS) and the use of some antiparkinsonian drugs (e.g., pergolide [Permax]).

Clinical manifestations of valvular heart disease are presented in Table 84.

Table 84 Manifestations of Valvular Heart Disease

Type	Manifestations
Mitral valve stenosis	Dyspnea on exertion, hemoptysis; fatigue. Atrial fibrillation on ECG, palpitations, stroke. Loud, accentuated S_1. Low-pitched, diastolic murmur.
Mitral valve regurgitation	*Acute:* Generally poorly tolerated. New systolic murmur with pulmonary edema and cardiogenic shock developing rapidly. *Chronic:* Weakness, fatigue, exertional dyspnea, palpitations. An S_3 gallop, holosystolic murmur.
Mitral valve prolapse	Palpitations, dyspnea, chest pain, activity intolerance, syncope. Holosystolic murmur.
Aortic valve stenosis	Angina, syncope, dyspnea on exertion, heart failure. Normal or soft S_1, diminished or absent S_2, systolic murmur, prominent S_4.
Aortic valve regurgitation	*Acute:* Abrupt onset of profound dyspnea, chest pain, left ventricular failure and cardiogenic shock. *Chronic:* Fatigue, exertional dyspnea, orthopnea, PND. Water-hammer pulse. Heaving precordial impulse. Diminished or absent S_1, S_3, or S_4. Soft high-pitched diastolic murmur, Austin-Flint murmur.
Tricuspid and pulmonic stenosis	*Tricuspid:* Peripheral edema, ascites, hepatomegaly. Diastolic low-pitched murmur with increased intensity during inspiration. *Pulmonic:* Fatigue, loud midsystolic murmur.

PND, Paroxysmal nocturnal dyspnea.

Mitral Valve Stenosis

Pathophysiology

Most cases of adult mitral valve stenosis result from rheumatic heart disease. Less common causes include congenital mitral stenosis, rheumatoid arthritis, and systemic lupus erythematosus (SLE).

- Rheumatic endocarditis causes scarring of valve leaflets and chordae tendineae. Contractures and adhesions develop between the commissures (the junctional areas).
- The stenotic mitral valve takes on a "fish mouth" shape because of the thickening and shortening of mitral valve structures. Flow obstruction increases left atrial pressure and volume, resulting in higher pulmonary vasculature pressure and eventually involving the right ventricle.

Clinical Manifestations

The primary symptom is exertional dyspnea due to reduced lung compliance. Fatigue and palpitations from atrial fibrillation may also occur. Heart sounds include a loud first heart sound and a low-pitched, rumbling diastolic murmur (best heard at the apex with the stethoscope bell). Other clinical manifestations are identified in Table 84.

Mitral Valve Regurgitation

Pathophysiology

Mitral valve function depends on the integrity of mitral leaflets, chordae tendineae, papillary muscles, left atrium (LA), and left ventricle (LV). A defect in any of these structures can result in regurgitation. Myocardial infarction with left ventricular failure increases the risk for rupture of the chordae tendineae and acute mitral regurgitation (MR).

- Most cases of MR are caused by myocardial infarction, chronic rheumatic heart disease, mitral valve prolapse, ischemic papillary muscle dysfunction, and infective endocarditis.
- MR allows blood to flow backward from the LV to the LA because of incomplete valve closure during systole. Both chambers of the left side of the heart must work harder to preserve an adequate cardiac output (CO).
- In acute MR, abrupt dilation of the LA or LV does not occur. The sudden increase in pressure and volume is transmitted to the pulmonary bed, resulting in pulmonary edema and cardiogenic shock.
- In chronic MR, the additional volume load results in left atrial enlargement and left ventricular dilation and hypertrophy, and finally a decrease in CO.

Clinical Manifestations

Patients with acute MR have thready peripheral pulses and cool, clammy extremities. A low CO may mask a new systolic murmur.

Rapid assessment (e.g., cardiac catheterization) and intervention (e.g., valve repair or replacement) are critical for a positive outcome.

Patients with chronic MR may remain asymptomatic for many years until the development of some degree of left ventricular failure. Manifestations are identified in Table 84.

Mitral Valve Prolapse

Pathophysiology

Mitral valve prolapse (MVP) is an abnormality of the mitral valve leaflets and papillary muscles or chordae that allows the leaflets to prolapse, or buckle, back into the left atrium during systole. It is the most common form of valvular heart disease in the United States.

- MVP is usually benign, but serious complications can occur, including mitral regurgitation, infective endocarditis, sudden cardiac death, and cerebral ischemia.
- There is an increased familial incidence in some patients resulting from a connective tissue defect affecting only the valve, or as part of Marfan's syndrome or other hereditary conditions that influence the structure of collagen in the body.

Clinical Manifestations

MVP encompasses a broad spectrum of severity. Most patients are asymptomatic and remain so for their entire lives. Clinical manifestations may include those identified in Table 84.

- Patients may or may not have chest pain. If chest pain occurs, episodes tend to occur in clusters, especially during periods of emotional stress. Chest pain may occasionally be accompanied by dyspnea, palpitations, and syncope and does not respond to antianginal treatment (e.g., nitrates).

Patients with MVP generally have a benign, manageable course unless problems related to MR develop. Table 85 provides a teaching plan for patients with MVP.

Aortic Valve Stenosis

Pathophysiology

Congenital aortic stenosis is generally found in childhood, adolescence, or young adulthood. In older patients, aortic stenosis is a result of rheumatic fever or degeneration similar to that of coronary artery disease.

- In rheumatic valve disease, fusion of the commissures and secondary calcification cause the valve leaflets to stiffen and retract, resulting in stenosis. Isolated aortic valve stenosis is usually nonrheumatic in origin.
- Aortic stenosis causes obstruction of flow from the left ventricle to the aorta during systole. The effect is left ventricular hypertrophy and increased myocardial oxygen consumption because of the increased myocardial mass.

Table 85	Patient and Caregiver Teaching Guide
	Mitral Valve Prolapse

When teaching the patient and/or caregiver how to manage mitral valve prolapse, teach the patient the following:

- Take medications as prescribed (e.g., β-adrenergic blockers to control palpitations, chest pain).
- Adopt healthy eating habits and avoid caffeine because it is a stimulant and may exacerbate symptoms.
- If you use diet pills or other over-the-counter drugs, check for common ingredients that are stimulants (e.g., caffeine, ephedrine), since these can exacerbate symptoms.
- Begin (or maintain) an exercise program to achieve optimal health.
- Contact the health care provider or emergency medical services (EMS) if symptoms develop or worsen (e.g., palpitations, fatigue, shortness of breath, anxiety).

- As the disease progresses and compensatory mechanisms fail, reduced CO leads to pulmonary hypertension and heart failure.

Clinical Manifestations

Symptoms of aortic stenosis develop when the valve orifice becomes about one third of its normal size. Symptoms include the classic triad of angina, syncope, and exertional dyspnea, reflecting left ventricular failure. Common manifestations are presented in Table 84. Prognosis is poor for a patient with symptoms and whose valve obstruction is not relieved.

Aortic Valve Regurgitation

Pathophysiology

Aortic regurgitation may be the result of primary disease of the aortic valve leaflets, the aortic root, or both.

- Acute aortic regurgitation is caused by infective endocarditis, trauma, or aortic dissection and constitutes a life-threatening emergency.
- Chronic aortic regurgitation is generally the result of rheumatic heart disease, a congenital bicuspid aortic valve, syphilis, or chronic arthritic conditions such as ankylosing spondylitis or reactive arthritis.
- Aortic regurgitation causes retrograde blood flow from the ascending aorta into the LV, resulting in volume overload.
- Myocardial contractility eventually declines, and blood volume increases in the LA and pulmonary bed. This leads to pulmonary hypertension and right ventricular failure.

Clinical Manifestations

Clinical manifestations of acute and chronic aortic valve regurgitation are presented in Table 84.

Tricuspid and Pulmonic Valve Disease

Diseases of the tricuspid and pulmonic valves are uncommon, with stenosis occurring more frequently than regurgitation. Tricuspid stenosis results in right atrial enlargement and elevated systemic venous pressures. Pulmonic stenosis results in right ventricular hypertension and hypertrophy. Table 84 presents clinical manifestations of these valve diseases.

Diagnostic Studies: Valvular Heart Disease

- CT scan of the chest with contrast is the gold standard for evaluating aortic disorders.
- ECG shows variations in heart rate (HR), rhythm, and possible ischemia or chamber enlargement.
- Echocardiogram reveals valve structure, function, and heart chamber size.
- Transesophageal echocardiography and Doppler color-flow imaging help diagnose and monitor valvular heart disease progression.
- Real-time 3-D echocardiography helps assess mitral valve and congenital heart disease.
- Chest x-ray reveals heart size, altered pulmonary circulation, and valve calcification.
- Cardiac catheterization detects chamber pressure changes and pressure gradients (differences) across the valves.

Collaborative Care: Valvular Heart Disease

An important aspect of conservative therapy is the prevention of recurrent rheumatic fever and infective endocarditis. Treatment depends on the valve involved and the severity of disease. It focuses on preventing exacerbations of heart failure, acute pulmonary edema, thromboembolism, and recurrent endocarditis. Heart failure is treated with vasodilators, positive inotropes, β-adrenergic blockers, diuretics, and a low-sodium diet.

- Anticoagulant therapy prevents and treats systemic or pulmonary emboli, and it is also used as a prophylactic measure in patients with atrial fibrillation.
- Atrial dysrhythmias are common and treated with calcium channel blockers, β-adrenergic blockers, digoxin, antidysrhythmic drugs, or electrical cardioversion.
- An alternative treatment for some patients with valvular heart disease is the *percutaneous transluminal balloon valvuloplasty*

(PTBV) procedure. Balloon valvuloplasty is used more often for pulmonic, aortic, and mitral stenosis. PTBV is done in the cardiac catheterization laboratory. It involves threading a balloon-tipped catheter from the femoral artery to the stenotic valve so that the balloon may be inflated in an attempt to separate valve leaflets.

- The PTBV procedure is generally indicated for older adult patients and patients who are poor surgical candidates.

Surgical Therapy

The type of surgery used depends on the valves involved, the pathology and severity of the disease, and the patient's clinical condition.

- Valve repair is usually the surgical procedure of choice. It is often used in mitral or tricuspid valvular heart disease.

Mitral *commissurotomy* (valvulotomy) is the procedure of choice for patients with pure mitral stenosis. The open method of commissurotomy (which has largely replaced the older, less precise closed method) requires the use of cardiopulmonary bypass, removal of thrombi from the atrium, and a commissure incision. Next the fused chordae are separated by splitting the papillary muscle and debriding the calcified valve.

- Open surgical *valvuloplasty* involves repairing the valve by suturing the torn leaflets, chordae tendineae, and papillary muscles. It is primarily used to treat mitral regurgitation or tricuspid regurgitation.
- Further repair or reconstruction of the valve may be necessary and can be achieved by *annuloplasty*, a procedure also used in cases of mitral or tricuspid regurgitation. Annuloplasty involves reconstruction of the annulus, with or without the aid of prosthetic rings (e.g., Carpentier ring).

Valve Replacement. Valve replacement may be required for mitral, aortic, tricuspid, and, occasionally, pulmonic valvular disease.

- Prosthetic valves are categorized as *mechanical* or *biologic (tissue) valves.* Mechanical valves are made of combinations of metal alloys, pyrolite carbon, and Dacron. Biologic valves are constructed from bovine, porcine, and human (cadaver) cardiac tissue. Mechanical prosthetic valves are more durable and last longer than biologic tissue valves, but they have an increased risk of thromboembolism and require long-term anticoagulant therapy. Biologic valves do not require anticoagulant therapy because of their low thrombogenicity. However, they are less durable and tend to cause early calcification, tissue degeneration, and stiffening of leaflets.
- Long-term anticoagulation is needed for those patients with biologic valves who have atrial fibrillation. Some patients with biologic valves or annuloplasty with prosthetic rings may need

anticoagulation the first few months after surgery until the suture lines are covered by endothelial cells (endothelialized).

- The choice of valves depends on many factors. For example, if a patient cannot take anticoagulant therapy (e.g., women of childbearing age), a biologic valve is considered. A mechanical valve may be best for a younger patient because it is more durable. For patients older than 65 years, durability is less important than the risks of bleeding from anticoagulants, so most receive a biologic valve.

Nursing Management
Goals
The patient with valvular heart disease will have normal cardiac function, improved activity tolerance, and an understanding of the disease process and maintenance measures.
Nursing Diagnoses
- Activity intolerance
- Excess fluid volume
- Decreased cardiac output
Nursing Interventions
Diagnosing and treating streptococcal infection and providing prophylactic antibiotics for patients with a history of rheumatic fever are critical to prevent acquired rheumatic valve disease. The patient at risk for endocarditis and any patient with certain high-risk cardiac conditions must also receive prophylactic antibiotics.

- The patient must adhere to recommended therapies. The individual with a history of rheumatic fever, endocarditis, and congenital heart disease should know the symptoms of valvular heart disease so early medical treatment may begin. Your role is to implement and evaluate the effectiveness of therapeutic interventions.
- Design activities considering the patient's limitations. An appropriate exercise plan can increase cardiac tolerance, but activities that cause fatigue and dyspnea should be restricted.
- Your patient's activities of daily living plan should have an emphasis on conserving energy, setting priorities, and taking planned rest periods.
- Referral to a vocational counselor may be necessary if the patient has a physically or emotionally demanding job.
- Perform ongoing cardiac assessments to monitor the effectiveness of medications. Teaching regarding the actions and side effects of drugs is important to achieve adherence.
- The patient on anticoagulation therapy (e.g., warfarin [Coumadin]) after surgery for valve replacement must have the international normalized ratio (INR) checked regularly to determine adequacy of therapy.

V

▼ **Patient and Caregiver Teaching**
- Teach the patient when to seek medical care. Any manifestations of infection, heart failure, and signs of bleeding require the patient to notify the health care provider.
- Discourage tobacco use.
- Encourage patients to wear a Medic Alert bracelet.

VARICOSE VEINS

Description
Varicose veins (varicosities) are dilated (3 mm or larger in diameter), tortuous subcutaneous veins commonly found in the saphenous vein system. They may be small and innocuous or large and bulging.
- *Primary* varicose veins (idiopathic) are caused by a congenital weakness of the veins and are more common in women.
- *Secondary* varicosities typically result from a previous venous thromboembolism (VTE). Secondary varicose veins may also occur in the esophagus as varices, in the anorectal area as hemorrhoids, and as abnormal arteriovenous (AV) connections.

Pathophysiology
The etiology of varicose veins is multifactorial. Risk factors include family history of venous disease, weakness of the vein structure, female gender, use of oral contraceptives or hormone therapy, tobacco use, increasing age, obesity, pregnancy, history of VTE, or occupations that require prolonged standing or sitting.
- Although the exact etiology remains unknown, it is thought that the vein valve leaflets are stretched and become incompetent (do not fit together properly). Incompetent vein valves allow retrograde blood flow, particularly when standing, resulting in increased venous pressure and further venous distention.

Clinical Manifestations
Discomfort from varicose veins varies dramatically among people and tends to be worsened after episodes of superficial thrombophlebitis. The most common varicose vein symptoms include a heavy, achy pain after prolonged standing/or sitting, which is relieved by walking or limb elevation. Some patients feel pressure or a cramplike, burning sensation. Swelling and/or nocturnal leg cramps may also occur.

Superficial thrombophlebitis is the most frequent complication of varicose veins and may occur spontaneously or after trauma, surgical procedures, or pregnancy.

Diagnostic Studies

- Superficial varicose veins can be diagnosed by appearance.
- Duplex ultrasound detects obstruction and reflux in the venous system.

Collaborative Care

Treatment is usually not indicated if varicose veins are only a cosmetic problem. If chronic venous insufficiency develops, care involves rest with limb elevation, elastic compression stockings, and exercise, such as walking.

Venoactive drugs (e.g., diosmin, hesperidin, rutosides [Venoruton]) with compression therapy are recommended for patients with varicose veins who experience pain and swelling.

Sclerotherapy involves the injection of a substance that obliterates venous telangiectasias (i.e., spider veins) and small superficial varicose veins. Direct IV injection of a sclerosing agent such as hypertonic saline induces inflammation and results in eventual thrombosis of the vein. After injection, a thigh-high elastic compression stocking is worn or an elastic bandage is applied to the leg for several days to maintain pressure over the vein. Long-term compression therapy is advised to help prevent further varicosities.

- Other noninvasive options for the treatment of isolated, small venous telangiectasias include laser therapy and high-intensity pulse-light therapy.

Surgical intervention is indicated for recurrent superficial vein thrombosis or when chronic venous insufficiency cannot be controlled with conservative therapy. Traditional surgical intervention involves ligation of the entire vein (usually the greater saphenous) and removal of its incompetent branches. An alternative, but time-consuming, technique is ambulatory phlebectomy, which involves pulling the varicosity through a "stab" incision followed by excision of the vein. A less invasive procedure is endovenous ablation of the saphenous vein. Ablation involves the insertion of a catheter that emits energy. This causes collapse and sclerosis of the vein.

Nursing Management

Prevention is a key factor related to varicose veins. Instruct the patient to avoid sitting or standing for long periods, maintain ideal body weight, take precautions against injury to the extremities, avoid wearing constrictive clothing, and walk daily.

After vein ligation surgery, check extremities regularly for color, movement, sensation, temperature, presence of edema, and pedal pulses. Some bruising and discoloration are considered normal.

- Postoperatively elevate the patient's legs 15 degrees to decrease edema.
- Apply elastic compression stockings and remove every 8 hours for short periods, and then reapply.

Long-term management of varicose veins is directed toward improving circulation, relieving discomfort, improving cosmetic appearance, and avoiding complications such as superficial thrombophlebitis and ulceration. Varicose veins can recur in other veins after surgery.

▼ **Patient and Caregiver Teaching**
- Teach the patient the proper use and care of custom-fitted elastic compression stockings. The patient should apply stockings in bed, before rising in the morning.
- Stress the importance of periodic positioning of the legs above the heart.
- The overweight patient may need assistance with weight loss.
- Patients with a job that requires long periods of standing or sitting need to frequently flex and extend their hips, legs, and ankles and change positions.

VENOUS THROMBOSIS

Description

Venous thrombosis involves the formation of a thrombus in association with inflammation of the vein. It is the most common disorder of the veins and is classified as either superficial vein thrombosis or deep vein thrombosis.

Superficial vein thrombosis (SVT) is the formation of a thrombus in a superficial vein, usually the greater or lesser saphenous vein. Risk factors for SVT include increased age, pregnancy, obesity, malignancy, thrombophilia, estrogen therapy, recent sclerotherapy (e.g., treatment for varicose veins), long-distance travel, and a history of SVT or venous thromboembolism. SVT also can occur in people with endothelial alterations (e.g., Buerger's disease).

Deep vein thrombosis (DVT) is a disorder involving a thrombus in a deep vein, most commonly the iliac and femoral veins. *Venous thromboembolism* (VTE) is the preferred terminology and represents the spectrum of pathology from DVT to pulmonary embolism (PE). Table 86 compares SVT and VTE.

Pathophysiology

Three important factors *(Virchow's triad)* in the etiology of venous thrombosis are venous stasis, damage of the endothelium (inner

Table 86	Comparison of Superficial Vein Thrombosis and Venous Thromboembolism	
	Superficial Vein Thrombosis (SVT)	**Venous Thromboembolism (VTE)**
Usual location	Typically, superficial leg veins (e.g., varicosities). Occasionally superficial arm veins.	Deep veins of arms (e.g., axillary, subclavian), legs (e.g., femoral), pelvis (e.g., iliac, inferior or superior vena cava), and pulmonary system.
Clinical findings	Tenderness, itchiness, redness, warmth, pain, inflammation, and induration along the course of the superficial vein. Vein appears as a palpable cord. Edema rarely occurs.	Tenderness to pressure over involved vein, induration of overlying muscle, venous distention. Edema. May have mild to moderate pain, deep reddish color to area caused by venous congestion. Note: Some patients may have no obvious physical changes in the affected extremity.
Sequelae	If untreated, clot may extend to deeper veins and VTE may occur.	Embolization to lungs (pulmonary embolism) may occur and may result in death.* Pulmonary hypertension and post-thrombotic syndrome with or without venous leg ulceration may develop.

*See Chapter 28 in Lewis et al.: *Medical-Surgical Nursing*, 9e, p. 552, for clinical manifestations related to pulmonary embolism.

lining of the vein), and hypercoagulability of the blood. The patient at risk for the development of VTE usually has predisposing conditions to these three disorders.

Venous stasis occurs when the valves are dysfunctional or the muscles of the extremities are inactive. Venous stasis occurs more frequently in people who are obese, have chronic heart failure or atrial fibrillation, have been on long trips without regular exercise, undergo a prolonged surgical procedure, or are immobile for long periods (e.g., with spinal cord injuries or fractured hips).

Damage to the endothelium of the vein may be caused by direct (e.g., surgery, intravascular catheterization, trauma, fracture, burns) or indirect (chemotherapy, vasculitis, sepsis, diabetes) injury to the vessel. Damaged endothelium has decreased fibrinolytic properties, which predisposed the patient to thrombus development.

Hypercoagulability of the blood occurs in many disorders, including severe anemias, polycythemia, sepsis, malignancies (e.g., cancers of the breast, brain, pancreas, and gastrointestinal tract), and nephrotic syndrome.

- Women who use tobacco, use oral contraceptives or hormone therapy, are over age 35 years, and have a family history of VTE are at extremely high risk to develop a thrombotic event.

Localized platelet aggregation and fibrin entrap RBCs, WBCs, and more platelets to form a thrombus. A frequent site of thrombus formation is the valve cusps of veins.

- As the thrombus enlarges, blood cells and fibrin collect behind it, producing a larger clot with a "tail" that eventually occludes the lumen of the vein.
- If a thrombus only partially blocks the vein, the thrombus becomes covered by endothelial cells and the thrombotic process stops.
- If the thrombus does not become detached, it undergoes lysis or becomes firmly organized and adherent within 5 to 7 days.
- The organized thrombus may detach and result in an embolus that flows through the venous circulation to the heart and lodges in the pulmonary circulation, becoming a pulmonary embolism (PE).

SUPERFICIAL VEIN THROMBOSIS
Clinical Manifestations

The patient may have a palpable, firm, subcutaneous cordlike vein. The surrounding area may be itchy, tender to the touch, reddened, and warm. A mild temperature elevation and leukocytosis may be present. Edema of the extremity may occur.

Duplex ultrasound is used to confirm the diagnosis (clot 5 cm or larger) and to rule out clot extension to a deep vein.

Collaborative Care

For patients with lower leg SVT, treatment consists of low–molecular-weight heparin (LMWH) for 45 days or a prophylactic dose of fondaparinux (Arixtra). If the SVT affects a very short vein segment (less than 5 cm) and is not near the saphenofemoral junction, anticoagulants may not be necessary and oral nonsteroidal antiinflammatory drugs (NSAIDs) can ease symptoms.

- Additional interventions to relieve SVT symptoms include telling the patient to wear elastic compression stockings, apply topical NSAIDs, and perform mild exercise such as walking.

VENOUS THROMBOEMBOLISM
Clinical Manifestations

The patient with lower extremity VTE may have unilateral leg edema, pain, tenderness with palpation, dilated superficial veins, a sense of fullness in the thigh or the calf, paresthesias, warm skin, erythema, or a systemic temperature greater than 100.4° F (38° C).

- If the inferior vena cava is involved, both legs may be edematous and cyanotic. If the superior vena cava is involved, similar symptoms may occur in the arms, neck, back, and face.

Diagnosis of an initial VTE is based on clinical assessment combined with D-dimer testing and duplex ultrasound.

Complications

The most serious complications of VTE are PE, post-thrombotic syndrome, and phlegmasia cerulea dolens.

- *Post-thrombotic syndrome* (PTS) can result from chronic venous hypertension caused by valvular destruction (from inflammation and scarring), stiff noncompliant vein walls, and persistent venous obstruction. Symptoms include pain, aching, heaviness, swelling, cramps, itching, and tingling. Clinical signs include persistent edema, increased pigmentation, eczema, secondary varicosities, and lipodermatosclerosis. Sequential compression devices may be used for patients with severe PTS.
- *Phlegmasia cerulea dolens* (swollen, blue, painful leg), a rare complication, may develop in a patient in the advanced stages of cancer. It results from severe lower extremity VTE(s) that involve the major leg veins causing near-total occlusion of venous outflow. Patients typically experience sudden, massive swelling, deep pain, and intense cyanosis of the extremity.

Diagnostic Studies

- Platelet count, hemoglobin (Hgb), hematocrit (Hct), D-dimer testing, and coagulation tests (bleeding time, prothrombin time [PT], and partial thromboplastin time [PTT]) may be altered if underlying blood dyscrasias are present.
- Venous compression ultrasound evaluates deep femoral, popliteal, and posterior tibial veins.
- Duplex ultrasound and color flow Doppler determine the location and extent of venous thrombi.

- Venogram (phlebogram) can determine the extent and location of the clot.

Collaborative Care

In patients at risk for VTE, a variety of interventions are used. Patients on bed rest need to change position every 2 hours. Unless contraindicated, teach patients to flex and extend their feet, knees, and hips every 2 to 4 hours while awake. Patients who are able to get out of bed need to be in a chair for meals and ambulate at least four to six times per day as tolerated. Explain to the patient and caregiver the importance of these measures.

- Elastic compression (antiembolism) stockings, when fitted correctly (both size and length) and worn properly and consistently from admission until discharge or full mobility, decrease VTE risk.
- Sequential compression devices (SCDs) apply external pressure to the lower extremities by means of an electric pump. SCDs may be used with elastic compression stockings. SCDs are not worn when a patient has an active VTE because of the risk of PE.

Anticoagulants are used routinely for VTE prevention and treatment. The goal of anticoagulant therapy for VTE prophylaxis is to prevent clot formation. The goals for treatment of a confirmed VTE are to prevent new clot development, spread of the clot, and embolization.

Three major classes of anticoagulants are available: (1) vitamin K antagonists, (2) thrombin inhibitors (both indirect and direct), and (3) factor Xa inhibitors. Anticoagulant therapy does not dissolve the clot. Clot lysis begins naturally through the body's intrinsic fibrinolytic system (see Table 38-10 on anticoagulant therapy, Lewis et al.: *Medical-Surgical Nursing,* ed. 9, p. 851).

Although most patients are managed medically, a small number of patients undergo surgery. Surgical options include open venous thrombectomy and inferior vena cava interruption. Venous thrombectomy involves the removal of a thrombus through an incision in the vein.

Nursing Management

Goals

The patient with VTE will have pain relief, decreased edema, no skin ulceration, no bleeding complications, and no evidence of PE.

Nursing Diagnoses/Collaborative Problems

- Acute pain
- Ineffective health maintenance
- Risk for impaired skin integrity
- Potential complication: bleeding related to anticoagulant therapy
- Potential complication: PE

Nursing Interventions

Focus your nursing care for the patient with VTE on the prevention of embolus formation and reduction of inflammation. Review with the patient any medications, vitamins, minerals, and dietary and herbal supplements being taken that may interfere with anticoagulant therapy.

- Always check the results of appropriate tests before initiating, administering, or adjusting anticoagulant therapy.
- Monitor for and reduce the risk of bleeding that may occur with anticoagulant therapy.
- Bed rest with limb elevation may be prescribed for patients with an acute VTE. Early ambulation after VTE results in a more rapid decrease in edema and limb pain. Teach the patient and caregiver the importance of exercise and assist the patient in ambulating several times a day.

▼ **Patient and Caregiver Teaching**

Focus discharge teaching on modification of VTE risk factors, use of elastic compression stockings, importance of monitoring laboratory values, medication instructions, and guidelines for follow-up.

- Once the edema is resolved, measure the patient for custom-fit, elastic compression stockings. Stocking use (or sleeves in the case of an upper extremity VTE) is recommended for at least 2 years after a VTE.
- If appropriate, advise the patient to stop smoking and avoid all nicotine products. Instruct the patient to avoid constrictive clothing.
- Teach patients to avoid standing or sitting in a motionless, leg-dependent position. Encourage frequent exercise of the calf muscles, active walking, and sitting in an aisle seat during long flights. For those at high risk for VTE who are planning a long trip, recommend properly fitted, knee-high elastic compression stockings during travel to decrease edema and VTE risk.
- Teach the patient and caregiver about signs and symptoms of PE such as sudden onset of dyspnea, tachypnea, and pleuritic chest pain.
- Instruct the patient and caregiver need about drug dosage, actions, and side effects; the need for routine blood tests; and what symptoms need immediate medical attention.
- Teach patients taking warfarin (Coumadin) to follow a consistent diet of foods containing vitamin K (e.g., dark green leafy vegetables) and to avoid any supplements containing vitamin K. Encourage proper hydration to prevent additional hypercoagulability of the blood, which may occur with dehydration.
- Help the patient develop an exercise program with an emphasis on walking and swimming. Water exercise is particularly beneficial because of the gentle, even pressure of the water.

V

WARTS, GENITAL

Description

Genital warts (condylomata acuminata) are caused by the human papillomavirus (HPV). HPV is a highly contagious sexually transmitted infection (STI) seen frequently in young, sexually active adults.

Pathophysiology

There are more than 100 types of papillomaviruses, with many of these types sexually transmitted. Ninety percent of genital warts are caused by HPV types 6 and 11. Although genital warts are not malignant, other HPV types (e.g., types 16 and 18) are oncogenic and associated with cervical, vaginal, vulvar, anal, and penile cancers.

Minor trauma during intercourse can cause abrasions that allow HPV to enter the body. The epithelial cells infected with HPV undergo transformation and proliferation to form a warty growth. The incubation period of the virus is generally 3 to 4 months.

Clinical Manifestations

Most individuals who have HPV do not know they are infected because symptoms are often not present.

- Genital warts are discrete, single, or multiple papillary growths that are white to gray and pink-flesh colored.
- They may grow and join together to form large, cauliflower-like masses. Most patients have 1 to 10 lesions.
- In men, the warts may occur on the penis and scrotum, around the anus, or in the urethra.
- In women, the warts may be located on the vulva, vagina, and cervix and in the perianal area.
- Itching may occur with anogenital warts. Bleeding on defecation may occur with anal warts.
- An infected mother may transmit the condition to her newborn. Cesarean delivery is not routinely indicated unless the birth canal becomes blocked by massive warts.

Diagnostic Studies

- A diagnosis can be made based of the gross appearance of the lesions.
- The HPV DNA test can determine if women with abnormal Pap test results need further follow-up.
- HPV cannot currently be confirmed by culture.
- Serologic and cytologic testing can be used to rule out carcinomas, secondary syphilis, or benign neoplasms.

Collaborative Care

The primary goal when treating visible genital warts is the removal of symptomatic warts. Genital warts are difficult to treat and often require multiple office visits. Therapy may be modified if a patient has not improved after three treatments or if the warts have not completely disappeared after six treatments.

- A common treatment is the use of 80% to 90% trichloroacetic acid (TCA) or bichloroacetic acid (BCA) applied directly to the wart surface.
- Podophyllin resin (10% to 25%), a cytotoxic agent, is recommended for small external genital warts.
- Podofilox (Condylox) liquid or gel can be applied by the patient for 3 successive days followed by 4 days of no treatment.
- Imiquimod cream (Aldara), an immune response modifier, can be applied three times per week for up to 16 weeks.

If warts do not regress with these therapies, treatments such as cryotherapy with liquid nitrogen, electrocautery, laser therapy, intralesional use of α-interferon, and surgical excision may be indicated.

Because treatment does not destroy the virus, recurrences and reinfection are possible, and careful long-term follow-up care is advised.

Vaccines (i.e., Gardasil, Cervarix) are available to protect against HPV types 6, 11, 16, and 18. The vaccine is given in three intramuscular (IM) doses over a 6-month period and has few side effects. These vaccines do not treat active HPV infection. Ideally, individuals should receive the vaccine before the start of sexual activity. The HPV vaccine reduces the risk of anal cancer and may also protect against oropharynx cancer.

Nursing Management: Genital Warts

See Nursing Management: Sexually Transmitted Infections, p. 564.

W

PART TWO

Treatments and Procedures

AMPUTATION

Description

An *amputation* is the removal of a body extremity by trauma or surgery. An estimated 2 million people in the United States are living with limb loss. The middle and older age groups have the highest incidence of amputation because of the effects of peripheral vascular disease, atherosclerosis, and vascular changes related to diabetes mellitus.

The most common reasons for amputations are peripheral vascular disease (PVD), trauma and thermal injuries, tumors, osteomyelitis, and congenital limb disorders. Most amputations performed are for PVD, especially in older patients with diabetes mellitus. These patients often experience peripheral neuropathy that progresses to trophic ulcers and subsequent gangrene. Although pain is often present, it is not usually the primary reason for an amputation.

- The goal of amputation surgery is to preserve extremity length and function while removing all infected, pathologic, or ischemic tissue. (See Fig. 63-22 for the levels of amputation of the upper and lower extremities, Lewis et al.: *Medical-Surgical Nursing,* ed. 9, p. 1531.)

Nursing Management

Control of causative illnesses such as peripheral vascular disease, diabetes mellitus, chronic osteomyelitis, and skin ulcers can eliminate or delay the need for amputation.

- Teach patients with these conditions to carefully examine the lower extremities daily and report problems to the health care provider, such as changes in skin color or temperature, decrease or absence of sensation, tingling, burning pain, or the presence of a lesion.
- Instruct people in proper safety precautions in recreational activities and the performance of potentially hazardous work. This is an especially important role for the occupational health nurse.

It is important for you to recognize the tremendous psychologic and social implications of an amputation. The disruption in body image caused by an amputation often results in a patient going through the grieving process. Use therapeutic communication to assist the patient and caregiver through this process to arrive at a realistic attitude about the future.

Preoperative Care

Before surgery, reinforce information that the patient and caregiver have received about the reasons for the amputation, the proposed prosthesis, and the mobility-training program.

- Instruct the patient in the performance of upper extremity exercises such as push-ups in bed or the wheelchair to promote arm strength. This instruction is essential for crutch walking and gait training.
- If a compression bandage is to be used after surgery, instruct the patient about its purpose and how it will be applied. If an immediate prosthesis is planned, discuss general ambulation expectations.

Tell the patient that the amputated limb may feel like it is still present after surgery. This phenomenon, termed *phantom limb sensation,* occurs in many amputees.

- As recovery and ambulation progress, phantom limb sensation and pain usually subside, although the pain can become chronic.
- The patient may also complain of shooting, burning, or crushing pain and feelings of coldness, heaviness, and cramping.

Postoperative Care

Prevention and detection of complications are important during the postoperative period. Carefully monitor the patient's vital signs and dressing for hemorrhage in the operative area. Careful attention to sterile technique during dressing changes reduces the potential for wound infection.

- If an immediate postoperative prosthesis has been applied, careful surveillance of the surgical site is required. A surgical tourniquet must always be available for emergency use. If excessive bleeding occurs, notify the surgeon immediately.
- Not all patients are candidates for prostheses. The seriously ill or debilitated patient may not have the upper body strength or energy required to use a prosthesis. Mobility with a wheelchair may be the most realistic goal for this type of patient.

Flexion contractures may delay the rehabilitation process. The most common and debilitating contracture is hip flexion. Patients should avoid sitting in a chair for more than 1 hour with hips flexed or having pillows under the surgical extremity.

▼ **Patient and Caregiver Teaching**

As the patient's overall condition improves, an exercise regimen is normally started under the supervision of the health care provider and physical therapist.

- Active range-of-motion exercises of all joints should be started as soon after surgery as the patient's pain level and medical status permit.

| Table 87 | Patient and Caregiver Teaching Guide *Following an Amputation* | A |

After an amputation, include the following instructions when teaching the patient and caregiver.

- Inspect the residual limb daily for signs of skin irritation, especially erythema, excoriation, and odor. Pay particular attention to areas prone to pressure.
- Discontinue use of the prosthesis if irritation develops. Have the area checked before resuming use of the prosthesis.
- Wash the residual limb thoroughly each night with warm water and a bacteriostatic soap. Rinse thoroughly and dry gently. Expose the residual limb to air for 20 min.
- Do not use any substance such as lotions, alcohol, powders, or oil on residual limb unless prescribed by the health care provider.
- Wear only a residual limb sock that is in good condition and supplied by the prosthetist.
- Change residual limb sock daily. Launder in a mild soap, squeeze, and lay flat to dry.
- Use prescribed pain management techniques.
- Perform range of motion (ROM) to all joints daily. Perform general strengthening exercises, including the upper extremities, daily.
- Do not elevate the residual limb on a pillow.
- Lie prone with hip in extension for 30 min three or four times daily.

- Crutch walking is started as soon as the patient is physically able. After an immediate postsurgical fitting, orders related to weight bearing must be carefully followed to avoid disruption of the skin flap and delay of the healing process.
- Before discharge, instruct the patient and caregiver about residual limb care, ambulation, prevention of contractures, recognition of complications, exercise, and follow-up care. Table 87 outlines patient and caregiver teaching after an amputation.

ARTIFICIAL AIRWAYS: ENDOTRACHEAL TUBES

Description

An artificial airway is created by inserting a tube into the trachea, bypassing upper airway and laryngeal structures. The tube is placed into the trachea through the mouth or nose past the larynx *(endotracheal [ET] intubation)* or through a stoma in the neck *(tracheostomy)*. ET intubation is more common in ICU patients than a tracheostomy. It is performed quickly and safely at the bed-side. Figure 18 shows the parts of an ET tube.

- Indications for ET intubation include upper airway obstruction, apnea, high risk of aspiration, ineffective clearance of secretions, and respiratory distress.

In *oral ET intubation,* the ET tube is passed through the mouth and vocal cords and into the trachea with the aid of a laryngoscope or bronchoscope. Oral ET intubation is preferred for most emergencies because the airway can be secured rapidly and a larger-diameter tube is used.

- Compared with the nasal route, a larger-diameter tube can be used for oral intubation. A larger-bore ET tube provides less airway resistance and easier performance of suctioning and fiberoptic bronchoscopy if needed.
- There are risks associated with oral ET intubation. It is difficult to place an oral tube if head and neck mobility is limited (e.g., suspected spinal cord injury). Teeth can be chipped or accidentally removed during the procedure. Salivation is increased and swallowing is difficult. Patients can obstruct the ET tube by biting down on it. Sedation along with a bite block or oropharyngeal airway can be used to avoid this. The ET tube and bite block (if used) should be secured (separately) to the face. Mouth care is a challenge.

In *nasal ET intubation,* the ET is placed blindly (i.e., without seeing the larynx) through the nose, nasopharynx, and vocal cords.

- Nasal intubation is contraindicated in patients with facial fractures, suspected fractures at the base of the skull, and postoperatively after cranial surgeries.
- Nasal ET tubes are more likely to kink than oral tubes. The work of breathing is greater because the longer, narrower tube offers more airflow resistance; suctioning and secretion removal are more difficult. Nasal tubes have been linked with increased incidence of sinus infection and ventilator-associated pneumonia (VAP).

Unless ET intubation is emergent, consent for the procedure is obtained. Tell the patient and caregiver the reason for ET intubation, the steps that will occur in the procedure, and the patient's role in the procedure (if indicated). It is also important to explain that while intubated, the patient will not be able to speak, but that you will provide other means of communication. Also explain that the patient's hands may be briefly restrained for safety purposes.

You need to have a self-inflating bag-valve-mask (BVM) (e.g., Ambu bag) available and attached to O_2, suctioning equipment ready at the bedside, and IV access. ET intubation is described in Lewis et al.: *Medical-Surgical Nursing,* ed. 9, pp. 1614 to 1615.

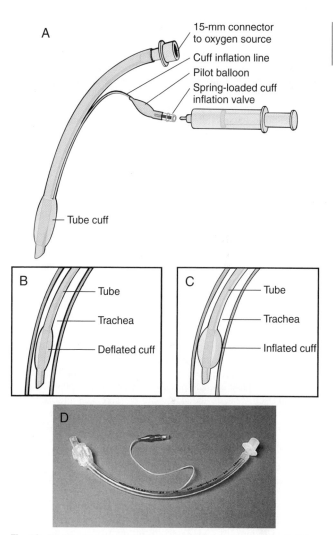

Fig. 18. Endotracheal tube. **A,** Parts of an endotracheal tube. **B,** Tube in place with cuff deflated. **C,** Tube in place with the cuff inflated. **D,** Photo of tube before placement.

Management of a patient with an artificial airway is often a shared responsibility between you and the respiratory therapist with specific management tasks determined by agency policy. Nursing responsibilities for the patient with an artificial airway may include some or all of the following: (1) maintaining correct tube placement, (2) maintaining proper cuff inflation, (3) monitoring oxygenation and ventilation, (4) maintaining tube patency, (5) assessing for complications, (6) providing oral care and maintaining skin integrity, and (7) fostering comfort and communication.

Continuously monitor the patient with an ET tube for proper placement. Observe for symmetric chest wall movement and auscultate to confirm bilateral breath sounds.

- It is an emergency if the ET tube is not positioned properly. If this occurs, stay with the patient, maintain the airway, support ventilation, and secure the appropriate assistance to immediately reposition the tube.
- It may be necessary to ventilate the patient with a BVM device (Ambu bag) and 100% O_2. If a malpositioned tube is not repositioned, no oxygen will be delivered to the lungs or the entire tidal volume will be delivered to one lung, placing the patient at risk for pneumothorax.

The cuff is an inflatable, pliable sleeve encircling the outer wall of the ET tube. The cuff stabilizes and seals the ET tube within the trachea and prevents the escape of ventilating gases.

Excess volume in the cuff can cause tracheal damage. To avoid this, inflate the cuff with air, and measure and monitor the cuff pressure. Normal arterial tracheal perfusion is estimated at 30 mm Hg. To ensure adequate tracheal perfusion, maintain cuff pressure at 20 to 25 cm H_2O. Measure and record cuff pressure after intubation and on a routine basis (e.g., every 8 hours) using the minimal occluding volume (MOV) technique or the minimal leak technique (MLT).

- The steps in the MOV technique for cuff inflation are as follows: (1) for the mechanically ventilated patient, place a stethoscope over the trachea and inflate the cuff to MOV by adding air until no air leak is heard at peak inspiratory pressure (end of ventilator inspiration); (2) for the spontaneously breathing patient, inflate until no sound is heard after a deep breath or after inhalation with a BVM; (3) use a manometer to verify that cuff pressure is between 20 and 25 mm Hg; and (4) record cuff pressure in the chart.
- If adequate cuff pressure cannot be maintained or larger volumes of air are needed to keep the cuff inflated, the cuff could be leaking or there could be tracheal dilation at the cuff site. In these situations, notify the physician to reposition or change the ET tube.

The procedure for MLT is similar with one exception. Remove a small amount of air from the cuff until a slight air leak is auscultated at peak inflation. Both techniques aim to prevent the risks of tracheal damage resulting from high cuff pressures.

- Vigilantly monitor the patient with an ET for adequate oxygenation and ventilation by assessing clinical findings, arterial blood gases (ABGs), and other indicators of oxygenation status.
- Do not routinely suction a patient. Routinely assess the patient to determine a need for suctioning. Indications for suctioning include (1) visible secretions in the ET tube, (2) sudden onset of respiratory distress, (3) suspected aspiration of secretions, (4) increase in peak airway pressures, (5) auscultation of adventitious breath sounds over the trachea and/or bronchi, (6) increase in respiratory rate and/or sustained coughing, and (7) sudden or gradual decrease in PaO_2 and/or SpO_2. See Table 88 for suctioning the patient with an artificial airway.

Table 88	Suctioning Procedures for Patient on Mechanical Ventilator

General Measures

1. Gather all equipment.
2. Wash hands and don personal protective equipment.
3. Explain procedure and patient's role in assisting with secretion removal by coughing.
4. Monitor patient's cardiopulmonary status (e.g., vital signs, SpO_2, SvO_2, $ScvO_2$, ECG, level of consciousness) before, during, and after the procedure.
5. Turn on suction and set vacuum to 100-120 mm Hg.
6. Pause ventilator alarms.

Open-Suction Technique

1. Open sterile catheter package using the inside of the package as a sterile field. Note: Suction catheter should be no wider than half the diameter of the ET tube (e.g., for a 7-mm ET tube, select a 10-F suction catheter).
2. Fill the sterile solution container with sterile normal saline or water.
3. Don sterile gloves.
4. Pick up sterile suction catheter with dominant hand. Using nondominant hand, secure the connecting tube (to suction) to the suction catheter.
5. Check equipment for proper functioning by suctioning a small volume of sterile saline solution from the container. *(Go to step 7.)*

Adapted from Chulay M, Seckel M: Suctioning: endotracheal or tracheostomy tube. In Wiegand DL-M, editor: *AACN procedure manual for critical care,* ed. 6, St Louis, 2011, Saunders.

Continued

Table 88	Suctioning Procedures for Patient on Mechanical Ventilator—cont'd

Closed-Suction Technique

6. Connect the suction tubing to the closed suction port.
7. Hyperoxygenate the patient for 30 sec using one of the following methods:
   - Activate the suction hyperoxygenation setting on the ventilator using nondominant hand.
   - Increase FIO_2 to 100%. NOTE: Remember to return FIO_2 to baseline level at the completion of the procedure if not done automatically after preset time by ventilator.
   - Disconnect the ventilator tubing from the ET tube and manually ventilate the patient with 100% O_2 using a BVM device.* Administer 5-6 breaths over 30 sec. NOTE: Use of a second person to deliver the manual breaths significantly increases the tidal volume delivered.
8. With suction off, gently and quickly insert the catheter using the dominant hand. When you meet resistance, pull back ½ in.
9. Apply continuous or intermittent suction using the nondominant thumb. Withdraw the catheter over 10 sec or less.
10. Hyperoxygenate for 30 sec as described in step 7.
11. If secretions remain and the patient has tolerated the procedure, perform two or three suction passes as described in steps 8 and 9. NOTE: Rinse the suction catheter with sterile saline solution between suctioning passes as needed.
12. Reconnect patient to ventilator (open-suction technique).
13. At the completion of ET tube suctioning, rinse the catheter and connecting tubing with the sterile saline solution.
14. Suction oral pharynx. NOTE: Use a separate catheter for this step when using the closed-suction technique.
15. Discard the suction catheter and rinse the connecting tubing with the sterile saline solution (open-suction technique).
16. Reset FIO_2 (if necessary) and ventilator alarms.
17. Reassess patient for signs of effective suctioning.

*Attach a PEEP valve to the BVM for patients on >5 cm H_2O PEEP.
BVM, Bag-valve-mask; *ET,* endotracheal; *FIO_2,* fraction of inspired oxygen; *PEEP,* positive end-expiratory pressure.

- With an oral ET tube in place, the patient's mouth is always open. Moisten the lips, tongue, and gums with saline or water swabs to prevent mucosal drying. Proper oral care provides comfort and prevents injury to the gums and plaque formation.
- Meticulous care is required to prevent skin breakdown on the face, lips, tongue, and/or nares because of pressure from the ET tube and/or bite block or from the method used to secure the ET

tube to the patient's face. Reposition and retape the ET tube every 24 hours and as needed.

For the nasally intubated patient, remove the old tape or ties and clean the skin around the ET tube with saline-soaked gauze or cotton swabs. For the orally intubated patient, remove the bite block (if present) and the old tape or ties. Provide oral hygiene and then reposition the ET tube to the opposite side of the mouth. Replace the bite block (if appropriate) and reconfirm proper cuff inflation and tube placement. Secure the ET tube again per agency policy.

- If the patient is anxious or uncooperative, it is recommended that two staff members should perform the repositioning procedure to prevent accidental dislodgement. Monitor the patient for any signs of respiratory distress throughout the procedure.

BASIC LIFE SUPPORT FOR HEALTH CARE PROVIDERS

Description

The steps of basic life support (BLS) consist of a series of actions and skills performed by the rescuer or rescuers based on assessment findings.

- The first actions the rescuer performs on finding an adult victim is to assess for responsiveness and to look for signs of breathing. If the victim does not respond, there is no breathing or abnormal breathing (e.g., agonal gasps), and the rescuer is alone, the rescuer shouts for help. If someone responds, the rescuer sends him/her to activate the *emergency response system* (ERS) and get an *automatic external defibrillator* (AED) (if available). If no one responds, the rescuer activates the ERS, gets an AED (if available), returns to the victim, and begins *cardiopulmonary resuscitation* (CPR) and defibrillation if necessary.

CPR

The current approach for CPR is the chest *compressions-airway-breathing (CAB)* sequence. Survival from cardiac arrest is the highest when immediate CPR is provided and defibrillation occurs within 3 to 5 minutes.

- The first step in CPR is to perform a pulse check by palpating the carotid pulse for at least 5 but no more than 10 seconds. While maintaining a head-tilt position with one hand on the forehead, locate the victim's trachea using two or three fingers of the other hand. If a pulse is felt, give one rescue breath every 5 to 6 seconds (10 to 12 breaths per minute) and recheck the pulse every 2 minutes. If no pulse is felt, initiate CAB.

- Chest compression technique consists of fast and deep applications of pressure on the sternum. The victim must be in the supine position when the compressions are performed. Chest compressions are combined with rescue breathing for an effective resuscitation effort of the victim of cardiac arrest. The compression-ventilation ratio for one- or two-rescuer CPR is 30 compressions to 2 breaths (Table 89). To maintain the quality and rate of compressions, rescuers should change roles every 2 minutes.

- When the AED or advanced cardiovascular life support (ACLS) team arrives, assess the victim's rhythm. If the victim has a shockable rhythm (e.g., ventricular tachycardia, ventricular fibrillation), deliver one shock followed by five cycles of CPR before checking the rhythm. If the rhythm is not a shockable rhythm, resume CPR and recheck the rhythm every five cycles.

- If a victim has a pulse but is gasping (e.g., agonal breathing) or not breathing, establish an open airway and begin rescue breathing. Open an adult's airway by hyperextending the head. Use the *head tilt–chin lift maneuver.* This involves tilting the head back with one hand and lifting the chin forward with the fingers of the other hand. Use the *jaw-thrust maneuver* if you suspect a cervical spine injury. Attempt to ventilate the victim using a mouth-to-barrier (recommended) device (e.g., face mask or bag-valve-mask) or mouth-to-mouth resuscitation. Give ventilations with the victim's nostrils pinched. Take a regular (not deep) breath and tightly seal your lips around the victim's mouth. Give one breath and watch for a rise in the victim's chest. Continue rescue breaths at a rate of 10 to 12 per minute.

- If the victim cannot be ventilated, proceed with CPR. When providing the next rescue breaths, look for any objects in the victim's mouth and remove them if visible (Table 90 and Figure 19).

Hands-Only CPR

Hands-only CPR can be used to help adult victims who suddenly collapse from cardiac arrest outside of a health care setting. If you witness this event (as a bystander), you can choose to provide chest

Table 89 — Adult One- and Two-Rescuer Basic Life Support with Automatic External Defibrillator (AED)

Assess
- Determine unresponsiveness: tap or shake victim's shoulder; shout, "Are you all right?"
- Check for no breathing or abnormal breathing (e.g., gasping).

Activate Emergency Response System (ERS)
- Activate ERS (e.g., call 911) and get the AED (if available) (outside of hospital).
- Call a code and ask for the AED or crash cart (in hospital).

Check for Pulse
- Feel for carotid pulse (5-10 sec).
- If victim has a pulse but is not breathing or not breathing adequately, begin rescue breathing at a rate of 1 breath every 5-6 sec (see Fig. A-1, Lewis et al.: *Medical-Surgical Nursing*, ed. 9, p. 1696) and recheck circulation every 2 min.

Begin High-Quality CPR
- If there is no pulse, expose the victim's chest and immediately begin chest compressions (see Fig. A-2, Lewis et al.: *Medical-Surgical Nursing*, ed. 9, p. 1697).
- Deliver compressions at a rate of at least 100/min.
- Compress the chest at least 2 in.
- Allow for complete chest recoil after each compression.
- Deliver a compression-ventilation ratio of 30 compressions to 2 breaths.
- Minimize interruptions in compressions by delivering the 2 breaths in <10 sec.

Deliver Effective Breaths
- Open airway adequately (see Fig. A-1, *A*, Lewis et al.: *Medical-Surgical Nursing*, ed. 9, p. 1696).
- Deliver breath to produce a visible chest rise (see Fig. A-1, *B*, and *C*, Lewis et al.: *Medical-Surgical Nursing*, ed. 9, p. 1696).
- Avoid excessive ventilation.

Integrate Prompt Use of the AED
- Use AED as soon as possible.
- If rhythm is shockable, deliver one shock and then resume chest compressions immediately after delivery of shock.
- If the rhythm is not shockable, resume CPR and recheck rhythm every five cycles.

Continue CPR
- Continue CPR between rhythm checks and shocks, and until ACLS providers arrive or the victim shows signs of movement.

Source: American Heart Association: *BLS for healthcare providers—student manual*, Dallas, 2011, The Association.
ACLS, Advanced cardiovascular life support; *CPR*, cardiopulmonary resuscitation.

Table 90	Management of the Adult Choking Victim

Conscious Adult Choking Victim

Assess Victim for Severe Airway Obstruction

Look for any of the following signs:

- Poor or no air exchange
- Clutching the neck with the thumb and fingers, making the universal choking sign
- Weak, ineffective cough or no cough at all
- High-pitched noise while inhaling or no noise at all
- Increased respiratory difficulty
- Possible cyanosis

Ask the victim if he or she is choking. If the victim nods yes and cannot talk or has any of the symptoms noted above, severe airway obstruction is present and you must take immediate action.

Abdominal Thrusts (Heimlich Maneuver) with Standing or Sitting Victim

1. Stand or kneel behind victim and wrap arms around the victim's waist.
2. Make fist with one hand.
3. Place thumb side of fist against victim's abdomen. Position fist midline, slightly above navel and well below breastbone.
4. Grasp fist with other hand and press fist into victim's abdomen with a quick, forceful upward thrust.
5. Repeat thrusts until object is expelled or victim becomes unresponsive.
6. Give each new thrust with a separate, distinct movement to relieve the obstruction. Caution: If victim is pregnant or obese, give chest thrusts instead of abdominal thrusts. Position hands (as described) over lower portion of the breastbone and apply quick backward thrusts.

Unconscious Adult Choking Victim

Assessment

If you see a choking victim collapse and become unresponsive:

1. Activate the emergency response system.
2. Lower the victim to the ground and begin CPR, starting with compressions (do not check for a pulse).
3. Open the victim's mouth wide each time you prepare to give breaths. Look for the object. If you see the object and can easily remove it, do so with your fingers. If you do not see the object, continue with CPR using the chest compression–airway-breathing sequence.
4. If efforts to ventilate are unsuccessful, continue with CPR.

Source: American Heart Association: *BLS for healthcare providers—student manual,* Dallas, 2011, The Association.

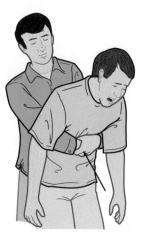

B

Fig. 19. Abdominal thrusts *(Heimlich maneuver)* administered to a conscious (standing) choking victim.

compressions only (push fast and deep in the center of the chest) or conventional CPR (described previously). Both methods are effective when done in the first few minutes of an out-of-hospital cardiac arrest.

BIOLOGIC AND TARGETED THERAPY

Description

Biologic and targeted therapy is used as a type of cancer treatment modality that can be effective alone or in combination with surgery, chemotherapy, and radiation therapy.

- *Biologic therapy (biologic response modifier therapy)* consists of agents that modify the relationship between the host and tumor by altering the biologic response of the host to the tumor cell (Table 91).
- *Targeted therapy* interferes with cancer growth by targeting specific cellular receptors and pathways that are important in tumor growth (see Table 91). Targeted therapies are more selective for specific molecular targets than chemotherapy (cytotoxic anticancer drugs). Thus they are able to kill cancer cells with less damage to normal cells compared with chemotherapy.

Table 91 Drug Therapy
Biologic and Targeted Therapy*

Drug	Mechanism of Action	Indications
α-interferon (Roferon-A, Intron A)	Inhibits DNA and protein synthesis Suppresses cell proliferation Increases cytotoxic effects of natural killer (NK) cells	Hairy cell leukemia, chronic myelogenous leukemia, malignant melanoma, renal cell carcinoma, ovarian cancer, multiple myeloma, Kaposi sarcoma
interleukin-2 (aldesleukin [Proleukin])	Stimulates proliferation of T and B cells Activates NK cells	Metastatic renal cell cancer, metastatic melanoma
BCG vaccine (TheraCys)	Induces an immune response that prevents angiogenesis of tumor	In situ bladder cancer
Epidermal Growth Factor Receptor (EGFR)–Tyrosine Kinase (TK) Inhibitors		
cetuximab (Erbitux)	Inhibits EGFR	Colorectal cancer, head and neck cancer
panitumumab (Vectibix)	Inhibits EGFR	Colorectal cancer
erlotinib (Tarceva)	Inhibits EGFR-TK	Non–small cell lung cancer, advanced pancreatic cancer
lapatinib (Tykerb)	Inhibits EGFR-TK and binds HER-2	Advanced breast cancer that is HER-2 positive
BCR-ABL Tyrosine Kinase Inhibitors		
imatinib (Gleevec)	Inhibits BCR-ABL TK	Chronic myeloid leukemia, GI stromal tumors (GIST)
nilotinib (Tasigna)	Inhibits BCR-ABL TK	Chronic myeloid leukemia
dasatinib (Sprycel)	Inhibits BCR-ABL TK	Chronic myeloid leukemia

B

CD20 Monoclonal Antibodies

rituximab (Rituxan)	Binds CD20 antigen, causing cytotoxicity	Non-Hodgkin's lymphoma (B cell)
ofatumumab (Arzerra)	Binds CD20 antigen, causing cytotoxicity	Chronic lymphocytic leukemia
ibritumomab tiuxetan/yttrium-90 (Zevalin)	Binds CD20 antigen, causing cytotoxicity and radiation injury	Non-Hodgkin's lymphoma (B cell)
tositumomab/[131I] tositumomab (Bexxar)	Binds CD20 antigen, causing immune attack and radiation injury	Non-Hodgkin's lymphoma (B cell)

Angiogenesis Inhibitors

bevacizumab (Avastin)	Binds vascular endothelial growth factor (VEGF), thereby inhibiting angiogenesis	Colorectal cancer, non–small cell lung cancer, and renal cell carcinoma
pazopanib (Votrient)	Binds VEGF, thereby inhibiting angiogenesis	Advanced renal cell carcinoma

Proteasome Inhibitors

bortezomib (Velcade)	Inhibits proteasome activity, which functions to regulate cell growth	Multiple myeloma
carfilzomib (Kyprolis)	Inhibits proteasome activity, which functions to regulate cell growth	Multiple myeloma

*An enhanced version of this table listing side effects (eTable 16-7, Lewis et al., *Medical-Surgical Nursing*, ed. 9) is available on the website.
BRAF, B-type Raf; *CTLA-4,* cytotoxic T lymphocyte antigen 4; *HER-2,* human epidermal growth factor receptor 2.

Continued

Drug Therapy
Biologic and Targeted Therapy—cont'd

Table 91

Drug	Mechanism of Action	Indications
Other Targeted Therapies		
alemtuzumab (Campath)	Binds CD52 antigen (found on T and B cells, monocytes, NK cells, neutrophils)	Chronic lymphocytic leukemia (B cell), GIST
trastuzumab (Herceptin)	Binds HER-2	Breast cancer (HER-2 positive)
pertuzumab (Perjeta)	Binds HER-2	Breast cancer (HER-2 positive)
sorafenib (Nexavar)	Inhibits multiple TKs	Advanced renal cell carcinoma
sunitinib (Sutent)	Inhibits multiple TKs	Advanced renal cell carcinoma, GIST
axitinib (Inlyta)	Inhibits multiple TKs	Advanced renal cell carcinoma
vandetanib (Caprelsa)	Inhibits multiple TKs	Medullary thyroid cancer
temsirolimus (Torisel)	Inhibits a specific protein known as the mammalian target of rapamycin (mTOR)	Advanced renal cell carcinoma
everolimus (Afinitor)	Inhibits a specific protein known as the mammalian target of rapamycin (mTOR)	Advanced renal cell carcinoma, advanced breast cancer
vemurafenib (Zelboraf)	Inhibits BRAF serine threonine kinase	BRAF V600E mutated metastatic melanoma
ipilimumab (Yervoy)	Binds with CTLA-4 causing an antitumor mediated immune response	Metastatic melanoma or unresectable melanoma
crizotinib (Xalkori)	Inhibits anaplastic lymphoma kinase (ALK)	Locally advanced or metastatic non–small cell lung cancer that is ALK positive

Targeted therapies include various tyrosine kinase inhibitors, monoclonal antibodies, angiogenesis inhibitors, and proteasome inhibitors.

- *Tyrosine kinase inhibitors* block an important enzyme that activates the signaling pathways that regulate cell proliferation and survival.
- *Monoclonal antibodies* bind to specific target cells and inhibit the internalization of receptor-antibody complexes and signaling pathways. They may also stimulate an immunologic response in the patient.
- *Angiogenesis inhibitors* work by preventing the mechanisms and pathways necessary for vascularization of tumors.
- *Proteasome inhibitors* promote an accumulation of proteins because they interfere with proteasomes (intracellular multienzyme complexes that degrade proteins). Thus they cause altered cell function.

Indications and side effects of biologic and targeted therapy are included in Table 91.

Nursing Management

The effects of biologic and targeted therapy occur acutely and are dose limited. Capillary leak syndrome and pulmonary edema are problems that require critical care nursing. Bone marrow depression that occurs with biologic therapy is usually more transient and less severe than that observed with chemotherapy.

- Fatigue associated with biologic therapy can be so severe that it can constitute a dose-limiting toxicity. As these agents are increasingly combined with chemotherapy, therapy-related effects increase.
- Acetaminophen administered before treatment and every 4 hours after treatment can help relieve the flulike syndrome associated with biologic agents. IV meperidine (Demerol) has been used to control the severe chills associated with some biologic agents.

Other nursing measures include monitoring vital signs and temperature, planning for periods of rest for the patient, assisting with activities of daily living (ADLs), and monitoring for adequate oral intake.

CHEMOTHERAPY

Description

Chemotherapy is the use of chemicals as a systemic therapy for cancer. It is a mainstay of cancer treatment for most solid tumors and hematologic malignancies (e.g., leukemias, lymphomas).The goal of chemotherapy is to eliminate or reduce the number of malignant cells present in the primary tumor and metastatic tumor site(s).

- The two major categories of chemotherapeutic drugs are *cell cycle phase–nonspecific* and *cell cycle phase–specific*. These agents are often administered in combination to maximize effectiveness by using agents that function by differing mechanisms and throughout the cell cycle.

Classification of Chemotherapeutic Drugs

Chemotherapy drugs are generally classified according to their molecular structure and mechanisms of action (Table 92).

Methods of Administration

The IV route is the most common route for chemotherapy administration. Major concerns associated with the IV administration of antineoplastic drugs include venous access difficulties, device- or catheter-related infection, and *extravasation* (infiltration of drugs into tissues surrounding the infusion site). Many chemotherapy drugs are either irritants or vesicants.

- *Irritants* will damage the intima of the vein, causing phlebitis and sclerosis and limiting future peripheral venous access.
- *Vesicants* may cause severe local tissue breakdown and necrosis if inadvertently infiltrated into the skin.

To minimize these problems, a central vascular access device may be placed in large blood vessels to permit frequent, continuous, or intermittent administration of chemotherapy, thus avoiding multiple venipunctures. (See pp. 309 to 311, Lewis et al.: *Medical-Surgical Nursing,* ed. 9.)

Regional chemotherapy delivers the drug directly to the tumor site. Examples of this type of administration include intraarterial, intraperitoneal, intrathecal (intraventricular), and intravesical bladder chemotherapy.

Effects of Chemotherapy

Chemotherapeutic agents cannot selectively distinguish between normal cells and cancer cells. Chemotherapy-induced side effects are caused by the destruction of normal cells that are rapidly proliferating such as those in the bone marrow, the lining of the

| Table 92 | Drug Therapy |
| | *Chemotherapy Drugs* |

Mechanisms of Action	**Examples**
Alkylating Agents	
Cell Cycle Phase–Nonspecific Agents	
Damage DNA by causing breaks in the double-stranded helix. If repair does not occur, cells will die immediately (cytocidal) or when they attempt to divide (cytostatic).	bendamustine (Treanda), busulfan (Myleran), chlorambucil (Leukeran), cyclophosphamide (Cytoxan, Neosar), dacarbazine (DTIC-Dome), ifosfamide (Ifex), mechlorethamine (Mustargen), melphalan (Alkeran), temozolomide (Temodar), thiotepa (Thioplex)
Nitrosoureas	
Cell Cycle Phase–Nonspecific Agents	
Like alkylating agents, break DNA helix, interfering with DNA replication. Cross blood-brain barrier.	carmustine (BiCNU, Gliadel), lomustine (CeeNU), streptozocin (Zanosar)
Platinum Drugs	
Cell Cycle Phase–Nonspecific Agents	
Bind to DNA and RNA, miscoding information and/or inhibiting DNA replication, and cells die.	carboplatin (Paraplatin), cisplatin (Platinol-AQ), oxaliplatin (Eloxatin)
Antimetabolites	
Cell Cycle Phase–Specific Agents	
Mimic naturally occurring substances, thus interfering with enzyme function or DNA synthesis. Primarily act during S phase. Purine and pyrimidine are building blocks of nucleic acids needed for DNA and RNA synthesis.	

C

NOTE: Many of these drugs are irritants or vesicants that require special attention during administration to avoid extravasation. It is important to know this information about a drug before administering it.

Continued

Table 92	Drug Therapy Chemotherapy Drugs—cont'd

Mechanisms of Action	Examples
Antimetabolites—cont'd *Cell Cycle Phase–Specific Agents—cont'd*	
■ Interfere with purine metabolism	cladribine (Leustatin), clofarabine (Clolar), fludarabine (Fludara), mercaptopurine (Purinethol), nelarabine (Arranon), pentostatin (Nipent), thioguanine
■ Interfere with pyrimidine metabolism	capecitabine (Xeloda); cytarabine (ara-C [Cytosar-U, DepoCyt]), floxuridine (FUDR), 5-fluorouracil (5-FU [Adrucil]), gemcitabine (Gemzar)
■ Interfere with folic acid metabolism	methotrexate (Rheumatrex, Trexall), pemetrexed (Alimta)
■ Interferes with DNA synthesis	hydroxyurea (Hydrea, Droxia)
Antitumor Antibiotics *Cell Cycle Phase–Nonspecific Agents*	
Bind directly to DNA, thus inhibiting the synthesis of DNA and interfering with transcription of RNA.	bleomycin (Blenoxane), dactinomycin (Cosmegen), daunorubicin (Cerubidine, DaunoXome), doxorubicin (Adriamycin, Rubex, Doxil), epirubicin (Ellence), idarubicin (Idamycin), mitomycin (Mutamycin), mitoxantrone (Novantrone), plicamycin (Mithracin), valrubicin (Valstar)
Mitotic Inhibitors *Cell Cycle Phase–Specific Agents* **Taxanes**	
Antimicrotubule agents that interfere with mitosis. Act during the late G_2 phase and mitosis to stabilize microtubules, thus inhibiting cell division.	albumin-bound paclitaxel (Abraxane), docetaxel (Taxotere), paclitaxel (Taxol)

Table 92	Drug Therapy Chemotherapy Drugs—cont'd

Mechanisms of Action	Examples
Vinca Alkaloids	
Act in M phase to inhibit mitosis.	vinblastine (Velban), vincristine (Oncovin), vinorelbine (Navelbine)
Others	
Microtubular inhibitors.	estramustine (Emcyt), ixabepilone (Ixempra), eribulin (Halaven)
Topoisomerase Inhibitors *Cell Cycle Phase–Specific Agents*	
Inhibit topoisomerases (normal enzymes) that function to make reversible breaks and repairs in DNA that allow for flexibility of DNA in replication.	etoposide (VePesid), irinotecan (Camptosar), teniposide (Vumon), topotecan (Hycamtin)
Corticosteroids *Cell Cycle Phase–Nonspecific Agents*	
Disrupt the cell membrane and inhibit synthesis of protein. Decrease circulating lymphocytes, inhibit mitosis, depress immune system, increase sense of well-being.	cortisone (Cortone), dexamethasone (Decadron), hydrocortisone (Cortef), methylprednisolone (Medrol), prednisone
Hormone Therapy *Cell Cycle Phase–Nonspecific Agents* **Antiestrogens**	
Selectively attach to estrogen receptors, causing down-regulation of them and inhibiting tumor growth. Also known as selective estrogen receptor modulators (SERMs).	fulvestrant (Faslodex), raloxifene (Evista), tamoxifen (Nolvadex), toremifene (Fareston)
Estrogens	
Interfere with hormone receptors and proteins.	estradiol (Estrace), estramustine (Emcyt), estrogen (Menest)
Aromatase Inhibitors	
Inhibit aromatase, an enzyme that converts adrenal androgen to estrogen.	anastrozole (Arimidex), exemestane (Aromasin), letrozole (Femara)

Continued

Table 92	Drug Therapy
	Chemotherapy Drugs—cont'd

Mechanisms of Action	Examples
Miscellaneous	
Enzyme derived from the yeast *Erwinia* used to deplete the supply of asparagine (amino acid) for leukemic cells that are dependent on an exogenous source of this amino acid. Inhibits protein synthesis.	*Erwinia asparaginase*, L-asparaginase (Elspar)
Causes changes in DNA in leukemia cells and leads to cell death.	arsenic trioxide (Trisenox)
Suppresses mitosis. Appears to alter DNA, RNA, and protein.	procarbazine (Matulane, Natulan)

gastrointestinal system, and the integumentary system (skin, hair, and nails). Effects of chemotherapy are caused by general cytotoxicity and organ-specific drug toxicities.

The adverse effects of these drugs can be classified as acute, delayed, or chronic.

- *Acute toxity* includes anaphylactic and hypersensitivity reactions, extravasation or a flare reaction, anticipatory nausea and vomiting, and dysrhythmias.
- *Delayed effects* are numerous and include delayed nausea and vomiting, mucositis, alopecia, skin rashes, bone marrow depression, altered bowel function, and a variety of neurotoxicities.
- *Chronic toxicities* involve damage to organs such as the heart, liver, kidneys, and lungs.

An extensive list of side effects and problems caused by chemotherapy and radiation therapy is provided in Table 16-11, Lewis et al.: *Medical-Surgical Nursing*, ed. 9, pp. 266 to 267.

Nursing Management: Chemotherapy and Radiation Therapy

You have an important role in helping patients deal with the side effects of chemotherapy and radiation.

- Myelosuppression is one of the most common effects of chemotherapy and to a lesser extent it can also occur with radiation. It can result in life-threatening and distressing effects, including infection, hemorrhage, and overwhelming fatigue. Monitor the CBC, particularly the neutrophil, platelet, and RBC counts.

- Fatigue is a nearly universal symptom, affecting most patients with cancer. You can help patients recognize that fatigue is a common effect of therapy. Ignoring fatigue may lead to an increase in symptoms. However, maintaining exercise and activity within tolerable limits is often helpful in managing fatigue. Guidelines for the evaluation and management of cancer-related fatigue are available online at *www.nccn.org*.

The intestinal mucosa is one of the tissues that are most sensitive to chemotherapy and radiation, resulting in nausea and vomiting, diarrhea, mucositis, and anorexia. These problems can affect the patient's hydration and nutritional status and sense of well-being.

- Assess patients with nausea and vomiting for signs and symptoms of dehydration and metabolic alkalosis. Nausea and vomiting can be successfully managed with antiemetic regimens, dietary modification, and other nondrug interventions.
- Both radiation- and chemotherapy-induced diarrhea are best managed with diet modification, antidiarrheals, antimotility agents, and antispasmodics (see Table 43-2, Lewis et al.: *Medical-Surgical Nursing,* ed. 9, p. 963).
- Mucositis can be alleviated by systemic and/or topical analgesics and antibiotics if infection is present. Monitor and get prompt treatment for oral candidiasis (which often occurs with mucositis). Frequent cleansing with saline and water and topical application of anesthetic gels directly to the lesions are standard care.
- Monitor the patient with anorexia during and after treatment to ensure weight loss does not become excessive. Also observe for dehydration. Small, frequent meals of high-protein, high-calorie foods are better tolerated than large meals.

Skin changes with chemotherapy range from mild erythema and hyperpigmentation to more distressing effects such as acral erythema. Alopecia caused by chemotherapy is usually reversible. Hair generally begins to grow back 3 to 4 weeks after the drugs are discontinued.

- With radiation, skin effects locally occur only in the treatment field. Basic skin care instructions are presented in Table 16-12, Lewis et al.: *Medical-Surgical Nursing,* ed. 9, p. 270. Verify these guidelines with your institution's radiation oncology department before using.

▼ **Patient and Caregiver Teaching**

Teaching is an important part of your role related to chemotherapy and radiation.

- To decrease the fear and anxiety often associated with chemotherapy and radiation, tell the patient what to expect during a course of treatment.

- Explore the patient's attitude toward treatment so that misconceptions or fear can be discussed.
- Inform patients of the possible treatment side effects that they may experience. Good nursing judgment is essential to determine the amount of information that the patient and caregiver can assimilate.

CHEST TUBES AND PLEURAL DRAINAGE

Description

Whenever fluid or air accumulates in the pleural space, the pressure becomes positive instead of negative and the lungs collapse. Chest tubes are inserted to drain the pleural space and reestablish negative pressure, allowing for proper lung expansion. Tubes may also be inserted in the mediastinal space to drain air and fluid postoperatively.

Chest Tube Insertion

Chest tubes can be inserted in the emergency department (ED), at the patient's bedside, or in the operating room. The patient is positioned with the arm raised above the head on the affected side to expose the midaxillary area, the standard site for insertion.

- The area is cleansed with antiseptic solution and the chest wall is prepared with a local anesthetic. A small incision is made over a rib. The chest tube is then advanced up and over the top of the rib to avoid the intercostal nerves and blood vessels (Fig. 20).
- Once inserted, the tube is connected to a pleural drainage system (Fig. 21). Two tubes may be connected to the same drainage unit with a Y-connector.
- The incision is closed with sutures and the chest tube is secured. The wound is covered with an occlusive dressing.
- Insertion of a chest tube and its presence in the pleural space is painful. Monitor patient comfort at frequent intervals and use appropriate pain-relieving interventions.

Pleural Drainage

There are two types of pleural drainage systems. The first type is a flutter valve, which consists of a one-way rubber valve within a rigid plastic tube. It is attached to the external end of the chest tube. The valve opens whenever pressure in the chest is greater than atmospheric pressure, such as during expiration, and it closes when intrathoracic pressure is less than atmospheric pressure, such as during inspiration. The flutter valve can be used

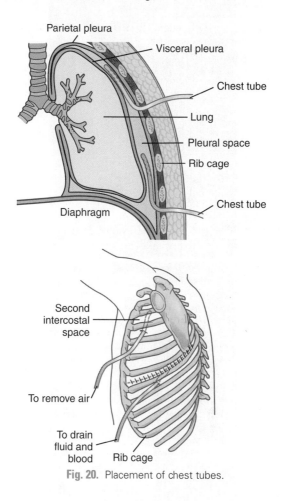

Parietal pleura

Visceral pleura

Chest tube

Lung

Pleural space

Rib cage

Chest tube

Diaphragm

Second
intercostal
space

To remove air

To drain
fluid and
blood   Rib cage

Fig. 20. Placement of chest tubes.

for emergency transport and for a small- to moderate-sized pneumothorax.

The second type of pleural drainage is larger and has three basic compartments (chambers).

■ The first compartment, or collection chamber, receives fluid and air from the pleural space. The drained fluid stays in this chamber while the air vents to the second chamber, called the water-seal chamber. This chamber contains 2 cm of water and

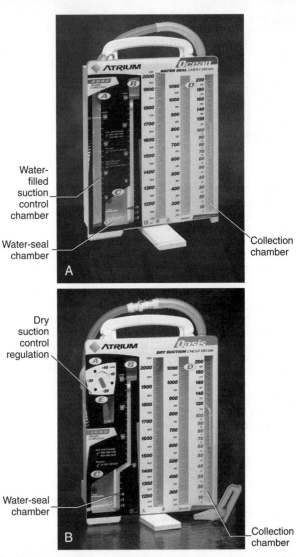

Fig. 21. Chest drainage unit. Both units have three chambers: (1) collection chamber; (2) water-seal chamber; and (3) suction control chamber. Suction control chamber requires a connection to a wall suction source that is dialed up higher than the prescribed suction for the suction to work. **A,** Water suction. This unit uses water in the suction control chamber to control the wall suction pressure. **B,** Dry suction. This unit controls wall suction by using a regulator control dial. (From Atrium Medical Corporation, Hudson, NH.)

acts as a one-way valve. Air enters from the collection chamber and bubbles up through the water. The water prevents backflow of air into the patient from the system.

- A third compartment, the suction control chamber, applies suction to the chest drainage.
- Initially, brisk bubbling of air occurs in this chamber when a pneumothorax is evacuated. During normal use, there will be intermittent bubbling during exhalation, coughing, or sneezing because of an increase in the patient's intrathoracic pressure. Eventually, the air leak seals and the lung is fully expanded.

A variety of commercial, disposable, plastic chest drainage systems are available. One system is the Pleur-evac (see Fig. 21).

Nursing Management: Chest Drainage

General guidelines for nursing care of the patient with chest tubes and water-seal drainage systems are presented in Table 28-21, Lewis et al.: *Medical-Surgical Nursing,* ed. 9, p. 546.

Drainage System

- Keep all tubing coiled loosely below chest level. Do not let it be compressed.
- Keep all connections among the chest tubes, drainage tubing, and drainage collector tight, and tape at connections.
- Observe for air fluctuations (tidaling) and bubbling in the water-seal chamber.
- Mark the time of measurement and the fluid level on the chamber according to the unit standards. Any change in the quantity or characteristics of drainage should be reported to the physician.
- Observe for air fluctuations and bubbling in the water-seal chamber. If tidaling is not observed, the drainage system is blocked, the lungs are reexpanded, or the system is attached to suction. If bubbling increases, there may be an air leak.
- Suspect a leak when bubbling is continuous. Retape tubing connections and ensure the dressing is air occlusive. If a leak persists, briefly clamp the chest tube at the patient's chest. If the leak stops, then the air is coming from the patient.
- High fluid levels in the water seal indicate residual negative pressure. The chest system may need to be vented by using the high-negativity release valve available on the drainage system to release residual pressure from the system.
- Never elevate the drainage system to the level of the patient's chest because this will cause fluid to drain back into the lungs.
- If the drainage system is overturned and the water seal is disrupted, return it to an upright position and encourage the patient to take a few deep breaths, followed by forced exhalations and cough maneuvers.

Do not strip or milk chest tubes, as this dangerously increases intrapleural pressures. If a physician orders the tubes to be milked or stripped, do so *gently*.

Milking: Alternately fold or squeeze and then release drainage tubing. Take 15-cm strips of the chest tube and squeeze and release starting close to the chest and repeating down the tube distally.

Stripping: Squeeze drainage tube with thumb and forefinger and use gentle pulling motion down tube with other hand, then release the tubing.

Patient's Clinical Status

- Monitor the patient's clinical status. Assess vital signs, lungs sounds, and pain level.
- Assess for manifestations of reaccumulation of air and fluid in the chest (decreased or absent breath sounds), significant bleeding (>100 mL/hr), chest drainage site infection (drainage, erythema, fever, increased WBC count), or poor wound healing. Notify the physician for a management plan. Evaluate for subcutaneous emphysema at the chest tube site.
- Encourage the patient to cough and breathe deeply periodically to facilitate lung expansion and encourage range-of-motion exercises to the shoulder on the affected side. Encourage use of incentive spirometry every hour while the patient is awake to prevent atelectasis or pneumonia.
- Clamping of chest tubes during transport or when the tube is accidentally disconnected is no longer advocated. If a chest tube becomes disconnected, immediately reestablish the water-seal system and attach a new drainage system as soon as possible.
- Closely monitor the patient for complications associated with chest tube placement and drainage. If volumes from 1 to 1.5 L of pleural fluid are removed rapidly, reexpansion pulmonary edema or a vasovagal response with symptomatic hypotension can occur.
- Use meticulous sterile technique during dressing changes to reduce the incidence of infected sites.

Chest Tube Removal

Chest tubes are removed when the lungs are reexpanded and fluid drainage has ceased or is minimal. Suction is usually discontinued and gravity drainage is used for 24 hours before tube removal.

- The tube is removed by cutting the suture, then having the patient take a deep breath, exhale, and bear down (Valsalva maneuver). Then the tube is removed.
- The site is immediately covered with an airtight dressing, the pleura will seal off, and the wound heals in several days.
- A chest x-ray is done to evaluate for pneumothorax or fluid reaccumulation.

DIALYSIS

Description

Dialysis is a technique in which substances move from the blood through a semipermeable membrane and into a dialysis solution (dialysate). It is used to correct fluid and electrolyte imbalances and remove waste products in renal failure. It can also be used to treat drug overdoses.

The two methods of dialysis are *peritoneal dialysis* (PD) and *hemodialysis* (HD) (Table 93).

- In PD the peritoneal membrane acts as the semipermeable membrane.

- In HD an artificial membrane (usually made of cellulose-based or synthetic materials) is used as the semipermeable membrane and is in contact with the patient's blood.

Dialysis is begun when the patient's uremia can no longer be adequately treated with conservative medical management. Generally dialysis is initiated when the glomerular filtration rate (GFR) (or creatinine clearance) of the patient with kidney disease is <15 mL/min. This criterion can vary widely in different clinical situations, and the physician determines when to start dialysis based on the patient's clinical status. Certain uremic complications, including encephalopathy, neuropathies, uncontrollable hyperkalemia, pericarditis, and accelerated hypertension, indicate a need for immediate dialysis.

Most patients with end-stage kidney disease (ESKD) are treated with dialysis because (1) there is a lack of donated organs, (2) some patients are physically or mentally unsuitable for transplantation, or (3) some patients do not want transplants.

- An increasing number of individuals, including older adults and those with complex medical problems, are receiving maintenance dialysis. A patient's chronologic age is not a factor in determining candidacy for dialysis. Factors that are important are the patient's ability to cope and the existing support system.

Dialysis is discussed in Lewis et al.: *Medical-Surgical Nursing,* ed. 9, pp. 1117 to 1118.

| Table 93 | Comparison of Peritoneal Dialysis and Hemodialysis |

Advantages	Disadvantages
Peritoneal Dialysis (PD)	
■ Immediate initiation in almost any hospital	■ Bacterial or chemical peritonitis
■ Less complicated than hemodialysis	■ Protein loss into dialysate
■ Portable system with CAPD	■ Exit site and tunnel infections
■ Fewer dietary restrictions	■ Self-image problems with catheter placement
■ Relatively short training time	■ Hyperglycemia
■ Usable in patient with vascular access problems	■ Surgery for catheter placement
■ Less cardiovascular stress	■ Contraindicated in patient with multiple abdominal surgeries, trauma, unrepaired hernia
■ Home dialysis possible	■ Requires completion of education program
■ Preferable for diabetic patient	■ Catheter can migrate
	■ Best instituted with willing partner
Hemodialysis (HD)	
■ Rapid fluid removal	■ Vascular access problems
■ Rapid removal of urea and creatinine	■ Dietary and fluid restrictions
■ Effective potassium removal	■ Heparinization may be necessary
■ Less protein loss	■ Extensive equipment necessary
■ Lowering of serum triglycerides	■ Hypotension during dialysis
■ Home dialysis possible	■ Added blood loss that contributes to anemia
■ Temporary access can be placed at bedside	■ Specially trained personnel necessary
	■ Surgery for permanent access placement
	■ Self-image problems with permanent access

CAPD, Continuous ambulatory peritoneal dialysis.

EMERGENCY PATIENT: PRIMARY AND SECONDARY SURVEY

Recognition of life-threatening illness or injury is one of the most important goals of emergency nursing. Initiation of interventions to reverse or prevent a crisis often is a priority before a diagnosis is made. This process begins with your first contact with the patient. Prompt identification of patients requiring immediate treatment and determination of appropriate interventions are essential nurse competencies.

- A *triage system* identifies and categorizes patients so the most critical are treated first.
- The process is based on the premise that patients with a threat to life must be treated before other patients.

Initially, assess the patient for any threats to life (e.g., Is the patient dying?) or presence of a high-risk situation (e.g., Is this a patient who should not wait to be seen?). After you complete the initial focused assessment to determine the presence of actual or potential threats to life, proceed with a more detailed assessment. A systematic approach to this assessment decreases the time required to identify potential threats to life and minimizes the risk of overlooking a life-threatening condition. A primary survey and a secondary survey are the approaches to use with all trauma patients.

The *primary survey* focuses on airway, breathing, circulation (ABC), disability, and exposure/environmental control. It aims to identify life-threatening conditions so that appropriate interventions can be initiated. You may identify life-threatening conditions related to ABCs (Table 94) at any point during the primary survey. When this occurs, start interventions immediately and before moving to the next step of the survey.

The *secondary survey* begins after addressing each step of the primary survey and starting any lifesaving interventions. The secondary survey is a brief, systematic process that aims to identify *all* injuries (see Table 69-5, Lewis et al.: *Medical Surgical Nursing* ed. 9, p. 1679).

Intervention and Evaluation

Regardless of the patient's chief complaint, ongoing monitoring and evaluation of interventions are critical. You are responsible for providing appropriate interventions and assessing the patient's

Table 94	Potential Life-Threatening Conditions Found During Primary Survey*

Airway
- Inhalation injury (e.g., fire victim)
- Obstruction (partial or complete) from foreign bodies, debris (e.g., vomitus), or tongue
- Penetrating wounds and/or blunt trauma to upper airway structures

Breathing
- Anaphylaxis
- Flail chest with pulmonary contusion
- Hemothorax
- Pneumothorax (e.g., open, tension)

Circulation
- Direct cardiac injury (e.g., myocardial infarction, trauma)
- Pericardial tamponade
- Shock (e.g., massive burns, hypovolemia)
- Uncontrolled external hemorrhage
- Hypothermia

Disability
- Head injury
- Stroke

*List is not all inclusive.

response. The evaluation of airway patency and the effectiveness of breathing will always be the highest priority.
- Monitor respiratory rate and rhythm, O_2 saturation, and arterial blood gases (ABGs) (if ordered) to evaluate the patient's respiratory status.
- Closely monitor level of consciousness, vital signs, quality of peripheral pulses, urine output, and skin temperature, color, and moisture for key information about circulation and perfusion.

Depending on the patient's injuries and/or illness, the patient may be (1) transported for diagnostic tests (e.g., CT scan) or to the operating room for immediate surgery; (2) admitted to an ICU, telemetry, or general unit; or (3) transferred to another facility. You may go with critically ill patients on transports. You are responsible for monitoring the patient during transport, notifying the health care team should the patient's condition become unstable, and initiating basic and advanced life-support measures as needed.

ENTERAL NUTRITION

Enteral nutrition (EN, also known as *tube feeding*) is nutrition (e.g., a nutritionally balanced liquefied food or formula) provided through the GI tract via a tube, catheter, or stoma that delivers nutrients distal to the oral cavity. EN may be ordered for the patient who has a functioning GI tract but is unable to take any or enough oral nourishment, or when it is unsafe to do so.

EN is considered to be easily administered, safer, more physiologically efficient, and typically less expensive than parenteral nutrition. Figure 22 shows the location of commonly used enteral feeding tubes. These include:

- Nasally and orally placed tubes (orogastric, nasogastric [NG], nasoduodenal, or nasojejunal) are most commonly used for short-term feeding (<4 weeks).

E

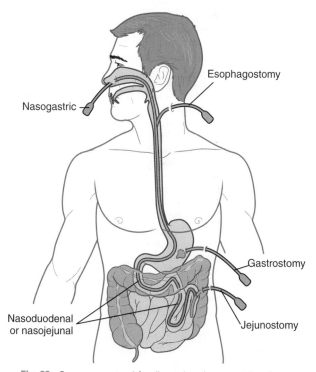

Fig. 22. Common enteral feeding tube placement locations.

- Nasoduodenal and nasojejunal tubes are transpyloric tubes. These tubes are used when pathophysiologic conditions such as risk of aspiration warrant feeding the patient below the pyloric sphincter.

If the feedings are necessary for an extended time, other tubes are placed in the stomach or small bowel by surgical, endoscopic, or fluoroscopic procedures.

Common delivery options are continuous infusion by pump, intermittent infusion by gravity, intermittent bolus by syringe, and cyclic feedings by infusion pump. Continuous infusion is most often used with critically ill patients. Intermittent feeding may be preferred as the patient improves or is receiving EN at home.

Tube Feedings and Safety

Aspiration and dislodged tubes are two important safety concerns. You have a critical role to ensure that tube feedings are administered safely.

Patient Position. Elevate head of bed to a minimum of 30 degrees, but preferably 45 degrees to prevent aspiration. Check institution policy for suspending feeding while the patient is supine. If intermittent delivery is used, the head should remain elevated for 30 to 60 minutes after feeding.

Aspiration Risk. Evaluate all enterally fed patients for risk of aspiration. Before starting tube feedings, ensure that the tube is in the proper position. Maintain head-of-bed elevation as described above. With increased residual volume there is increased risk for aspiration of formula into the lungs.

- Check gastric residual volumes every 4 hours during the first 48 hours for gastrically fed patients. After the enteral feeding goal rate is achieved, gastric residual monitoring may be decreased to every 6 to 8 hours in non–critically ill patients or continued every 4 hours in critically ill patients.

Tube Position. Confirm tube position of newly inserted nasal or orogastric tubes before feeding or administering medications. X-ray confirmation may be needed. Maintain proper placement of tube after feedings are started.

- To determine if a feeding tube has maintained the proper position, mark the exit site of the feeding tube at the time of the initial x-ray and observe for a change in the external tube length during feedings. Recheck the tube insertion length at regular intervals.

The types of problems encountered in patients receiving tube feedings and corrective measures are presented in Table 40-11, Lewis et al.: *Medical-Surgical Nursing,* ed. 9, p. 899.

Patient teaching includes skin care, care of the tube, and complete information about feeding administration and potential complications.

MECHANICAL VENTILATION

Description

Mechanical ventilation is the process by which room air or oxygen-enriched air is moved in and out of the lungs by a mechanical ventilator. Mechanical ventilation is not curative. It is a means of supporting patients until they recover the ability to breathe independently, as a bridge to long-term mechanical ventilation, or until a decision is made to withdraw ventilatory support. Indications for mechanical ventilation include (1) apnea or an impending inability to breathe, (2) acute respiratory failure, (3) severe hypoxia, and (4) respiratory muscle fatigue.

Types of Mechanical Ventilators

The two major types of mechanical ventilation are negative pressure and positive pressure ventilation.

- *Negative pressure ventilation* involves the use of chambers that encase the chest or body and surround it with intermittent subatmospheric or negative pressure. Intermittent negative pressure around the chest wall causes the chest to be pulled outward. This reduces intrathoracic pressure. Air rushes in through the upper airway, which is outside the sealed chamber. Expiration is passive; the machine cycles off, allowing chest retraction. This type of ventilation is similar to normal ventilation in that decreased intrathoracic pressures produce inspiration and expiration is passive. Negative pressure ventilation delivers noninvasive ventilation and does not require an artificial airway.
- Several portable negative pressure ventilators are available for home use for patients with neuromuscular diseases, central nervous system disorders, diseases and injuries of the spinal cord, and severe chronic obstructive pulmonary disease (COPD). Negative pressure ventilators are not used extensively for acutely ill patients.
- *Positive pressure ventilation* (PPV) is the primary method used with acutely ill patients. During inspiration, the ventilator pushes air into the lungs under positive pressure. Unlike spontaneous ventilation, intrathoracic pressure is raised during lung inflation rather than lowered. Expiration occurs passively as in normal expiration. PPVs are categorized into volume and pressure ventilators.

See the nursing care plan for the patient receiving mechanical ventilation in eNCP 66-1, available on the website for Lewis et al.: *Medical-Surgical Nursing,* ed. 9.

M

OSTOMIES

Description

An *ostomy* is a surgical procedure that allows intestinal contents to pass from the bowel through an opening in the skin on the abdomen. The opening is called a *stoma,* and it is created when the intestine is brought through the abdominal wall and sutured to the skin. The intestinal contents then empty through the hole on the surface of the abdomen rather than being eliminated through the anus.

An ostomy is used when the normal elimination route is no longer possible. For example, if the person has colorectal cancer, the diseased portion is removed together with a certain margin of healthy tissue. Sometimes the tumor can be resected, leaving enough healthy tissue to immediately *anastomose* (reconnect) the two remaining ends of healthy bowel, and no ostomy is necessary. If the tumor involves the rectum and is large enough to necessitate the removal of the anal sphincters, the anus is sutured shut and a permanent ostomy is created.

Types of Ostomies

Ostomies are described according to location and type (Fig. 23). An ostomy in the ileum is called an *ileostomy* and an ostomy in the colon is called a *colostomy*. The ostomy is further characterized by its anatomic site (e.g., sigmoid or transverse colostomy). The more distal the ostomy, the more the intestinal contents resemble feces that is eliminated from an intact colon and rectum. A comparison of colostomies and ileostomies is shown in Table 95.

The major types of ostomies are end stoma, loop, and double-barrel ostomies.

- An *end stoma* is created by dividing the bowel and bringing the proximal end as a single stoma. The distal portion of the GI tract is surgically removed, or the distal segment is oversewn and left in the abdominal cavity. If the distal bowel is removed, then the stoma is permanent.

- A *loop stoma* is constructed by bringing a loop of bowel to the abdominal surface and then opening the anterior part of the bowel to provide fecal diversion. This results in one stoma with a proximal and distal opening and an intact posterior bowel wall that separates the two openings. A loop stoma is usually temporary.

- In a *double-barrel stoma* the bowel is divided, and both the proximal and distal ends are brought through the abdominal wall as two separate stomas. The proximal one is the functioning stoma; the distal, nonfunctioning stoma is referred to as the mucus fistula. The double-barreled stoma is usually temporary.

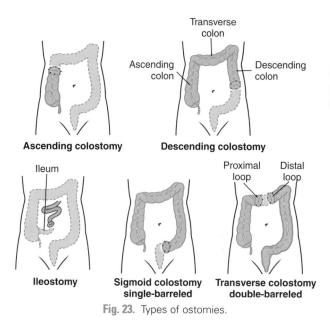

Fig. 23. Types of ostomies.

The procedures used to perform ostomy surgeries are further discussed in Lewis et al.: *Medical-Surgical Nursing,* ed. 9, pp. 990 to 991.

Nursing Management
Preoperative Care
Preoperative care that is unique to ostomy surgery includes (1) psychologic preparation for the ostomy; (2) selection of a flat site on the abdomen that allows secure attachment of the collection bag; and (3) selection of a stoma site that will be clearly visible to the patient to facilitate self-care. Psychologic preparation and emotional support are important as the person copes with the change in body image and a loss of control over elimination and its odors.

- A wound, ostomy, and continence (WOC) nurse should select the site where the ostomy will be positioned and mark the abdomen preoperatively. Stomas placed outside the rectus muscle increase the chance of developing a hernia. A flat site makes it much easier to create a good seal and avoid leakage from the bag.

Postoperative Care
Postoperative nursing care includes assessment of the stoma and provision of an appropriate pouching system that protects the skin and contains drainage and odor. The stoma should be dark pink to red.

Table 95   Comparison of Ileostomy and Colostomy

Characteristic	Ileostomy	Colostomy		
		Ascending	Transverse	Sigmoid
Stool consistency	Liquid to semiliquid	Semiliquid	Semiliquid to semiformed	Formed
Fluid requirement	Increased	Increased	Possibly increased	No change
Bowel regulation	No	No	No	Yes (if there is a history of a regular bowel pattern)
Pouch and skin barriers	Yes	Yes	Yes	Dependent on regulation
Irrigation	No	No	No	Possibly every 24-48 hr (if patient meets criteria)
Indications for surgery	Ulcerative colitis, Crohn's disease, diseased or injured colon, familial polyposis, trauma, cancer	Perforating diverticulum in lower colon, trauma, rectovaginal fistula, inoperable tumors of colon, rectum, or pelvis	Same as for ascending	Cancer of the rectum or rectosigmoidal area, perforating diverticulum, trauma

A dusky blue stoma indicates ischemia, and a brown-black stoma indicates necrosis. Assess and document stoma color every 4 hours. Teach the patient that the stoma is mildly to moderately swollen the first 2 to 3 weeks after surgery.

All pouching systems consist of an adhesive skin barrier and a bag or pouch to collect the feces. The skin barrier is a piece of pectin-based or karaya wafer that has a measurable thickness and hydrocolloid adhesive properties.

▼ Patient and Caregiver Teaching

- Teach the patient to perform a pouch change, provide appropriate skin care, control odor, care for the stoma, and identify signs and symptoms of complications.
- Instruct the patient about the importance of fluids and a healthy diet. Provide the names and addresses of United Ostomy Associations of America, and instruct the patient on when to seek health care.
- Home care and outpatient follow-up by a WOC nurse are highly recommended. Patients should be discharged with written information about their particular ostomy, instructions for pouch changes, a list of supplies and where to purchase them (including names and phone numbers of retailers), and outpatient follow-up appointments with the surgeon and WOC nurse.
- Emotional support, interventions from skillful WOC nurses, and visits from people who have successfully learned to manage their ostomies will help patients learn to cope with and manage the new stoma.
- See Table 43-29 for ostomy teaching guidelines, Lewis et al.: *Medical-Surgical Nursing,* ed. 9, p. 993.

Colostomy Care

A colostomy in the ascending and transverse colon has semiliquid stools. Instruct the patient to use a drainable pouch. A colostomy in the sigmoid or descending colon has semiformed or formed stools and sometimes can be regulated by the irrigation method. The patient may or may not wear a drainage pouch. A well-balanced diet and adequate fluid intake are important.

Colostomy irrigations may be used to stimulate emptying of the colon. Regularity is possible only when the stoma is in the distal colon or rectum. If bowel control is achieved, there should be little or no spillage between irrigations, and the patient may need to wear only a pad or cover over the stoma. The procedure for colostomy irrigation is presented in Table 96.

Ileostomy Care

- Because regularity cannot be established, a pouch must be worn at all times. An open-ended, drainable pouch is preferable so drainage can be easily emptied. The drainable pouch is usually worn for 4 to 7 days before being changed unless leakage occurs.

Table 96	**Patient and Caregiver Teaching Guide**
	Colostomy Irrigation

Include the following instructions when teaching the patient and caregiver to perform a colostomy irrigation.

Equipment*
- Lubricant
- Irrigation set (1000- to 2000-mL container, tubing with irrigating stoma cone, clamp)
- Irrigating sleeve with adhesive or belt
- Toilet tissue to clean around the stoma
- Disposal sack for soiled dressing

Procedure
1. Place 500 to 1000 mL of lukewarm water (not to exceed 105° F [40.5° C]) in container. Titrate the volume for the individual; use enough irrigant to distend the bowel but not enough to cause cramping pain. Most adults use 500 to 1000 mL of water.
2. Ensure a comfortable position. Patient may sit in chair in front of toilet or on the toilet if the perineal wound is healed.
3. Clear tubing of all air by flushing it with fluid.
4. Hang container on hook or IV pole (18 to 24 in) above stoma (about shoulder height).
5. Apply irrigating sleeve and place bottom end in toilet bowl.
6. Lubricate stoma cone, insert cone tip gently into the stoma, and hold tip securely in place. The cone is designed to prevent perforation, control the depth of insertion, and prevent water from coming out of the stoma.
7. Allow irrigation solution to flow in steadily for 5 to 10 min.
8. If cramping occurs, stop the flow of solution for a few seconds, leaving the cone in place.
9. Clamp the tubing and remove irrigating cone when the desired amount of irrigant has been delivered or when the patient senses colonic distention.
10. Allow 30 to 45 min for the solution and feces to be expelled. Initial evacuation is usually complete in 10 to 15 min. Close off the irrigating sleeve at the bottom to allow ambulation.
11. Clean, rinse, and dry peristomal skin well.
12. Replace the colostomy drainage pouch or desired stoma covering.
13. Wash and rinse all equipment and hang to dry.

*Commercial sets usually have all the equipment that you will need.

- In the first 24 to 48 hours after surgery, the amount of drainage from the stoma may be negligible. Once peristalsis returns, the patient may experience a period of high volume output of 1000 to 1800 mL/day. Later, the average amount can be 500 mL/day.

▼ **Patient and Caregiver Teaching**

Instruct the patient to drink at least 2 to 3 L/day when there are excessive fluid losses from heat and sweating. Patients must learn signs and symptoms of fluid and electrolyte imbalance so they can take appropriate action.

- A low-fiber diet is ordered initially. Fiber-containing foods are reintroduced gradually. A return to a normal, presurgical diet is the goal.
- The stoma bleeds easily when it is touched because it has a high vascular supply. Tell the patient that minimal oozing of blood is normal.
- Encourage the patient to share concerns and ask questions, provide information in a manner that is easily understood, recommend support services, and assist patients to develop confidence and competence in managing the stoma.
- Help the patient understand that sexual function or sexual activity may be affected.

OXYGEN THERAPY

Description

Oxygen (O_2) therapy is frequently used in the treatment of chronic obstructive pulmonary disease (COPD) and other problems associated with hypoxemia. Long-term continuous O_2 therapy (LTOT) increases survival and improves exercise capacity and mental status in hypoxemic patients.

Goals for O_2 therapy are to keep the SaO_2 above 90% during rest, sleep, and exertion, or PaO_2 greater than 60 mm Hg. O_2 is usually administered to treat hypoxemia caused by (1) respiratory disorders such as COPD, pulmonary hypertension, cor pulmonale, pneumonia, atelectasis, lung cancer, and pulmonary emboli; (2) cardiovascular disorders such as myocardial infarction, dysrhythmias, angina pectoris, and cardiogenic shock; and (3) central nervous system disorders such as overdose of opioids, head injury, and sleep disorders (sleep apnea).

Methods of Administration

Various methods of O_2 administration are used (Table 97). The method selected depends on factors such as the fraction of inspired O_2 concentration (FIO_2), the patient's mobility and cooperation, humidification required, comfort, and cost.

Table 97   Methods of Oxygen Administration

Description	Nursing Interventions
Low-Flow Delivery Devices *Nasal Cannula* ▪ Most commonly used device. ▪ O_2 delivered via plastic nasal prongs. ▪ Safe and simple method that allows some freedom of movement; patient can eat, talk, or cough while wearing device. ▪ Useful for a patient requiring low O_2 concentrations. ▪ O_2 concentrations of 24% (at 1 L/min) to 44% (at 6 L/min) can be obtained.	▪ Stabilize nasal cannula when caring for a restless patient. ▪ Amount of O_2 inhaled depends on room air and patient's breathing pattern. ▪ Most patients with COPD can tolerate 2 L/min via cannula. ▪ Assess patient's nares and ears for skin breakdown; may need to pad cannula where it sits on ears. ▪ If flow rates are >5 L/min, nasal membranes may dry and may cause pain in frontal sinuses. 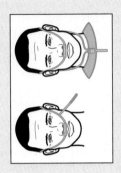

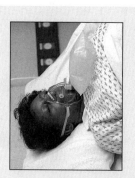

Simple Face Mask

- Covers patient's nose and mouth.
- Used only for short periods, especially when transporting patients.
- Longer use is typically not tolerated because of tight seal and heat generated around nose and mouth from mask.
- O_2 concentrations of 35%-50% can be achieved with flow rates of 6-12 L/min.
- Mask provides adequate humidification of inspired air.
- Wash and dry under mask q2hr.
- Mask must fit snugly.
- Nasal cannula may be provided while patient is eating.
- Watch for pressure necrosis at top of ears from elastic straps if patient wears for a longer time. (Gauze or other padding may alleviate this problem.)

Partial and Non-Rebreather Masks

- Useful for short-term (24 hr) therapy for patients needing higher O_2 concentrations (60%-90% at 10-15 L/min).
- O_2 flows into reservoir bag and mask during inhalation.
- This bag allows patient to rebreathe about first third of exhaled air (rich in O_2) in conjunction with flowing O_2.
- Vents remain open on partial mask only. Some facilities prefer this over non-rebreather as a safety issue.
- O_2 flow rate must be sufficient to keep bag from collapsing during inspiration to avoid CO_2 buildup.
- If deflation occurs, increase liter flow to keep bag inflated.
- Mask should fit snugly.
- With non-rebreather masks, make sure valves are open during expiration and closed during inhalation to prevent drastic decrease in FIO_2.
- Monitor patient closely, since more advanced interventions may be required such as CPAP, BiPAP, or intubation with mechanical ventilation.

Continued

Table 97   Methods of Oxygen Administration—cont'd

Description	Nursing Interventions
Oxygen-Conserving Cannula ■ Generally indicated for long-term O_2 therapy at home vs. during hospitalization (e.g., pulmonary fibrosis, pulmonary hypertension). ■ May be "moustache" (Oxymizer) or "pendant" type. ■ Cannula has a built-in reservoir that ↑ O_2 concentration and allows patient to use lower flow, usually 30%–50%, which increases comfort, lowers cost, and can be increased with activities. ■ Can deliver up to 8 L/min O_2.	■ May cause necrosis over tops of ears. Can be padded. ■ Cannula cannot be cleaned. Manufacturer recommends changing cannula every week. ■ It is more expensive than standard cannulas and requires evaluation with ABGs and oximetry to determine correct flow for patient. ■ Cannula is highly visible.

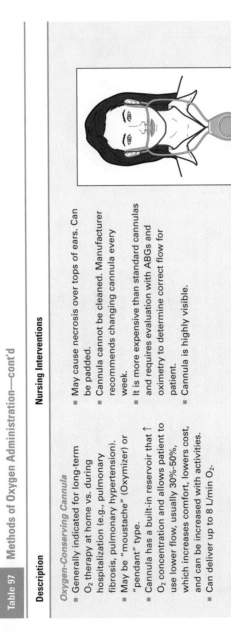

Pendant-type O_2-conserving cannula

High-Flow Delivery Devices

Tracheostomy Collar

- Collar attaches to neck with elastic strap and can deliver high humidity and O_2 via tracheostomy.
- O_2 concentration is lost into atmosphere because collar does not fit tightly.
- Venturi device can be attached to flowmeter and thus can deliver exact amounts of O_2 via collar.

- Secretions collect inside collar and around tracheostomy. Remove collar and clean at least q4hr to prevent aspiration of fluid and infection.
- Because condensation occurs in tubing, periodically drain distally to tracheostomy.

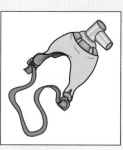

Tracheostomy T Bar

- Almost identical to tracheostomy collar, but it has a vent and a T connector that allow an inline catheter (e.g., Ballard catheter) to be connected for suctioning.
- Tight fit allows better O_2 and humidity delivery than tracheostomy collar.

- Empty as necessary.
- Because T bars disconnect easily, monitor closely.
- T bar may pull on a patient's tracheostomy tube, causing irritation and potential tissue damage. Monitor this closely.
- See tracheostomy collar above.

Continued

0

Table 97 Methods of Oxygen Administration—cont'd

Description	Nursing Interventions
Venturi Mask	■ Entrainment device on mask must be changed to deliver higher concentrations of O_2.
■ Mask can deliver precise, high-flow rates of O_2.	■ Air entrainment ports must not be occluded.
■ Lightweight plastic, cone-shaped device is fitted to face.	■ Mask is uncomfortable. Remove when patient eats.
■ Masks are available for delivery of 24%, 28%, 31%, 35%, 40%, and 50% O_2.	■ Patient can talk but voice may be muffled.
■ Method is especially helpful for administering low, constant O_2 concentrations to patients with COPD.	■ See other applicable nursing interventions under simple face mask above.
■ Adaptors can be applied to increase humidification.	

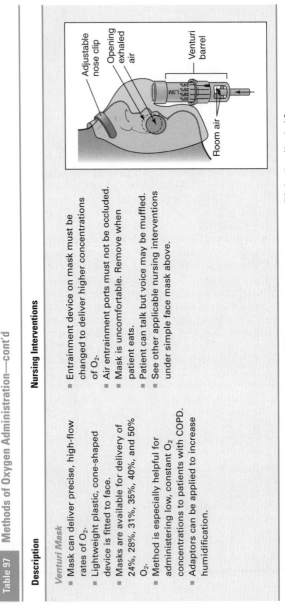

ABGs, Arterial blood gases; *BiPAP*, biphasic positive airway pressure; *CPAP*, continuous positive airway pressure; *FIO₂*, fraction of inspired O_2.

- O_2 obtained from cylinders or wall systems is dry. Dry O_2 has an irritating effect on the mucous membranes and dries secretions. Therefore it is important that a high flow of O_2 delivering greater than 35% to 50% oxygen be humidified when administered.

Complications

O_2 supports combustion and increases the rate of burning, so it is important to prohibit smoking in the area in which O_2 is being used. A "No Smoking" sign should be prominently displayed on the patient's door. Also caution the patient against smoking cigarettes with an O_2 cannula in place.

The chemoreceptors in the respiratory center that control the drive to breathe respond to CO_2 and O_2. Normally CO_2 accumulation is the major stimulant of the respiratory center. Over time some COPD patients develop a tolerance for high CO_2 levels (the respiratory center loses its sensitivity to the elevated CO_2 levels). Theoretically, for these individuals the "drive" to breathe is hypoxemia.

- It is critical to start O_2 at low flow rates until levels of arterial blood gases (ABGs) can be obtained. ABGs are used as a guide to determine what FIO_2 level is sufficient and can be tolerated. Assess the patient's mental status and vital signs before starting O_2 therapy and frequently thereafter.

Pulmonary oxygen toxicity may result from prolonged exposure to a high level of O_2 (PaO_2). High concentrations of O_2 can result in a severe inflammatory response because of oxygen radicals and damaged alveolar-capillary membranes resulting in severe pulmonary edema, shunting of blood, and hypoxemia. These individuals develop acute respiratory distress syndrome (ARDS).

- To prevent toxicity, the amount of O_2 administered should be just enough to maintain the PaO_2 within a normal or acceptable range for the patient.

Infection can be a major hazard of O_2 administration. Heated nebulizers present the highest risk. Constant use of humidity supports bacterial growth, with *Pseudomonas aeruginosa* the most common infecting organism. Disposable equipment that operates as a closed system should be used. Each hospital has a policy on the required frequency of equipment changes based on the type of equipment used.

Chronic Oxygen Therapy at Home

Improved survival occurs in patients with COPD who receive LTOT (more than 15 hours/day) to treat hypoxemia. The improved prognosis results from preventing disease progression and subsequent cor pulmonale. The benefits of LTOT include improved mental acuity, lung mechanics, sleep, and exercise tolerance; decreased hematocrit; and reduced pulmonary hypertension.

- Periodic reevaluations are necessary for the patient who is using chronic supplemental O_2. Generally the patient should be reevaluated every 30 to 90 days during the first year of therapy and annually after that, as long as the patient remains stable.

▼ **Patient and Caregiver Teaching**

A home care guide for teaching the patient and family about home O_2 use is given in Table 98.

Table 98	**Patient and Caregiver Teaching Guide** *Home Oxygen Use*

The company that provides the prescribed O_2 therapy equipment will instruct the patient on equipment care. The following are some general instructions that you may include when teaching the patient and caregiver about the use of home O_2.

Decreasing Risk for Infection

- Brush teeth or use mouthwash several times a day.
- Wash nasal cannula (prongs) with a liquid soap and thoroughly rinse once or twice a week.
- Replace cannula every 2-4 wk.
- If you have a cold, replace the cannula after your symptoms pass.
- Always remove secretions that are coughed out.
- If you use an O_2 concentrator, every day unplug the unit and wipe down the cabinet with a damp cloth and dry it.
- Ask the company providing the equipment how often to change the filter.

Safety Issues

- Post "No Smoking" warning signs outside the home.
- O_2 will not "blow up," but it will increase the rate of burning because it is a fuel for the fire.
- Do not allow smoking in the home, and do not smoke yourself while wearing O_2. Nasal cannulas and masks can catch fire and cause serious burns to face and airways.
- Do not use flammable liquids such as paint thinners, cleaning fluids, gasoline, kerosene, oil-based paints, or aerosol sprays while receiving O_2.
- Do not use blankets or fabrics that carry a static charge, such as wool or synthetics.
- Inform your electric company if you are using a concentrator. In case of a power failure, the company will know the medical urgency of restoring your power.

Adapted from *www.YourLungHealth.org.*

PACEMAKERS

Description

The artificial cardiac pacemaker is an electronic device used to pace the heart when the normal conduction pathway is damaged. The basic pacing circuit consists of a power source (battery-powered pulse generator), one or more conducting leads (pacing leads), and the myocardium. The electrical signal (stimulus) travels from the pacemaker, through the leads, to the wall of the myocardium. The myocardium is "captured" and stimulated to contract.

Demand pacemakers, which are the most common, have the ability to sense the heart's electrical activity and fire only when the heart rate (HR) drops below a preset rate. Demand pacemakers have two distinct features: (1) a sensing device that inhibits the pacemaker when the HR is adequate and (2) a pacing device that triggers the pacemaker when no QRS complexes occur within a preset time.

Permanent pacemakers are implanted entirely within the patient's body. The power source is implanted subcutaneously, usually over the pectoral muscle on the patient's nondominant side. It is attached to pacer leads, which are threaded transvenously (through a vein) to the right atrium and one or both ventricles. Indications for insertion of a permanent pacemaker are listed in Table 99.

A *temporary pacemaker* is one that has the power source outside the body. There are three types of temporary pacemakers: transvenous,

Table 99	Indications for Permanent Pacemakers

- Acquired AV block
- Second-degree AV block
- Third-degree AV block
- Atrial fibrillation with a slow ventricular response
- Bundle branch block
- Cardiomyopathy
    - Dilated
    - Hypertrophic
- Heart failure
- SA node dysfunction
- Tachydysrhythmias (e.g., ventricular tachycardia)

AV, Atrioventricular; *SA,* sinoatrial.

epicardial, and transcutaneous. Table 100 lists common reasons for temporary pacing.

- A *transvenous pacemaker* consists of a lead or leads that are threaded transvenously to the right atrium and/or right ventricle and attached to the external power source.
- In *epicardial pacemakers,* atrial and ventricular pacing leads are attached to the epicardium during heart surgery. The leads are passed through the chest wall and attached to the external power source.
- A *transcutaneous pacemaker* is used to provide adequate heart rate and rhythm to the patient in an emergency situation. This type of pacemaker involves the use of external electrode pads that are connected to the external power source.

Patient Monitoring

Patients with temporary or permanent pacemakers are monitored by ECG to evaluate the status of the pacemaker. Pacemaker malfunction primarily involves a failure to sense or a failure to capture.

- *Failure to sense* occurs when the pacemaker fails to recognize spontaneous atrial or ventricular activity and fires inappropriately. Failure to sense is caused by pacer lead fracture (breakage), battery failure, sensing set too high, or electrode displacement.
- *Failure to capture* occurs when the electrical charge to the myocardium is insufficient to produce atrial or ventricular contraction. This can result in serious bradycardia or asystole.

Table 100	Indications for Temporary Pacemakers*

- Maintenance of adequate HR and rhythm during special circumstances such as surgery and postoperative recovery, during cardiac catheterization or coronary angioplasty, during drug therapy that may cause bradycardia, and before implantation of a permanent pacemaker
- As prophylaxis after open heart surgery
- Acute anterior MI with second- or third-degree AV block or bundle branch block
- Acute inferior MI with symptomatic bradycardia and AV block
- Electrophysiologic studies to evaluate patient with bradydysrhythmias and tachydysrhythmias

*List is not all-inclusive.
AV, Atrioventricular.

Failure to capture may be caused by pacer lead fracture, battery failure, electrode displacement, electrical charge set too low, or fibrosis at the electrode tip.

Nursing Management

After the pacemaker has been inserted, the patient can be out of bed once stable. Have the patient limit arm and shoulder activity on the operative side to prevent dislodging the newly implanted pacing leads.

- Observe the insertion site for signs of bleeding, and check that the incision is intact. Note any temperature elevation or pain at the insertion site and treat as ordered. Most patients are discharged the same day or the next day if stable.
- After discharge, patients need to check pacemaker function on a regular basis. This can include outpatient visits to a pacemaker clinic or home monitoring using telephone transmitter devices.
- The goals of pacemaker therapy include enhancing physiologic functioning and quality of life. Emphasize this to the patient and the caregiver, and provide specific advice on activity restrictions. Table 101 outlines patient and caregiver teaching for the patient with a pacemaker.

Table 101	Patient and Caregiver Teaching Guide *Pacemaker*

Include the following instructions when teaching the patient and caregiver management of a pacemaker.

- Maintain follow-up care with your cardiologist to begin regular pacemaker function checks.
- Report any signs of infection at incision site (e.g., redness, swelling, drainage) or fever to your cardiologist immediately.
- Keep incision dry for 4 days after implantation, or as ordered.
- Avoid lifting arm on pacemaker side above shoulder until approved by your cardiologist.
- Avoid direct blows to pacemaker site.
- Avoid close proximity to high-output electric generators, because these can interfere with the function of the pacemaker.
- You should not have a MRI scan unless the pacemaker is approved as MRI safe or there is a protocol in place for patient safety during the procedure.
- Microwave ovens are safe to use and do not interfere with pacemaker function.
- Avoid standing near antitheft devices in doorways of department stores and public libraries. You should walk through them at a normal pace.

Continued

Table 101	Patient and Caregiver Teaching Guide *Pacemaker*—cont'd

- Air travel is not restricted. Inform airport security of presence of pacemaker because it may set off the metal detector. If hand-held screening wand is used, it should not be placed directly over the pacemaker. Manufacturer information may vary regarding the effect of metal detectors on the function of the pacemaker.
- Monitor pulse and inform cardiologist if it drops below predetermined rate.
- Carry pacemaker information card and a current list of your medications at all times.
- Obtain and wear a Medic Alert ID or bracelet at all times.

PARENTERAL NUTRITION

Description

Parenteral nutrition (PN) is the administration of nutrients by a route (e.g., bloodstream) other than the GI tract. It is used when the GI tract cannot be used for the ingestion, digestion, and absorption of essential nutrients (Table 102).

Administration of PN

PN may be administered as central PN or peripheral parenteral nutrition. Both central and peripheral PN are used in a patient who is not a candidate for enteral nutrition (EN). The patient receiving PN must be able to tolerate a large volume of fluid.

- *Central PN* is indicated when long-term nutritional support is necessary or when the patient has high protein and caloric requirements. Central PN may be given through a central venous catheter that originates at the subclavian or jugular vein and whose tip lies in the superior vena cava. Central PN may also be administered using peripherally inserted central catheters (PICCs) that are placed into the basilic or cephalic vein and then advanced into the distal end of the superior vena cava.
- *Peripheral parenteral nutrition* (PPN) is administered through a large, peripherally inserted catheter or vascular access device that uses a large vein. PPN is used when (1) nutritional support is needed for only a short time, (2) protein and caloric requirements are not high, (3) the risk of a central catheter is too great, or (4) parenteral support is used to supplement inadequate oral intake.

Commercially prepared PN base solutions are available. These base solutions contain dextrose and protein in the form of amino acids. The pharmacy adds the prescribed electrolytes (e.g., sodium, chloride,

Table 102	Indications for Parenteral Nutrition*

- Chronic severe diarrhea and vomiting
- Complicated surgery or trauma
- GI obstruction
- Intractable diarrhea
- Severe anorexia nervosa
- Severe malabsorption
- Short bowel syndrome
- GI tract anomalies and fistulae

*This list is not all inclusive.

P

calcium, magnesium, phosphate), vitamins, and trace elements (e.g., zinc, copper, chromium, manganese) to prepare the solution to meet the patient's needs.

A three-in-one or total nutrient admixture containing an IV fat emulsion, dextrose, and amino acids is widely used.

Refeeding syndrome is a complication of PN that is characterized by fluid retention and electrolyte imbalances (hypophosphatemia, hypokalemia, hypomagnesemia). Conditions predisposing patients to refeeding syndrome include long-standing malnutrition states such as chronic alcoholism, vomiting and diarrhea, chemotherapy, and major surgery.

- Refeeding syndrome can occur any time a malnourished patient is started on aggressive nutritional support. Hypophosphatemia is the hallmark of refeeding syndrome and is associated with serious outcomes, including cardiac dysrhythmias, respiratory arrest, and neurologic disturbances (e.g., paresthesias).

Other complications of PN are listed in Table 103.

Home Nutritional Support

Home PN or enteral nutrition is an accepted mode of nutritional therapy for the person who does not require hospitalization but who requires continued nutritional support. Some patients have been successfully treated at home for many months and even years.

- Teach the patient and caregiver about catheter or tube care, proper technique in mixing and handling of the solutions and tubing, and side effects and complications.
- Tell the family about support groups such as the Oley Foundation *(www.oley.org)* that provide peer support and advocacy.

Home nutritional therapies are expensive. For patients to be reimbursed for expenses, specific criteria must be met. The discharge planning team needs to be involved early in the admission to help

Table 103	Complications of Parenteral Nutrition

Infection
- Fungus
- Gram-positive bacteria
- Gram-negative bacteria

Metabolic Problems
- Hyperglycemia, hypoglycemia
- Altered renal function
- Essential fatty acid deficiency
- Electrolyte and vitamin excesses and deficiencies
- Trace mineral deficiencies
- Hyperlipidemia

Catheter-Related Problems
- Air embolus
- Pneumothorax, hemothorax, and hydrothorax
- Hemorrhage
- Dislodgment
- Thrombosis of vein
- Phlebitis

plan for such issues. Home nutritional support may also be a burden on the patient and the caregivers and may affect quality of life.

RADIATION THERAPY

Description

Radiation therapy is one of the oldest methods of cancer treatment. Delivery of high-energy beams, when absorbed into tissue, produces ionization of atomic particles. The energy in ionizing radiation acts to break the chemical bonds in DNA. The DNA is damaged, resulting in cell death.

Different types of ionizing radiation are used to treat cancer, including electromagnetic radiation (i.e., x-rays, gamma rays) and particulate radiation (alpha particles, electrons, neutrons, protons). High-energy x-rays (photons) are generated by an electric machine, such as a linear accelerator.

- The nomenclature for radiation dose is gray (Gy) or centigray (cGy). A centigray is equivalent to 1 rad, and 100 centigray equals 1 gray.
- Once the total dose to be delivered is determined, that dose is divided into daily fractions. Doses between 180 and 200 cGy/day are considered standard fractionation, typically delivered

once a day Monday through Friday for a period of 2 to 8 weeks (depending on the desired total dose).

- Radiation only has an effect on tissues within the treatment field. It is not appropriate as the primary treatment for systemic disease. However, radiation may be used by itself in combination with chemotherapy or surgery to treat primary tumors, or for palliation of metastatic lesions.
- Radiation can be delivered externally (known as *teletherapy* or *external beam radiation therapy*) or internally *(brachytherapy)*.

Rapidly dividing cells in the GI tract, oral mucosa, and bone marrow die quickly and exhibit early acute responses to radiation. Tissues with slowly proliferating cells, such as cartilage, bone, and kidneys, manifest later responses to radiation. Some cancers are more susceptible to radiation than others (Table 104).

R

Table 104	Tumor Radiosensitivity*

High Radiosensitivity
- Ovarian dysgerminoma
- Testicular seminoma
- Hodgkin's lymphoma
- Non-Hodgkin's lymphoma
- Wilms' tumor
- Neuroblastoma

Moderate Radiosensitivity
- Oropharyngeal carcinoma
- Esophageal carcinoma
- Breast adenocarcinoma
- Uterine and cervical carcinoma
- Prostate carcinoma
- Bladder carcinoma

Mild Radiosensitivity
- Soft tissue sarcomas (e.g., chondrosarcoma)
- Gastric adenocarcinoma
- Renal adenocarcinoma
- Colon adenocarcinoma

Poor Radiosensitivity
- Osteosarcoma
- Malignant melanoma
- Malignant glioma
- Testicular nonseminoma

*Radiosensitivity is the relative susceptibility of cells and tissues to the effects of radiation.

Nursing Management: Chemotherapy and Radiation Therapy
See Chemotherapy, p. 694.
▼ **Patient and Caregiver Teaching**
See Chemotherapy, pp. 699 to 700.

TRACHEOSTOMY

Description

A *tracheostomy* is a surgically created stoma (opening) in the trachea to establish an airway. It is used to (1) bypass an upper airway obstruction, (2) facilitate removal of secretions, or (3) permit long-term mechanical ventilation.

Most surgical tracheostomies are done in the operating room using general anesthesia. These are typically done electively on patients already intubated who require prolonged mechanical ventilation. When swelling, trauma, or upper airway obstruction prevents endotracheal intubation, an emergent surgical tracheostomy may be performed at the bedside.

A *minimally invasive percutaneous tracheostomy* can also be performed at the bedside using local anesthesia and sedation and analgesia. A needle is placed into the trachea, followed by a guide wire. The opening is progressively dilated until it is large enough for insertion of a tracheostomy tube.

- A tracheostomy provides a more secure airway, is less likely to be displaced, and allows more freedom of movement than an endotracheal tube. There is less risk of long-term damage to the vocal cords. Airway resistance and work of breathing are decreased, facilitating independent breathing. Patient comfort may be increased because no tube is present in the mouth.
- The patient can eat with a tracheostomy because the tube enters lower in the airway (Fig. 24). Speaking is also permitted once the tracheostomy cuff can be deflated.

When the patient can adequately exchange air and expectorate secretions, the tracheostomy tube can be removed. Close the stoma with tape strips and cover it with an occlusive dressing. Instruct the patient to splint the stoma with the fingers when coughing, swallowing, or speaking.

- Epithelial tissue begins to form in 24 to 48 hours, and the opening closes in several days. Surgical intervention to close a tracheostomy is not required.

Nursing Management

Before the tracheotomy, explain to the patient and family the purpose of the procedure and inform them that the patient will not be

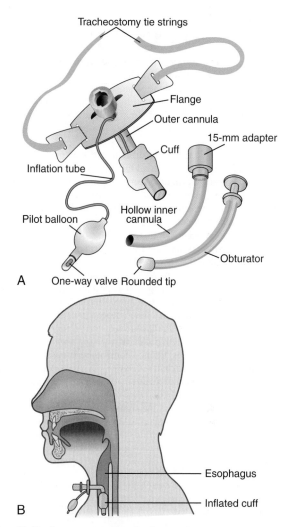

Fig. 24. Tracheostomy tube. **A,** Parts of a tracheostomy tube. **B,** Tracheostomy tube inserted in airway with inflated cuff.

able to speak if an inflated cuff is used. A variety of tubes are available to meet patient needs (see Fig. 25). Characteristics and nursing management of tracheostomies are described in Table 27-5, Lewis et al.: *Medical-Surgical Nursing*, ed. 9, p. 508.

Care should be taken not to dislodge the tracheostomy tube during the first 5 to 7 days when the stoma is not mature (healed).

- Retention sutures may be placed in the tracheal cartilage when the tracheotomy is performed. Tape the free ends of the sutures to the skin in a place and manner that leaves them accessible if the tube is dislodged.
- Because tube replacement is difficult, several precautions are required: (1) keep a replacement tube of equal or smaller size at the bedside, readily available for emergency reinsertion, (2) do not change tracheostomy tapes for at least 24 hours after the insertion procedure, and (3) let a physician perform the first tube change, usually no sooner than 7 days after the tracheotomy.
- If the tube is accidentally dislodged, immediately attempt to replace it. See the discussion of tube replacement techniques on p. 510 of Lewis et al.: *Medical-Surgical Nursing,* ed. 9.

Care of the patient with a tracheostomy involves suctioning the airway to remove secretions, cleaning around the stoma, changing tracheostomy ties, and inner cannula care if a nondisposable inner cannula is used. See Table 105 for a detailed description of tracheostomy care.

▼ **Patient and Caregiver Teaching**

- Assess ability of the patient and caregiver to provide care at home.
- Include instructions for tracheostomy tube care, stoma care, suctioning, airway care, and responding to emergencies.
- Make a referral to a home health care nurse to provide ongoing assistance and support.
- Teach patient and caregiver the signs and symptoms to report to health care professionals, such as changes in secretions (color and consistency) and elevated temperature.

Table 105	Tracheostomy Care

1. Explain procedure to patient.
2. Use tracheostomy care kit or collect necessary sterile equipment (e.g., suction catheter, gloves, water basin, drape, tracheostomy ties, tube brush or pipe cleaners, 4 × 4 gauze pads, sterile water or normal saline, and tracheostomy dressing [optional]).
   NOTE: Clean rather than sterile technique is used at home.
3. Position patient in semi-Fowler's position.
4. Assemble needed materials on bedside table next to patient.
5. Wash hands. Put on goggles and clean gloves.

Table 105	Tracheostomy Care—cont'd

6. Auscultate chest sounds. If rhonchi or coarse crackles are present, suction the patient if unable to cough up secretions (see Table 27-6, Lewis, et al.: *Medical-Surgical Nursing*, ed. 9, p. 509). Remove soiled dressing and clean gloves.

7. Open sterile equipment, pour sterile H_2O or normal saline into two compartments of sterile container or two basins, and put on sterile gloves. NOTE: Hydrogen peroxide (3%) is no longer recommended unless an infection is present. If it is used, rinse the inner cannula and skin with sterile H_2O or normal saline afterward to prevent trauma to tissue.

8. Unlock and remove inner cannula, if present. Many tracheostomy tubes do not have inner cannulas. Care for these tubes includes all steps except for inner cannula care.

9. If disposable inner cannula is used, replace with new cannula. If a nondisposable cannula is used:
   - Immerse inner cannula in sterile solution and clean inside and outside of cannula using tube brush or pipe cleaners.
   - Rinse cannula in sterile solution. Remove from solution and shake to dry.
   - Insert inner cannula into outer cannula with the curved part downward, and lock in place.

10. Remove dried secretions from stoma using 4 × 4 gauze pad soaked in sterile water or saline. Gently pat area around the stoma dry. Be sure to clean under the tracheostomy faceplate, using cotton swabs to reach this area.

11. Maintain position of tracheal retention sutures (if present) by taping above and below the stoma.

12. Change tracheostomy ties. Use two-person change technique or secure new ties to flanges before removing the old ones. Tie tracheostomy ties securely with room for two fingers between ties and skin (see Fig. 27-5, Lewis, et al.: *Medical-Surgical Nursing*, ed. 9, p. 510). To prevent accidental tube removal, secure the tracheostomy tube by gently applying pressure to the flange of the tube during the tie changes. *Do not change tracheostomy ties for 24 hr after the tracheostomy procedure.*

13. As an alternative, some patients prefer tracheostomy ties made of Velcro, which are easier to adjust.

14. If drainage is excessive, place dressing around tube (see Fig. 27-5, Lewis, et al.: *Medical-Surgical Nursing*, ed. 9, p. 510). A tracheostomy dressing or unlined gauze should be used. Do not cut the gauze because threads may be inhaled or wrap around the tracheostomy tube. Change the dressing frequently. Wet dressings promote infection and stoma irritation.

15. Repeat care three times a day and as needed.

T

URINARY CATHETERIZATION

Indications for short-term urinary catheterization are listed in Table 106. Two unacceptable reasons are (1) routine acquisition of a urine specimen for laboratory analysis and (2) convenience of the nursing staff or the patient's family.

- Possible complications of long-term use (>30 days) of indwelling catheters include hospital-acquired infections (HAIs), bladder spasms, periurethral abscess, pain, urinary tract infections (UTIs), urosepsis, urethral trauma/erosion, fistula/stricture formation, and stones.

Catheterization for sterile urine specimens may occasionally be indicated when patients have a history of complicated UTI. A catheter should be the final means of providing the patient with a dry environment for the prevention of skin breakdown and protection of dressings or skin lesions.

Table 106 **Indications for Urinary Catheterization**

Indwelling Catheter
- Relief of urinary retention caused by lower urinary tract obstruction, paralysis, or inability to void
- Bladder decompression preoperatively and operatively for lower abdominal or pelvic surgery
- Facilitation of surgical repair of urethra and surrounding structures
- Splinting of ureters or urethra to facilitate healing after surgery or other trauma in area
- Accurate measurement of urine output in critically ill patient
- Measurement of residual urine after urination (postvoid residual [PVR]) if portable ultrasound not available
- Contamination of stage III or IV pressure ulcers with urine that has impeded healing, despite appropriate personal care for the incontinence (indwelling)
- Terminal illness or severe impairment, which makes positioning or clothing changes uncomfortable, or which is associated with intractable pain (indwelling)

Straight (In-and-Out) Catheter
- Study of anatomic structures of urinary system
- Urodynamic testing
- Collection of sterile urine sample in selected situations
- Instillation of medications into bladder

Strict aseptic technique is mandatory when a urinary catheter is inserted. After insertion, nursing actions include maintenance and protection of the closed drainage system. Do not routinely irrigate the catheter, as this should only be done if ordered. While the patient has a catheter in place, maintain patency of the catheter, manage fluid intake, provide for the patient's comfort and safety, and prevent infection. Address the psychologic implications of urinary drainage. Patient concerns can include embarrassment related to exposure of the body, an altered body image, and fear that care of the catheter will result in increased dependency.

- Catheters vary in construction materials, tip shape, and lumen size. Catheters are sized according to the French scale. Each French unit equals 0.33 mm of diameter. The diameter listed is the internal diameter of the catheter. The size used varies with the patient's size and the purpose for catheterization.

The most common route of catheterization is insertion of the catheter through the external meatus into the urethra, past the internal sphincter, and into the bladder.

Suprapubic catheterization is the simplest and oldest method of urinary diversion. The two methods of insertion of a suprapubic catheter into the bladder are (1) through a small incision in the abdominal wall and (2) by the use of a trocar. A suprapubic catheter is placed while the patient is under general anesthesia for another surgical procedure or at the bedside with a local anesthetic. The catheter may be sutured into place.

- The suprapubic catheter is used in temporary situations, such as bladder, prostate, and urethral surgery, and also used long term in selected patients.

- Tape the catheter to prevent dislodgement. The care of the tube and catheter is similar to that of the urethral catheter. A pectin-base skin barrier (e.g., Stomahesive) is effective in protecting the skin around the insertion site from breakdown.

- A suprapubic catheter is prone to poor drainage because of mechanical obstruction of the catheter tip by the bladder wall, sediment, and clots. To ensure patency of the tube include (1) preventing tube kinking by coiling the excess tubing and maintaining gravity drainage, (2) having the patient turn from side to side, and (3) milking the tube. If these measures are not effective, obtain a physician's order to irrigate the catheter with sterile technique.

- If the patient experiences bladder spasms that are difficult to control, urinary leakage may result. Oxybutynin (Ditropan) or other oral antispasmodics or belladonna and opium (B&O) suppositories may be prescribed to decrease bladder spasms.

An alternative approach to a long-term indwelling catheter is *intermittent catheterization,* also referred to as "straight" or "in-and-out" catheterization. It is used in conditions such as neurogenic bladder (e.g., spinal cord injuries, chronic neurologic diseases) or bladder outlet obstruction in men. This type of catheterization may also be used in the oliguric and anuric phases of acute kidney injury to reduce the possibility of infection from an indwelling catheter. Intermittent catheterization is also used postoperatively, often after a surgical procedure to treat urinary incontinence.

- The main goal of intermittent catheterization is to prevent urinary retention, stasis, and compromised blood supply to the bladder caused by prolonged pressure.
- The technique consists of inserting a urethral catheter into the bladder every 3 to 5 hours. Some patients perform intermittent catheterization only once or twice each day to measure residual urine and ensure an empty bladder.
- Instruct patients to wash and rinse the catheter and their hands with soap and water before and after catheterization. Lubricant is necessary for men and may make catheterization more comfortable for women.
- The catheter may be inserted by the patient, caregiver, or the health care provider.
- In general, patients should change the catheter every 7 days.
- In the hospital or long-term care facility, sterile technique is used for catheterizations. For home care, a clean technique that includes good hand washing with soap and water is used.
- Teach the patient to observe for signs of UTI so that treatment can be instituted early. If indicated, some patients are placed on a regimen of prophylactic antibiotics.

PART THREE

Reference Appendix

ABBREVIATIONS

ABG	arterial blood gas
ACE	angiotensin-converting enzyme
ACLS	advanced cardiac life support
ACS	acute coronary syndrome
ACTH	adrenocorticotropic hormone
ADH	antidiuretic hormone
AED	automatic external defibrillator
AIDS	acquired immunodeficiency syndrome
AKA	above-knee amputation
AKI	acute kidney injury
ALI	acute lung injury
ALL	acute lymphocytic leukemia
ALS	amyotrophic lateral sclerosis
AMI	acute myocardial infarction
ANA	antinuclear antibody
ANS	autonomic nervous system
AORN	Association of periOperative Registered Nurses
APD	automated peritoneal dialysis
aPTT	activated partial thromboplastin time
ARDS	acute respiratory distress syndrome
ATN	acute tubular necrosis
BCLS	basic cardiac life support
BKA	below-knee amputation
BMI	body mass index
BMR	basal metabolic rate
BMT	bone marrow transplantation
BPH	benign prostatic hyperplasia
BSE	breast self-examination
BUN	blood urea nitrogen
CABG	coronary artery bypass graft
CAD	coronary artery disease, circulatory assist device
CAPD	continuous ambulatory peritoneal dialysis
CAVH	continuous arteriovenous hemofiltration
CBC	complete blood count
CCU	coronary care unit; critical care unit
CDC	Centers for Disease Control and Prevention
CIS	carcinoma in situ
CKD	chronic kidney disease
CLL	chronic lymphocytic leukemia
CML	chronic myelocytic leukemia
CMP	cardiomyopathy

Continued

ABBREVIATIONS—cont'd

CN	cranial nerve
CNS	central nervous system
CO	cardiac output
COPD	chronic obstructive pulmonary disease
CPAP	continuous positive airway pressure
CPR	cardiopulmonary resuscitation
CRRT	continuous renal replacement therapy
CRNA	certified registered nurse anesthetist
CSF	cerebrospinal fluid
CT	computed tomography
CVA	cerebrovascular accident; costovertebral angle
CVAD	central venous access device
CVI	chronic venous insufficiency
CVP	central venous pressure
D&C	dilation and curettage
DDD	degenerative disc disease
DI	diabetes insipidus
DIC	disseminated intravascular coagulation
DJD	degenerative joint disease
DKA	diabetic ketoacidosis
DM	diabetes mellitus; diastolic murmur
DRE	digital rectal examination
DVT	deep vein thrombosis
ECF	extracellular fluid
ECG	electrocardiogram
ED	emergency department, erectile dysfunction
EEG	electroencephalogram
EMG	electromyogram
EMS	emergency medical services
ENT	ear, nose, and throat
ERCP	endoscopic retrograde cholangiopancreatography
ESR	erythrocyte sedimentation rate
ESKD	end-stage kidney disease
ET	endotracheal
FEV	forced expiratory volume
FRC	functional residual capacity
FUO	fever of unknown origin
GCS	Glasgow Coma Scale
GERD	gastroesophageal reflux disease
GFR	glomerular filtration rate
GH	growth hormone
GI	glycemic index
GTT	glucose tolerance test

ABBREVIATIONS—cont'd

GU	genitourinary
GYN, Gyn	gynecological
H&P	history and physical examination
HAV	hepatitis A virus
HBV	hepatitis B virus
Hgb	hemoglobin
Hct	hematocrit
HCV	hepatitis C virus
HD	hemodialysis, Huntington's disease
HDL	high-density lipoprotein
HF	heart failure
HIV	human immunodeficiency virus
HPV	human papillomavirus
HSCT	hematopoietic stem cell transplantation
I&D	incision and drainage
IABP	intraaortic balloon pump
IBS	irritable bowel syndrome
ICP	intracranial pressure
IE	infective endocarditis
IFG	impaired fasting glucose
IGT	impaired glucose tolerance
INR	international normalized ratio
IOP	intraocular pressure
IPPB	intermittent positive pressure breathing
ITP	idiopathic thrombocytopenic purpura
IUD	intrauterine device
IV	intravenous
IVP	intravenous push; intravenous pyelogram
JVD	jugular venous distention
KUB	kidney, ureters, and bladder (x-ray)
KS	Kaposi sarcoma
KVO	keep vein open
LAD	left anterior descending
LDL	low-density lipoprotein
LGV	lymphogranuloma venereum
LLQ	left lower quadrant
LMN	lower motor neuron
LMP	last menstrual period
LOC	level of consciousness
LP	lumbar puncture
LUQ	left upper quadrant
LVH	left ventricular hypertrophy
MAP	mean arterial pressure

Continued

ABBREVIATIONS—cont'd

MD	muscular dystrophy
MDS	myelodysplastic syndrome
MG	myasthenia gravis
MI	myocardial infarction
MICU	medical intensive care unit
MODS	multiple organ dysfunction syndrome
MRB	manual resuscitation bag
MS	multiple sclerosis
MVP	mitral valve prolapse
NAFLD	nonalcoholic fatty liver disease
NANDA-I	North American Nursing Diagnosis Association–International
NASH	nonalcoholic steatohepatitis
NG	nasogastric
NHL	non-Hodgkin's lymphoma
NIDDM	non–insulin-dependent diabetes mellitus
NPO	nothing by mouth
NS	normal saline
NSR	normal sinus rhythm
OA	osteoarthritis
OD	right eye; optical density; overdose
OL	left eye
OOB	out of bed
OR	operating room
ORIF	open reduction and internal fixation
OSA	obstructive sleep apnea
OTC	over-the-counter
PA	posteroanterior; physician's assistant
PAC	premature atrial contraction
$PaCO_2$	partial pressure of carbon dioxide in arterial blood
PaO_2	partial pressure of oxygen in arterial blood
PACU	postanesthesia care unit
PAD	peripheral artery disease
PAP	pulmonary artery pressure
PAWP	pulmonary artery wedge pressure
PCA	patient-controlled analgesia
PCI	percutaneous coronary intervention
PCO_2	partial pressure of carbon dioxide
PCWP	pulmonary capillary wedge pressure
PD	Parkinson's disease, peritoneal dialysis
PE	pulmonary embolism; physical examination
PEEP	positive end-expiratory pressure
PEFR	peak expiratory flow rate

ABBREVIATIONS—cont'd

PERRLA	pupils equal, round, and reactive to light and accommodation
PET	positron emission tomography
PICC	percutaneously inserted central catheter
PID	pelvic inflammatory disease
PKD	polycystic kidey disease
PMH	past medical history
PMI	point of maximal impulse
PMS	premenstrual syndrome
PN	parenteral nutrition
PND	paroxysmal nocturnal dyspnea; postnasal drip
PNS	peripheral nervous system
PO, po	orally
POC	point-of-care
PPD	purified protein derivative
PSA	prostate-specific antigen
PSS	progressive systemic sclerosis
PT	prothrombin time
PTT	partial thromboplastin time
PVC	premature ventricular contraction
PUD	peptic ulcer disease
R/O	rule out
RA	rheumatoid arthritis
REM	rapid eye movement
RF	rheumatic fever
RHD	rheumatic heart disease
RLQ	right lower quadrant
RLS	restless legs syndrome
ROM	range of motion
ROS	review of systems
RUQ	right upper quadrant
SA	sinoatrial
SCI	spinal cord injury
SCD	sickle cell disease, sudden cardiac death
SDP	sleep-disordered breathing
SICU	surgical intensive care unit
SIRS	systemic inflammatory response syndrome
SLE	systemic lupus erythematosus
SNS	sympathetic nervous system
SOB	shortness of breath
STI	sexually transmitted infection
STSG	split-thickness skin graft
SVR	systemic vascular resistance

Continued

ABBREVIATIONS—cont'd

SVT	superficial vein thrombosis
TAH	total abdominal hysterectomy
TB	tuberculosis
TBSA	total body surface area
TCDB	turn, cough, and deep breathe
TENS	transcutaneous electrical nerve stimulation
THR	total hip replacement
TIA	transient ischemic attack
TJC	The Joint Commission
TKO	to keep open
TPR	temperature, pulse, and respirations
TURP	transurethral resection of the prostate
UA	unstable angina
UAP	unlicensed assistive personnel
UGI	upper gastrointestinal
UI	urinary incontinence
UMN	upper motor neuron
URI	upper respiratory infection
UTI	urinary tract infection
VAD	venous access device, ventricular assist device
VDH	valvular disease of the heart
VF	ventricular fibrillation
VS	vital signs
VT	ventricular tachycardia
VTE	venous thromboembolism
WHR	waist-to-hip ratio
WNL	within normal limits

THE JOINT COMMISSION
OFFICIAL "DO NOT USE" LIST*

Do Not Use	Potential Problem	Use Instead
U, u (unit)	Mistaken for "0" (zero), the number "4" (four) or "cc"	Write "unit"
IU (International Unit)	Mistaken for IV (intravenous) or the number "10" (ten)	Write "International Unit"
Q.D., QD, q.d., qd (daily)	Mistaken for each other	Write "daily"
Q.O.D, QOD, q.o.d., qod (every other day)	Period after the Q mistaken for "I" and "O" mistaken for "I"	Write "every other day"
Trailing zero (X.0 mg)†	Decimal point is missed	Write "X mg"
Lack of leading zero (.X mg)		Write "0.X mg"
MS	Can mean morphine sulfate or magnesium sulfate	Write "morphine sulfate"
MSO_4 and $MgSO_4$	Confused for one another	Write "magnesium sulfate"

*Applies to all order and all medication-related documentation that is handwritten (including free-text computer entry) or on pre-printed forms
†**Exception:** A "trailing zero" may be used only where required to demonstrate the level of precision of the value being reported, such as for laboratory results, imaging studies that report size of lesions, or catheter/tube sizes. It may not be used in medication orders or other medication-related documentation.

Additional Abbreviations, Acronyms, and Symbols

Abbreviation	Preferred Term
μg (for microgram)	Write "mcg"
HS or hs (for bedtime or half-strength)	Write "at bedtime" or "half-strength"
TIW (for three times per week)	Write "3 times weekly" or "three times weekly"
SC or SQ (for subcutaneous)	Write "Sub-Q," "subQ," or "subcutaneously"
D/C (for discharge)	Write "discharge"
cc (for cubic centimeter)	Write "mL" for milliliters
AS, AD, AU (left, right, or both ears)	Write "left ear," "right ear," or "both ears"

BLOOD GASES, ARTERIAL

Normal Values

	Arterial (Sea Level)
pH	7.35-7.45
PaO$_2$*	80-100 mm Hg
PaCO$_2$	35-45 mm Hg
HCO$_3$	22-26 mEq/L
O$_2$ saturation	>95%

*In a patient >60 years old, PaO$_2$ is equal to 80 mm Hg minus 1 mm Hg for every year over 60. Expected PaO$_2$ = FIO$_2$ × 5.

Interpreting Arterial Blood Gases (ABGs)

1. Check pH
   ↑ = Alkalosis; ↓ = acidosis
2. Check PaCO$_2$
   ↑ = CO$_2$ retention (hypoventilation); respiratory acidosis or compensating for metabolic alkalosis
   ↓ = CO$_2$ blown off (hyperventilation); respiratory alkalosis or compensating for metabolic acidosis
3. Check HCO$_3$
   ↑ = Nonvolatile acid is lost; HCO$_3$ is gained (metabolic alkalosis or compensating for respiratory acidosis)
   ↓ = Nonvolatile acid is added; HCO$_3$ is lost (metabolic acidosis or compensating for respiratory alkalosis)
4. Determine imbalance
5. Determine if compensation exists

Determining the Imbalance in ABGs

If	pH ↑ and PaCO$_2$ ↓ or pH ↓ and PaCO$_2$ ↑	Then respiratory disorder
If	pH ↑ and HCO$_3$ ↑ or pH ↓ and HCO$_3$ ↑	Then metabolic disorder
If	PaCO$_2$ ↑ and HCO$_3$ ↑ or PaCO$_2$ ↓ and HCO$_3$ ↓	Then compensation is occurring
If	PaCO$_2$ ↑ and HCO$_3$ ↓ or PaCO$_2$ ↓ and HCO$_3$ ↑	Then mixed imbalance

LABORATORY VALUES

Test	Conventional Units	SI Units
Complete Blood Count		
Red blood cells (RBCs)	*Male:* 4.3-5.7 × 10⁶/μL *Female:* 3.8-5.1 × 10⁶/μL	*Male:* 4.3-5.7 × 10¹²/L *Female:* 3.8-5.1 × 10¹²/L
White blood cells (WBCs)	4.0-11.0 × 10³/μL	4.0-11.0 × 10⁹/L
Hemoglobin (Hgb)	*Male:* 13.2-17.3 g/dL *Female:* 11.7-15.5 g/dL	*Male:* 132-173 g/L *Female:* 117-155 g/L
Hematocrit (Hct)	*Male:* 39%-50% *Female:* 35%-47%	*Male:* 0.39-0.50 *Female:* 0.35-0.47
Chemistry		
Alanine aminotransferase (ALT)	10-40 U/L	0.17-0.68 μkat/L
Albumin	3.5-5 g/dL	35-50 g/L
Alkaline phosphatase	38-126 U/L	0.65-2.14 μkat/L
Aspartate aminotransferase (AST)	10-30 U/L	0.17-0.51 μkat/L
Ammonia	15-45 mcg N/dL	11-32 μmol N/L
Amylase	30-122 U/L	0.51-2.07 μkat/L
Bilirubin		
▪ Total	0.2-1.2 mg/dL	3.4-21.0 μmol/L
▪ Direct	0.1-0.3 mg/dL	1.7-5.1 μmol/L
▪ Indirect	0.1-1.0 mg/dL	1.7-17 μmol/L
Blood urea nitrogen (BUN)	10-30 mg/dL	1.8-7.1 mmol/L
Calcium (total)	8.6-10.2 mg/dL	2.15-2.55 mmol/L
Cholesterol	<200 mg/dL	<5.2 mmol/L
▪ HDL	*Male:* >40 mg/dL *Female:* >50 mg/dL	>1.04 mmol/L >1.3 mmol/L

HDL, High-density lipoprotein.

Continued

LABORATORY VALUES—cont'd

Test	Conventional Units	SI Units
Cholesterol—cont'd		

▪ LDL	*Recommended:*
	  <100 mg/dL
	Near optimal:
	  100-129 mg/dL
	  (2.6-3.34
	  mmol/L)
	Moderate risk for
	  CAD: 130-159
	  mg/dL (3.37-4.12
	  mmol/L)
	High risk for CAD:
	  >160 mg/dL
	  (>4.14 mmol/L)
		Recommended:
		  <2.6 mmol/L
		Near optimal:
		  2.6-3.34 mmol/L
		Moderate risk for
		  CAD: 3.37-4.12
		  mmol/L
		High risk for CAD:
		  >4.14 mmol/L

Chloride	96-106 mEq/L	96-106 mmol/L
CO_2	23-29 mEq/L	23-29 mmol/L
Creatinine	0.5-1.5 mg/dL	44-133 μmol/L
Glucose	70-120 mg/dL	3.89-6.66 mmol/L
Iron	50-175 mcg/dL	9.0-31.3 μmol/L
Lactate dehydrogenase (LDH)	140-280 U/L	0.83-2.5 μkat/L
Lipase	31-186 U/L	0.5-3.2 μkat/L
Magnesium	1.5-2.5 mEq/L	0.75-1.25 mmol/L
Osmolality	275-295 mOsm/kg	275-295 mmol/kg
Phosphorus (phosphate)	2.4-4.4 mg/dL	0.78-1.42 mmol/L
Potassium	3.5-5.0 mEq/L	3.5-5.0 mmol/L
Protein (total)	6.4-8.3 g/dL	64-83 g/L
Sodium	135-145 mEq/L	135-145 mmol/L
Triglyceride	<150 mg/dL	<1.7 mmol/L
Coagulation		
Platelets	150-400 × 10^3/μL	150-400 × 10^9/L
PT	11-16 sec	Same as conventional unit
aPTT	25-35 sec	Same as conventional unit
FSP	<10 mcg/mL	<10 mg/L

aPTT, Activated partial thromboplastin time; *FSP,* fibrin split products; *LDL,* low-density lipoprotein; *PT,* prothrombin time.

BLOOD PRODUCTS*

Description	Special Considerations	Indications for Use
Packed RBCs Packed RBCs are prepared from whole blood by sedimentation or centrifugation. One unit contains 250-350 mL. They can be stored up to 35 days depending on processing.	Use of RBCs for treatment allows remaining components of blood (e.g., platelets, albumin, plasma) to be used for other purposes. There is less danger of fluid overload. Packed RBCs are preferred RBC source because they are more component specific. Leukocyte depletion (leukoreduction) by filtration, washing, or freezing frequently used. Decreases hemolytic febrile or mild allergic reactions in patients who receive frequent transfusions.	Severe or symptomatic anemia, acute blood loss. One unit of RBCs can be expected to increase Hgb by 1 g/dL or Hct by 3% in a typical adult. One unit of RBC can replace a blood loss of 500 mL.
Frozen RBCs Frozen RBCs are prepared from RBCs using glycerol for protection and frozen. They can be stored for 10 yr.	Must be used within 24 hr of thawing. Successive washings with saline solution remove majority of WBCs and plasma proteins.	Autotransfusion. Stockpiling or rare donors for patients with alloantibodies.

Continued

BLOOD PRODUCTS—cont'd

Description	Special Considerations	Indications for Use
Platelets		
Platelets are prepared from fresh whole blood. One donor unit contains 30-60 mL of platelet concentrate (from whole blood). Platelets also pooled from multiple donors. An apheresed single donation contains 200-400 mL of platelets.	Multiple units of platelets can be obtained from one donor by plateletpheresis. They can be kept at room temperature for 1-5 days depending on type of collection and storage bag used. Bag should be agitated periodically. For patients who receive frequent transfusions and become refractory, may give leukocyte reduced, HLA, or type specific to prevent alloimmunization to HLA antigens.	Bleeding caused by thrombocytopenia; may be contraindicated in thrombotic thrombocytopenic purpura and heparin-induced thrombocytopenia except in life-threatening hemorrhage. Expected increase is 10,000/μL/U. Failure to have an increase may be due to fever, sepsis, splenomegaly, or DIC or development of antibodies (*refractory*).
Fresh Frozen Plasma		
Liquid portion of whole blood is separated from cells and frozen. One unit contains 200-250 mL. Plasma is rich in clotting factors but contains no platelets. May be stored for ≥1 yr, depending on storage. Must be used within 24 hr after thawing.	Use of plasma in treating hypovolemic shock is being replaced by pure preparations such as albumin and plasma expanders.	Bleeding caused by deficiency in clotting factors (e.g., DIC, hemorrhage, massive transfusion, liver disease, vitamin K deficiency, excess warfarin).

Albumin

Albumin is prepared from plasma. It can be stored for 5 yr. It is available in 5% or 25% solution.

Albumin 25 g/dL is osmotically equal to 500 mL of plasma. Hyperosmolar solution acts by moving water from extravascular to intravascular space. It is heat treated and does not transmit viruses.

Hypovolemic shock, hypoalbuminemia.

Cryoprecipitates and Commercial Concentrates

Cryoprecipitate is prepared from fresh frozen plasma, with 10-20 mL/bag. It can be stored for 1 yr. Once thawed, must be used within 5 days.

See Table 31-19 in Lewis et al.: *Medical-Surgical Nursing,* ed. 9, p. 656.

Replacement of clotting factors, especially factor VIII, von Willebrand factor, and fibrinogen.

DIC, Disseminated intravascular coagulation; *HLA,* human leukocyte antigen.

*Component therapy has replaced the use of whole blood, which accounts for <10% of all transfusions. Granulocyte transfusions are not included here because they are rarely used.

BREATH SOUNDS

Normal Sounds

Type	Normal Site	Duration, I/E Ratio	Characteristics
Vesicular	Peripheral lung	I > E 3:1	Soft, low-pitched, gentle, rustling sounds; heard over all lung areas except major bronchi; abnormal when heard over the large airways
Broncho vesicular	Sternal border of the major bronchi	I = E 1:1	Medium pitch and intensity; heard anteriorly over the mainstem bronchi on either side of the sternum and posteriorly between the scapulae; abnormal if heard over peripheral lung fields
Bronchial	Trachea and bronchi	I < E 2:3	Louder, higher pitched; resembles air blowing through a hollow pipe; abnormal if heard over peripheral lung

Adventitious Sounds (Abnormal Sounds)

Characteristics	Possible Clinical Condition
Fine Crackles (Formerly Called Rales) Series of short-duration, discontinuous, high-pitched sounds heard just before the end of inspiration; similar sound to that made by rolling hair between fingers just behind ear	Idiopathic pulmonary fibrosis, interstitial edema (early pulmonary edema), alveolar filling (pneumonia), loss of lung volume (atelectasis), early phase of heart failure

Coarse Crackles

Series of long-duration, discontinuous, low-pitched sounds caused by air passing through airway intermittently occluded by mucus, unstable bronchial wall, or fold of mucosa; evident on inspiration and, at times, expiration

Heart failure, pulmonary edema, pneumonia with severe congestion, chronic obstructive pulmonary disease (COPD)

Rhonchi

Continuous rumbling, snoring, or rattling sounds from obstruction of large airways with secretions; most prominent on expiration

COPD, cystic fibrosis, pneumonia, bronchiectasis

Wheezes

Continuous high-pitched squeaking or musical sound caused by rapid vibration of bronchial walls; first evident on expiration but possibly evident on inspiration as obstruction of airway increases

Bronchospasm (caused by asthma), airway obstruction (caused by foreign body, tumor), COPD

Pleural Friction Rub

Creaking or grating sound from roughened, inflamed surfaces of the pleura rubbing together; evident during inspiration, expiration, or both

Pleurisy, pneumonia, pulmonary infarct

E, Expiration; *I,* inspiration.

COMMONLY USED FORMULAS

Parameter	Formula	Normal Range
Anion gap	$Na - (HCO_3^+ + Cl)$	8-16 mEq/L
Body mass index (BMI)	$\dfrac{\text{Weight in pounds}}{\text{Height in inches}^2} \times 703$	18.5-24.9 kg/m²
Cardiac index (CI)	CO/Body surface area (BSA)	2.2-4.0 L/min/m²
Cardiac output (CO)	$HR \times SV$	4-8 L/min
Cerebral perfusion pressure (CPP)	$MAP - ICP$	80-100 mm Hg
Ejection fraction (EF)	$\dfrac{SV}{\text{End-diastolic volume}} \times 100$	60% or greater
Heart rate (HR)		60-80 beats/min
Mean arterial pressure (MAP)	$\dfrac{2(DBP) + SBP}{3}$	70-105 mm Hg
Stroke volume (SV)	$\dfrac{CO}{HR}$	60-150 mL/beat

DBP, Diastolic blood pressure; *ICP*, intracranial pressure; *SBP*, systolic blood pressure.

COMMONLY USED HERBS

Name	Uses Based on Scientific Evidence	Comments
Aloe	Constipation	■ Short-term use only. ■ May cause electrolyte imbalances. ■ May lower blood glucose.
Cranberry	Prevention of urinary tract infection	■ Drinking cranberry juice appears to be safe. ■ Excessive amounts can lead to gastrointestinal upset or diarrhea.
Echinacea	May reduce incidence and duration of upper respiratory tract infections	■ Short-term use is recommended. ■ Use with caution in patients with conditions affecting immune system. ■ Use cautiously in patients with asthma because of increased risk of allergic reaction.
Evening primrose	Eczema, skin irritation	■ Contraindicated in individuals with seizure disorders.
Feverfew	Migraine headache prevention	■ May increase risk of bleeding. ■ Long-term users may experience withdrawal symptoms.
Garlic	May decrease cholesterol and low-density lipoproteins (studies have been inconsistent)	■ May increase risk of bleeding. ■ May lower blood glucose.

Continued

COMMONLY USED HERBS—cont'd

Name	Uses Based on Scientific Evidence	Comments
Ginger	Nausea and vomiting of pregnancy	■ May increase risk of bleeding. ■ May lower blood glucose. ■ Use in pregnancy should not exceed 1 g/day. ■ Supervision by health care provider is recommended for pregnant women considering use of ginger.
Ginkgo biloba	Symptoms of claudication	■ Generally well tolerated in recommended dosages for up to 6 months. ■ May increase risk of stroke. ■ May increase risk of bleeding. ■ May affect blood glucose levels.
Ginseng (*Panax* species)	Improves mental performance Enhances immune system Lowers blood glucose in healthy individuals	■ May increase or decrease blood pressure. ■ May increase risk of bleeding. ■ Avoid in patients with hormone-sensitive conditions such as breast cancer.
Hawthorn	Mild to moderate heart failure	■ May add to the effects of cardiac glycosides, antihypertensives, and cholesterol-lowering agents.

Kava	Anxiety	▪ FDA has issued warning of severe liver damage linked to use. ▪ Avoid in patients with liver problems and patients taking medications that affect liver. ▪ May increase drowsiness. ▪ Use cautiously with herbs or supplements that are metabolized by kidneys.
St. John's wort	Short-term treatment of depression (studies on benefits of use are contradictory)	▪ Well tolerated in recommended doses for 1-3 months. ▪ May lead to serious interactions with herbs, supplements, OTC drugs, or prescription drugs. ▪ Interferes with metabolism of drugs that use cytochrome P450 enzyme system. ▪ May lead to increased side effects when taken with other antidepressants. ▪ Advise patients to consult health care professional before self-medicating with St. John's wort.
Zinc	Upper respiratory tract infections	▪ Relatively safe. ▪ Should not be taken with dairy products or caffeine, which will reduce its absorption.

Source: Data from *www.naturalstandard.com*.

FDA, Food and Drug Administration; *OTC*, over-the-counter.

*Advise patients who are pregnant or lactating to consult a health care practitioner before using any herbs. There is limited scientific evidence for the use of most herbs during pregnancy or lactation.

CHARACTERISTICS OF COMMON DYSRHYTHMIAS

Pattern	Rate and Rhythm	P Wave	PR Interval	QRS Complex
Normal sinus rhythm	60-100 beats/min and regular	Normal	Normal	Normal
Sinus bradycardia	<60 beats/min and regular	Normal	Normal	Normal
Sinus tachycardia	101-200 beats/min and regular	Normal	Normal	Normal
Premature atrial contraction	Usually 60-100 beats/min and irregular	Abnormal shape	Normal	Normal (usually)
Paroxysmal supraventricular tachycardia	150-220 beats/min and regular	Abnormal shape, may be hidden in the preceding T wave	Normal or shortened	Normal (usually)
Atrial flutter	*Atrial:* 200-350 beats/min and regular *Ventricular:* > or <100 beats/min and may be regular or irregular	Flutter (F) waves (sawtoothed pattern); more flutter waves than QRS complexes; may occur in a 2:1, 3:1, 4:1, etc., pattern	Not measurable	Normal (usually)

	Rate	P/Fibrillatory (f) waves	PR interval	QRS complex
Atrial fibrillation	*Atrial:* 350-600 beats/min and irregular; *Ventricular:* > or <100 beats/min and irregular	Fibrillatory (f) waves	Not measurable	Normal (usually)
Junctional dysrhythmias	40-180 beats/min and regular	Inverted, may be hidden in QRS complex	Variable	Normal (usually)
First-degree AV block	Normal and regular	Normal	>0.20 sec	Normal
Second-degree AV block				
■ Type I (Mobitz I, Wenckebach heart block)	*Atrial:* Normal and regular; *Ventricular:* Slower and irregular	Normal	Progressive lengthening	Normal QRS width, with pattern of one nonconducted (blocked) QRS complex
■ Type II (Mobitz II heart block)	*Atrial:* Usually normal and regular; *Ventricular:* Slower and regular or irregular	More P waves than QRS complexes (e.g., 2:1, 3:1)	Normal or prolonged	Widened QRS, preceded by ≥2 P waves, with nonconducted (blocked) QRS complex

Continued

CHARACTERISTICS OF COMMON DYSRHYTHMIAS—cont'd

Pattern	Rate and Rhythm	P Wave	PR Interval	QRS Complex
Third-degree AV block (complete heart block)	*Atrial:* Regular but may appear irregular due to P waves hidden in QRS complexes *Ventricular:* 20-60 beats/min and regular	Normal, but no connection with QRS complex	Variable	Normal or widened, no relationship with P waves
Premature ventricular contraction (PVC)	Underlying rhythm can be any rate; regular or irregular rhythm; PVCs occur at variable rates	Not usually visible, hidden in the PVC	Not measurable	Wide and distorted
Ventricular tachycardia	150-250 beats/min and regular or irregular	Not usually visible	Not measurable	Wide and distorted
Accelerated idioventricular rhythm	40-100 beats/min and regular	Not usually visible	Not measurable	Wide and distorted
Ventricular fibrillation	Not measurable and irregular	Absent	Not measurable	Not measurable

AV, Atrioventricular.

ELECTROCARDIOGRAM (ECG) MONITORING

Waveform and Normal Sinus Rhythm

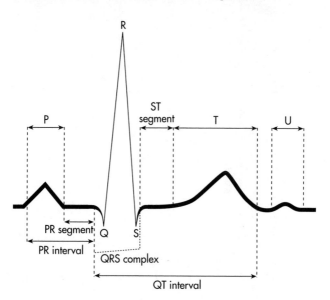

ECG MONITORING: DEFINITION AND SOURCES OF VARIATION IN ECG WAVEFORMS AND INTERVALS*

Description	Normal Duration (sec)	Source of Possible Variation
P Wave Represents time for the passage of the electrical impulse through the atrium, causing atrial depolarization (contraction); should be upright	0.06–0.12	Disturbance in conduction within atria
PR Interval Measured from beginning of P wave to beginning of QRS complex; represents time taken for impulse to spread through the atria, AV node and bundle of His, the bundle branches, and Purkinje fibers, to a point immediately preceding ventricular contraction	0.12–0.20	Disturbance in conduction usually in AV node, bundle of His, or bundle branches but can be in atria as well
QRS Interval Measured from beginning to end of QRS complex; represents time taken for depolarization (contraction) of both ventricles (systole)	<0.12	Disturbance in conduction in bundle branches or in ventricles

ST Segment

Measured from the S wave of the QRS complex to the beginning of the T wave; represents the time between ventricular depolarization and repolarization (diastole); should be isoelectric (flat)

0.12

Disturbances usually caused by ischemia or infarction

T Wave

Represents time for ventricular repolarization; should be upright

0.16

Disturbances usually caused by electrolyte imbalances, ischemia, or infarction

QT Interval

Measured from beginning of QRS complex to end of T wave; represents time taken for entire electrical depolarization and repolarization of the ventricles

0.34-0.43

Disturbances usually affecting repolarization more than depolarization and caused by drugs, electrolyte imbalances, and changes in heart rate

AV, Atrioventricular.

*Heart rate influences the duration of these intervals, especially those of the PR and QT intervals (e.g., QT interval decreases in duration as HR increases).

GLASGOW COMA SCALE

Appropriate Stimulus	Response	Score
Eyes Open		
Approach to bedside	Spontaneous response.	4
Verbal command	Opening of eyes to name or command.	3
Pain	Lack of opening of eyes to previous stimuli but opening to pain.	2
	Lack of opening of eyes to any stimulus.	1
	Untestable.*	U
Best Verbal Response		
Verbal questioning with maximum arousal	Appropriate orientation, conversant. Correct identification of self, place, yr, and mo.	5
	Confusion. Conversant, but disorientation in one or more spheres.	4
	Inappropriate or disorganized use of words (e.g., cursing), lack of sustained conversation.	3
	Incomprehensible words, sounds (e.g., moaning).	2
	Lack of sound, even with painful stimuli.	1
	Untestable.*	U
Best Motor Response		
Verbal command (e.g., "raise your arm, hold up two fingers")	Obedience of command.	6
	Localization of pain, lack of obedience but presence of attempts to remove offending stimulus.	5
Pain (pressure on proximal nail bed)	Flexion withdrawal,* flexion of arm in response to pain without abnormal flexion posture.	4
	Abnormal flexion, flexing of arm at elbow and pronation, making a fist.	3
	Abnormal extension, extension of arm at elbow usually with adduction and internal rotation of arm at shoulder.	2
	Lack of response.	1
	Untestable.*	U

*Added to the original scale by some centers.

HEART SOUNDS

Auscultatory Sites

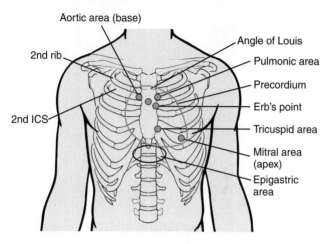

HEART SOUNDS—cont'd

Characteristics of Heart Sounds

Sound	Auscultation Site	Clinical Occurrence
S_1 (M_1 T_1)	Apex	Closing of mitral and tricuspid valves; signals the beginning of systole
S_2 (A_2 P_2)	A_2 at second ICS, RSB; P_2 at second ICS, LSB	Closing of aortic and pulmonic valves; signals the beginning of diastole
S_2 physiologic split	Second ICS, LSB (pulmonic area)	Can be normal and is a split sound that corresponds with the respiratory cycle caused by a normal delay of pulmonic valve during inspiration; can be abnormal if heard during expiration or if it is constant during the respiratory cycle; accentuated during exercise or in individuals with thin chest walls; heard most often in children and young adults
S_3 (ventricular gallop)	Apex	Low-intensity vibration of the ventricular wall usually associated with decreased compliance of the ventricles during filling; heard closely after S_2; common in children and young adults and during last trimester of pregnancy

S₄ (atrial gallop)	Apex	Low-frequency vibration caused by atrial filling and contraction against increased resistance in ventricle; precedes S₁ of next cycle; may be normal in infants, children, and athletes; pathologic in patients with heart disease
Murmurs	Heard with stethoscope lifted just off chest wall	Produced by turbulent blood flow across diseased heart valves. They are graded on a 6-point Roman numeral scale of loudness and recorded as a ratio. The numerator is the intensity of the murmur and the denominator is always VI, which indicates that the six-point scale is being used. A I/VI indicates a murmur that is barely audible, heard only in a quiet room and then not easily; a VI/VI indicates a murmur that can be heard with stethoscope lifted off chest wall.
Pericardial friction rubs	Usually heard best at the apex, with patient upright and leaning forward, and following expiration	Caused by friction that occurs when inflamed surfaces of pericardium (pericarditis) move against each other. They are high-pitched, scratchy sounds that may be transient or intermittent and may last several hours to days.

ICS, Intercostal space; *LSB*, left sternal border; *RSB*, right sternal border.

INTRACRANIAL PRESSURE MONITORING

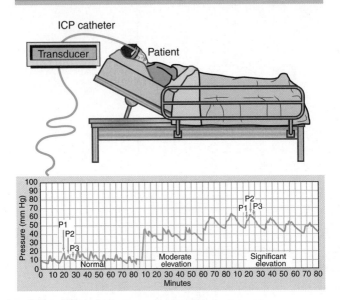

Intracranial pressure monitoring can be used to continuously measure ICP. The ICP tracing shows normal, elevated, and plateau waves. At high ICP the P2 peak is higher than the P1 peak, and the peaks become less distinct and plateau.

LUNG VOLUMES AND CAPACITIES

Parameter	Definitions	Normal Values*
Volumes		
Tidal volume (V_T)	Volume of air inhaled and exhaled with each breath. Only a small proportion of total capacity of lungs.	0.5 L
Expiratory reserve volume (ERV)	Additional air that can be forcefully exhaled after normal exhalation is complete.	1.0 L
Residual volume (RV)	Amount of air remaining in lungs after forced expiration. Air available in lungs for gas exchange between breaths.	1.5 L
Inspiratory reserve volume (IRV)	Maximum volume of air that can be inhaled forcefully after normal inhalation.	3.0 L
Capacities		
Total lung capacity (TLC)	Maximum volume of air that lungs can contain (TLC = IRV + V_T + ERV + RV).	6.0 L
Functional residual capacity (FRC)	Volume of air remaining in lungs at end of normal exhalation (FRC = ERV + RV). Increase or decrease possible with lung disease.	2.5 L
Vital capacity (VC)	Maximum volume of air that can be exhaled after maximum inspiration (VC = IRV + V_T + ERV); higher VC for men (generally).	4.5 L
Inspiratory capacity (IC)	Maximum volume of air that can be inhaled after normal expiration (IC = V_T + IRV).	3.5 L

*Normal values vary with patient's height, weight, age, race, and gender.

MEDICATION ADMINISTRATION

Equivalent Weights and Measures

Metric	Apothecary	Household
Weight		
1 kg	2.2 pounds	
1000 mg = 1 g	gr xv	
60 or 65 mg	gr i	
30 mg	gr ss (one half)	
0.4 mg	1/150 gr	
1 mcg = 0.0001 mg		
Volume		
1000 mL = 1 L	Approx. 1 quart	Approx. 1 quart
1 L distilled water weighs	1 kg	
500 mL	Approx. 1 pint	16 ounces
240 or 250 mL	viii (8 ounces)	1 cup
30 mL	i (1 fluid ounce)	2 tbs
15 mL	iv (4 fluid drams)	1 tbs
4 to 5 mL	i (1 fluid dram)	1 tsp
1 mL	Minims xv or xvi	

Drug Calculations
Ratio and Proportion
1. To set up a ratio and proportion, put on the right-hand side what you already have or what you already know (e.g., 1000 mg: 1 mL).
2. On the left-hand side put X, or what you want to know (e.g., 750 mg: X).
3. The equation should look like this: 750 mg: X = 1000 mg: 1 mL
4. Multiply the two inside numbers. Multiply the two outside numbers.

$$1000X = 750$$

5. Solve for X:

$$X = \frac{750}{1000} = 0.75 \text{ mL}$$

IV Drip Rate

$$\frac{\text{Total number of milliliters to be infused}}{\text{Total number of minutes infusion}} \times \frac{\text{Drop factor}}{} = \frac{\text{Rate}}{\text{(Drops per minute)}}$$

Techniques of Administration
Angles of Injection

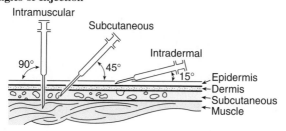

Injection Sites
Subcutaneous

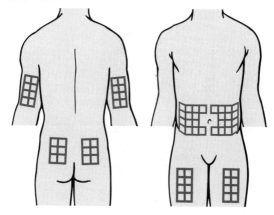

Intramuscular: Deltoid Muscle

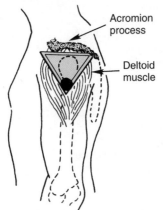

Intramuscular: Dorsogluteal Muscle

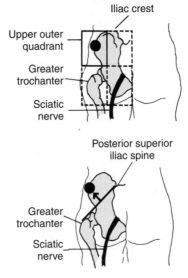

Intramuscular: Vastus Lateralis Muscle

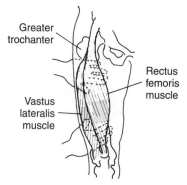

Intramuscular: Ventrogluteal Muscle

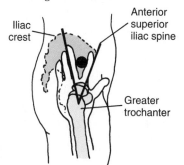

Z-*Track Technique*

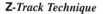

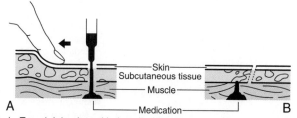

A, In Z-track injection, skin is pulled laterally, then injection is administered. **B,** After needle is withdrawn, skin is released. This technique helps prevent medication from leaking.

Intermittent IV Drug Administration

Peripheral Vein Intermittent Infusion Device
1. Irrigate device with 1 mL of normal saline.
2. Administer prescribed medication.
3. Irrigate device with 1 mL of normal saline after medication administration is completed.
4. If policy, perform a final irrigation with 1 mL of heparin solution (100 units of heparin per milliliter).

Central Vein Intermittent Infusion Device
1. Irrigate device with 2 to 5 mL of normal saline (volume depends on type of infusion catheter and agency policy).
2. Administer prescribed medication.
3. Irrigate device with 2 to 5 mL of normal saline when medication administration is completed.
4. Irrigate device with 2 to 5 mL of heparin solution (100 units of heparin per milliliter).

IV Site Complications

	Infiltration	Phlebitis
Assessment		
Color	Pale	Red
Temperature	Cool to cold	Warm to hot
Swelling	Rounded	Cordlike vein path
Pain	Yes, usually	Yes
Flow	Slowed or stopped	No change or may be slowed
Nursing Actions	Tourniquet proximally (flow continues—infiltration)	Discontinue IV; usually call IV team
	Lower bag (blood in tubing—no infiltration)	Note irritating solution (diazepam [Valium], cephalothin sodium Keflin], potassium chloride [KCl] running too fast)
	Discontinue IV	
	Call IV team	
	Get order for warm compresses and elevate part	Warm compresses; elevate and immobilize part

TEMPERATURE CONVERSION FACTORS

°C	°F	°C	°F	°C	°F
34.0	93.2	37.2	99.0	40.2	104.4
34.2	93.6	37.4	99.3	40.4	104.7
34.4	93.9	37.6	99.7	40.6	105.2
34.6	94.3	37.8	100.0	40.8	105.4
34.8	94.6	38.0	100.4	41.0	105.9
35.0	95.0	38.2	100.8	41.2	106.1
35.2	95.4	38.4	101.1	41.4	106.5
35.4	95.7	38.6	101.5	41.6	106.8
35.6	96.1	38.8	101.8	41.8	107.2
35.8	96.4	39.0	102.2	42.0	107.6
36.0	96.8	39.2	102.6	42.2	108.0
36.2	97.2	39.4	102.9	42.4	108.3
36.4	97.5	39.6	103.3	42.6	108.7
36.6	97.9	39.8	103.6	42.8	109.0
36.8	98.2	40.0	104.0	43.0	109.4
37.0	98.6				

°C = Temperature in Celsius (centigrade) degrees. (°C × 9/5) + 32 = °F.
°F = Temperature in Fahrenheit degrees. (°F − 32) × 5/9 = °C.

TNM CLASSIFICATION SYSTEM

Primary Tumor (T)

T_0	No evidence of primary tumor
T_{is}	Carcinoma in situ
T_{1-4}	Ascending degrees of increase in tumor size and involvement
T_x	Tumor cannot be measured or found

Regional Lymph Nodes (N)

N_0	No evidence of disease in lymph nodes
N_{1-4}	Ascending degrees of nodal involvement
N_x	Regional lymph nodes unable to be assessed clinically

Distant Metastases (M)

M_0	No evidence of distant metastases
M_{1-4}	Ascending degrees of metastatic involvement, including distant nodes
M_x	Cannot be determined

NOTE: For examples of TNM classification system applied to diseases, see Fig. 31-14 and Table 28-17 in Lewis et al.: *Medical-Surgical Nursing*, ed. 9, pp. 671 and 538.

ENGLISH/SPANISH COMMON MEDICAL TERMS

Hints for Pronunciation of Spanish Words

1. h is silent.
2. j is pronounced as h.
3. ll is pronounced as a y sound.
4. r is pronounced with a trilled sound, and rr is trilled even more.
5. v is pronounced with a b sound.
6. A y by itself is pronounced with a long e sound.
7. Accent marks over the vowel indicate the syllable that is to be stressed.

Introductory

I am _____.	Soy _____.
What is your name?	¿Cómo se llama usted?
I would like to examine you now.	Quisiera examinarlo (a) ahora.

General

How do you feel?	¿Cómo se siente?
Good	Bien
Bad	Mal
Do you feel better today?	¿Se siente mejor hoy?
Where do you work?	¿Dónde trabaja? (Cuál es su profesión o trabajo?) (¿Qué hace usted?)
Are you allergic to anything?	¿Es usted alérgico(a) a algo?
Medications, foods, insect bites?	¿Medicinas, alimentos, picaduras de insectos?
Do you take any medications?	¿Toma usted algunas medicinas?
Do you have any drug allergies?	¿Es usted alérgico(a) a algún médicamento?
Do you have a history of	¿Ha sufrido antes:
heart disease?	del corazón?
diabetes?	de diabetes?
epilepsy?	de epilepsia?
bronchitis?	de bronquitis?
emphysema?	de enfisema?
asthma?	de asma?

Pain

Have you any pain?	¿Tiene dolor?
Where is the pain?	¿Dónde le duele?
Do you have any pain here?	¿Le duele aquí?
How severe is the pain?	¿Qué tan fuerte es el dolor?
Mild, moderate, sharp, or severe?	¿Ligero, moderado, agudo, severo?

ENGLISH/SPANISH COMMON MEDICAL TERMS—cont'd

What were you doing when the pain started?	¿Qué estaba haciendo cuando le comenzó el dolor?
Have you ever had this pain before?	¿Ha tenido este dolor antes?
Do you have a pain in your side?	¿Tiene usted dolor en el costado?
Is it worse now?	¿Es peor ahora?
Does it still pain you?	¿Le duele todavía?
Did you feel much pain at the time?	¿Sintió mucho dolor entonces?
Show me where.	Muéstreme dónde.
Does it hurt when I press here?	¿Le duele cuando aprieto aquí?

Head

Head	La cabeza
Face	La cara

Eyes

Eye	El ojo

Ears/Nose/Throat

Ears	Los oídos
Eardrum	El tímpano
Laryngitis	La laringitis
Lip	El labio
Mouth	La boca
Nose	La naríz
Tongue	La lengua

Cardiovascular

Heart	El corazón
Heart attack	El ataque del corazón
Heart disease	La enfermedad del corazón
Heart murmur	El soplo del corazón
High blood pressure	Presión alta

Respiratory

Chest	El pecho
Lungs	Los pulmones

Gastrointestinal

Abdomen	El abdomen
Intestines/bowels	Los intestinos
Liver	El hígado

Continued

ENGLISH/SPANISH COMMON MEDICAL TERMS—cont'd

Gastrointestinal—cont'd

Nausea	Náusea
Gastric ulcer	La úlcera gástrica
Stomach	El estómago, la panza, la barriga
Stomachache	El dolor de estómago

Genitourinary

Genitals	Los genitales
Kidney	El riñón
Penis	El pene, el miembro
Urine	La orina

Musculoskeletal

Ankle	El tobillo
Arm	El brazo
Back	La espalda
Bones	Los huesos
Elbow	El codo
Finger	El dedo
Foot	El pie
Fracture	La fractura
Hand	La mano
Hip	La cadera
Knee	La rodilla
Leg	La pierna
Muscles	Los músculos
Rib	La costilla
Shoulder	El hombro
Thigh	El muslo

Neurologic

Brain	El cerebro
Dizziness	El vértigo, el mareo
Epilepsy	La epilepsia
Fainting spell	El desmayo
Unconsciousness	Pérdida del conocimiento (inconsciente, sin sentido)

Endocrine/Reproductive

Uterus	El útero, la matríz
Vagina	La vagina

URINALYSIS

Test	Normal	Abnormal Finding	Possible Etiology and Significance
Color	Amber yellow	Dark, smoky color	Hematuria.
		Yellow-brown to olive green	Excessive bilirubin.
		Orange-red or orange-brown	Phenazopyridine (Pyridium).
		Cloudiness of freshly voided urine	Infection.
		Colorless urine	Excessive fluid intake, renal disease, or diabetes insipidus.
Odor	Aromatic	Urine allowed to stand	Becomes ammonia-like in odor.
		Unpleasant odor	Urinary tract infection.
Protein	Random protein (dipstick): 0-trace	Persistent proteinuria	Characteristic of acute and chronic renal disease, especially involving glomeruli; heart failure.
	24-hr protein (quantitative): <150 mg/day		In absence of disease: high-protein diet, strenuous exercise, dehydration, fever, emotional stress, contamination by vaginal secretions.
Glucose	None	Glycosuria	Diabetes mellitus, low renal threshold for glucose reabsorption (if blood glucose level is normal). Pituitary disorders.
Ketones	None	Present	Altered carbohydrate and fat metabolism in diabetes mellitus and starvation; dehydration, vomiting, severe diarrhea.
Bilirubin	None	Present	Liver disorders. May appear before jaundice is visible.

Continued

URINALYSIS—cont'd

Test	Normal	Abnormal Finding	Possible Etiology and Significance
Specific gravity	1.003-1.030 Maximum concentrating ability of kidney in morning urine (1.025-1.030)	Low High Fixed at about 1.010	Dilute urine; excessive diuresis; diabetes insipidus. Dehydration, albuminuria, glycosuria. Renal inability to concentrate urine; end-stage renal disease.
Osmolality	300-1300 mOsm/kg (300-1300 mmol/kg)	<300 mOsm/kg >1300 mOsm/kg	Tubular dysfunction. Kidney lost ability to concentrate or dilute urine. (Not part of routine urinalysis.) Urinary tract infection; urine allowed to stand at room temperature (bacteria decompose urea to ammonia).
pH	4.0-8.0 (average, 6.0)	>8.0 <4.0	Respiratory or metabolic acidosis
RBC	0-4/hpf	>4/hpf	Calculi, cystitis, neoplasm, glomerulonephritis, tuberculosis, kidney biopsy, trauma.
WBC	0-5/hpf	>5/hpf	Urinary tract infection or inflammation.
Casts	None Occasional hyaline	Present	Molds of the renal tubules that may contain protein, WBCs, RBCs, or bacteria. Noncellular casts (hyaline in appearance) occasionally found in normal urine.
Culture for organisms	No organisms in bladder <10⁴ organisms/mL result of normal urethral flora	Bacteria counts >10⁵/mL	Urinary tract infection. Most common organisms are *Escherichia coli*, enterococci, *Klebsiella*, *Proteus*, and streptococci.

hpf, High-powered field.